*H*ealth: *The Basics*

Canadian Edition

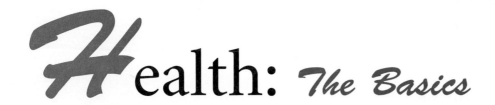

Health: The Basics

Canadian Edition

Rebecca J. Donatelle
Oregon State University

Lorraine G. Davis
University of Oregon

Anne J. Munroe
Sheridan College

Alex Munroe
Wilfrid Laurier University

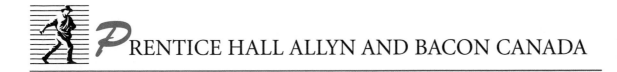

PRENTICE HALL ALLYN AND BACON CANADA

SCARBOROUGH, ONTARIO

Canadian Cataloguing in Publication Data

Health : the basics
Includes index.
ISBN 0-205-28374-8
1. Health   I. Donatelle, Rebecca J., 1950-
RA776.H42 1998   613   C97-931869-6

© 1998 Prentice-Hall Canada Inc., Scarborough, Ontario
A Division of Simon & Schuster/A Viacom Company

Allyn and Bacon, Inc., Needham Heights, MA

Prentice-Hall, Inc., Upper Saddle River, New Jersey
Prentice-Hall International (UK) Limited, London
Prentice-Hall of Australia, Pty. Limited, Sydney
Prentice-Hall Hispanoamericana, S.A., Mexico City
Prentice-Hall of India Private Limited, New Delhi
Prentice-Hall of Japan, Inc., Tokyo
Simon & Schuster Southeast Asia Private Limited, Singapore
Editora Prentice-Hall do Brasil, Ltda., Rio de Janeiro

ISBN 0-205-28374-8

Vice-President, Editorial Director: Laura Pearson
Vice-President, Acquisitions: Cliff Newman
Associate Developmental Editor: Carol Steven
Marketing Manager: Kris Begic
Production Editor: Andrew Winton
Copy Editor: Gilda Mekler
Editorial Assistant: Sharon Loeb
Production Coordinator: Wendy Moran
Permissions/Photo Research: Susan Wallace-Cox
Cover Design: Julia Hall
Cover Image: José Ortega Inc./SIS
Page Layout: Zofia Moczulak

Original English Language edition published by Allyn and Bacon, Inc.,
Needham Heights, MA. Copyright © 1997, 1995.

1 2 3 4 5   02 01 00 99 98

Printed and bound in the United States of America.

Visit the Prentice Hall Canada web site! Send us your comments, browse our catalogues, and
more at **www.phcanada.com**. Or reach us through e-mail at **phabinfo_pubcanada@prenhall.com**.

Every reasonable effort has been made to obtain permissions for all articles and data used in this
edition. If errors or omissions have occurred, they will be corrected in future editions provided
written notification has been received by the publisher.

$\mathcal{B}$rief Contents

${\cal C}$ontents

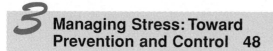

3 Managing Stress: Toward Prevention and Control 48

4 Violence and Abuse: Societal Challenges 67

2: Creating Healthy and Caring Relationships

5 Healthy Relationships and Sexuality: Making Commitments 85

3: Building Healthy Lifestyles

5: Preventing and Fighting Disease

12 Cardiovascular Disease and Cancer: Reducing Your Risks 283

13 Infectious and Noninfectious Conditions: Risks and Responsibilities 314

6: Facing Life's Challenges

14 Life's Transitions: The Aging Process 353

15 Environmental Health: Thinking Globally, Acting Locally 379

16 Consumerism: Selecting Health-Care Products and Services 398

$\mathcal{P}$reface

Chances are that if your students are like most of today's university and college students, they already know more than any previous generation about health. Contrary to what most of us think, because health information changes quickly and there is so much to know, none of us can ever really know enough. Even if we have the basic facts, translating them into a meaningful plan of action that is personally relevant can be a difficult task. But today students have the opportunity to choose from health alternatives that were not available a few short years ago. With so many choices available, how can students be sure their everyday decisions will ultimately lead to good health? With this in mind, we have placed increasing emphasis on developing skills to help students make informed, responsible health decisions.

Achieving good health includes recognizing the importance of a particular health outcome, understanding the factors that contribute to the positive and negative aspects of health, contemplating how actions affect health, and choosing to change or modify risky behaviours and develop new and improved behaviours. *Health: The Basics* can be an important source of reliable health information. As you use the latest health information, the special features, and the learning aids in the book, as well as the supplements, we hope to make your students' access to health fun and enlightening with long-term results of improved overall health.

In setting out to adapt the text for Canadian students, we listened to the comments and concerns of Canadian personal health educators. We learned that we share the following goals for a personal health text:

- To prepare students to lead healthy lives long after they have left the classroom by providing tools and strategies to effect positive behaviour change.

- To include coverage of "high interest" topics that have traditionally been left out of health texts, such as material that exposes students to multicultural and gender-specific perspectives on health.

- To provide current Canadian material that includes the latest health research and citations.

- To recognize that students learn visually and require strong pedagogical elements to help them synthesize information and build healthy behaviour skills.

- To include practical, real-life applications to the material presented in the text that encourage students to apply the material to their own lives.

New to The Canadian Edition:

While maintaining the format and organizational style of the U.S. second edition, we have made several changes to reflect issues and policies in Canadian society. There have been revisions to Chapter 1 to reflect the Canadian context of gender issues and health, as well as the broader view of health outlined in policy. Chapter 4, "Violence and Abuse," has been rewritten, focusing on the often subtle role that violence plays in our society. Chapters 10 and 11, which deal with addiction, have also been largely rewritten to highlight the greater reliance in Canada on education in combatting addiction, rather than the heavily legislative approach described in the U.S. second edition. Chapter 16, "Consumerism," has been totally rewritten as well to describe the unique mix of public and private initiatives in the provision of health care in Canada.

Throughout the text, we have endeavoured to include current Canadian statistics and sources.

Organization

- Beginning with the introduction of the **DECIDE model for decision-making and Prochaska and DiClemente's Stages of Change model** in Chapter 1, decision making through critical thinking now forms the cornerstone of every chapter, from the "What Do You Think?" scenarios and reflective questions throughout the chapter to the boxed features, and the "Taking Charge" section at the end of each chapter.

- **Cancer and heart disease coverage** emphasizes prevention and treatment of the major killing diseases. Coverage includes options that women face in light of improved technological advances in the area of cancer treatment. In addition, a section on women and heart disease includes coverage of risk factors, symptoms of heart disease in postmenopausal women, and why women's heart symptoms are often neglected.

- **Coverage of gender issues in health** is integrated throughout the text. Topics include gender bias in mental health treatment, women and heart disease, and how gender roles may affect stress levels and a person's ultimate health status.

- **The role of community in health** demonstrates how to improve a community's health. Community coverage is integrated throughout the text and in special "Checklist for Change: Making Community Decisions" parts within the "Taking Charge" section at the end of each chapter.

- **Prevention** is emphasized in the context of changing health behaviours. For example, the text covers how early intervention allows more options, how prevention eases the burden on the health-care system, and how prevention affects lifetime decisions.

- A **pedagogical framework** emphasizing building health skills is integrated consistently throughout the text. Students will learn specific applications in every chapter through "Rate Yourself" boxes, "Skills for Behaviour Change" boxes, "Building Communication Skills" boxes, and in the "Taking Charge" section.

Special Features

Each chapter of *Health: The Basics* includes the following special feature boxes designed to help build health behaviour skills as well as encouraging students to think about and apply the concepts:

 "Skills for Behaviour Change" boxes offer specific skills students can use in improving their health behaviour.

"Building Communication Skills" boxes in every chapter strengthen the emphasis on using communication as a tool to better health. These boxes provide practical suggestions for improving communication behaviours, interpersonal relations, and social interactions, all essential components of good health.

"Global Perspectives" boxes are designed to promote acceptance of diversity on and help students adjust to an increasingly diverse world. These boxes increase awareness that people of differing backgrounds can have different perspectives, concerns, and solutions related to current health issues.

"Focus on Canada" boxes highlight the particular characteristics of health situations and practices in our own unique environment.

"Rate Yourself" (self-assessment) boxes give students the chance to examine their behaviours and determine ways to improve their health. Additional assessments are available in the self-assessment manual.

"Taking Charge" sections at the end of each chapter encourage students to apply the chapter material to their own lives. This highly acclaimed feature, expanded to include more directed activities, now includes the following sections: *Making Decisions for You*, which outlines steps and strategies for making and implementing health decisions; *Checklists for Change*, which outline specific actions to be taken to change unhealthy behaviours, on both a personal and community level; *Critical Thinking* situations, which present a hypothetical situation in which students must make a decision—we encourage the use of the DECIDE model to make this decision.

"Weblinks" give students a list of useful Web sites relating to each chapter. The sites have been researched and tested for quality and relevance.

Learning Aids

Chapter Objectives: Each chapter begins with a list of objectives tied to the major sections of the chapter to emphasize important topics. These objectives can serve as a helpful tool for you to use when presenting the key concepts in the chapter.

"What Do You Think" chapter opening scenarios: These scenarios prompt stimulating discussions that introduce the concepts presented in the chapters.

"What Do You Think" reflective questions: These questions appear in major sections of every chapter to encourage you to think critically about important concepts as they read through the chapter.

Margin Glossary of Key Terms: For convenience and added emphasis, Key Terms are boldfaced in the text and defined in the margin on the page where they are first introduced.

Chapter Summary: Linked to the chapter opening learning objectives, these summaries provide a quick, at-a-glance review of key points presented in each chapter.

Discussion Questions: Tied to major sections of the chapter, these new questions encourage consideration of important concepts from varying angles.

Application Exercises: These new exercises are linked to the chapter opening scenarios and expand your discussion on these points.

References: Extensive listings of major sources used in researching each chapter are provided in the Reference section at the end of the text.

Supplements

Available with *Health: The Basics, Canadian Edition,* is a comprehensive set of ancillary material designed to facilitate your classroom preparation and enhance student learning.

Instructor's Resource Manual, Canadian Edition This comprehensive resource manual, filled with material to enhance your course includes the following: what's new in this edition, chapter objectives, detailed chapter outlines, discussion questions, student activities including individual, community, and diverse population/non-traditional categories, additional references, for further information, and a list of applicable media resources for classroom presentation.

Student Resource Manual, Canadian Edition This practical study aid is packed with activities and exercises that give students a chance to improve their understanding of the concepts they learn in the text. They will also see how they can apply these concepts to their lives. Included are critical thinking activities and a unique Language Enrichment Glossary.

Test Item File, Canadian Edition Our Test Item File is composed of over 1600 questions made up of factual, applied and conceptual multiple-choice each rated for difficulty level, true/false, fill-in-the-blank, matching and essay formats. Answers and page references to the text are provided with each question.

Computerized Testing Program, Canadian Edition ESATEST III, the best-selling, state-of-the-art test generation software program, is available free to adopters. Designed to operate on IBM (Windows) and Macintosh computers, this program allows you to quickly create and print tests, add your own questions, edit questions, scramble questions, create multiple versions of tests and much more.

Health Transparencies Accentuate your lectures with this set of full-color transparencies representing charts and illustrations found in *Health: The Basics,* as well as diagrams and artwork from other sources. Large type format is perfect for presentations in large classrooms.

AIDS and STIs Slide Set Containing photos and charts depicting the problem of AIDS and sexually transmitted infections, this set of 50 slides enables you to present in-depth discussions about these topics in the classroom. It comes complete with a 16-page booklet that will help you create an informative round-table that gets your students discussing these very serious issues. Ask your representative about restrictions on this item.

CNN Video Through an exclusive arrangement with Cable News Network (CNN), this specially edited videotape offers two hours of footage culled from recent CNN programming. With the latest news and information on health, this videotape provides an excellent vehicle for launching lectures, showing additional examples and sparking classroom discussion. A video user's guide containing a summary of each CNN video segment, along with questions for discussions, is also available.

***Take Charge of Your Health!* Self-Assessment Workbook with Review and Practice Tests** Using this self-assessment workbook along with *Health: The Basics* will encourage students to acquire a broader understanding of health issues, evaluate their attitudes and behaviours, and gain a clearer picture of their health overall. Included are general review questions and two practice tests (with solutions) for each chapter.

Acknowledgments

We would like to thank the following people at Prentice Hall Allyn and Bacon for their part in the Canadian edition of *Health: The Basics*: Acquisitions Editor, Cliff Newman; Developmental Editor, Carol Steven; Production Editor, Andrew Winton; Production Coordinator, Deborah Starks; and Copy Editor, Gilda Mekler.

In addition, we would like to thank the following reviewers, who provided many constructive recommendations:

Patricia Wainright, University of Waterloo; Deborah Holts, Sir Sandford Fleming College; Coreen Fleming, Centennial College; Lorne Adams, Brock University; Joan Krohn, University of Saskatchewan.

Contributors:

Patricia Ketcham, Health Educator and Director of Student Health Education and Student Services at the University of Iowa, contributed greatly to the chapter on "Alcohol, Tobacco, and Caffeine." She was also responsible for significant revisions and ideas to the chapters "Birth Control, Pregnancy, and Childbirth," "Licit and Illicit Drugs," and the "Injury Prevention and Emergency Care" appendix. Her help in the development of the content and her ideas have been invaluable.

Rod Harter, Associate Professor in the Department of Exercise and Sport Science at Oregon State University, utilized his expertise in human physiology, training, human performance, and strength and conditioning in writing his exceptional chapter, "Personal Fitness."

Chris Hafner-Eaton, Assistant Professor in the Department of Public Health at Oregon State University and RAND corporation-policy analyst, used her considerable background in health services and public policy to provide a major revision of Chapter 16, "Consumerism."

Donna Champeau, Health Educator and Assistant Professor at Oregon State University, offered her expertise in the areas of health policy and the rights of the dying to provide excellent revisions and updates to Chapter 14, "Life's Transitions."

Peggy Pederson, Health Educator and Assistant Professor at Northern Illinois University, used her background in sexuality education to submit significant editorial comment and revisions for Chapter 5, "Healthy Relationships and Sexuality."

$\mathcal{P}$romoting Healthy Behaviour Change

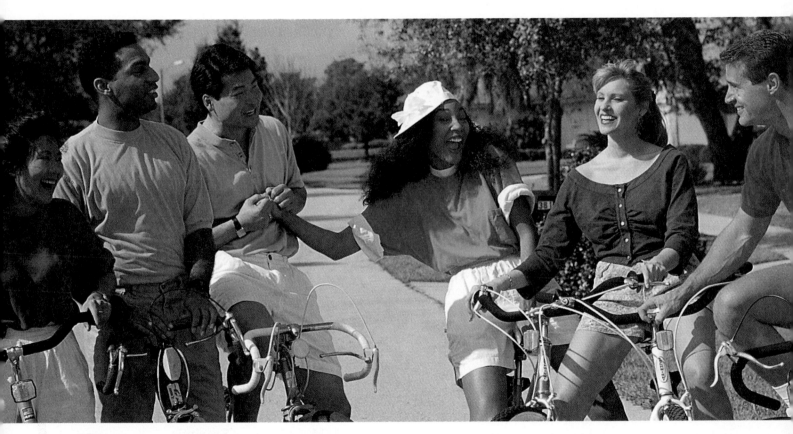

$\mathcal{C}$HAPTER OBJECTIVES

◆ Define health and wellness, and explain the interconnected roles of the physical, social, intellectual, emotional, environmental, and spiritual dimensions of health.

◆ Discuss the health status of Canadians, the factors that contribute to health, and national goals for promoting health and preventing premature death and disability.

◆ Evaluate the role of gender in health status, health research, and health training.

◆ Identify the leading causes of death and the lifestyle patterns associated with the reduction of risks.

◆ Examine how predisposing factors, beliefs, attitudes, and significant others affect your behaviour changes.

◆ Survey behaviour, change techniques and learn how to apply them to personal situations.

◆ Apply decision-making techniques to behaviour changes.

Tim is a 22-year-old second-year university student who is 35 kilograms overweight and does not like exercising. A sensitive, caring young man, he has many close friends and is a volunteer at many health-related agencies that help people in need. He likes to enjoy nature and the inner peace he derives from a walk on the beach or a quiet night by a campfire in the wilderness. He is a strong advocate for human rights, animal rights, and the preservation of the environment.

Kim is a 20-year-old first-year student who lives off campus. She tries to eat healthful foods some of the time, feels she is about 5 kilograms overweight, and walks 2 to 4 kilometres per day. She is shy and hasn't made many friends since coming to college. During a typical day, she goes to class, studies, watches TV, and writes letters to her high school friends and family. She likes bicycle riding, but she only finds time to get out for a short ride on weekends. She is tired much of the time and wonders why she is in school. After a checkup, her doctor says, "Everything looks good. Keep up whatever you're doing, and you should be fine."

■ Do you know people who are like either of these individuals? Who do you think is the healthier? The more unhealthy? What factors may have contributed to their current behaviours? What actions could you take to help these people achieve a more balanced "healthstyle"? Where else could they go for help?

If you and your close friends were to list the most important things in your lives, you might be surprised at the differences in the responses. Some of you would probably list family, love, financial security, significant others, and happiness. Others might also list health. Raised on a steady diet of clichés—"If you have your health, you have everything," "Be all that you can be," "Use it or lose it," "Just do it"—most of us readily acknowledge that good health is a desirable goal. But what does it really mean to be healthy? How can you "get healthy" if you aren't doing so well now? How can you maintain and enhance the good health behaviours you may already have?

This text offers fundamental information that will provide you an *Access to Health* consistent with who you are and what you want to become. Health is not an entity that is always totally within your control, but there are many changes you can make in your behaviour that may significantly affect your risk factors. For those risk factors beyond your control, you must learn to react, adapt, and make optimal use of your resources to create the best situation for yourself. By making informed, rational decisions, you will be able to improve both the quality and the length of your life.

𝒲HAT IS HEALTH?

The current definition of **health** has evolved over several periods of world and Canadian history.

Health and Sickness: Defined by Extremes

Prior to the late 1800s, people viewed health as the opposite of sickness. A person was healthy if he or she wasn't suffering from a life-threatening infectious disease. When deadly epidemics such as bubonic plague, pneumonic plague, influenza, tuberculosis, and cholera killed millions of people, survivors were considered healthy and congratulated themselves on their good fortune. In the late 1800s and early 1900s, researchers slowly began to discover that victims of these epidemics were not simply unhealthy people. Rather, they were the victims of microorganisms found in contaminated water, air, and human wastes. Public health officials moved swiftly to sanitize the environment and, as a result, many people began to think of health as *good hygiene*. Practices such as sanitary disposal of wastes and other behaviours that promoted hygiene were the harbingers of good health.

Health: More Than a Statistic

Once scientists began to learn about the microorganisms that cause infectious diseases, dramatic changes occurred in the sickness profile of the Canadian public. In the early 1900s, the leading causes of death were infectious diseases such as tuberculosis, pneumonia, and influenza. The average life expectancy was only 58.84 for males and 60.60 for females.[1] Improvements in sanitation brought about dramatic changes in life expectancy; the development of vaccines and antibiotics added even more years to the average life span. According to **mortality** (death rate) sta-

Responsiveness to the physical, emotional, social, spiritual, intellectual, and environmental dimensions of life—not merely the presence or absence of illness—determines health status.

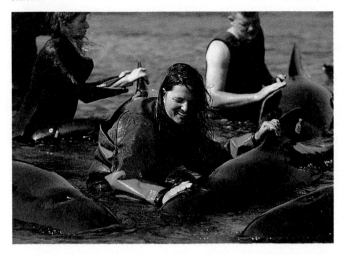

tistics, people are now living longer than in any previous time in our history. **Morbidity** (illness) rates also indicate that people are sick less often from the common infectious diseases that devastated previous generations. Today, because most childhood diseases are curable and because multiple public health efforts are aimed at reducing the spread of infectious diseases, many people are living well into their 70s and 80s.

However, just because we're living longer and not getting sick as often doesn't mean we're necessarily healthier. If you and your classmates were asked to define the term *health*, there would be many different views. One body that attempted to clarify what the term meant was the World Health Organization (WHO), created in the 1940s to link with national and international health organizations. Its objective was "the attainment by all peoples of the highest possible level of health."[2]

The mandate of the World Health Organization was broad in scope and included helping governments strengthen health services, improving standards of health teaching and training for the professions, providing health information, promoting cooperation with other specialized agencies and professional and scientific groups, promoting maternal and child health, fostering activities that enhance mental health, coordinating and promoting research, and reporting on social and administrative interventions that affect health. WHO's definition of health reflects its broad mandate. "Health is the state of complete physical, mental, and social well-being, not merely the absence of disease or infirmity."[3] Health officials viewed this as a landmark definition because it said for the first time that health was more than the absence of disease. The WHO definition also implied that health was more than just a vital statistic indicating low mortality or morbidity rates.

Although the WHO definition of health maintained currency well into the 1960s, critics argued that health is not a state that people somehow manage to achieve; rather, it is an ever-changing dimension of life. They also argued that complete health was much more than just a measure of physical, intellectual, and social aspects of life given growing recognition of the contributions of environmental, intellectual, and spiritual health to the quality of life as well as to the number of years a person lives.

Health as Wellness: Putting Quality into Years

René Dubos, biologist and philosopher, expanded the WHO definition of health. We have adapted Dubos's definition: "Health involves social, emotional, intellectual, spiritual, and biological fitness on the part of the individual, which results from adaptations to the environment."[4] Note that we use the term *intellectual health* rather than *mental health* because the latter is often used interchangeably with *emotional health* or as the counterpart to *physical health*. The term *intellectual health* more accurately reflects the reasoning abilities and cognitive processes that we can bring to bear as thinking beings.

As more people considered the term *health,* the concept began to include many different components and encompass many different aspects of life. Eventually the term **wellness** came to refer to the achievement of the highest level of health in each of several key dimensions. Today, *health* and *wellness* are often used interchangeably to mean the dynamic, ever-changing process of trying to achieve one's individual potential in each of several interrelated dimensions. These dimensions typically include those presented in Figure 1.1.

■ **Physical Health.** Includes physical characteristics such as body size and shape, sensory acuity, susceptibility to disease and disorders, body functioning, and recuperative ability.

■ **Social Health.** Refers to the ability to have satisfying interpersonal relationships, to interact with others, and to adapt to various social situations, and to daily behaviours.

■ **Intellectual Health.** Refers to the ability to learn, the ability to grow from experience, and intellectual capabilities.

Health: Dynamic, ever-changing process of trying to achieve your individual potential in the physical, social, emotional, intellectual, spiritual, and environmental dimensions.

Mortality: Death rate.

Morbidity: Illness rate.

Wellness: The achievement of the highest level of health possible in each of several dimensions.

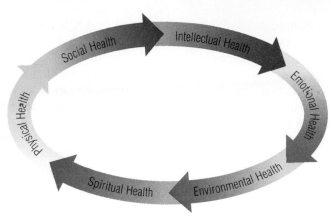

FIGURE 1.1

The Six Dimensions of Health

Decision making is a vital component of one's mental health.

- **Emotional Health.** Refers to the feeling component and to the ability to express emotions when appropriate and to control inappropriate expressions of emotion. Feelings of self-esteem, self-confidence, self-efficacy, trust, love, and many other emotional reactions and responses are all part of emotional health.

- **Environmental Health.** Refers to an appreciation of the external environment and the role individuals play in preserving, protecting, and improving environmental conditions.

- **Spiritual Health.** May involve a belief in a supreme being or a specified way of living prescribed by a particular religion. Spiritual health also includes the feeling of unity with the environment—a feeling of oneness with others and with nature—and a guiding sense of meaning or value in life. It also may include the ability to understand and express one's purpose in life; to feel a part of a greater spectrum of existence; to experience love, joy, pain, sorrow, peace, contentment, and wonder over life's experiences; and to care about and respect all living things.

Whether contemporary definitions are of health or wellness, they focus on individual attempts to achieve optimal well-being within a realistic framework of individual potential.

In Figure 1.2, a continuum from illness to optimal well-being describes health and wellness. Where you are on this continuum may vary from day to day as you are buffeted by life's ups and downs. But if you persist in your attempts to change behaviours to reduce risk, your chances of remaining on the positive end of the continuum will greatly improve. The current definition of health acknowledges that each of us must attempt to achieve this optimal level of being in a sometimes hostile environment. Each of us must come to terms with the obstacles obstructing the

way to optimal health in our own way by focussing on our positive attributes whenever possible, changing those negative aspects of ourselves that we can, and learning to recognize and deal with those that we cannot.

Well individuals take an honest look at their personal capabilities and limitations and make an effort to change those factors that are within their control. They try to achieve a balance in each of the health/wellness dimensions while trying to achieve a positive wellness position on an imaginary continuum. Many people believe that wellness can best be achieved by the adoption of a holistic approach in which a person emphasizes the integration of and balance between mind, body, and spirit. Persons on the illness and disability end of the continuum have failed to achieve this integration and balance and may be seriously deficient in one or more of the wellness dimensions.

But the disability component of the wellness continuum does not imply that a person with physical handicaps cannot achieve wellness. Such a person may in fact be very healthy in terms of relationships with others, level of self-confidence, environmental sensitivity, and overall attitude toward life. In contrast, a person who spends hours in front of a mirror lifting weights to perfect the size and

---

Having the motivation to improve the quality of your life within the framework of your unique capabilities and limitations is crucial to achieving health and wellness.

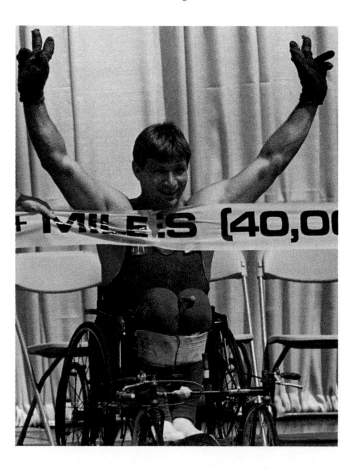

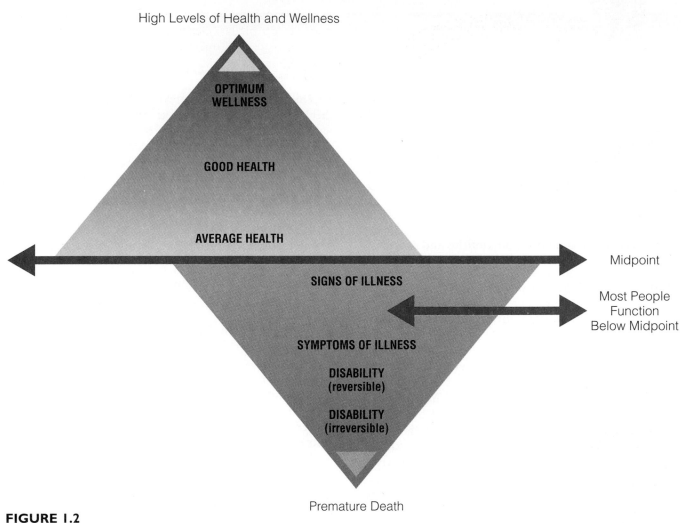

High Levels of Health and Wellness

OPTIMUM
WELLNESS

GOOD HEALTH

AVERAGE HEALTH

Midpoint

SIGNS OF ILLNESS

Most People
Function
Below Midpoint

SYMPTOMS OF ILLNESS

DISABILITY
(reversible)

DISABILITY
(irreversible)

Premature Death

FIGURE 1.2

The Continuum from Illness to Wellness

shape of each muscle may be unhealthy in these same terms. Although we often place a premium on physical attractiveness and external trappings, appearance and physical performance indicators are actually only two signs of a person's overall health.

Typically, the closer you get to your potential in the six components of health, the more well you will be. Both health and wellness are ongoing, active processes that include those positive attitudes and behaviours that continually improve the quality of your life. By completing the appraisal in the Rate Yourself box, you may gain a better perspective on how you measure up in each of the health dimensions discussed above.

Health Promotion:
Helping You Stay Healthy

In discussions of health and wellness, the term **health promotion** is often used. Health promotion programs combine educational, organizational, procedural, environ-

mental, and financial supports to help individuals and groups change negative health behaviours. In other words, health promotion programs don't just tell people to lose weight and to eat better food: they help them learn more (*educational supports*), provide programs and services that encourage them to participate (*organizational supports*), establish rules governing their behaviours and supporting their decisions to change (*environmental supports*), and provide monetary incentives to motivate them toward healthful decision making (*financial supports*). In short, health promotion programs enhance the likelihood that, once a person decides to change a behaviour, conditions are optimal for his or her success. Health promotion programs identify healthy people who are at risk for disease

> **Health promotion:** Combines educational, organizational, policy, financial, and environmental supports to help people change negative health behaviours.

Healthy Public Policy in Canada

A 1974 paper written by Marc Lalonde, the Minister of Health, titled *A New Perspective on the Health of Canadians: A Working Document,* marked a change in the definition of health in Canada that had implications for health policy. Lalonde saw *health* as having four components: human biology (physical, mental, and genetic), the environment (external; largely out of the control of the individual), lifestyle (the aggregate of individual decisions affecting health), and the health care organization. Health was linked to economic opportunities and social justice. Social change, alienation, and crumbling values were seen as potentially a greater threat to health than the inadequacy of the health care system. Lalonde's definition of health went beyond formal medical care to regard modifying behaviour and environment as central to improved health.

Further, Lalonde noted that the nature of illness had changed since the turn of the century. The major causes of death were no longer infectious diseases, but accidents. Illness was more often chronic rather than acute. He also stated that mental health had been neglected in Canada for years and that most health care dollars went to the health care organization rather than biology, environment, and lifestyle. Using the expanded *health field* concept, Lalonde's primary objective was to increase the number of disability-free days for Canadians.

Lalonde saw a need to prevent mental illness, to use health research to explore environmental, lifestyle, and service delivery issues, to control abusive advertising, and to consider the effects of recreation, labour and social organizations, and retirement on health. His recommendations included:

- increasing the efficiency of health care
- developing research strategies
- enhancing the role of the federal government as a regulatory body
- supporting health promotion
- setting health goals

Although *A New Perspective* was regarded by some critics as a "world class" document, the recommendation to set specific and measureable goals has been left to other countries. An example of such a specific goal might be "to reduce the numbers of adolescent smokers by 25% by the year 2000." The United States, for example, has developed such specific health targets as part of a program titled *Healthy People* 2000.

Source: M. Lalonde, *A New Perspective on the Health of Canadians: A Working Document* (Ottawa: Government of Canada, 1974).

and attempt to motivate them to improve their health status. They encourage those whose health and wellness behaviours are already sound to maintain and improve them. But health promotion goes one step further by modifying behaviours, attitudes, and values and by introducing health-enhancing activities.

In 1986 Jake Epp, Minister of Health and Welfare, laid out his concept of health promotion in *Achieving Health for All: A Framework for Health Promotion.*[5] He identified three health challenges as part of his framework: reducing inequities, increasing prevention, and enhancing coping. Self-care, mutual aid, and healthy environments were identified as the mechanisms of health promotion. Implementation strategies included fostering public participation, strengthening community health services, and coordinating healthy public policy.

The Canadian government conducted a Health Promotion Survey (1990)[6] to provide a better understanding of the health status of Canadians. This national research initiative explored a wide range of topics such as social relationships, worker health, environment, smoking, alcohol use, nutrition, exercise, heart disease prevention, sexual health and STD prevention, and dental health practices.

Whether we use the term *health* or *wellness,* we are talking about a person's overall responses to the challenges of living. Occasional dips into the ice cream bucket and other dietary slips, failure to exercise every day, flare-ups of anger, and other deviations from optimal behaviour should not be viewed as major failures to maintain wellness. Actually, an ability to recognize that each of us is an imperfect being attempting to adapt in an imperfect world signals individual well-being.

We must also remember to be tolerant of others who are attempting to improve their health. Rather than being warriors against pleasure in our zeal to change the health behaviours of others, we need to be supportive, understanding, and nonjudgemental in our interactions with them. *Health bashing*—intolerance or negative feelings, words, or actions aimed at people who fail to meet our own expectations of health—may indicate our own defi-

How Healthy Are You?

Although many of us recognize the importance of healthy behaviours, we are often negligent in maintaining a healthy regimen. Rate your health status in each of the following dimensions by circling the number that best describes you.

	Very Unhealthy	Somewhat Unhealthy	Somewhat Healthy	Very Healthy
Physical Health	1	2	3	4
Social Health	1	2	3	4
Emotional Health	1	2	3	4
Intellectual Health	1	2	3	4
Environmental Health	1	2	3	4
Spiritual Health	1	2	3	4

After completing the above section, how healthy do you think you are? Which area(s), if any, do you think you should work on improving?

Now answer the following set of questions regarding each dimension of health. Indicate how often you think the statements describe you.

Physical Health

	Rarely, If Ever	Sometimes	Most of the Time	Always
1. I maintain a desirable weight.	1	2	3	4
2. I engage in vigorous exercises such as brisk walking, jogging, swimming, or running for at least 30 minutes per day, 3–4 times per week.	1	2	3	4
3. I do exercises designed to strengthen my muscles and joints.	1	2	3	4
4. I warm up and cool down by stretching before and after vigorous exercise.	1	2	3	4
5. I feel good about the condition of my body.	1	2	3	4
6. I get 7–8 hours of sleep each night.	1	2	3	4
7. My immune system is strong and I am able to avoid most infectious diseases.	1	2	3	4
8. My body heals itself quickly when I get sick or injured.	1	2	3	4
9. I have lots of energy and can get through the day without being overly tired.	1	2	3	4
10. I listen to my body; when there is something wrong, I seek professional advice.	1	2	3	4

(continued)

ciencies in the psychological, social, and/or spiritual dimensions of the health continuum.

Prevention: Actions or behaviours designed to keep you from getting sick.

Primary prevention: Actions designed to stop problems before they start.

Prevention: The Key to Future Health

Prevention means taking positive actions now to avoid becoming sick later. Getting immunized against diseases such as polio, never starting to smoke cigarettes, practising safer sex, and taking similar preventive measures constitute **primary prevention**—actions designed to stop health problems before they start. Another form of prevention is

Social Health

	Rarely, If Ever	Sometimes	Most of the Time	Always
1. When I meet people I feel good about the impression I make on them.	1	2	3	4
2. I am open, honest, and get along well with other people.	1	2	3	4
3. I participate in a wide variety of social activities and enjoy being with people who are different from me.	1	2	3	4
4. I try to be a "better person" and work on behaviours that have caused problems in my interactions with others.	1	2	3	4
5. I get along well with the members of my family.	1	2	3	4
6. I am a good listener.	1	2	3	4
7. I am open and accessible to a loving and responsible relationship.	1	2	3	4
8. I have someone I can talk to about my private feelings.	1	2	3	4
9. I consider the feelings of others and do not act in hurtful or selfish ways.	1	2	3	4
10. I consider how what I say might be perceived by others before I speak.	1	2	3	4

Emotional Health

	Rarely, If Ever	Sometimes	Most of the Time	Always
1. I find it easy to laugh about things that happen in my life.	1	2	3	4
2. I avoid using alcohol as a means of helping me forget my problems.	1	2	3	4
3. I can express my feelings without feeling silly.	1	2	3	4
4. When I am angry, I try to let others know in non-confrontational and non-hurtful ways.	1	2	3	4
5. I am a chronic worrier and tend to be suspicious of others.	4	3	2	1
6. I recognize when I am stressed and take steps to relax through exercise, quiet time, or other activities.	1	2	3	4
7. I feel good about myself and believe others like me for who I am.	1	2	3	4
8. When I am upset, I talk to others and actively try to work through my problems.	1	2	3	4
9. I am flexible and adapt or adjust to change in a positive way.	1	2	3	4
10. My friends regard me as a stable, emotionally well-adjusted person.	1	2	3	4

(continued)

Secondary prevention: Intervention early in the development of a health problem.

secondary prevention, or the recognition of a health problem early in its development and intervention to eliminate its underlying causes before serious illness develops. Attending health education seminars in order to

Environmental Health

	Rarely, If Ever	Sometimes	Most of the Time	Always
1. I am concerned about environmental pollution and actively try to preserve and protect natural resources.	1	2	3	4
2. I report people who intentionally hurt the environment.	1	2	3	4
3. I recycle my garbage.	1	2	3	4
4. I reuse plastic and paper bags and tin foil.	1	2	3	4
5. I vote for pro-environmental candidates in elections.	1	2	3	4
6. I write my elected leaders about environmental concerns.	1	2	3	4
7. I consider the amount of packaging covering a product when I buy groceries.	1	2	3	4
8. I try to buy products that are recyclable.	1	2	3	4
9. I use both sides of the paper when taking class notes or doing assignments.	1	2	3	4
10. I try not to leave the tap running too long when I brush my teeth, shave, or bathe.	1	2	3	4

Spiritual Health

	Rarely, If Ever	Sometimes	Most of the Time	Always
1. I believe life is a precious gift that should be nurtured.	1	2	3	4
2. I take time to enjoy nature and the beauty around me.	1	2	3	4
3. I take time alone to think about what's important in life—who I am, what I value, where I fit in, and where I'm going.	1	2	3	4
4. I have faith in a greater power, be it a God-like force, nature, or the connectedness of all living things.	1	2	3	4
5. I engage in acts of caring and goodwill without expecting something in return.	1	2	3	4
6. I feel sorrow for those who are suffering and try to help them through difficult times.	1	2	3	4
7. I feel confident that I have touched the lives of others in a positive way.	1	2	3	4
8. I work for peace in my interpersonal relationships, in my community, and in the world at large.	1	2	3	4
9. I am content with who I am.	1	2	3	4
10. I go for the gusto and experience life to the fullest.	1	2	3	4

(continued)

stop cigarette smoking is an example of secondary prevention.

Because two of every three deaths and one of every three hospitalizations are linked to largely preventable behaviours—tobacco use, alcohol abuse, sedentary activities, and overeating, for example—primary and secondary prevention are essential to reducing the *incidence* (number of new cases) and *prevalence* (number of existing cases) of

Intellectual Health

	Rarely, If Ever	Sometimes	Most of the Time	Always
1. I tend to act impulsively without thinking about the consequences.	4	3	2	1
2. I learn from my mistakes and try to act differently the next time.	1	2	3	4
3. I follow directions or recommended guidelines and act in ways likely to keep myself and others safe.	1	2	3	4
4. I consider the alternatives before making decisions.	1	2	3	4
5. I am alert and ready to respond to life's challenges in ways that reflect thought and sound judgement.	1	2	3	4
6. I tend to let my emotions get the better of me and I act without thinking.	4	3	2	1
7. I actively try to learn all I can about products and services before making decisions.	1	2	3	4
8. I manage my time well, rather than time managing me.	1	2	3	4
9. My friends and family trust my judgement.	1	2	3	4
10. I think about my self-talk (the things I tell myself) and then examine the real evidence for my perceptions and feelings.	1	2	3	4

Personal Checklist

Now, total your scores in each of the health dimensions and compare it to the ideal score. Which areas do you need to work on? How does your score compare with how you rated yourself in the first part of the questionnaire?

	Ideal Score	Your Score
Physical Health	40	_____
Social Health	40	_____
Emotional Health	40	_____
Environmental Health	40	_____
Spiritual Health	40	_____
Intellectual Health	40	_____

What Your Scores Mean

Scores of 35–40: Outstanding! Your answers show that you are aware of the importance of this area to your health. More importantly, you are putting your knowledge to work for you by practising good health habits. As long as you continue to do so this area should not pose a serious health risk. It's likely that you are setting an example for your family and friends to follow. Although you received a very high score on this part of the test, you may want to consider other areas where your scores could be improved.

Scores of 30–35: Your health practices in this area are good, but there is room for improvement. Look again at the items you answered that scored one or two points. What changes could you make to improve your score? Even a small change in behaviour can often help you achieve better health.

Scores of 20–30: Your health risks are showing! Would you like more information about the risks you are facing and why it is important for you to change these behaviours? Perhaps you need help in deciding how to make the changes you desire. In either case, help is available from this book, from your professor, and from your student health services.

Scores below 20: You may be taking serious and unnecessary risks with your health. Perhaps you are not aware of the risks and what to do about them. In this book you will find the information you need to help you improve your scores and your health.

Source: Adapted from the U.S. Health and Human Services, *Health Style: A Self Test* (Washington, DC: Public Health Service, 1981).

diseases and disabilities.[7] Historically, the government has underfunded health education and health promotion activities; less than 5 percent of the total health care expenditure in Canada focusses on these preventive areas. Instead, government money has been allocated primarily for research and **tertiary prevention,** treatment and/or rehabilitation efforts made after a person has become sick. This form of prevention is both more costly and less effective in promoting health than is any other prevention method.

> **Tertiary prevention:** Treatment and/or rehabilitation efforts.

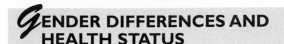

GENDER DIFFERENCES AND HEALTH STATUS

You don't have to be a health expert to know that there are physiological differences between men and women. Although much of male and female anatomy is identical, it's clear that many major medical differences exist. Many diseases—osteoporosis, thyroid disease, lupus, and Alzheimer's disease, for example—are far more common in women than in men. Diseases may show up differently in men than in women—research suggests that hypertension treatment for men may not be beneficial to Caucasian women, for example. Finally, although women live longer than men, they don't necessarily have a better quality of life.[8]

GLOBAL PERSPECTIVES

Disparities in Health: Real or Imagined?

While arguments currently rage over the best system of health care for Canada, it is useful to remember the vast differences between the haves and the have-nots when it comes to certain health indicators. Achieving a healthier Canada depends on significant improvements in the health of population groups now at higher risk for premature death, disease, and disability.

1. Of all the death rates listed, which shows the greatest disparity between status Indians and other Canadians? Which rates are worse for other Canadians than for status Indians?

2. What factors do you believe have contributed to these disparities?

3. What actions could be taken to improve each of the above health indicators? Which indicators may be modified by individual actions? Which ones must be modified by community (legislative, economic, environmental, or health care system) measures? By both individual and community actions?

Source: L. Lemchuk-Favel, Health Canada, *Trends in First Nations Mortality, 1979–1993,* Minister of Public Works and Government Services Canada, 1996, Cat. No. 34-79/1993E.

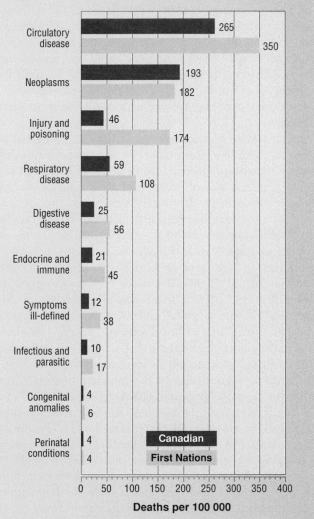

Leading Causes of Death Canadian and First Nations Populations, 1991–1993

Gender bias has been identified as a serious weakness in medical research. In one study, Eichler, Reisman, and Borins[9] reviewed medical journals in both Canada and the United States. They identified four factors in gender bias: androcentricity, overgeneralization, gender insensitivity, and double standards. *Androcentricity* means viewing the world from a male perspective. *Overgeneralization* occurs when a study explores issues for one sex but presents findings as though they apply to both sexes. In order to determine the precise effects of a drug or treatment, researchers have not wanted to deal with variations caused by women's menstrual cycles.

Of course, men and women do vary physiologically, and the elimination of women from many studies means that the results from these studies cannot be applied to women directly. According to social psychologist Carol Tavris, "If you want to know the effects of Drug X and you throw women out of your study because the menstrual cycle affects their responses to medication, you cannot then extrapolate from your study of men to women, precisely because the menstrual cycle affects their responses to medication."[10]

Gender insensitivity means overlooking sex as an important variable. Double standards refers to the "evaluation, treatment or measurement of the identical behaviours, traits or situations by different means".[11] A new policy on clinical trials as of 1996 stated that any testing has to be done on women if it is likely to be used by women. An example of such a trial might be an investigation of the use of angioplasty, a procedure to treat heart disease.

There has been increasing pressure placed on government to provide a more balanced approach to funding women's health programs. One example of increased activism is in the area of breast cancer. In Canada, one in nine women will be diagnosed with breast cancer; yet, until recently, there has been little research on the causes, treatments, and social and psychological concerns of women diagnosed with this illness. Women's increasing awareness of this serious health concern led to the National Forum on Breast Cancer, held in Montreal in November 1993. The Forum was a gathering of researchers, volunteers, policy makers, activists, and women who had a diagnosis of breast cancer, and their families. The participants developed a list of recommendations and pressured government to implement them. In 1996, $6.5 million was awarded by the Canadian Breast Cancer Initiative to fund 29 breast cancer research projects in Canada.[12] Health Canada is also funding research into communication with respect to breast cancer. The Breast Cancer Initiative has been extended for another five years as of April 1997 and the new government has pledged $35 million for this purpose. Further, a new women's health strategy is being developed and a National Population Health Institute is to be created in the near future.

IMPROVING YOUR HEALTH

Benefits of Achieving Optimal Health

Figure 1.3 provides an overview of the leading causes of death in Canada today. Risks for each of these leading killers can be reduced significantly by the practice of specific lifestyle patterns—for example, consuming a diet low in saturated fat and cholesterol, exercising regularly, reducing sodium intake, and managing stress. Individual behaviour is believed to be a major determinant of good health, but heredity, access to health care, the social influences of family and friends, community resources designed to promote health, and the environment are other factors that influence health status. When these factors are combined, the net effect on health can be great.

For example, you may be predisposed to a less healthy lifestyle if medical services are scarce in your area, if your family doesn't believe in mainstream medicine, or if family members or friends smoke, drink heavily, and/or take drugs. While you can't change your genetic history, and while improving your environment and the health care system can be difficult, you can influence your future health status by the behaviours you choose today.

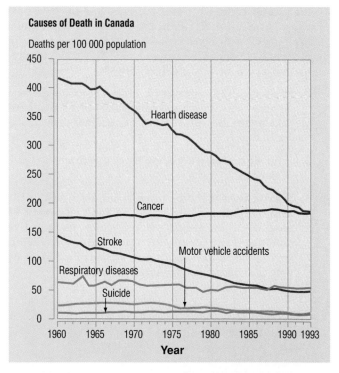

FIGURE 1.3

Causes of Death in Canada

Source: Canada Year Book, 1997, p. 95.

As Figure 1.3 shows, heart disease and cancer are the leading causes of death in Canada. Reduction in risk for these and other major diseases is just one of the benefits that you can hope to achieve when choosing healthy behaviours. Among the others are

- improved quality of life, in addition to an increased life span
- greater energy levels and increased capacity for and interest in having fun
- a stronger immune system, which enhances your ability to fight infections
- improved self-confidence, self-concept and self-esteem, and self-efficacy
- enhanced relationships with others due to better communication and "quality" time spent with them
- an improved ability to control and manage stress
- a reduced reliance on the health care system
- improved cardiovascular functioning
- increased muscle tone, strength, flexibility, and endurance, which results in improved physical appearance, performance, and self-esteem
- a more positive outlook on life, fewer negative thoughts, and an ability to view life as challenging and negative events as an opportunity for growth
- improved environmental sensitivity, responsibility, and behaviours
- enhanced levels of spiritual health, awareness, and feelings of oneness with yourself, others, and the environment

Making Health-Wise Choices

Although mounting evidence indicates that there are significant benefits to being healthy, many people find it difficult to become and remain healthy. Most experts believe that there are several key behaviours that will help people live longer, such as:

- getting a good night's sleep (minimum of seven hours)
- maintaining healthy eating habits
- weight management
- physical recreational activities
- avoiding tobacco products
- practising safe sex
- limiting intake of alcohol
- scheduling regular self-exams and medical checkups

Although health professionals can statistically assess the health benefits of these behaviours, there are several other actions that may not cause quantifiable "years added to life," but may significantly result in "life added to years," such as

- controlling the real and imaginary stressors in life
- forming and maintaining meaningful relationships with family and friends
- making time for oneself
- participating in at least one fun activity each day
- respecting the environment and the people in it
- considering alternatives when making decisions and assessing how actions affect others
- valuing each day and making the best of each opportunity
- viewing mistakes as opportunities to learn and grow
- being as kind to oneself as to others
- understanding the health care system and using it wisely

While it's easy to list things that one should do and even that one may really want to do, change is not easy. All people, no matter where they are on the health/wellness continuum, have to start somewhere. The key is to decide what needs to change, determine the major actions necessary for the accomplishment of goals, set up a plan of action, and get started. But first, it is important to take a close look at those factors that may contribute to current behaviours.

PREPARING FOR BEHAVIOUR CHANGE

Mark Twain said that "habit is habit, and not to be flung out the window by anyone, but coaxed downstairs a step at a time." Changing negative behaviour patterns into healthy ones is often a time-consuming and difficult process. The chances of successfully changing negative behaviour problems improve when you make gradual changes that give you time to unlearn negative patterns and to substitute positive ones. We have not yet developed a foolproof method for effectively changing behaviour, but we do know that certain behaviour changes can benefit both individuals and society. To understand how the process of behaviour change works, we must first identify specific behaviour patterns and attempt to understand the reasons for them.

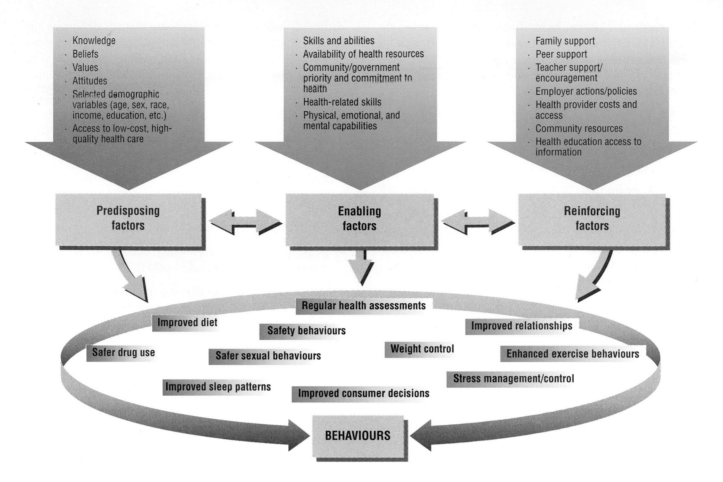

FIGURE 1.4

Factors That Influence Your Behaviour-Change Decisions

Factors Influencing Behaviour Change

Figure 1.4 identifies the major factors that influence behaviour and behaviour-change decisions. These factors can be divided into three general categories: predisposing, enabling, and reinforcing factors.

Predisposing Factors. Our life experiences, knowledge, cultural and ethnic inheritance, and current beliefs and values are all *predisposing factors* influencing behaviour and behaviour change. Factors that may predispose us to certain conditions include our age, sex, race, income, family background, educational background, and access to health care. For example, if your parents smoked, you are 90 percent more likely to start smoking than someone whose parents didn't. If your peers smoke, you are 80 percent more likely to smoke than someone whose friends don't.

Enabling Factors. Skills or abilities; physical, emotional, and mental capabilities; and resources and accessible facilities that make health decisions more convenient or difficult are *enabling factors*. Positive enablers encourage you to carry through on your intentions. Negative enablers work against your intentions to change. For example, if you would like to join a local fitness centre but discover that the closest one is 10 kilometres away and that the membership fee is $500, those negative enablers may convince you to stay home. On the other hand, if your school's fitness centre is two blocks away, is open until midnight, and has a special student membership deal, those positive enablers will probably convince you to join the centre. Identifying these positive and negative enabling factors and devising alternative plans when the negative factors outweigh the positive are part of a necessary planning strategy for behavioural change.

Reinforcing Factors. The presence or absence of support, encouragement, or discouragement that significant people in your life bring to a situation is a *reinforcing factor*. For example, if you decide to stop smoking and your family and friends smoke in your presence, you may be tempted to start smoking again. In other words, your smoking behaviour was reinforced. Reinforcing factors also include policies and services that make it easier for you to maintain a particular behaviour. If, however, you are overweight and you lose a few pounds and all your friends tell you how terrific you look, your positive behaviour will be reinforced and you will be more likely to continue. Reinforcing factors, which may influence you toward positive and/or negative behaviours, include money, popularity, support and appreciation from friends, and family interest and enthusiasm for what you are doing.

The manner in which you reward or punish yourself for your own successes and failures may affect your chances of adopting healthy behaviours. Learning to accept small failures and to concentrate on your successes may foster further successes. Berating yourself because you binged on ice cream, argued with a friend, or didn't jog because it was raining may create an internal environment in which failure becomes almost inevitable. Telling yourself that you're worth the extra time and effort and giving yourself a pat on the back for small accomplishments is an often-overlooked factor in positive behaviour change.

It is not our intention to blame you if you are struggling with personal health behaviours or to suggest that all the variables that affect health are within your control. Our goal is to help you realize which factors are within your personal control and to show you how to maximize your decision-making powers to maintain your current good health, improve your current health, or prevent premature deterioration of your health status.

Major changes in health behaviour are not made by following easy, one-step recipes. Lasting behaviour changes that ultimately improve your overall health and well-being require careful thought, individual analysis, and considerable effort. Changing beliefs, attitudes, values, actions, and behaviours that have been developing from infancy is difficult. Not surprisingly, even the most strong-willed people discover that willpower alone is not enough to get them through the many adjustments usually needed to change behaviour.

Wanting to change is a prerequisite of the change process, but there is much more to the process than motivation. Motivation must be combined with common sense, commitment, and a realistic understanding of how best to move from point A to point B. *Readiness* is the state of being that precedes behaviour change. People who are ready to change possess the knowledge, attitudes, skills, and internal and external resources that make change a likely reality. For someone to be ready for change, certain basic steps and adjustments in thinking must occur.

𝒲HAT DO YOU THINK?

Who do you think you could ask to help support you in your behaviour change effort? What factors could make this change difficult? What can you do to avoid these difficulties?

Your Beliefs and Attitudes

Even if you know why you should make a specific behaviour change, your beliefs and attitudes about the value of your actions in making a difference will significantly affect what you do. We often assume that when rational people realize there is a risk in what they are doing, they will act to reduce that risk. But this is not necessarily true. Consider the number of physicians and other health professionals who smoke, fail to manage stress, consume high-fat diets, and act in other unhealthy ways. They surely know better, but their "knowing" is disconnected from their "doing." Why is this so? Two strong influences on our actions are beliefs and attitudes.

A **belief** is an appraisal of the relationship between some object, action, or idea (for example, smoking) and some attribute of that object, action, or idea (for example, smoking is expensive, dirty, and causes cancer—or it is relaxing). Beliefs may develop from direct experience (for example, if you have trouble breathing after smoking for several years) or from secondhand experience or knowledge conveyed by other people (for example, if you see your grandfather die of lung cancer after he has smoked for years).[13] Although most of us have a general idea of what constitutes a belief, we may be a bit uncertain about what constitutes an attitude. We often hear or make such comments as, "He's got a rotten attitude," or, "She needs an attitude adjustment," but may still be unable to define *attitude*. An **attitude** is a relatively stable set of beliefs, feelings, and behavioural tendencies in relation to something or someone.

Do Beliefs and Attitudes Influence Behaviour?

It seems logical to conclude that your beliefs will influence your behaviour. If you believe (make the appraisal) that taking drugs (an action) is harmful for you (attribute of that action), you will not use drugs. If you believe that drinking and driving are incompatible, you will never drink and drive. Or will you?

Psychologists studying the relationship between beliefs and health behaviours have determined that although beliefs may subtly influence behaviour, these beliefs may not actually cause people to change behaviour. In 1966, psychologist I. Rosenstock developed a model for explaining

Belief: Appraisal of the relationship between some object, action, or idea and some attribute of that object, action, or idea.

Attitude: Relatively stable set of beliefs, feelings, and behavioural tendencies in relation to something or someone.

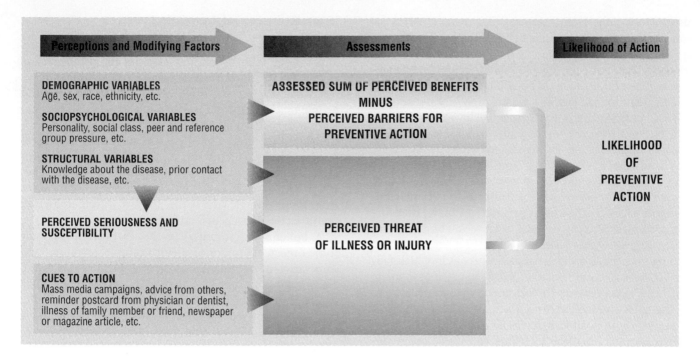

FIGURE 1.5

Health Belief Model

Source: Adapted by permission from Edward P. Sarafino, *Health Psychology: Biopsychosocial Interactions* (New York: John Wiley & Sons, 1990), p. 190. © 1990 by John Wiley & Sons.

how beliefs may or may not influence subsequent behaviours.[14] His **Health Belief Model (HBM)** provides a means to show when beliefs affect behaviour change (see Figure 1.5). Although many other models attempt to explain the influence of beliefs on behaviours, the HBM is one of the most widely accepted models. According to the HBM, several factors must support a belief in order for change to be likely to occur:

- *Perceived seriousness of the health problem.* First, a person needs to consider how severe the medical and social consequences would be if the health problem was to develop or was left untreated. The more serious a person believes the effects will be, the more likely he or she is to take action.

- *Perceived susceptibility to the health problem.* Next, a person needs to evaluate the likelihood of developing the health problem. Those who perceive themselves as more likely to develop the health problem are more likely to take preventive action.

- *Cues to action.* Those who are reminded or alerted about a potential health problem are more likely to take preventive action.

Three other factors are linked to perceived risk for health problems: *demographic variables,* including age, gender,

race, and ethnic background; *sociopsychological variables,* including personality traits, social class, and social pressure; and *structural variables,* including knowledge about or prior contact with the health problem.

The Health Belief Model is followed many times every day. Take, for example, smokers. Older smokers are likely to know other smokers who have developed serious heart or lung problems as a result of smoking. They are thus more likely to perceive a threat to their health connected with the behaviour of smoking than is a young person who has just begun smoking. The greater the perceived threat of health problems caused by smoking, the greater the chance a person will quit smoking. However, many chronic smokers know that they have serious health problems, yet they continue to smoke. Why do people fail to take actions to avoid further harm? According to Rosenstock, some people do not believe that they will be affected by a severe problem—they act as if they believe they have some kind of immunity—and are unlikely to change their behaviours. In some cases, they may think that, even if they get cancer or have a heart attack, the health care system will cure them.

Health Belief Model (HBM): Model for explaining how beliefs may influence behaviours.

Are You "Staged" for Change?

Have you ever come up with a great New Year's or Monday morning resolution about something you "are going to do differently" only to have your good intention fall by the wayside a few days later? As most of people have discovered at one time or another, changing established behaviours is not an easy task. Much of what we do is influenced by an entire host of variables, including our past history, reward systems, values, and culture. If you are in your 20s, you've been doing them for years and they seem to be a natural part of who you are. Changing that part of you will usually not be easy.

A number of theories/models help explain why some people are successful at their attempts at behaviour change and others are not. One that has gained attention in recent years is the Stages of Change or Transtheoretical model from researchers James Prochaska and Carlo DiClemente in the early 1980s. Developed from research on smoking cessation and drug and alcohol addiction, the Stages of Change model has been applied to a wide range of health behaviours over the years, including HIV prevention. Essentially, the Stages of Change model asks:

Are you ready for change?

and

Where are you on the readiness scale?

This probably sounds a bit familiar to you. Like other behavioural models discussed in this chapter, the Stages of Change model indicates that the more ready you are to change and the higher your motivation, the greater your chances of success. From their research, Prochaska and DiClemente concluded that an individual proceeds through five distinctive stages during the change process. Those stages are:

1. The Pre-Contemplation Stage, in which you probably aren't aware that you have a problem and, therefore, haven't even considered making any changes. Others around you, however, often do recognize the need for change.

2. The Contemplation Stage, in which you acknowledge the problem and begin to think about the need to change. Acknowledgement usually results from increased awareness, often in the form of feedback from family and friends or access to information. Although you may not know how to proceed, you start to examine the issue.

3. The Decision/Determination Stage (also called Preparation), during which you actually decide to make a change and begin to make plans about how to proceed.

4. The Action Stage, wherein you begin to follow the specific action plan you've created.

5. The Maintenance Stage, in which you keep up or maintain your behaviour changes. During this stage, you need to be aware of the potential for relapses and develop strategies for dealing with such challenges.

How Staged Are You?

To understand the Stages of Change model, try the following exercise:

- Think about one health behaviour you would consider changing.

  _____

  Just the fact that you are aware of it puts you in the Contemplative Stage. Now take it a bit further.

- How serious are you about the change? What are the possible actions you could take to make it work? What are potential barriers that could interfere with success? What or who will help motivate you?

  _____

  _____

  _____

- When will you start? What actions will you take? Have you set realistic, gradual goals? Who will help support your efforts? Have you verbalized your intentions to anyone?

  _____

  _____

  _____

- Have you identified some ongoing reinforcements to help you follow the plan? List actions you will take on a daily basis. How will you reward yourself? What will you do if you slip and don't meet the goals for a particular day? What alternative actions can you take? What will you use as motivation to stay on target?

  _____

  _____

  _____

Other HBM factors that affect the likelihood of behaviour change are assessments about whether the benefits outweigh the costs and whether actions will actually work. If you are so addicted to smoking that the thought of quitting is not acceptable to you, or if you enjoy smoking too much, you will probably keep smoking, particularly if the consequences won't be felt for some time and the pleasure is there for the moment.

Your Intentions to Change

Our attitudes tend to reflect our emotional responses to
situations and also tend to follow from our beliefs. According to the **Theory of Reasoned Action,** our behaviours result from our intentions to perform actions. An
intention is a product of our attitude toward an action
and our beliefs about what others may want us to do.[15] A
behavioural intention, then, is a written or stated commitment to perform an action.

If, for example, you are out of shape and your health is
important to you, you may take steps to improve your fitness level. But if your best friends tell you that you really do
need to get into shape and you want to gain their respect or
admiration, your intention to begin an exercise program
may become stronger. In brief, the more consistent and
powerful your attitudes about an action are and the more
you are influenced by others to take that action, the greater
will be your stated intention to do so—in this example, to
exercise. The more you verbalize your commitment to exercising, the more likely it is that you will exercise.

Significant Others as Change Agents

Many people are highly influenced by the approval or disapproval (real or imagined) of close friends and loved
ones and of the social and cultural groups to which they
belong. Such influences can offer support for health actions, making healthy behaviour all the more possible to
attain; they can also affect behaviour negatively, interfering with even the best intentions of making a positive
change.

Your Family.   From the time of your birth, your parents
have influenced your behaviours by giving you strong
cues about which actions are socially acceptable and
which are not. Brushing your teeth, bathing, wearing deodorant, and chewing food with your mouth closed are
probably all behaviours that your family instilled in you
long ago. Your family culture influenced your food
choices, your religious beliefs, your political beliefs, and
all your other values and actions. If you deviated from
your family's norms, your mother or father probably let
you know fairly quickly.

Family can mean many things to a child growing up.
For those who have two parents present, it may mean a
mother and a father who take the time to teach respect for
property and for others, and to provide the social support
and comfort that a child needs to feel loved and secure.
For others, it may mean a single mom or dad who uses the
support of friends and relatives to create a loving and nurturing atmosphere for growth. In some cases, family is the
group of loved ones that a person lives with, whether relatives, friends, or a group brought together by common
bonds. No two family structures are exactly alike. What
good family units have in common is a dedication to the
healthful development of all family members, unconditional trust, and a commitment to work out difficulties.

When the loving family unit does not exist, when it
does not provide for basic human needs, or when dysfunctional, irresponsible individuals try to build a family
under the influence of drugs or alcohol, it becomes difficult for a child to learn positive health behaviours.
Healthy behaviours get their start in healthy homes; unhealthy homes breed unhealthy habits. Healthy families
provide the foundation for a clear and necessary understanding of what is right and wrong, what is positive and
negative. Without this fundamental grounding, many
young people have great difficulties.

Social Bonds.   Like family, hometown environments
also mold behaviours. If you deviated from the actions expected in your hometown, you probably suffered strange
looks, ostracism by some high school cliques, and other
negative social reactions. The more you value the opinions of other people, the more likely you are to change a
behaviour that offends them. If you couldn't care less
what they think, you probably brush off their negative reactions or suggested changes. How often have you told
yourself, "I don't care what so-and-so thinks. I'll do what
I darn well please"? Although most of us have thought or
said these words, we in fact all too often care too much
about what even the insignificant people in our lives
think. We say certain things, act in a prescribed manner,
and respond in a specific way because our culture, our
upbringing, and our need to be liked by others pressure
us to do what we believe they think is the right thing. In
general, the lower your level of self-esteem and self-efficacy, the higher the chances that others will influence your
actions.

Sometimes, the influence of others can be a powerful
social support for our positive behaviour changes. At other
times, we are influenced to drink too much, party too hard,
eat too much, or engage in some other negative action because we don't want to be left out or because we fear criticism. Learning to understand the subtle and not-so-subtle
ways in which our families, friends, and other people have
influenced and continue to influence our behaviours is an
important step toward changing our behaviours.

BEHAVIOUR CHANGE TECHNIQUES

Once you have analyzed all the factors influencing your current behaviour and all the factors that may influence the direction and potential success of the behaviour change you are considering, you must decide which of several possible behaviour change techniques will work best for you.

Shaping: Developing New Behaviours in Small Steps

Regardless of how motivated and committed you are to change, some behaviours are almost impossible to change immediately. To reach your goal, you may need to take a number of individual steps, each designed to change one small piece of the larger behaviour. This process is known as **shaping.**

Whatever the desired behaviour change, all shaping involves

- starting slowly and trying not to cause undue stress during the early stages of the program

- keeping the steps small and achievable

- being flexible and ready to change if the original plan proves uncomfortable

- refusing to skip steps or to move to the next step until the previous step has been mastered; behaviours don't develop overnight, so they won't change overnight

Visualizing: The Imagined Rehearsal

Mental practice and rehearsal can help change unhealthy behaviours into healthy ones. Athletes and others have used a technique known as **imagined rehearsal** to reach their goals. By visualizing their planned action ahead of time, they were better prepared when they put themselves to the test.

Modelling

Modelling, or learning behaviours through careful observation of other people, is one of the most effective strategies for changing behaviour. If you carefully observe behaviours you admire and isolate their components, you can model the steps of your behaviour change strategy on a proven success.

Controlling the Situation

Sometimes, putting yourself in the right setting or with the right group of people will positively influence your behaviours directly or indirectly. Many situations and occasions trigger similar behaviours by different people. For example, in libraries, churches, and museums, most peo-ple talk softly. Few people laugh at funerals. The term **situational inducement** refers to an attempt to influence a behaviour by using situations and occasions that are structured to exert control over that behaviour.

Reinforcement: "Different Strokes for Different Folks"

A **positive reinforcement** seeks to increase the likelihood that a behaviour will occur by presenting something positive as a reward for that behaviour. Each of us is motivated by different reinforcers. While a special T-shirt may be a positive reinforcer for young adults entering a race, it may not be for a 50-year-old runner who dislikes message-bearing T-shirts, or for someone with a drawer full of them.

Most positive reinforcers can be classified under five headings: consumable, activity, manipulative, possessional, and social reinforcers.

- *Consumable reinforcers* are delicious edibles such as candy, cookies, or gourmet meals.

- *Activity reinforcers* are opportunities to watch TV, to go on a vacation, to go swimming, or to do something else enjoyable.

- *Manipulative reinforcers* are such incentives as lower rent in exchange for mowing the lawn or the promise of a better grade for doing an extra-credit project.

- *Possessional reinforcers* are tangible rewards such as a new TV or a sports car.

- *Social reinforcers* are such things as loving looks, affectionate hugs, and praise.

When choosing reinforcers to help you maintain a healthy behaviour or change an unhealthy behaviour, you need to determine what would motivate you to act in a particular way. Your rewards or reinforcers may initially come from others (extrinsic rewards), but as you see positive changes in yourself, you will begin to reward and reinforce yourself (intrinsic rewards). Keep in mind that reinforcers

---

Theory of Reasoned Action: Model for explaining the importance of our intentions in determining behaviours.

Shaping: Using a series of small steps to get to a particular goal gradually.

Imagined rehearsal: Practising through mental imagery, to become better able to perform an event in actuality.

Modelling: Learning specific behaviours by watching others perform them.

Situational inducement: Attempt to influence a behaviour by using situations and occasions that are structured to exert control over that behaviour.

Positive reinforcement: Presenting something positive following a behaviour that is being reinforced.

How to Help Someone Make a Change

In our quest to help loved ones change unhealthy behaviours, we sometimes become self-righteous. We then become "warriors against pleasure" to our loved ones and all our brilliant advice falls on deaf ears.

Why do our good intentions go up in smoke? Probably because of the way we communicate our advice. Ask yourself the following questions before offering your words of wisdom:

- Did your friend ask for your advice or help?

- Did your friend give any indication of being dissatisfied about something? Is there something that your friend indicated needed a change?

- Are you in a position to offer advice? Are you practising what you preach?

- If you were in need of advice or help, how would you want someone to approach the subject with you?

- How honest can you be? How well do you know your friend's reactions? Can your friend take constructive advice? Is your friend very sensitive or defensive about his or her problem?

After you've asked yourself these questions,

- **Go slow.** Wait for some suggestion that your friend wants to talk. Don't just meet him or her in class and say, "Hey, have you thought about getting rid of that weight?"

- **If your friend doesn't initiate a conversation about the problem, try to ease into it slowly.** You could say, "Boy, I sure put on weight over the holidays. I really need to start working out to get rid of these extra pounds. I hate to go alone. Would you be interested in going swimming with me sometime this week?"

- **If your friend brings up the problem, be supportive.** "I know how hard it is to lose weight. I've struggled with it myself over the years, but have found that such and such works for me. I need to lose some weight myself. Let's work on it together. It'd really help me to have someone help me stay motivated."

- **If your friend is successful in getting started, regularly compliment his or her persistence in sticking to the diet/exercise program.** Don't overdo the compliments, particularly with someone who isn't comfortable with a cheerleader approach. Treat him or her as you'd normally do. Don't go overboard.

- **If your friend has a setback, say it's okay.** Say you understand, but also encourage him or her to get back on track and stay motivated.

- **Help your friend stay interested.** Try to think of new things to do, new exercise routines, and new eating habits that will make behaviour change a lifestyle change rather than an obstacle to be overcome.

- **Keep positive and offer support whenever it's asked for.** If you are brushed off or if your friend becomes angry, be patient and try another method.

---

should immediately follow a behaviour. But beware of overkill. If you reward yourself with a movie on the VCR every time you go jogging, this reinforcer will soon lose its power. It would be better to give yourself this reward after, say, a full week of adherence to your jogging program.

ᗯHAT DO YOU THINK?

What type of consumable reinforcers (food or drink) would be a healthy reward for your new behaviour? If you could choose one activity reinforcer to reward yourself after you've been successful for one day in your new behaviour, what would it be? If you could obtain/buy something for yourself (possessional reinforcer) after you reach your goal, what would it be? If you maintain your behaviour for one week, what type of social reinforcer would you like to receive from your friends?

Changing Self-Talk

Self-talk, or the way you think and talk to yourself, can also play a role in modifying your health-related behaviours. Here are some cognitive procedures for changing self-talk.

Rational-Emotive Therapy. This form of cognitive therapy or self-directed behaviour change is based on the premise that there is a close connection between what people say to themselves and how they feel. According to psychologist Albert Ellis, most everyday emotional problems and related behaviours stem from irrational statements that people make to themselves when events in their lives are different from what they would like them to be.[16]

Meichenbaum's Self-Instructional Methods. In Meichenbaum's behavioural therapies, clients are encouraged to give "self-instructions" ("Slow down, don't rush") and "positive affirmations" ("My speech is going fine— I'm almost done!") to themselves instead of thinking self-defeating thoughts ("I'm talking too fast—my speech is terrible") whenever a situation seems to be getting out of control. Meichenbaum is perhaps best known for a process known as stress inoculation, in which clients are subjected to extreme stressors in a laboratory environment. Before a stressful event (e.g., going to the doctor), clients practise individual coping skills (e.g., deep breathing exercises) and self-instructions (e.g., "I'll feel better once I know what's causing my pain"). Meichenbaum

The success of efforts to change unhealthy behaviours often depends on conscious decisions to choose the right friends and to put oneself in constructive situations.

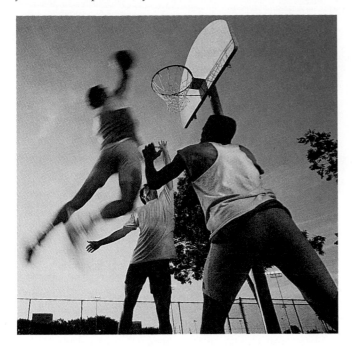

demonstrated that clients who practised coping techniques and self-instruction were less likely to resort to negative behaviours in stressful situations.

Blocking/Thought Stopping. By purposely blocking or stopping negative thoughts, a person can concentrate on taking positive steps toward necessary behaviour change. For example, suppose you are preoccupied with your ex-partner, who has recently deserted you for someone else. In blocking/thought stopping, you consciously stop thinking about the situation and force yourself to think about something more pleasant (e.g., dinner tomorrow with your best friend). By refusing to dwell on negative images and by forcing yourself to focus elsewhere, you can save wasted energy, time, and emotional resources and move on to positive change.

MAKING BEHAVIOUR CHANGE

Self-Assessment: Antecedents and Consequences

Behaviours, thoughts, and feelings always occur in a context—the situation. Situations can be divided into two components: the events that come before and those that come after a behaviour. *Antecedents* are the setting events for a behaviour; they cue or stimulate a person to act in certain ways. Antecedents can be physical events,

thoughts, emotions, or the actions of other people. *Consequences*—the results of behaviour—affect whether a person will repeat a behaviour.[17] Consequences can also be physical events, thoughts, emotions, or the actions of other people.

Learning to recognize the antecedents of a behaviour and acting to modify them is one method of changing behaviour. A diary noting your undesirable behaviours and identifying the settings in which they occur can be a useful tool. For example, if you are gaining weight because you are snacking too much, keep a diary of when, where, and with whom you snack. If you are shovelling in the potato chips while studying, you may need to study in the library, where food isn't allowed, or to keep only low-calorie snacks in the house. If you eat more when you are angry, upset, depressed, or stressed, try to deal directly with your stressors. The positive consequences of these changes will be that you will maintain your weight. In the Skills for Behaviour Change box, you may recognize several factors that can make behaviour change more difficult.

Analyzing the Behaviour You Want to Change

Successful behaviour change requires a careful assessment of exactly what it is that you want to change. All too often we berate ourselves by using generalities: "I am not a good person, I'm lousy to my friend, I need to be a better person." Before you can begin to change a negative behaviour, you must take a hard look at its specifics. Determining the specific behaviour you would like to change—in contrast to the general problem—will allow you to set clear goals for change. What are you doing that makes you a lousy friend? Are you gossiping about your friend? Are you lying to your friend? Have you been a "taker" rather than a "giver" in the friendship? Or are you really a good friend most of the time?

Let's say the problem is gossiping. You can now analyze this behaviour by examining the following components:

- *Frequency.* How often are you gossiping? All the time, or only once in a while?

- *Duration.* Have you been gossiping about your friend for a long period of time? How long?

- *Seriousness.* Is your gossiping just idle chatter, or are you really getting down and dirty and trying to injure the other person? What are the consequences for you? For your friend? For your friendship?

- *Basis for problem behaviour.* Is your gossip based on facts, on your perceptions of facts, or on deliberate embellishments of facts?

- *Antecedents.* What kinds of situations trigger your gossiping? Do some settings or people bring out the gossip in you more than other settings and people? What triggers your feelings of dislike for or irritation toward your friend? Why are you talking behind your friend's back?

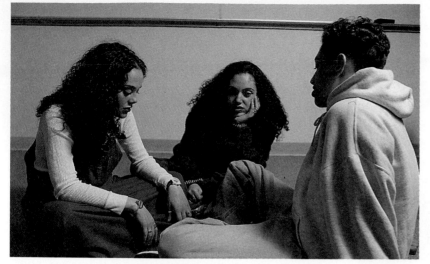

Talking with friends who have similar values can help you clarify your thinking about behaviours you want to change and provide ongoing support as you attempt to reach your goals.

Decision Making: Choices for Change

You've assessed the antecedents and consequences of the behaviour you want to change and analyzed its components. Now comes the real crunch: deciding what to do when faced with choices. Decision making is a skill that you must consciously develop. Choosing among alternatives is difficult when you are consciously and unconsciously pressured by internal and external influences. For example, "just saying no" is, of course, one choice when you are handed a glass of beer at a party. However, if you are trying desperately not to be considered a dweeb, if people with whom you identify are all drinking, or if you like the taste of beer, the decision becomes harder. By practising the following decision-making skills prior to having that drink put into your hands, you will increase your chances of making the choice you really want to make. This set of skills, referred to as DECIDE, can be applied to many situations in which you have to make a decision.[18]

D *Decide in advance what the problem is.* By defining the problem in advance, you will have time to decide how important it is. If you have really decided that drinking is not for you, or that drinking in certain situations could put you at risk, you will have set your basic criteria for acting in specific situations.

E *Explore the alternatives.* List the possible alternatives, ranging from not drinking to drinking heavily. If any of these alternatives is unacceptable to you, cross it off and work with those remaining.

C *Consider the consequences.* Think about each of the alternatives remaining. What are the possible positive and negative consequences of each? Think about what will probably happen, not just what may happen in the best and worst scenarios. How risky is each alternative? Are the consequences of losing the friendship of a group because you refuse to drink as serious as of drinking heavily and getting into trouble sexually or of

drinking and driving? Is there another alternative that could reduce your risks?

I *Identify your values.* Your beliefs and feelings about certain behaviours represent your values, and your values influence the vast majority of your behaviours. When choosing to drink or not to drink in a social setting, or when choosing how much to drink, you should base your choice on an analysis of your values.

D *Decide and take action.* If you have seriously thought about the first four DECIDE skills and decided that it's okay to have one or two drinks over the course of the evening and that that is the absolute limit, this may be a reasonable decision for you. Now you must take action based upon your decision—you must actively resist temptation and stick to your limit.

E *Evaluate the consequences.* A key component of the decision-making process is a careful look backward at your decision and your resulting behaviour, how you felt about them, and whether you want to do anything differently in the future. You may add other alternatives at step 2, for instance. The secret to success is to think about the problem in advance, consider your values and wants, and anticipate the choices you will have.

🖊 WHAT DO YOU THINK?

Why is it sometimes hard for you to make decisions? What things influence your decisions?

Setting Goals

There are several steps you can take to develop behaviour-change goals that are realistic for you. For example, suppose that you are gaining weight. Rather than saying, "I eat too much and my goal is to not eat so much," you need to be specific about your current behaviour. Are you eating too many sweets? Are you gorging yourself at dinner and not eating breakfast? Perhaps a better statement of the

Managing Your Behaviour-Change Strategies

Having read this chapter, you should realize that health involves many dimensions of your life. Changing negative health-related behaviours is a complicated, multifaceted process requiring a great deal of commitment, personal insight, and knowledge. Very few of us could ever "just do it" as the advertisements may lead you to believe (at least not on the first try). As you read this book, you will find that each chapter lists specific activities and choices that enable you to adopt or maintain healthy behaviours. It may be helpful for you to consider the following activities and questions as you begin planning your best course of action.

Making Decisions for You

1. List the specific behaviour that you want to change.
2. Outline the steps you will take to achieve this change.
3. What reinforcers can you give yourself along the way? Who could you call upon to help keep you motivated? Are they willing to help?
4. What techniques do you think will be most useful (positive reinforcement, shaping, modelling, imagined rehearsal, situational inducement, changes in self-talk, others)?

Checklist for Change: Making Personal Choices

✓ Are you ready to make this change? Are you in a healthy emotional state? Are you doing it for you or to please someone else?

✓ Have you completed a personal health history to assess your risks from various sources?

✓ Have you developed an action plan with short- and long-term goals? Have you set priorities?

✓ Have you assessed your personal resources? Who can you call on to help you? Where can you go for support and advice?

✓ Have you planned alternative actions in case you run into obstacles or begin to self-sabotage?

✓ Have you set up a list of reinforcers and supports that will keep you motivated along the way?

✓ Have you established a set of guidelines for success? Will you have small goals to achieve at selected intervals or will you only consider yourself successful if you have met your ultimate goal?

Checklist for Change: Making Community Choices

✓ Have you taken time to become educated about issues/concerns affecting others in your community?

✓ Have you prioritized the actions that you can take to make a difference in changing community behaviours? Do you have a particular goal?

✓ Do you act responsibly to preserve the environment by consuming fewer resources? Using fewer packaged items? Reusing, recycling, and reducing consumption whenever possible?

✓ Do you analyze what is happening in your school, community, state, and nation by reading about issues, actively discussing problems and possible solutions, and developing personal opinions?

✓ Do you listen carefully to what your elected officials say and let them know in writing or by calling if you disagree with them?

✓ Do you vote for elected officials whose policies, rhetoric, and past histories have indicated that they support improvements in health care, the environment, education, and minority health?

✓ Do you volunteer your time to help others who are less fortunate at least once during every term?

✓ Do you purchase products and services from companies that have proven records of protecting the environment, providing safe foods and products, and supporting the health and well-being of others through their organizational practices?

Critical Thinking

Each chapter of this text will end with a decision-making situation. You may wish to use the DECIDE model introduced in this chapter to develop decision-making skills. For your first decision, let's return to the situation described when we introduced the DECIDE model: To drink or not to drink. Let's assume that you are attending a major dorm party tonight where alcohol will be served—and you have a test tomorrow afternoon. Using the decision-making model, will you drink? If so, will you set a limit? How will you respond if offered more than your limit?

---

problem would be, "I eat too many high-fat foods, particularly at dinner." A realistic goal that could follow from that statement is, "I am going to try to eat less fat during dinner every day." What strategies could you use to reach this goal? Recording all the foods you eat every day may show, for instance, that the greatest source of fat in your meals is condiments. You could reach your goal by buying low-fat dressings and other condiments, by limiting your use of condiments, or by finding fat-free substitutes. You may find you've been eating too many fried and sautéed foods. In that case, your goal would be to bake or broil as many foods as possible, thereby reducing your fat intake.

Another antecedent for your diet choices may be with whom you're eating. Do you eat as much or the same type of foods when you are with your dieting, fitness-conscious friends as you do when you are with your overweight, food-loving friends? Or do you eat more fattening foods in greater quantity when you are alone? Why? Answering these kinds of questions will give you valuable insights into your behaviours.

Summary

◆ Health is defined as a dynamic process of trying to achieve your individual potential in the physical, social, emotional, intellectual, spiritual, and environmental dimensions. Wellness means achieving the highest level of health possible along several dimensions.

◆ Although Canadians have increased average life span, we need to increase our span of quality life.

◆ Gender continues to play a major role in health status and care. Women have longer lives but more medical problems than do men. The recent political support to include women in medical research and training attempts to close the gap in health care.

◆ The leading causes of death are heart disease, cancer, and stroke. Many of the risks associated with the leading killers can be reduced through lifestyle changes.

◆ Several factors contribute to your health status, but not all of them are within your control. Your beliefs and attitudes, your intentions to change, support from significant others, and your readiness to change are all factors over which you have some degree of control. Access to health care, genetic predisposition, health policies that are supportive of your actions, and other factors are all potential reinforcing, predisposing, and enabling factors that may influence your health decisions.

◆ Applying behaviour change techniques such as shaping, visualizing, modelling, controlling the situation, reinforcing, and changing self-talk to your personal situations will help you to be successful in making behaviour changes.

◆ Decision making has several key components: Defining the problem, Exploring alternatives, Considering consequences, Identifying your values, Deciding and acting, and Evaluating the consequences of your choices. Following the DECIDE model can assist you to make behaviour changes.

Discussion Questions

1. How are the terms *health* and *wellness* similar? What, if any, are important distinctions between these terms?

2. How healthy are Canadians today? How will health promotion and illness and accident prevention improve both life span and quality of life?

3. What are some of the major differences in the way males and females are treated in the health care system? Why do you think these differences exist?

4. What are the leading causes of death when you look at all ages and races? What lifestyle changes can you make to lower your risks for major diseases?

5. What is the Health Belief Model? The Theory of Reasoned Action? How may each of these models be working when a young woman decides to smoke her first cigarette? Her last cigarette?

6. Explain the predisposing, reinforcing, and enabling factors influencing the decision of a young welfare mother who is deciding to sell drugs to support her children.

7. Describe how you could use each of the behaviour change techniques to change your couch-potato behaviour and start an exercise program.

8. What are the key components of the decision-making process? Why is it important that you be ready to change before you try to start changing?

Application Exercise

Reread the *What Do You Think?* scenarios at the beginning of the chapter and answer the following questions.

1. From what you learned in this chapter, what steps would each of the people discussed here have to take to change their behaviours?

2. On your campus, where could students having similar problems go for help?

3. As a friend, what can you do to be more supportive of the health of someone you know who is trying to make a change?

Health on the Net

Canadian Association for Quality in Health Care
highlander.cbnet.ns.ca/cbnet/healthca/caqhc/

Healthyway
www1.sympatico.ca:80/healthyway/

World Health Organization
www.who.ch/

Psychosocial Health

Achieving Intellectual, Emotional, Social, and Spiritual Wellness

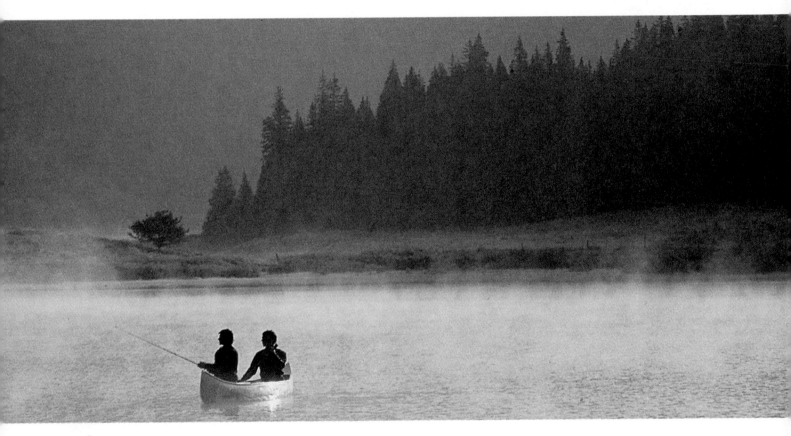

CHAPTER OBJECTIVES

◆ Define psychosocial health in terms of its intellectual, emotional, social, and spiritual components, and identify the basic elements shared by psychosocially healthy people.

◆ Identify the internal and external factors influencing psychosocial health.

◆ Discuss the positive steps you can take to enhance your psychosocial health.

◆ Identify and describe common psychosocial problems, and explain their causes and available treatments.

◆ Illustrate the warning signs of suicide and what actions can be taken to help a suicidal individual.

◆ Evaluate the role gender plays in diagnoses of mental health.

◆ Identify the different types of mental health professionals and the most popular types of therapy.

Marisol is a 19-year-old first-year student majoring in liberal arts. She has become increasingly bored with her classes, finds little excitement in her days, and doesn't have the energy or desire to go out with friends. One recent weekend, she stayed in bed for two days "resting," and when she got up on Monday, she was still so tired that she could barely stay awake in class. She can't concentrate, she finds herself lounging on the couch watching TV every evening, and she doesn't care whether her apartment is a mess. She has gone to the student health centre, but after several tests, the doctor tells her that there is nothing physically wrong with her.

- Have you ever felt like Marisol? What do you think has contributed to her present condition? Do you have any friends who are showing similar characteristics? Why might a typical student health professional miss such obvious symptoms? What do you think Marisol should do to help herself get better? As a friend, what could you do to help her? What services and programs are available on your campus for helping someone like her?

Most of us have felt this "down" occasionally, but we are typically able to get through the day in a reasonably productive, if not altogether exciting, way. We eventually sort through seemingly overwhelming problems, suppress our anxieties, and use our social support system (families, friends, significant others, etc.) to help us get through the low times. But for some of us, these skirmishes with the blues become persistent, nagging experiences that vary from small "downers" to "black holes" that are increasingly difficult to emerge from. Whether caused by temporary setbacks or major blows, these miserable moods can sap our energy, reduce our physical reserves, waste our time, diminish our spirit, and take the joy out of our lives. They may even lead to serious mental illness. Eventually, they may result in a shortened life expectancy. Perhaps even more important, they will almost certainly result in diminished life experiences.

How we feel and think about ourselves, those around us, and our circumstances can tell us a lot about our psychosocial health. Just as important as our physical health, our psychosocial health can have a profound impact on the quality of our lives. And, just as with our physical health, we can enhance our psychosocial health by becoming aware of and working toward modifying our behaviours.

DEFINING PSYCHOSOCIAL HEALTH

Psychosocial health encompasses the intellectual, emotional, social, and spiritual dimensions of health. Psychosocially healthy people have managed to develop these dimensions to optimal levels (see Figure 2.1). They seem to have an endless reserve for facing life's ups and downs. They respond to challenges, disappointments, joys, frustrations, and pain by summoning up personal resources acquired through years of experience. Their resiliency is strong and they are actively involved in the process of living rather than being trapped in despondency caused by the negative events in their lives.

Psychosocial health is the result of a complex interaction between a person's history and conscious and unconscious thoughts about and interpretations of the past. Although definitions of psychosocial health vary, most authorities identify several basic elements shared by psychosocially healthy people.[1]

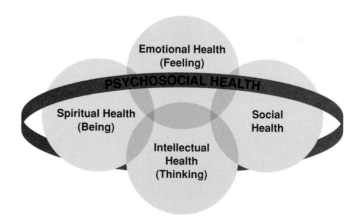

FIGURE 2.1

Psychosocial Health as a complex Interaction of Your Intellectual, Emotional, Social, and Spiritual Health.

- *They feel good about themselves.* Psychosocially healthy people are not overwhelmed by fear, love, anger, jealousy, guilt, or worry. They estimate their abilities accurately, take life's disappointments in stride, maintain their self-respect, and accept their personal shortcomings.

- *They feel comfortable with other people.* Psychosocially healthy people have satisfying and lasting personal relationships and do not take advantage of others, nor do they allow others to take advantage of them. They can give love, consider others' interests, respect personal differences, and feel responsible for their fellow human beings.

- *They control tension and anxiety.* Psychosocially healthy people recognize the underlying causes and symptoms of stress and anxiety in their lives and consciously struggle to avoid illogical or irrational thoughts, unnecessary aggression, hostility, excessive excuse making, and blaming others for their problems.

- *They are able to meet the demands of life.* Psychosocially healthy people try to solve problems as they arise, to accept responsibility, and to plan ahead. They set realistic goals, think for themselves, and make independent decisions. Acknowledging that change is inevitable, they welcome new experiences. They use their natural abilities to control their environment whenever possible and try to fit themselves into the environment whenever necessary.

- *They curb hate and guilt.* Psychosocially healthy people acknowledge and combat their tendencies to respond with hate, anger, thoughtlessness, selfishness, vengeful acts, or feelings of inadequacy. They do not try to knock others aside to get ahead but rather reach out to help others—even those they don't particularly care for.

- *They maintain a positive outlook.* Psychosocially healthy people try to approach each day with a presumption that things will go well. Since they believe that life is a gift, they are determined to enjoy it on a moment-to-moment basis rather than wander through it aimlessly. They block out most negative and cynical thoughts, give the good things in life star billing, and look to the future with enthusiasm.

- *They enrich the lives of others.* Psychosocially healthy people recognize that there are others whose needs are greater than their own. They seek to ease these others' burdens by doing such simple things as giving a ride to an elderly neighbour who can't drive, bringing flowers to someone who's in pain, making dinner for someone who's too grief-stricken to cook, volunteering at a community agency, and making charitable donations.

- *They cherish the things that make them smile.* Psychosocially healthy people make a special place in their lives for memories of the past. Family pictures, high school mementos, souvenirs of past vacations, and other reminders of good experiences brighten their day. Fun is an integral part of their lives. So is making time for themselves.

- *They value diversity.* Psychosocially healthy people don't fear difference. They do not feel threatened by people who are of a different race, gender, religion, sexual orientation, ethnicity, or political party. They appreciate creativity in others as well as in themselves.

- *They appreciate nature.* Psychosocially healthy people enjoy and respect natural beauty and wonders. They take the time to enjoy their surroundings and are conscious of their place in the universe.

Of course, few of us ever achieve perfection in these areas. Attaining psychosocial health and wellness involves many complex processes. You will see how the decisions you make today may significantly affect your future psychosocial health and learn how to defend yourself against some common and debilitating psychosocial problems.

*W*HAT DO YOU THINK?

In which of the elements of psychosocial health are you currently healthy? Which areas could use improvement? Are you willing to work today on these elements to improve your future psychosocial health?

Intellectual Health: The Thinking You

The term **intellectual health** is often used to describe the "thinking" part of psychosocial health. As a thinking being, you have the ability to reason, interpret, and remember events from a unique perspective; to sense, perceive, and evaluate what is happening; and to solve problems. In short, you are intellectually able to sort through the clutter of events, contradictory messages, and uncertainties of a situation and attach meaning (either positive or negative) to it. Your values, attitudes, and beliefs about your body, your family, your relationships, and life in general are usually—at least in part—a reflection of your intellectual health.

An intellectually healthy person is likely to respond in a positive way even when things do not go as expected. For

Psychosocial health: The intellectual, emotional, social, and spiritual dimensions of health.

Intellectual health: The "thinking" part of psychosocial health. Includes your values, attitudes, and beliefs.

example, an intellectually healthy student who receives a D on an exam may be very disappointed, but she will try to assess why she did poorly. Did she study enough? Did she attend class and ask questions about the things she didn't understand? Even though the test result may be very important to her, she will find a constructive way to deal with her frustration: she may talk to the instructor, plan to devote more time to studying before the next exam, or hire a tutor. In contrast, an intellectually unhealthy person may take a distorted view and respond in an irrational manner. She may believe that her instructor is out to get her or that other students cheated on the exam. She may allow her low grade to provoke a major crisis in her life. She may spend the next 24 hours getting wasted, decide to quit school, try to get back at her instructor, or even blame her roommate for preventing her from studying.

When a person's intellectual health begins to deteriorate, he or she may experience sharp declines in rational thinking ability and increasingly distorted perceptions. The person may become cynical and distrustful, experience volatile mood swings, or choose to be isolated from others. The person's negative reactions to events may threaten the life and health of others. People showing such signs of extreme abnormal behaviour or intellectual disorders are classified as having *mental illnesses,* discussed later in this chapter.

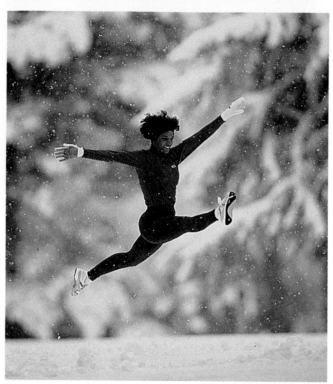

A joyful spirit and the resiliency to face life's ups and downs are measures of psychosocial health as defined in terms of intellectual, emotional, social, and spiritual wellness.

Emotional Health: The Feeling You

Emotional health refers to the "feeling," or subjective, side of psychosocial health. **Emotions** are intensified feelings or complex patterns of feelings that we experience on a minute-by-minute, day-to-day basis. Loving, caring, hating, hurt, despair, release, joy, anxiety, fear, frustration, and intense anger are some of the many emotions we experience.

Psychologist Richard Lazarus believes that there are four basic types of emotions: (1) emotions resulting from harm, loss, or threats; (2) emotions resulting from benefits; (3) borderline emotions, such as hope and compassion; and (4) more complex emotions, such as grief, disappointment, bewilderment, and curiosity.[2] Each of us may experience any of these emotions in any combination at any time. As rational beings, it is our responsibility to

evaluate our individual emotional responses, the environment that is causing these responses, and the appropriateness of our actions.

Emotionally healthy people are usually able to respond in a stable and appropriate manner to upsetting events. When they feel threatened, they are not likely to react in an extreme fashion, behave inconsistently, or adopt an offensive attack mode.

Emotionally unhealthy people are much more likely to let their feelings overpower them than are emotionally healthy people. Emotionally unhealthy people may be highly volatile and prone to unpredictable emotional outbursts and to inappropriate, sometimes frightening responses to events. An ex-boyfriend who becomes so angry that he begins to hit you and push you around in front of your friends because he is jealous of your new relationship is showing an extremely unhealthy and dangerous emotional reaction.

Emotional health also affects social interactions. Someone feeling hostile, withdrawn, or displaying other mood fluctuations may be avoided by others. People in the midst of emotional turmoil may be grumpy, nasty, irritable, or overly quiet; they may cry easily or demonstrate other disturbing emotional responses. Since they are not much fun to be around, their friends may avoid them at the very time they are most in need of emotional

Emotional health: The "feeling" part of psychosocial health. Includes your emotional reactions to life.

Emotions: Intensified feelings or complex patterns of feelings we constantly experience.

Learning to Trust: The Tie That Binds

What does the word *trust* really mean to you? How many people in your social group do you trust with your innermost thoughts? Would you trust your life with them? Lend them money? Lend them your notes the day before a big exam?

By indicating how much you agree with the following statements, you may find out how much you trust the significant people in your life:

1. I know how my partner (or friend) is going to act. My partner (or friend) can always be counted on to act as I expect.

2. I am very familiar with the patterns of behaviour my partner (or friend) has established, and he or she will behave in certain ways.

3. I have found that my partner (or friend) is a thoroughly dependable person, especially when it comes to things that are important.

4. My partner (or friend) has proven to be a faithful person. No matter with whom my partner (or friend) was involved in a relationship, he or she would never be unfaithful, even if there was absolutely no chance of being caught.

5. I am never concerned that unpredictable conflicts and serious tensions may damage our relationship because I know we can weather any storm.

6. I feel completely secure in facing unknown new situations because I know my partner (or friend) will never let me down.

Items 1 and 2 measure the component of *predictability,* your ability to foretell your partner's (or friend's) actions. Items 3 and 4 measure *dependability,* your feelings that your partner (or friend) is someone upon whom you can rely even when you feel vulnerable and afraid. Finally, items 5 and 6 measure *faith,* your confidence that, although the future may be uncertain and people can change, your partner (or friend) will continue to care for and respond to you.

Trust is hard-won but valuable in any relationship, intimate or not. As you face life's challenges, you learn how much you can depend on another person, not just how much you would like to expect of your relationship. Ironically, while trust may take a long time to develop, it can be utterly destroyed in moments. If you discover that your partner or best friend has betrayed you—by violating a confidence or cheating on you—your best efforts to forgive and forget may never make you completely trustful again. The pain of betrayal makes trust a risky venture.

How can trust be developed and strengthened from the start of a relationship? Here are some approaches:

- *When interpreting another's behaviour, be fair and realistic.* Try to understand the behaviour from his or her point of view rather than take it personally.

- *Beware of dwelling on negative memories.* Balance remembered disappointments by recalling the good and selfless things the other person has done.

- *Focus on the other person's actions instead of jumping to conclusions about his or her motives.* Many unpleasant actions are the result not of malice but of honest mistakes and human error.

- *Be trustworthy yourself.* In order to gain the trust of another person, it is important that you be a good model. Having double standards, being untrustworthy yourself, and then berating your friend or partner for slipups is an unhealthy response.

- *Finally, remember that trust is always risky.* However, intimacy in your social interactions is a desirable component of social and emotional health. To avoid all risk of lost trust is to lose an opportunity to grow and have meaningful interactions with others.

Taking Action

Think about how much you trust your parents, your partner, and your best friend. Why do you trust each of these people as much as you do? What things do you not trust about them? Have there been specific incidents to prove you can't trust them? Have you thought about why they may have acted as they did? What positive things have they done that may prove you can trust them? How trustworthy have you been to them? What actions can you take to be more trustworthy? What actions can you take to help your friend/partner become a more trustworthy person or to remain trustworthy in the future?

Source: Adapted from Charles G. Morris, *Understanding Psychology,* 2nd ed., © 1993, 569. Adapted by permission of Prentice-Hall, Inc., Englewood Cliffs, NJ.

support. Social isolation is just one of the many potential negative consequences of unstable emotional responses.

For students, a more immediate concern is the impact of emotional trauma or turmoil on academic perfor-mance. Have you ever tried to study for an exam after a fight with a close friend or family member? Emotional turmoil may seriously affect your ability to think, reason, or act in a rational way. Many otherwise rational people do ridiculous things when they are going through a major emotional upset. Intellectual functioning and emotional responses are indeed intricately connected.

Social Health: Interactions with Others

Social health is the part of psychosocial health dealing with our interactions with others and our ability to adapt to social situations. Socially healthy individuals have a wide range of social interactions with family, friends, acquaintances, and individuals with whom they may only occasionally come into contact. They are able to listen, to express themselves, to form healthy relationships, to act in socially acceptable and responsible ways, and to find a best fit for themselves in society.

Numerous studies have documented the importance of our social life in the achievement and maintenance of health, and two factors of social health have proven to be particularly important:[3]

- *Presence of strong social bonds.* **Social bonds,** or social linkages, reflect the general degree and nature of our interpersonal contacts and interactions. Social bonds generally have six major functions: (1) providing intimacy, (2) providing feelings of belonging to or integration with a group, (3) providing opportunities for giving or receiving nurturance, (4) providing reassurance of one's worth, (5) providing assistance and guidance, and (6) providing advice. In general, people who are more "connected" to others manage stress more effectively and are much more resilient when they are bombarded by life's crises.

- *Presence of key social supports.* **Social supports** refer to relationships that bring positive benefits to the individual. Social supports can be either expressive (emotional support, encouragement) or structural (housing, money). Families provide both structural and expressive support to children. Adults need to develop their own social supports. Psychosocially healthy people create a network of friends and family to whom they can give and receive support.

Social health also reflects the way we react to others around us. In its most extreme forms, a lack of social health may be represented by aggressive acts of prejudice and bias toward other individuals or groups. **Prejudice** is a negative evaluation of an entire group of people that is typically based on unfavourable (and often wrong) ideas about the group.[4] In its most obvious manifestations, prejudice is reflected in acts of discrimination against others, in overt acts of hate and bias, and in purposeful intent to harm individuals or groups.

Spiritual Health

Although intellectual and emotional health are key factors in your overall psychosocial functioning, it is possible for you to be intellectually and emotionally healthy and still not achieve optimal levels of psychosocial well-being. What is missing? For many people, that difficult-to-describe element that gives zest to life is the spiritual dimension. What does it mean to be spiritually healthy? Spiritual health refers to possession of a belief in some unifying force that gives purpose or meaning to life or to a sense of belonging to a scheme of existence greater than the merely personal. For some people, this unifying force is nature; for others, it is a feeling of connection to other people coupled with a recognition of the eternal nature of the human race; for still others, the unifying force is a god or other spiritual symbol.

Many of us live on a rather superficial material plane throughout the formative years of our lives. We have basic human needs that must be satisfied according to a set hierarchical order. We tend to be rather egocentric, or self-oriented, during these formative years and seek immediate material and emotional gratification while denying or ignoring the spiritual aspect of our selves. Worrying about the clothes you wear, the car you drive, the appearance of your apartment, and other material possessions are examples of this type of preoccupation. According to psychologists and psychoanalysts such as Carl Jung, our materialistic Western civilization leads us to deny our spiritual needs for much of our lives. But there comes a point, usually around midlife, when we discover that material possessions do not automatically bring a sense of happiness or self-worth.[5] Crisis may move us to this realization earlier. A failed relationship, the death of a close friend or family member, or other loss often prompts us to look for meaning in what is happening around us. We recognize that material things, prestige, money, power, and fame count for little in the larger scheme of existence, and that if we were to die tomorrow these would not give meaning to our lives. At this point, many people reach what is often called a midlife crisis, which is characterized by a sense of spiritual bankruptcy.[6] According to Jung,

> We need not be devastated by this sudden recognition, for with it comes the opportunity to reach deep within ourselves in order to resolve and integrate the polarities of our nature. Within our creative and collective unconscious we may discover a richness and a strength and a wisdom that we have not been able to utilize before.[7]

As we develop into spiritually healthy beings, we begin to recognize who we are as unique individuals. We reach a better understanding of our strengths and shortcomings and of our place in the universe. Many of us find that our families, the environment, animals, friends, strangers who are suffering, and religion assume greater significance in our lives. We become more willing to sacrifice for others or to improve the world around us. Many people do not have to wait until their middle years to experience spiritual growth. While the media regularly report horrible stories of hate, crime, violence, and global destruction, they frequently ignore the heartening stories of young people having humanistic concerns who volunteer to work with others in need and who are seriously searching for meaning in life.

Spiritual health takes time and experience to acquire. The longer you live, the more you experience. The more you ponder the meaning of your experiences, the greater your chances of achieving psychosocial health.

*W*HAT DO YOU THINK?

How do you feel about your intellectual health? Your emotional health? Your social health? Your spiritual health? Can you think of any areas of improvement? Is it important to you that you make improvement?

*F*ACTORS INFLUENCING PSYCHOSOCIAL HEALTH

Although it's relatively easy to say what psychosocial health is, it is much more difficult to assess why some people are psychosocially well virtually all the time, others are some of the time, and still others almost never are. What factors have influenced your own patterns of intellectual, emotional, social, and spiritual health? Are these factors changeable? Can you do anything to improve your health if you have problems? How can you enhance the positive qualities you already possess?

Most of our intellectual, emotional, and spiritual reactions to life are a direct outcome of our experiences and social and cultural expectations. Each of us is born with the innate capacity to experience emotions. Some of us apparently have a predisposition toward more emotionality than others. But how we express our emotions has a lot to do with our intellectual interpretations of events. These interpretations are often learned reactions to certain environmental and social stimuli.

External Influences

Our psychosocial health is based on how we perceive our life's experiences. While some experiences are under our control, others are not. External influences are those factors in our life that we do not control, such as who raised us and the physical environment in which we live.

Influences of the Family. Our families are a significant influence on our psychosocial development. Children raised in healthy, nurturing, happy families are more likely to become well-adjusted, productive adults. Children raised in families in which violence, sexual, physical, or emotional abuse, negative behaviours, distrust, anger, dietary deprivation, drug abuse, parental discord, or other

characteristics of **dysfunctional families** are present may have a harder time adapting to life. In dysfunctional families, love, security, and unconditional trust are so lacking that the children in such families are often confused and psychologically bruised. Yet, not all people raised in dysfunctional families become psychosocially unhealthy. Conversely, not all people from healthy family environments become well adjusted. There are obviously more factors involved in our "process of becoming" than just our family.

Influences of the Greater Environment. While isolated negative events may do little damage to psychosocial health, persistent stressors, uncertainties, and threats may cause significant problems. Children raised in environments where crime is rampant and daily safety is in question, for example, run an increased risk of psychosocial problems. Drugs, crime, violent acts, school failure, unemployment, and a host of other bad things can happen to good people. But it is believed that certain protective factors, such as having a positive role model in the midst of chaos or a high level of self-esteem, may help children from even the worst environments remain healthy and well adjusted.

Another important influence on psychosocial health is access to health services and programs designed to support the maintenance and/or enhancement of psychosocial health. Going to a support group or seeing a trained counsellor or therapist is often a crucial first step in prevention and intervention efforts. Individuals from poor socioeconomic environments who cannot afford such services often find it difficult to secure help in positively influencing their psychosocial health.

Internal Influences

Although your life experiences influence you in fairly obvious ways, many internal factors are also working more subtly to shape who you are and who you become. Some of these factors are your hereditary traits, your hormonal functioning, your physical health status (including neurological functioning), your physical fitness level, and

Social bonds: Degree and nature of our interpersonal contacts.

Social supports: Structural and functional aspects of our social interactions.

Prejudice: A negative evaluation of an entire group of people that is typically based on unfavourable and often wrong ideas about the group.

Dysfunctional families: Families in which there is violence; physical, emotional, or sexual abuse; parental discord; or other negative family interactions.

selected elements of your intellectual and emotional health. If problems occur with any of these factors, overall psychosocial health declines.

During our formative years, our successes and failures in school, in athletics, in friendships, in our intimate relationships, in our jobs, and in every other aspect of life subtly shape our perceptions and beliefs about our own personal worth and ability to act to help ourselves. These perceptions and beliefs in turn become internal influences on our psychosocial health. Psychologist Albert Bandura used the term **self-efficacy** to describe a person's belief about whether he or she can successfully engage in and execute a specific behaviour. If one has already been successful in academics, athletics, or achieving popularity, one will undoubtedly expect to be successful in these events in the future. If one has always been the last chosen to play basketball or volleyball or has never been able to make friends easily, one may tend to believe that failure is inevitable. In general, the more self-efficacious a person is and the more his or her past experiences have been positive, the more likely he or she will be to keep trying to execute a specific behaviour successfully. A person having low self-efficacy may give up easily or never even try to change a behaviour. People who have a high level of self-efficacy are also more likely to feel that they have **personal control** over situations, or, in other words, their own internal resources allow them to control events.

Psychologist Martin Seligman has proposed that people who continually experience failure may develop a pattern of responding known as **learned helplessness** in which they give up and fail to take any action to help themselves. Recently, Seligman's theory has been expanded; just as we may learn to be helpless, so may we learn to be optimistic. His learned optimism research provides growing evidence for the central place of intellectual health in overall positive development.[8]

Personality. Our personality is the unique mix of characteristics that distinguishes us from others. Hereditary, environmental, cultural, and experiential factors influence how we develop. For each of us, the amount of influence exerted by any of these factors differs. Our personality determines how we react to the challenges of life. It also determines how we interpret the feelings we experience and how we resolve the conflicts we feel on being denied the things we need or want.

The modern effort to understand the development of the human personality began with the teachings of Sigmund Freud (1856–1939), an Austrian physician.

To Freud, personality development was a psychosexual process based on the gratification of sexual impulses. He believed each person possessed three conflicting personality forces, which he labelled the id, ego, and superego. The **id** consists of our unconscious desire for immediate gratification of wants and needs without regard to laws, rules, customs, or the needs of others. The **ego** seeks to restrain the id and to delay gratification. In addition, it consciously attempts to satisfy the id in socially acceptable ways. Finally, the **superego** acts as our conscience, or moral monitor. The moral standards and values of our parents are often used by the superego to judge the ego's intentions. Freud believed that a healthy ego was one that had figured out how to satisfy most of the id's impulses in ways that did not greatly offend the superego.

Scientist B. F. Skinner developed one of the earliest branches of psychology. As part of the precepts of **behavioural psychology,** Skinner stated that all behaviour is learned through a system of rewards and punishments. According to Skinner, "right" behaviours could be encouraged through rewards, and "wrong" behaviours could be eliminated through punishments.

A third branch of psychology is **developmental psychology.** The originators of this school of thought include Carl Jung and Erik Erikson, who taught that the development of personality and emotional health was dependent on the successful completion of a series of developmental tasks at various stages of the life cycle.

Erikson identified eight stages of psychosocial development (see Figure 2.2). He believed that at each stage we must resolve particular crises in order to continue growth. Successful resolution of each crisis gives us a new building block for developing self-fulfillment and emotional health. Erikson identified these building blocks as hope, will, purpose, competence, fidelity, love, care, and wisdom.

Abraham H. Maslow led the movement known as **humanistic psychology.** Humanistic psychologists be-

---

Self-efficacy: Belief in your ability to perform a task successfully.

Personal control: Belief that your internal resources can allow you to control a situation.

Learned helplessness: Pattern of responding to situations by giving up because you have always failed in the past.

Id: Our unconscious desire for immediate gratification of wants and needs.

Ego: Personality force that seeks to restrain the id.

Superego: Personality force that serves as our conscience.

Behavioural psychology: Branch of psychology that posits that all behaviour is learned through a system of punishments and rewards.

Developmental psychology: Branch of psychology that focusses on the personality's development by means of progression through developmental tasks.

Humanistic psychology: Branch of psychology that posits that behaviour is motivated by the desire to grow and achieve by making rational decisions that meet our individual needs.

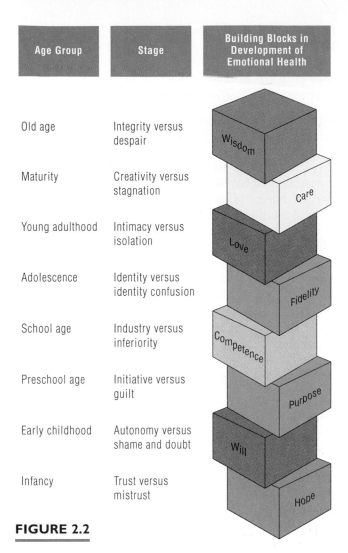

Age Group	Stage	Building Blocks in Development of Emotional Health
Old age	Integrity versus despair	Wisdom
Maturity	Creativity versus stagnation	Care
Young adulthood	Intimacy versus isolation	Love
Adolescence	Identity versus identity confusion	Fidelity
School age	Industry versus inferiority	Competence
Preschool age	Initiative versus guilt	Purpose
Early childhood	Autonomy versus shame and doubt	Will
Infancy	Trust versus mistrust	Hope

FIGURE 2.2

The Major Stages in Psychosocial Development as Defined by Erikson

lieve that behaviour is motivated by a desire for personal growth and achievement and that it involves free choice and the ability to make conscious, rational decisions. Maslow developed the theory that people achieve emotional well-being by meeting a hierarchy of needs: physiological needs (oxygen, food, water, sleep, sexual release, and exercise); security needs (a physically and emotionally safe and consistent environment); love and belonging needs (a family or other support group); self-esteem needs; and self-actualization needs (the achievement of self-fulfillment). Before achieving higher levels and eventually becoming "self-actualized," people must fulfill the needs of the previous levels (see Figure 2.3).

Most of the later schools of psychosocial theory promote the idea that we have the power not only to understand our behaviour but also to actively change it and thus to mold our own personalities. An accurate picture of personality development probably requires combining aspects of all the personality theories. We feel conflicts and guilt over our desires and social rules, as Freud believed, and we have the capacity to learn behaviourally as well.

Life Span and Maturity. Although the exact determinants of personality are impossible to define, researchers do know that our personalities are not static. Rather, they change as we move through the stages of our lives. Our temperaments also change as we grow, as is illustrated by the extreme emotions experienced by many people in early adolescence. Most of us learn to control our emotions as we advance toward adulthood.

FIGURE 2.3

Maslow's Hierarchy of Needs

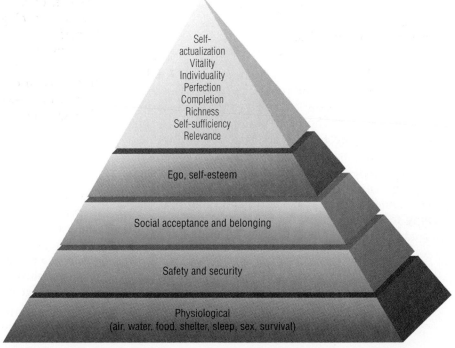

Self-actualization
Vitality
Individuality
Perfection
Completion
Richness
Self-sufficiency
Relevance

Ego, self-esteem

Social acceptance and belonging

Safety and security

Physiological
(air, water, food, shelter, sleep, sex, survival)

The college years mark a critical transition period for young adults and their parents. During this time, many of you move away from your families and establish yourselves as independent adults. For most, this step toward maturity entails changing the nature of your relationship with your parents. The transition to independence will be easier if you have successfully accomplished earlier developmental tasks such as learning how to solve problems, to make and evaluate decisions, to define and adhere to personal values, and to establish both casual and intimate relationships. Management of personal finances, career management strategies, interpersonal communication skills, and parenting skills (for those who choose to become parents) are among the developmental tasks college students must accomplish. Older students often have to balance the responsibilities of family, career, and school. Parents of students must accept their children's greater independence and, in some cases, adjust to being alone after years of family interaction.

If you have not fulfilled earlier tasks, you will continue to grow but may find your life interrupted by recurrent "crises" left over from earlier stages. For example, if you did not learn to trust others in childhood, you may have difficulty establishing intimate relationships in late adolescence or early adulthood.

*W*HAT DO YOU THINK?

Which factors of psychosocial health have had the greatest positive impact on your life? Any negative influences? Which are influencing your life most now?

*E*NHANCING PSYCHOSOCIAL HEALTH

You may believe that your psychosocial health is fairly well developed by the time you reach college. However, you can always take steps to change your behaviour and to improve your psychosocial health. Your well-being is largely determined by your ability to respond to life's challenges and can be defined by your level of self-fulfillment or self-actualization. Attaining self-fulfillment is a lifelong, conscious process that involves building self-esteem, understanding and controlling emotions, and learning to solve problems and make decisions. Before you read on, take a few minutes to find out where you are

Self-esteem: Sense of self-respect or self-confidence.

on your road to psychosocial health by completing the Rate Yourself box.

Developing and Maintaining Self-Esteem

Self-esteem refers to one's sense of self-respect or self-confidence. It can be defined as how much one likes oneself and values one's own personal worth as an individual. People with high self-esteem tend to feel good about themselves and have a positive outlook on life. People with low self-esteem often do not like themselves, constantly demean themselves, and doubt their ability to succeed.

Our self-esteem is a result of the relationships we have with our parents and family during our formative years, our friends as we grow older, our significant others as we form intimate relationships, and with our teachers, co-workers, and others throughout our lives. If we felt loved and valued as children, our self-esteem may allow us to believe that we are inherently lovable individuals as we reach adulthood. The love and support we received from our families in childhood constitute a resource that we call on to help us deal successfully with problems at all stages of our lives.

Finding a Support Group. The best way to maintain your self-esteem is through a support group. You need peers who share your values and offer you the nurturing that your family can no longer provide. The prime prerequisite for a support group is that it makes you feel good about yourself and forces you to take an honest look at your actions and the choices that you make. Members of the group should refrain from exerting negative pressures on one another.

Try to be a support for others. Become more interesting by being more interested (in people, current events, etc.). Send news clippings to friends. Join a discussion, political action, or recreational group. Write more postcards and "thinking of you" notes to people who matter. This will build both your own self-esteem and that of your friends.

Completing Required Tasks. Another way to boost your self-esteem is to learn how to complete required tasks successfully. You are not likely to succeed in your studies if you leave term papers until the last minute, fail to keep up with the reading for your courses, and do not ask for clarification of points that are confusing to you. Most college campuses provide study groups for various content areas. These groups offer tips for managing time, understanding assignments, dealing with professors, and preparing for test taking. Poor grades, or grades that do not meet a student's expectations, are major contributors to diminished self-esteem and to emotional distress among college students.

Forming Realistic Expectations. Having realistic expectations of yourself is another method of boosting

Respecting Who You Are

Look at each item on the scales below and write the letter *S* in the space that best represents your self-description of that trait. Use the number code 1–7 as your guide, as in the following example of the trait of fairness:

1 = extremely fair

2 = rather fair

3 = somewhat fair

4 = equally fair or unfair, or not sure

5 = somewhat unfair

6 = rather unfair

7 = extremely unfair

When you have completed your self-description, go back through each of the items and write the letter *I* in the space that best represents your ideal self, or who you think you ought to be. Using the number codes, determine the difference between your *S* score and *I* score on each trait. Your self-esteem is a measure of how well you like and respect yourself. Traits that have low discrepancy scores on this scale most likely make a positive contribution toward your self-esteem. Traits that have a large difference score may indicate areas you should work on to improve your self-esteem.

	1 2 3 4 5 6 7	
fair	___:___:___:___:___:___:___	unfair
independent	___:___:___:___:___:___:___	dependent
religious	___:___:___:___:___:___:___	irreligious
unselfish	___:___:___:___:___:___:___	selfish
self-confident	___:___:___:___:___:___:___	lacking confidence
competent	___:___:___:___:___:___:___	incompetent
important	___:___:___:___:___:___:___	unimportant
attractive	___:___:___:___:___:___:___	unattractive
educated	___:___:___:___:___:___:___	uneducated
sociable	___:___:___:___:___:___:___	unsociable
kind	___:___:___:___:___:___:___	cruel
wise	___:___:___:___:___:___:___	foolish
graceful	___:___:___:___:___:___:___	awkward
intelligent	___:___:___:___:___:___:___	unintelligent
artistic	___:___:___:___:___:___:___	inartistic
tall	___:___:___:___:___:___:___	short
obese	___:___:___:___:___:___:___	skinny

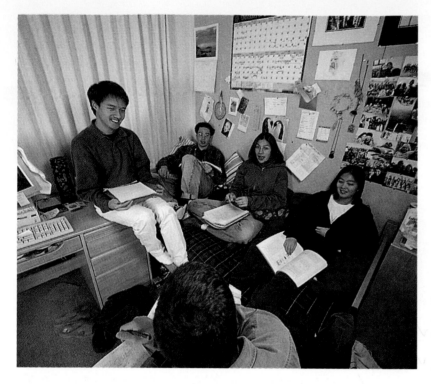

Past successes and happy experiences, which are often recalled through photos, mementos, and recollections, contribute to a person's psychosocial health.

self-esteem. College is a time to explore your potential. If you expect perfect grades, a steady stream of Saturday-night dates and a soap-opera-type romantic involvement, a good job, and a beautiful home and car, you may be setting yourself up for failure. Assess your current resources and the direction you are heading. Set small, incremental goals that are possible for you to meet. Don't decide, "I'm going to turn my life around and get better grades." Decide instead that tomorrow you will spend at least two hours studying for a class or going to the library to do research on a paper, or decide to talk to your professors to see what they recommend to help you better understand a topic.

Taking and Making Time for You. Taking time to enjoy yourself is another way to boost your self-esteem and psychosocial health. For some people, participating in a sport improves self-esteem by creating a sense of achievement. For others, meeting a new challenge, such as successfully auditioning for a university play or going to a party where they don't know anyone, is an important part of developing social skills. Viewing each new activity as something to look forward to and an opportunity to have fun is an important part of keeping the excitement in your life.

Maintaining Physical Health. Maintaining physical health also contributes to self-esteem. Regular exercise fosters a sense of well-being. Nourishing meals can help you avoid the weight gain experienced by many college students.

Examining Problems and Seeking Help. Examining your problems and seeking help when needed will also boost your self-esteem. Facing and solving problems can be one of life's most satisfying experiences. You do not necessarily have to deal with your problems alone. Help can come in the form of a friend, a group, or a mental health professional.

WHAT DO YOU THINK?

Which of the above tasks have you actively pursued in the past month, past six months, and past year? Are you becoming more active in enhancing your self-esteem? What steps could you take to improve your self-esteem?

Getting Adequate Amounts of Rest

Getting adequate sleep is a key contributor to positive physical and psychosocial functioning. Many of us never seem to get enough sleep. Either we don't have time to sleep or we can't seem to fall asleep once our heads hit the pillow. An estimated 20 to 40 percent of all adults have trouble sleeping. Known as *insomnia*, this sleep disorder afflicts almost everyone at one time or another. Insomnia is more common in women than in men, and its prevalence correlates with age and socioeconomic class. Though many people turn to over-the-counter sleeping pills, barbiturates, or tranquillizers to get some sleep, the following methods for conquering sleeplessness are less harmful:[9]

■ *If your sleeplessness arises from worry or grief, try to correct what's bothering you.* If you can't correct it yourself, confide in a friend, join a support group, or find a qualified counsellor to help you.

Making time for friends and activities that you enjoy and that bring laughter into your life is a powerful strategy for maintaining psychosocial health.

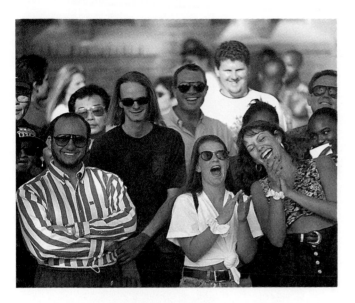

- *Don't drink alcohol or smoke before bedtime.* Alcohol can disrupt sleep patterns and make insomnia worse. Nicotine also makes you wakeful.

- *Avoid eating a heavy meal in the evening, particularly at bedtime.* Don't drink large amounts of liquids before retiring, either.

- *Eliminate or reduce consumption of caffeinated beverages except in the morning or early afternoon.*

- *Avoid daytime naps, even if you're tired.*

- *Spend an hour or more relaxing before retiring.* Read, listen to music, watch TV, or take a warm bath.

- *If you're unable to fall asleep, get up and do something rather than lie there.* Don't bring work to bed. If you wake up in the middle of the night and can't fall asleep again, try reading for a short time. Counting sheep or reconstructing a happy event or narrative in your mind may lull you to sleep.

- *Avoid reproaching yourself.* Don't make your sleeplessness a cause for additional worry. Insomnia is not a crime. Not everyone needs eight hours of sleep. You can feel well—and be quite healthy—on less. Don't worry that you have to make up lost sleep. One good night's sleep will reinvigorate you.

- *Don't watch the clock at night.* Turn it to the wall to avoid the temptation to worry about the night slipping away.

- *Go to bed and rise on a regular schedule.* Keep this schedule no matter how much you have or haven't slept in the recent past.

The Mind-Body Connection

Can negative emotions make a person physically sick and positive emotions boost the immune system? Researchers have explored the possible interaction between emotions and health, especially in conditions of uncontrolled, persistent stress. According to the simplest theory of this interaction, the brain of an emotionally overwrought person sends signals to the adrenal glands, which respond by secreting cortisol and epinephrine (adrenaline), the hormones that activate the body's stress response. These chemicals are also known to suppress immune functioning, so it has been surmised that the persistently overwrought person undergoes subtle immune changes. What remains to be shown is how these changes affect overall health, if they do at all. According to Marvin Stein, a professor of psychiatry at the Mount Sinai School of Medicine in New York City, "Work thus far on emotions and health adds up to little more than findings in search of meaning."[10] We still do not have conclusive proof of a relationship between emotions and health, he argues, but evidence for such a relationship is accumulating.

The notion that laughter can save your life gained wide acceptance with the 1979 publication of *Anatomy of an Illness,* by magazine editor Norman Cousins. In this book, Cousins recounted his recovery from a rheumatic disease of the spine—ankylosing spondylitis—with the aid of Marx Brothers movies and *Candid Camera* videos that made him laugh.[11] Similarly, in his 1988 best-seller, *Love, Medicine and Miracles,* surgeon Bernie Siegel argued that a fighting spirit and the determination to survive are vital adjuncts to standard cancer therapy.[12]

In the 1970s and 1980s, a number of widely publicized studies of the health of widowed and divorced people showed that their rates of illness and death are higher than those of married people. Moreover, their lab tests revealed below-normal immune-system functioning. Several follow-up studies have shown unusually high rates of cancer among depressed people.[13] But are these studies conclusive evidence of the mind-body connection? Probably not, because they do not account for many other factors known to be relevant to health. For example, some researchers suggest that people who are divorced, widowed, or depressed are more likely to drink and smoke, to use drugs, to eat and sleep poorly, and to fail to exercise—all of which may affect the immune system. Another possibly relevant factor is that such people may be less tolerant of illness and more likely to report their problems.[14]

Among the work most widely cited as proof that psychosocial treatment can help patients fight disease is an experiment involving women with advanced breast cancer. David Spiegel, professor of psychiatry at Stanford University, reported in 1989 that 50 women randomly assigned to a weekly support group lived an average of 18 months longer than 36 similarly afflicted women not in the support group. The implication of this finding is that the women in the support group cheered each other up while they endured agonizing therapy and that this allowed them to sleep and eat better, which promoted their survival. But a significant flaw in Spiegel's study was his failure to specifically measure immune functioning.[15]

In fact, the immune system changes measured in various other studies of the mind-body connection are relatively small. (They are nowhere near as large as the disruptions that occur in people with AIDS, for example.) The health consequences of such minute changes are difficult to gauge because the body can tolerate a certain amount of reduced immune function without illness resulting. The exact amount the body is able to tolerate and under what circumstances are still unresolved questions.[16]

In summary, although there is a large body of evidence pointing to at least a minor association between the emotions and physical health, there is still no definitive proof of such a relationship. Clearly, we still have a lot to learn in this area. In the meantime, however, maintaining an optimistic mindset is probably sound advice.

*W*HEN THINGS GO WRONG

In spite of our own best efforts to remain psychosocially healthy, circumstances and events in our lives sometimes prove to be more than we can handle. If we have the financial and educational resources to seek help, some of these difficulties can be prevented. But in the case of other difficulties, the road to recovery may be long.

Depression

Depression is the most common emotional disorder in Canada: 6 percent of Canadians aged 18 and over have experienced a Major Depressive Episode. Although depression is amenable to treatment, according to the 1994–1995 National Population Health Survey (NPHS) only 26 percent of those diagnosed with depression reported more than three consultations, a level of contact defined as "receiving treatment."[17]

There are two acknowledged forms of depression: endogenous and exogenous depression. **Endogenous depression** is of biochemical origin. Neurotransmitters (chemicals that transmit nerve impulses across synapses)

> **Endogenous depression:** A type of depression that has a biochemical basis, such as neurotransmitter imbalances.
>
> **Exogenous depression:** A type of depression that has an external cause, such as the loss of a loved one.

Without appropriate treatment, depression and anxiety can become overwhelming problems that affect not only psychosocial well-being, but also physical health.

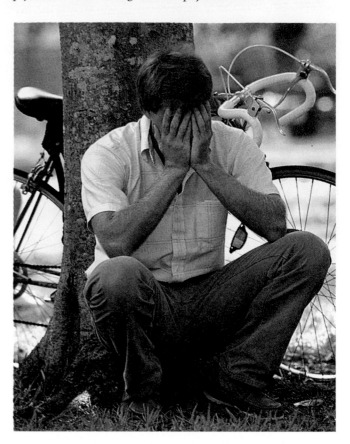

in the brain that are responsible for mood elevation become unbalanced for unknown reasons. A decrease in the amount of these neurotransmitters gives rise to outward expressions of depression. If not treated, endogenous depression may become chronic. **Exogenous depression,** on the other hand, is usually caused by an external event such as the loss of something or someone of great value. Victims of exogenous depression can slide into chronic depression if they are unable to work through the grieving process necessary for overcoming event-related depression.

Similar symptoms appear in the two types of depression: lingering sadness; inability to find joy in pleasure-giving activities; loss of interest in work; diminished or increased appetite; unexplainable fatigue; sleep disorders, including insomnia or early-morning awakenings; loss of sex drive; withdrawal from friends and family; feelings of hopelessness and worthlessness; and a desire to die. A depressed person may be unable to get out of bed in the morning or may find it impossible to leave the house.

A depressed person usually suffers from low self-esteem. He or she may feel alone, separated from, and unable to communicate with others. After a while, depression becomes a vicious circle. The person feels helpless and trapped, having no way out. He or she may feel that depression is a deserved punishment for real or imagined failings. Prolonged depression may cause a person to feel utterly worthless and to view suicide as the only way out.

Facts and Fallacies about Depression. Although depression appears to be one of the fastest-growing psychosocial health problems, the general public is uninformed about many aspects of the disease. Myth and misperception about the disease abound. Keeping the following points in mind may help you in discussions of this problem:[18]

1. *Real depression is* not *a natural reaction to crisis and loss.* Something has happened to the mood and thinking of depressed people so that they are afflicted by pervasive pessimism, helplessness, despair, and lethargy, sometimes coupled with agitation. Victims may have difficulty at work and have chronically negative interpersonal relationships. Symptoms may come and go and may get worse or stay stable but won't get better without treatment. Depressed people forget what it's like to feel normal.

2. *People will* not *snap out of depression by using a little willpower.* Telling a depressed person to snap out of it is like telling a diabetic to produce more insulin. Medical intervention in the form of antidepressant drugs

and therapy is often necessary for recovery. Depression also tends to recur—more than half of those afflicted once will experience a recurrence. And although most people survive depression, it can be fatal: depression is the leading cause of suicide in this country for both women and men.

3. *Frequent crying is* not *a hallmark of depression.* Some depressed people don't cry at all. In fact, biochemists theorize that crying may actually ward off depression by releasing chemicals that the body produces as a positive response to distress.

4. *Depression is* not *"all in the mind."* One of the best-known factors that makes one vulnerable to clinical depression is genetics. Studies of adopted children, as well as fraternal and identical twins, support the genetic link to depression. The data suggest that depressive illnesses originate with an inherited chemical imbalance in the brain. But do brain chemicals alter mood or does mood alter the balance of brain chemicals, and to what extent? Currently, no one knows for sure but it seems that each affects the other. Depression can also be a side-effect of certain physiological conditions, such as thyroid disorders, Lyme disease, diabetes, multiple sclerosis, hepatitis, mononucleosis, rheumatoid arthritis, and pancreatic cancer.

FOCUS ON CANADA

Depression Among Older Canadians

While the psychosocial and physical losses in later life are believed to predispose many elderly persons to depression, studies using strict diagnostic criteria have found low rates of depressive illness in persons over 65. A greater proportion of seniors experience dysphoria and depressive symptoms of a lesser severity than those associated with major depressive disorders. However, arguments

have been put forward that depression is qualitatively different in older adults and thus may be underdetected. While chronic illness and subsequent loss of independence among the aged may contribute to symptoms of depression, depression may also interfere with the motivation necessary to comply with drug therapy or rehabilitation programs.

Estimated Number of Depression Cases in Canada by 10-Year Age Intervals, 1981–2006

Age Group	Prevalence Rate (%)	1981	1986	1991	1996	2001	2006
65–74	8.8	130 038	145 209	165 273	182 442	189 809	200 174
75–84	10.5	72 387	86 069	105 053	122 609	142 916	159 170
85+	12.6	24 419	28 703	36 653	47 401	60 833	73 861
TOTAL CASES		226 844	259 981	306 979	352 452	393 556	433 205
TOTAL POPULATION 65+ ('000)		2361.0	2697.6	3169.6	3617.0	4000.8	4376.8
TOTAL PREVALENCE RATE (%)		9.6	9.6	9.7	9.7	9.8	9.9

Source: Adapted from K. L. McEwan, M. Donnelly, D. Robertson, and C. Hertzman, *Mental Health Problems Among Canada's Seniors: Demographic and Epidemiological Considerations* (Ottawa: Minister of Supply and Services), Cat. No. H39-203/1991E, 17.

5. *It is* not *true that only in-depth psychotherapy can cure long-term clinical depression.* No single psychotherapy method works for all cases of depression. But two methods are thought to be particularly well suited to this disorder, and neither of them requires years of treatment.

Treating Depression. Different types of depression require different types of treatment. Selecting the best treatment for a specific patient involves determining his or her type and degree of depression and its possible causes. Both psychotherapeutic and pharmacological modes of treatment are recommended for clinical (severe and prolonged) depression. Drugs often relieve the symptoms of depression, such as loss of sleep or appetite, while psychotherapy can improve a depressed person's social and interpersonal functioning. Treatment may be weighted toward one or the other mode depending on the specific situation. In some cases, psychotherapy alone may be the most successful treatment. The two most common psychotherapeutic therapies for depression are cognitive therapy and interpersonal therapy.

Cognitive therapy aims to help a patient look at life rationally and to correct habitually pessimistic thought patterns. It focusses on the here and now rather than analyzing a patient's past. To pull a person out of depression, cognitive therapists usually need 6 to 18 months of weekly sessions comprising reasoning and behavioural exercises.

Interpersonal therapy has also proved successful in the treatment of depression and is sometimes combined with cognitive therapy. It also addresses the present but differs from cognitive therapy in that its primary goal is to correct chronic human relationship problems. Interpersonal therapists focus on patients' relationships with their families and other people.

Antidepressant drugs relieve symptoms in nearly 80 percent of people with chronic depression. Several types of the antidepressant drugs known as tricyclics are available and work by preventing the excessive absorption of mood-lifting neurotransmitters. Tricyclics can take from six weeks to three months to become effective. Newer antidepressant drugs, called tetracyclics, work in one or two weeks.

Electroconvulsive therapy (ECT) is another treatment for depression. A patient given ECT is sedated under light general anesthesia and electric current is applied to the temples for five seconds at a time for a period of about 15 or 20 minutes. Between 10 and 20 percent of those with depression who do not respond to drug therapy are responsive to ECT, but because a major risk associated with ECT is permanent memory loss, some therapists do not recommend its use under any circumstances.

Clinics have been established in large metropolitan areas to offer group support for depressed people. Some clinics treat all types of depressed people; others restrict themselves to specific groups, such as widows, adolescents, or families and friends of people with depression.

Obsessive-Compulsive Disorders

An **obsessive-compulsive disorder (OCD)** is an illness in which people have obsessive thoughts or perform habitual behaviours that they cannot control. People with compulsions feel forced to engage in a repetitive behaviour, almost as if the behaviour controls them. Feeling an obsessive need for cleanliness and washing one's hands 20 times before eating, counting to a certain number while using the toilet, and checking and rechecking all the light switches in the house before leaving or going to bed are examples of compulsive behaviours. More harmful compulsive behaviours include pulling out one's hair and other forms of self-mutilation.

The causes of obsessive-compulsive disorders are difficult to isolate. Some theorists believe that sufferers engage in compulsive behaviours to distract themselves from more pressing problems. Until recently, behavioural therapy, which focusses on controlling and changing behaviours, was the common treatment for these disorders. However, research now indicates that some of these disorders may be caused by a lack of the neurotransmitter serotonin in the limbic system (an area of the brain concerned with emotion and motivation). In 1974, a drug called clomipramine (Anafranil), which researchers believe alters the way serotonin is used in the brain, was released in Canada for prescription use. Used in conjunction with behavioural therapy, clomipramine has been found to help alleviate symptoms of obsessive-compulsive disorders.

Anxiety Disorders

Rates of anxiety disorders do not fall far behind those for depression at about 12 to 13 percent of the population. **Anxiety disorders,** in which people are plagued by persistent feelings of threat and of anxiety about everyday problems of living, are characterized by fatigue, back pains, headaches, feelings of unreality, a sensation of weakness

---

Obsessive-compulsive disorder (OCD): A disorder characterized by obsessive thoughts or habitual behaviours that cannot be controlled.

Anxiety disorders: Disorders characterized by persistent feelings of threat and anxiety in coping with the everyday problems of living.

Phobia: A deep and persistent fear of a specific object, activity, or situation that results in a compelling desire to avoid the source of the fear.

Panic attack: The sudden, rapid onset of disabling terror.

Seasonal affective disorder (SAD): A type of depression that occurs in the winter months, when sunlight levels are low.

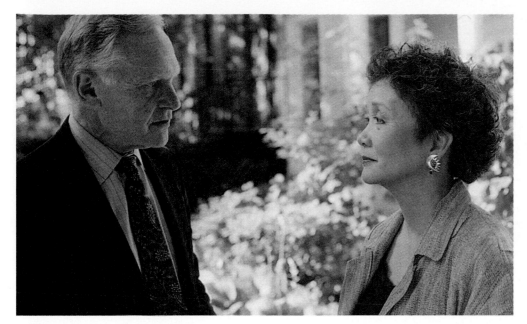

in the legs, and fear of losing control. Generalized anxiety disorders can last for more than six months and typically result in excessive worry about two or more personal problems. Three major types of anxiety disorders are phobias, panic attacks, and posttraumatic stress disorder.

Phobias. A **phobia** is a deep and persistent fear of a specific object, activity, or situation, and results in a compelling desire to avoid the source of fear. Phobias are thought to be more prevalent in women than in men. Simple phobias, such as fear of spiders, fear of flying, and fear of heights, can be treated successfully with behavioural therapy. Social phobias (fears that are related to interaction with others), such as fear of public speaking, fear of inadequate sexual performance, and fear of eating in public places, require more extensive therapy.

Panic Attacks. A **panic attack** is the sudden onset of disabling terror. Symptoms include shortness of breath, dizziness, sweating, shaking, choking, trembling, and heart palpitations. A victim of a panic attack may feel that he or she is having a heart attack. Panic attacks may have no obvious link to environmental stimuli, or they may be learned responses to environmental stimuli. Researchers believe that panic attacks are caused by some physiological change or biochemical imbalance in the brain and are still searching for the mechanisms that trigger such attacks.

Post-traumatic Stress Disorder. Post-traumatic stress disorder (PTSD) afflicts some victims of severe traumas such as rape, assault, war, or airplane crashes. PTSD manifests itself in terrifying flashbacks to the sufferer's trauma.

When correctly diagnosed, anxiety disorders are treatable, usually through a combination of methods. Because undiagnosed diabetes, heart conditions, and endocrine disorders can mimic anxiety disorders, doctors recommend a thorough physical examination to rule out physical causes. If it is established that the causes are not physical, treatment usually consists of psychotherapy combined with medication.

Seasonal Affective Disorder

Seasonal affective disorder (SAD), a type of depression, affects a number of Canadians. Others experience a milder form of the disorder known as the winter blues. SAD strikes during the winter months and is associated with reduced exposure to sunlight. People with SAD suffer from irritability, apathy, carbohydrate craving and weight gain, increases in sleep time, and general sadness. Researchers believe that SAD is caused by a malfunction in the hypothalamus, the gland responsible for regulating responses to external stimuli. Stress may also play a role in SAD.

Certain factors seem to put people at risk for SAD. Women are four times more likely to suffer from SAD than are men. Although SAD occurs in people of all ages, those between 20 and 40 appear to be most vulnerable. Certain families appear to be at risk. And people living in Canada are more at risk than are those living farther south. During the winter, there are fewer hours of sunlight in northern regions than in southern areas. An estimated 10 percent of the population in the United States experience SAD, whereas fewer than 2 percent of those living in southern states such as Florida and New Mexico suffer from the disorder.

There are some simple but effective therapies for SAD. The most beneficial appears to be light therapy, in which a patient is exposed to lamps that mimic sunlight. After being exposed to this lighting each day, 80 percent of patients experience relief from their symptoms within four days. Other forms of treatment for SAD are diet change (eating more foods high in complex carbohydrates), increased exercise, stress management techniques, sleep

Cultural Differences in Emotional Terms

If you live in Canada and speak Canadian English, your emotional life is categorized differently than if you come from Japan or Indonesia. Some words that describe emotions in the Canadian English language, and therefore reflect the Canadian experience, have no real equivalent in other languages. Are there emotions that exist in English that do not exist in German, Chinese, or Japanese? If such differences exist, what do they tell us about emotion?

According to James A. Russell, who has conducted extensive research into cross-cultural comparisons of emotional terms, such differences do exist. There are 2000 words to describe emotions in English, but only 1500 in Dutch, 750 in Taiwanese Chinese, and 230 in Malay. More important than the number of specific terms, however, are the categories of emotion different languages allow. Some English words have no real equivalent in other languages. Russell points out that English distinguishes between *terror, horror, dread, apprehension,* and *timidity* as types of fear. However in Gidjingali, an Australian aboriginal language, one word, *guradadj,* suffices. What English treats as different emotions—for example, *anger* and *sadness*—other languages treat as one emotion. Some languages do not make the English distinction between *shame* and *embarrassment*. In China, there exists no term for *anxiety*; in Sri Lanka, there exists no term for *guilt.*

These differences are important because they show researchers that emotional experience may not be the same across all cultures. Cultural differences in emotion are probably due to differences in the way each culture approaches, appraises, and responds to various life events. For example, the definition of *shameful events* among the Awlad 'Ali, a tribe of Egyptian Bedouins, is highly specific: shameful events are those that injure one's honour; therefore, how a person codes an event is a central element in that person's language. In addition, just because a language does not have a particular word does not mean that the concept does not exist; it might, for example, be expressed in a phrase rather than in a single word.

From psychologists' points of view, the use of language to describe emotion is important because any discussion of emotion that names emotions uses specific words in a specific language. A theory of emotion that is truly universal to all people in all languages must be cross-culturally valid—not bound by specific word entries in a dictionary. This is an enormous challenge. Most psychologists believe that all human beings experience the same emotions, but to prove their beliefs they must first find terminology that is consistent across cultures. Without such consistency, cross-cultural differences will be hard to separate from cross-cultural similarities.

Source: Adapted from Lester A. Lefton, *Psychology,* 5th ed., 377. © 1994 by Allyn & Bacon. Reprinted by permission.

restriction (limiting the number of hours slept in a 24-hour period), psychotherapy, and antidepressants.

Schizophrenia

Perhaps the most frightening of all mental disorders is **schizophrenia,** a disease that affects about 1 percent of the Canadian population. Schizophrenia is characterized by alterations of the senses (including auditory and visual hallucinations); the inability to sort out incoming stimuli and to make appropriate responses; an altered sense of self; and radical changes in emotions, movements, and behaviours. Victims of this disease often cannot function in society.

For decades, scientists believed that schizophrenia was an environmentally provoked form of madness. They blamed abnormal family interactions or early-childhood

Schizophrenia: A mental illness with that is characterized by irrational behaviour, severe alterations of the senses (hallucinations), and, often, an inability to function in society.

traumas. Since the mid-1980s, however, when magnetic resonance imaging (MRI) and positron emission tomography (PET) began to allow scientists to study brain function more closely, scientists have recognized that schizophrenia is a biological disease of the brain. It has become evident that the brain damage involved occurs very early in life, possibly as early as in the second trimester of fetal development. However, the disease most commonly has its onset in late adolescence.

Schizophrenia is treatable but not curable at present. Treatments usually include some combination of hospitalization, medication, and supportive psychotherapy. Supportive psychotherapy, as opposed to psychoanalysis, can help the patient acquire skills for living in society.

Even though the environmental theories of schizophrenia have been discarded in favour of biological theories, a stigma remains attached to the disease. Families of schizophrenics often experience anger and guilt associated with misunderstandings about the causes of the disease. They often need help in the form of information, family counselling, and advice on how to meet the schizophrenic's needs for shelter, medical care, vocational training, and social interaction.

Gender Issues in Psychosocial Health

Studies have shown that gender bias often gets in the way of correct diagnosis of psychosocial disorders. In one study, for instance, 175 mental health professionals, of both genders, were asked to diagnose a patient on the basis of a summarized case history. Some of the professionals were told that the patient was male, others that the patient was female. The gender of the patient made a substantial difference in the diagnosis given (though the gender of the clinician did not). When subjects thought the patient was female, they were more likely to diagnose hysterical personality, a "women's disorder." When they believed the patient to be male, the more likely diagnosis was antisocial personality, a "male disorder."

Depression and Gender. For reasons that are not well understood, two-thirds of all people suffering from depression are women. Researchers have proposed biological, psychological, and social explanations for this fact. The biological explanation rests on the observation that women appear to be at greater risk for depression when their hormone levels change significantly, as during the premenstrual period, the period following the birth of a child, and the onset of menopause. Men's hormone levels appear to remain more stable throughout life. Researchers therefore theorized that women were inherently more at risk for depression. Yet evidence relating to this theory is either inconsistent or contrary.

Depression is often preceded by a stressful event. Some psychologists therefore theorized that women might be under more stress than are men and thus more prone to become depressed. However, women do not report a greater occurrence of more stressful events than do men.

Finally, researchers have observed gender differences in coping strategies, or the response to certain events or stimuli, and have proposed the explanation that women's strategies put them at more risk for depression than do men's strategies. Results indicated that the men tried to distract themselves from a depressed mood whereas the women tended to focus attention on it. If focussing on depressed feelings intensifies these feelings, women's response style may make them more likely than men to become clinically depressed. This hypothesis has not been directly tested, but some supporting evidence suggests its validity.[19]

PMS: Physical or Mental Disorder? A major controversy regarding gender bias has been over the inclusion of a "provisional" diagnosis for premenstrual syndrome (PMS) in the American Psychiatric Association's *Diagnostic and Statistical Manual of Mental Disorders* (fourth edition; known as *DSM-IV*). The provisional inclusion, in an appendix to *DSM-IV*, signals that PMS should come in for further study and may be included as an approved diagnosis in future editions of the *DSM*.

SUICIDE: GIVING UP ON LIFE

There were 3749 suicides reported in Canada in 1994. Experts estimate that there may actually be many more cases; due to the difficulty in determining the causes of suspicious deaths, many suicides are not reflected in the statistics. Suicide is often a consequence of poor coping skills, lack of social support, lack of self-esteem, and the inability to see one's way out of a bad or negative situation.

University students are more likely than the general population to attempt suicide; suicide is the second leading cause of death in people between the ages of 15 and 24. The pressures, joys, disappointments, challenges, and changes of the college environment are believed to be in part responsible for these rates. However, young adults who choose not to go to university but who are searching for the directions to their career goals, relationship goals, and other life aspirations are also at risk for suicide.

Risk factors for suicide include a family history of suicide, previous suicide attempts, excessive drug and alcohol use, prolonged depression, financial difficulties, serious illness in the suicide contemplator or in his or her loved ones, and loss of a loved one through death or rejection. Although women attempt suicide at four times the rate of men, more than three times as many men as women actually succeed in ending their lives. The elderly, divorced people, former psychiatric patients, and Native Canadians have a higher risk of suicide than others. In 1986 those over 65 made up 13 percent of those who committed suicide.[20] Alcoholics also have a high rate of suicide.

Depression is often a precursor of suicide. People who have been suffering from depression are more likely to attempt suicide while they are recovering, when their energy level is higher, than while they are in the depths of depression. Although only 15 percent of depressed people are suicidal, most suicide-prone individuals are depressed.[21]

Due to the growing incidence of suicide, many of us will be touched by a suicide at some time. In most cases, the suicide does not occur unpredictably. In fact, between 75 and 80 percent of people who commit suicide give a warning of their intentions.

Warning Signals

Common warnings of a suicide intent include:

- a direct statement about committing suicide, such as "I can't take it anymore. I might as well end it all."

- an indirect statement about committing suicide, such as, "Soon this pain will be over," or, "You won't have to worry about me anymore."

- "final preparations," such as writing a will, repairing poor relationships with family or friends, giving away prized possessions, or writing revealing letters

- a preoccupation with themes of death
- a withdrawal from friends and family and from activities once found pleasurable
- change in eating and sleeping habits
- drug and alcohol use
- marked personality change
- frequent complaints about physical symptoms, often related to emotions, such as stomachaches, headaches, fatigue, etc.
- not tolerating praise or rewards
- a sudden and unexplained demonstration of happiness following a period of depression
- changes in personal appearance
- loss of interest in classes or work and an inability to concentrate
- failure to recover from a personal loss or crisis and deepening or prolonged depression
- excessive risk taking and an "I don't care what happens to me" attitude

Taking Action to Prevent a Suicide Attempt

If someone you know threatens suicide or displays any of the above warnings, take the following actions:

- *Monitor the warning signals.* Try to keep an eye on the person involved, or see that there is someone around the person as much as possible.
- *Take any threats seriously.*
- *Let the person know how much you care about him or her.* State that you are there if he or she needs help.
- *Listen.* Try not to be shocked by or to discredit what the person says to you. Empathize, sympathize, and keep the person talking.
- *Ask the person directly, "Are you thinking of hurting or killing yourself?"*
- *Do not belittle the person's feelings or say that he or she doesn't really mean it or couldn't succeed at suicide.* To some people, these comments offer the challenge of proving you wrong.
- *Help the person think about other alternatives.* Be ready to offer choices. Offer to go for help with the person. Call your local suicide hotline and use all available community and campus resources.
- *Make a contract to meet the person at a later time in their home.*
- *If the person has a plan, remove any pills or guns; get help.*

- *Remember that your relationships with others involve responsibilities.* If you need to stay with the person, take the person to a health care facility, or provide support, give of yourself and your time.
- *Tell your friend's spouse, partner, parents, brothers and sisters, or counsellor.* Do not keep your suspicions to yourself. Don't let a suicidal friend talk you into keeping your discussions confidential. Let your friend know you must share this information with a professional. If your friend is successful in a suicide attempt, you will have to live with the consequences of your inaction.

*W*HAT DO YOU THINK?

If your roommate showed some of the warning signs of suicide, what action would you take? Whom would you contact first? Where on campus might your friend get help? What if someone in your class that you hardly knew gave some of the warning signs? What would you then do?

*S*EEKING PROFESSIONAL HELP

Many Canadians feel that seeking professional help for psychosocial problems is an admission of personal failure they cannot afford to make. Typically, any physical health problem, such as abscessed tooth or prolonged severe pain, sends us to the nearest dentist or physician. On the other hand, we tend to ignore psychosocial problems until they pose a serious threat to our well-being—and even then, we may refuse to ask for the help we need. Despite this tradition, an increasing number of Canadians are turning to mental health professionals for help. Researchers believe that more people want help today because "normal" living has become more hazardous. Breakdown in support systems, high expectations of the individual by society, and dysfunctional families are cited as the three major reasons more people are asking for assistance than ever before.

You should consider seeking help under the following circumstances:

- if you think you need help
- if you experience wild mood swings
- if a problem is interfering with your daily life
- if your fears or feelings of guilt frequently distract your attention
- if you begin to withdraw from others
- if you have hallucinations
- if you feel that life is not worth living

- if you feel inadequate or worthless
- if your emotional responses are inappropriate to various situations
- if your daily life seems to be nothing but repeated crises
- if you feel you can't "get your act together"
- if you are considering suicide
- if you turn to drugs or alcohol to escape from your problems
- if you feel out of control

Types of Mental Health Professionals

Several types of mental health professionals, or providers, are available to help you. The most important criterion when choosing a provider is whether you feel you can work well with that person, not how many degrees he or she has.

Psychiatrist. A **psychiatrist** is a medical doctor. After obtaining an M.D. degree, a psychiatrist spends up to 12 years studying psychosocial health and disease. As a licensed physician, a psychiatrist can prescribe medications for various mental or emotional problems and may have admitting privileges at a local hospital. Some psychiatrists are affiliated with hospitals, while others are in private practice. Psychiatric fees are normally covered by provincial or territorial health insurance.

Psychoanalyst. A **psychoanalyst** is a psychiatrist or a psychologist having special training in psychoanalysis. Psychoanalysis is a type of therapy in which a patient is helped to remember early traumas that have blocked personal growth. Facing these traumas helps the patient to resolve the conflicts they have caused and to begin to lead a more productive life.

Psychologist. A **psychologist** usually has a Ph.D. degree in counselling or clinical psychology. In addition, all provinces require licensure. Psychologists are trained in various types of talk therapy. Most are trained to conduct both individual and group counselling sessions. Psychologists may also be trained in certain specialties, such as family counselling, sexual counselling, or counselling related to compulsive behaviours. Psychologists may be in private practice and may also work in publicly funded organizations. Some Employee Assistance Programs cover a certain number of psychologist visits annually, and the Extended Health Plan through your university may have some coverage for psychologists' fees.

Clinical/Psychiatric Social Worker. A **social worker** has at least a master's degree in social work (M.S.W.) and two years of experience in a clinical setting. The provinces require an examination for accreditation in the College of Clinical Social Work. Some social workers work in clinical settings, whereas others have private practices. Certified clinical social workers (C.S.W.) often work in private practices, and their patients are sometimes insured through employee assistance programs.

Counsellor. Persons having a variety of academic and experiential training call themselves counsellors. The **counsellor** often has a master's degree in counselling, psychology, educational psychology, or a related human service. Professional societies recommend at least two years of graduate coursework or supervised practice as a minimal requirement. Many counsellors are trained to do individual and group counselling. They often specialize in one type of counselling, such as family, marital, relationship, children, drug, divorce, behavioural, or personal counselling.

Psychiatric Nurse Specialist. Although all registered nurses can work in psychiatric settings, some have chosen to continue their education and specialize in psychiatric practice. The psychiatric nurse specialist can be certified by the Registered Psychiatric Nursing Association in some provinces.

Remember that, in Canada, anyone can use the title of therapist or counsellor. Before you begin treatment, you should consider the credentials of your counsellor, your desired outcomes, and the expectations of you and your counsellor.

What to Expect When You Begin Therapy

The first trip to a therapist can be extremely difficult. Most of us have misconceptions about what therapy is and about what it can do. That first visit is a verbal and mental sizing up between you and the therapist. You may not accomplish much in that first hour. If you decide that the therapist is not for you, you will at least have learned how to present your problem and what qualities you need in a therapist.

1. Before meeting a therapist, briefly explain your needs to the therapist or appointments secretary. Ask what the fee is. Arrive on time. Wear comfortable clothing.

Psychiatrist: A licensed physician who specializes in treating mental and emotional disorders.

Psychoanalyst: A psychiatrist or psychologist having special training in psychoanalysis.

Psychologist: A person with a Ph.D. degree and training in psychology.

Social worker: A person with an M.S.W. degree and clinical training.

Counsellor: A person having a variety of academic and experiential training who deals with the treatment of emotional problems.

Managing Your Psychosocial Health

Psychosocial health is a complex concept. Finding the best way to help yourself achieve optimal psychosocial health requires careful introspection and planned action. Remembering the following points and acting upon them whenever possible may help you along the way.

Making Decisions for You

Psychosocial health is influenced by many factors. Why is being psychosocially healthy important to you? To the people who are close to you?

What actions can you take today that will help improve your emotional health? What steps could you take right now that could help you improve your social health? What could you do to improve your spiritual health? Finally, if you felt that you had a psychosocial problem, would you seek help? Why or why not?

Checklist for Change

✓ Consider life a constant process of discovery and learning.

✓ Accept yourself as the best that you are able to be right now.

✓ Remember that nobody is perfect.

✓ Remember that the most difficult times in life occur during transitions and can be opportunities for growth even though they are painful.

✓ Remember that there are other perspectives than your own.

✓ Recognize the sources of your own anxiety and act to reduce them.

✓ Ask for help when you need it; discuss your problems with others.

✓ Become sensitive to and aware of your own body's signals—take care of yourself.

✓ Find a meaning for your life and work toward achieving your goals.

✓ Develop strategies to get through problem situations.

✓ Remain open to emotional experiences—give yourself to today rather than always reserving yourself for tomorrow.

✓ Even when you fail, be proud of yourself for trying.

✓ Keep your sense of humour—learn to laugh at yourself.

✓ Never quit trying to grow, to experience, to love, and to live life to its fullest.

Critical Thinking

Suppose that your roommate ended a long-term relationship last month. Ever since, your roommate no longer jogs every morning, no longer attends religious services, and doesn't even want to attend school mixers to meet someone else. Worse yet, even minor mistakes lead your roommate to self-berating.

You are concerned about your roommate's psychosocial health, but unsure of what to do. You know that your roommate has in the past said that anyone who needs therapy should be "locked up and the key thrown away." But your roommate's mood is beginning to affect you. Use the DECIDE model described in Chapter 1 to decide what you would do in this situation. Explain your decision. If the action you chose did not bring about the desired result, what would you do next? Then list some ways you can show support for a friend who shows signs of psychosocial illness.

Expect to spend about an hour with the therapist during your first visit.

2. The therapist may want to take down your history and details about the problems that have brought you to therapy. Answer as honestly as possible. Many therapists will ask how you feel about aspects of your life. Do not be embarrassed to acknowledge your feelings.

3. Therapists are not mind readers. They cannot tell what you are thinking. It is therefore critical to the success of your treatment that you have enough trust in your therapist that you can be open and honest.

4. Do not expect the therapist to tell you what to do or how to behave. Very few hand out behavioural prescriptions.

5. Find out if the therapist will allow you to set your own therapeutic goals and timetables. Also, find out if, later in therapy, your therapist will allow you to determine what is and what is not helping you.

6. If, after your first visit (or even after several visits), you feel you cannot work with a therapist, you must summon up the courage to say so. Do not worry about hurting the therapist's feelings. If there is a personality conflict or if you do not feel comfortable, the therapy will not be effective.

WHAT DO YOU THINK?

Have you ever thought about seeing a therapist? What made you decide to go—or not to go? If you didn't go, did things get better quickly? Do you think you might have worked out your problem faster if you saw a therapist?

Summary

- Psychosocial health is a complex phenomenon involving intellectual, emotional, social, and spiritual health.

- Many factors influence psychosocial health, including life experiences, family, the environment, other people, self-esteem, self-efficacy, and personality.

- Social bonds and social support networks contribute to the ability to cope with life's challenges.

- Common psychosocial problems include depression, obsessive-compulsive disorders, anxiety disorders (including phobias, panic attacks, and post-traumatic stress syndrome), seasonal affective disorder, and schizophrenia.

- Suicide is a result of negative psychosocial reactions to life. People intending to commit suicide often give warning signs of their intentions. Such people can often be helped.

- Mental health professionals include psychiatrists, psychoanalysts, psychologists, clinical/psychiatric social workers, counsellors, and psychiatric nurse specialists. Major types of therapy include behavioural, cognitive, family, and psychodynamic therapies.

Discussion Questions

1. What is psychosocial health? What indicates that you either are or aren't psychosocially healthy? Why do you think the college environment may provide a real challenge to your psychosocial health?

2. Discuss the factors that influence your overall level of psychosocial health. What factors can you change? Which ones may be more difficult to change?

3. What steps could you take today to improve your psychosocial health? Which steps require long-term effort?

4. What factors appear to contribute to psychosocial difficulties and illnesses? Which of the more common psychosocial illnesses is likely to affect people in your age group?

5. What are the warning signs of suicide? What would you do if you heard a stranger in the cafeteria say to no one in particular that he was going to "do the world a favour and end it all"?

6. Discuss the different types of health professionals and therapies. If you felt depressed about breaking off a long-term relationship, which professional and therapy do you think would be most beneficial? Explain your answer. What services are provided by your student health centre? Are fees charged to students?

7. What psychosocial areas do you need to work on? Which are most important? Why?

Application Exercise

1. How psychosocially healthy is the individual described in the scenario presented at the beginning of the chapter?

2. What factors may have contributed to Marisol's current health status?

3. What services on your campus would be available to help Marisol improve her psychosocial health?

4. As a friend, what could you do to help Marisol?

Health on the Net

Canadian Mental Health Association (Hamilton Wentworth Branch ... check here for a link to a branch in your area)
www.netaccess.on.ca/~cmhaham/

Child & Family Canada
www.cfc-efc.ca/startup/home_eng.htm

Health Promotion Online
www.hc-sc.gc.ca/hppb/hpoe.htm

3

Managing Stress
Toward Prevention and Control

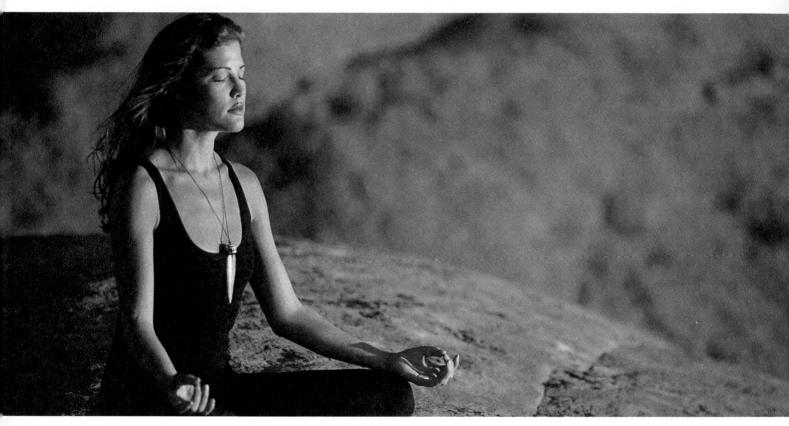

CHAPTER OBJECTIVES

◆ Define stress and examine how stress may have direct and indirect effects on your immune system and on your overall health status.

◆ Explain the three phases of the general adaptation syndrome and describe what happens physiologically when you perceive a threat.

◆ Discuss psychosocial, environmental, and self-imposed sources of stress.

◆ Examine how evolving societal expectations may cause new kinds of stress.

◆ Examine the special stressors that affect university students.

◆ Explore techniques for managing stress.

Erica is taking 20 credits this term: her parents are unable to help her financially, and she must graduate before her savings are depleted. She is also working ten hours per week and is involved in several student organizations. She finds that she is usually up until 1 A.M., wakes up at dawn, and must budget every minute of the day just to keep up. In spite of her efforts, she is falling farther and farther behind, has stopped seeing her friends, and is chronically tired. She recently developed a serious cold that has lingered for two weeks. She has also had a persistent headache and finds it difficult to get to sleep at night.

- Why is Erica so stressed? Why is she suffering from persistent illnesses? Is it possible to do everything right and still not have enough time to get everything done? What should Erica do to manage her stress? Where can she go for help?

Stress: it's hard to live with it, but it's almost impossible to live without it. We are bombarded by a host of subtle and not-so-subtle internal and external stresses from the moment we awake in the morning until we finally drift into deep sleep at day's end. Even during our sleeping moments, noise, temperature changes, and other activities can be sources of stress. Rarely does a day go by without someone you know talking about being under stress from homework, financial pressures, relationship demands, or other problems. Despite our best efforts to ignore it, stress cannot be run from, hidden from, or wished away. For some people, stress provides the stimulus for growth and higher levels of achievement. Yet for others, it increases the likelihood of dysfunctional or abnormal behaviour or illness.

Stress in itself is neither positive nor negative. Rather, our reactions to stress can be positive or negative. Whether we are aware of it or not, our reactions to stress can become the habits that lead us either to health-enhancing personal growth or to debilitation in the form of migraines, alcohol and drug addiction, circulatory disorders, asthma, gastrointestinal problems, and hypertension (high blood pressure). In addition, stress can lead to psychological and social problems, including dysfunctional relationships. In this chapter, we will explore why and how these reactions take place and how we may be able to control them.

*W*HAT IS STRESS?

Many things that have contributed to making you who you are also have influenced how you respond to stressful events in your life. Stress reactions—such as breaking out in a cold sweat before getting up in front of the class to speak, becoming anxious around people who speak too slowly or drive too cautiously, feeling nervous when meeting new people—are all unique by-products of past experiences. Your family, friends, environmental conditions, general health status, personality, and support systems affect how you respond to a given event.

Stress means different things to different people. Often, we think of stress as an externally imposed factor that threatens or makes a demand on our minds and bodies. If your hard-nosed instructor tells you that you must do a ten-page paper in the next week, that's an external stressor. But, actually, most stress is self-imposed and is usually the result of an internal state of emotional tension that occurs in response to the various demands of living. Stress may manifest itself in physiological responses to the demands placed upon us, and many researchers define *stress* as these responses.[1] Most current definitions state that **stress** is the mental and physical response of our bodies to the changes in our lives.

A **stressor** is any physical, social, or psychological event or condition that causes our bodies to have to adjust to a specific situation. Stressors may be tangible, such as an angry parent or a disgruntled roommate, or intangible, such as the mixed emotions associated with meeting your significant other's parents for the first time. **Adjustment** is our attempt to cope with a given situation.[2] As we try to adjust to a stressor, strain may develop. **Strain** is the

Stress: Our mental and physical responses to change.

Stressor: A physical, social, or psychological event or condition that causes us to have to adjust to a specific situation.

Adjustment: Our attempt to cope with a given situation.

Strain: The wear and tear our bodies and minds sustain as we adjust to or resist a stressor.

wear and tear our bodies and minds sustain during the process of adjusting to or resisting a stressor.

Stress and strain are associated with most of our daily activities. Generally, positive stress, or stress that presents the opportunity for personal growth and satisfaction, is called **eustress.** Getting married, starting school, beginning a career, developing new friendships, and learning a new physical skill all give rise to eustress. **Distress,** or negative stress, is caused by those events, such as financial problems, injury or illness, the death of a loved one, trouble at work, academic difficulties, and the breakup of a relationship, that result in debilitative stress and strain.

In many cases, we cannot prevent the occurrence of distress: like eustress, it is a part of life. However, we can train ourselves to recognize the events that cause distress and to anticipate the reactions we have to them. We can learn to practise prestress coping skills and to develop poststress management techniques. Development of both skills depends on our understanding of the major components of stress.

The Mind-Body Connection: Physiological Responses

Although much has been written about the negative effects of stress, researchers have only recently begun to untangle the complex web of physical and emotional interactions that actually cause the body to break down over time. As a result, stress is often described generically as a "disease of prolonged arousal" that often leads to other negative health effects. Nearly all systems of the body become potential targets for this onslaught, and the long-term effects may be devastating.

Much of the initial impetus for studying the health effects of stress came from indirect observations. Cardiologists in the Framingham Heart Study and other research projects noted that highly stressed individuals seemed to experience significantly greater risks for cardiovascular disease and hypertension.[3] Monkeys exposed to high levels of unpredictable stressors in studies showed signifi-

Stress is a positive factor in life when it creates opportunities for personal growth and satisfaction rather than psychological or physical wear and tear.

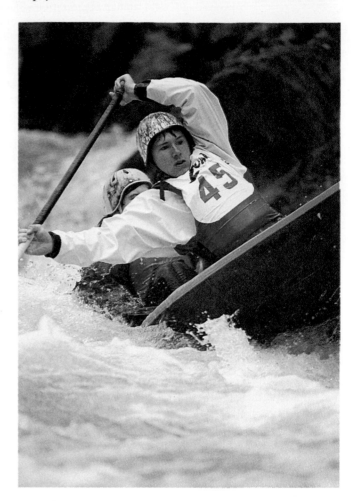

cantly increased levels of disease and mortality.[4] In a study of susceptibility to cold viruses, subjects inhaled high doses of the virus through the nose. Those subjects who reported recent high levels of stressors were much more likely to catch a cold following exposure to virus than were their low-stress counterparts.[5] While the battle over the legitimacy of these observations continues to be waged in research labs across the country, certain factors relating too much stress over long periods of time to selected ailments have gained credibility. What does repeated stress actually do to the body? Why are health experts so concerned about stress?

Psychoneuroimmunology (PNI). Although the health effects of prolonged stress provide dramatic evidence of the direct and indirect impact of stress on body organs, researchers continue to seek more definitive answers about the exact physiological mechanisms that lead to specific diseases. The science of **psychoneuroimmunology (PNI)** attempts to analyze the relationship between the mind's response to stress and the ability of the immune system to function effectively.

Eustress: Stress that presents opportunities for personal growth.

Distress: Stress that can have a negative effect on health.

Psychoneuroimmunology (PNI): Science of the interaction between the mind and the immune system.

Homeostasis: A balanced physical state in which all the body's systems function smoothly.

Adaptive response: Form of adjustment in which the body attempts to restore homeostasis.

General adaptation syndrome (GAS): The pattern followed by our physiological responses to stress, consisting of the alarm, resistance, and exhaustion phases.

Are Native Canadians More at Risk for Stress?

First Nations peoples are known to struggle with particular hardships such as poor sanitation, lack of opportunities for employment, and loss of band members due to early death. The figure in this box shows the eleven major determinants of health selected by the study population in a Canadian investigation of First Nations peoples. Death or loss, followed by unemployment, then poor housing, were the most frequently identified determinants. Physical and sexual abuse were the only conditions on which males and females differed, with females perceiving both to have a greater effect on their health.

A greater proportion of older respondents than younger respondents reported housing, water, sanitation, pollution, and poverty to have important effects on their health. While unemployment ranked second for the total study population, it ranked first for those aged 20 to 39, second for those aged 15 to 19, and eighth for those aged 40 and older. Death or loss was considered important by a greater proportion of respondents in both the 15-to-19 and 40-and-older age groups (41.1 percent and 50 percent respectively) than the middle age groups. Sexual, physical, and emotional abuse held relatively the same importance across age groups.

The question asked was: "Do you think that any of the following currently affect your social, mental, physical, or spiritual wellness?"

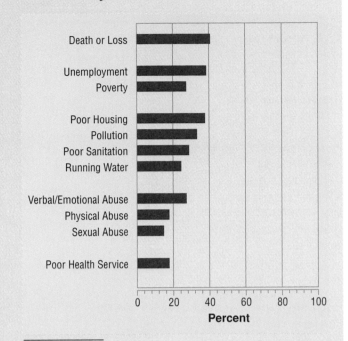

Source: Adapted from Ted Myers, et al., *Ontario First Nations AIDS Healthy Lifestyle Survey.* National AIDS Clearinghouse, Canadian Public Health Association, (Ottawa: 1993), 16.

Much of the preliminary PNI data on stress levels and immune functioning have focussed on the hypothesis that, during periods of prolonged stress, elevated levels of adrenal hormones destroy or reduce the ability of the white blood cells known as *natural killer T cells* to aid in the immune response. When killer Ts are suppressed, illnesses have a greater chance of gaining a foothold in the body. In addition to killer T suppression, many other bodily processes are disrupted and overall disease-fighting capacity is reduced. Although several studies have supported the hypothesis of a relationship between increased stress levels and greater risk of disease in times of grief, social disruption, poor mood, and so forth, there is much to be learned about possible mediating factors in this process.[6] Other studies have shown no increased risk for disease among people suffering from prolonged arousal by stressors.[7]

THE GENERAL ADAPTATION SYNDROME

Every living organism tends toward a state of balance known as **homeostasis.** In homeostasis, all physical and psychological systems function smoothly, and equilib-

rium is maintained. When a stressor disrupts homeostasis, the body adjusts with an **adaptive response,** or an attempt to restore homeostasis. This adaptive response to stress varies in intensity and physical manifestation from person to person and from stressor to stressor.

The physiological responses to stress follow a pattern that was first recognized in 1936 by Hans Selye. The three-stage response to stress Selye outlined is called the **general adaptation syndrome (GAS).** The phases of the GAS are alarm, resistance, and exhaustion.[8]

Alarm Phase

During the alarm phase, a stressor disturbs homeostasis. The brain subconsciously perceives the stressor and prepares the body either to fight or to run away, a response sometimes called the *fight or flight response.* The subconscious perceptions and appraisal of the stressor stimulate the areas in the brain responsible for emotions. Emotional stimulation, in turn, starts the physical reactions that we associate with stress (see Figure 3.1). This entire process usually takes only a few seconds.

When the mind perceives a stressor (either real or imaginary), such as a potential attacker, the *cerebral cortex,* the region of the brain that interprets the nature of an event, is called to attention. If the cerebral cortex consciously or

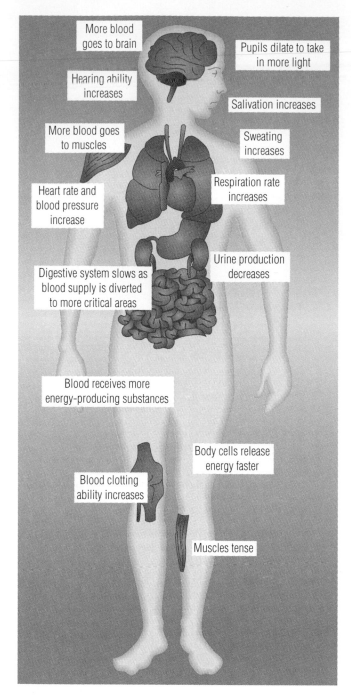

FIGURE 3.1

The General Adaptation Syndrome: Alarm Phase

ANS has two branches. The **sympathetic nervous system,** one branch, begins to energize the body for either fight or flight by signalling the release of several stress hormones that speed the heart rate, increase the breathing rate, and trigger many other stress responses. The **parasympathetic nervous system,** the other branch, functions to slow all the systems stimulated by the stress response. Thus, the parasympathetic branch of the ANS serves as a system of checks and balances on the sympathetic branch. In a healthy person, these two branches work together in a balance that controls the negative effects of stress. However, long-term stress can cause this balance to become strained, and chronic physical problems can occur as stress reactions become the dominant forces in a person's body.

The responses of the sympathetic nervous system to stress involve a complex series of biochemical exchanges between different parts of the body. The **hypothalamus,** a section of the brain, functions as the control centre of the sympathetic nervous system and determines the overall reaction to stressors. When the hypothalamus perceives that extra energy is needed to fight a stressor, it stimulates the adrenal glands, located near the top of the kidneys, to release the hormone **epinephrine,** also called adrenaline. Epinephrine causes more blood to be pumped with each beat of the heart, dilates the bronchioles (air sacs in the lungs) to increase oxygen intake, increases the breathing rate, stimulates the liver to release more glucose (which fuels muscular exertion), and dilates the pupils to improve visual sensitivity. The body is then poised to act immediately.

As epinephrine secretion increases, blood is diverted away from the digestive system, possibly causing nausea and cramping if the distress occurs shortly after a meal, and drying of nasal and salivary tissues, producing a dry mouth.

The stress response occurring during the alarm phase also provides for longer-term reaction to stress. The hypothalamus triggers the pituitary gland, which in turn releases another powerful hormone, **adrenocorticotrophic hormone (ACTH).** ACTH signals the adrenal glands to release **cortisol,** a hormone that makes stored nutrients more readily available to meet energy demands. Finally, other parts of the brain and body release endorphins, the body's naturally occurring opiates, which relieve pain that may be caused by a stressor.

Resistance Phase

The resistance phase of the GAS begins almost immediately after the alarm phase starts. In this phase, the body has reacted to the stressor and adjusted in a way that begins to allow the system to return to homeostasis. As the sympathetic nervous system is working to energize the body via the hormonal action of epinephrine, norepinephrine, cortisol, and other hormones, the parasympathetic nervous system is helping to keep these energy levels under control and returns the body to a normal level of functioning.

unconsciously perceives a threat, it triggers an instantaneous **autonomic nervous system (ANS)** response that prepares the body for action. The ANS is the portion of the central nervous system that regulates bodily functions that we do not normally consciously control, such as heart function, breathing, and glandular function. When we are stressed, the rate of all these bodily functions increases dramatically to give us the physical strength to protect ourselves against an attack, or to mobilize internal forces. The

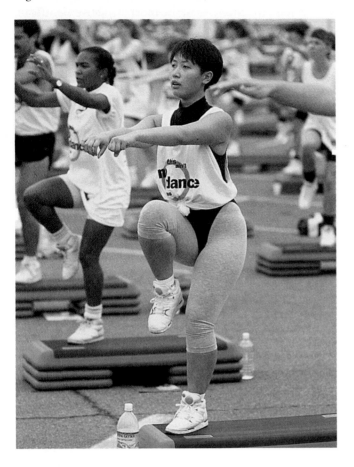

Aerobic exercise is one way to replenish the energy stores the body uses in adapting and adjusting to negative stressors.

Stress researchers theorize that when its deep adaptation energy stores are depleted, an organism dies. Stress management, then, is dependent on an ability to replenish superficial stores, and thereby to conserve deep stores. Superficial adaptation energy stores can be replenished by aerobic exercise (exercise that raises the heart rate), balancing work with relaxation, eliminating unnecessary drugs, maintaining a secure home environment, practising good nutritional habits, finding challenges and adventures instead of threats in stressors, setting realistic goals, and establishing and maintaining supportive relationships.

𝒲HAT DO YOU THINK?

What are the greatest sources of stress for you right now? What can you do to keep your superficial adaptation energy stores high and reduce your risks of becoming run down? Have you ever noticed that you tend to get sick more during certain times? Why might this occur?

𝒮OURCES OF STRESS

Both eustress and distress have many sources. These sources include psychosocial factors, such as changes, hassles, pressure, inconsistent goals and objectives, conflict, overload, and burnout; environmental stressors, such as natural and human-made disasters; and

Exhaustion Phase

In the exhaustion phase of the GAS, the physical and psychological energy used to fight a stressor has been depleted. Short-term stress would probably not deplete all of a person's energy reserves, but chronic stressors, such as the struggle to get straight As, financial worries, or fights with family and friends may create continuous states of alarm and resistance. When a person no longer has the adaptation energy stores for fighting a distressor, serious illness may result.

Adaptation Energy Stores. Many stress researchers believe that each of us possesses *adaptation energy stores.* In these researchers' model, these energy stores are the physical and mental foundations of our ability to cope with stress. Two levels of adaptation energy stores exist: *deep* and *superficial.* We apparently have little control over our deep adaptation energy stores: heredity seems to be the primary influence on them and some scientists speculate that their size is preset in each of our cells. Superficial adaptation energy stores surround the deep stores. These relatively easy-to-reach stores are used before the deep energy stores beneath them and they are renewable.

Autonomic nervous system (ANS): The portion of the central nervous system that regulates bodily functions that we do not normally consciously control.

Sympathetic nervous system: Branch of the autonomic nervous system responsible for stress arousal.

Parasympathetic nervous system: Part of the autonomic nervous system responsible for slowing systems stimulated by the stress response.

Hypothalamus: A section of the brain that controls the sympathetic nervous system and directs the stress response.

Epinephrine: Also called adrenaline, a hormone that stimulates body systems in response to stress.

Adrenocorticotrophic hormone (ACTH): A pituitary hormone that stimulates the adrenal glands to secrete cortisol.

Cortisol: Hormone released by the adrenal glands that makes stored nutrients more readily available to meet energy demands.

self-imposed stress. We'll look at each factor in more detail in this section.

Psychosocial Sources of Stress

As you learned in the previous chapter, psychosocial health relates to the intellectual, emotional, social, and spiritual dimensions of health. These dimensions define how we perceive our lives, relate to one another, and react to stress. Psychosocial stress refers to the factors in our daily lives that cause stress. Many factors in our daily lives cause us to be stressed. Our interactions with others, the subtle and not-so-subtle expectations we and others have of ourselves, and the social conditions we work in, play in, and live in all force us to adjust and readjust continually. Some of these stressors present very real threats to our mental and/or physical well-being; others cause us to worry about things that may never happen. Still other stressors result from otherwise good psychosocial events—being around someone you're attracted to, meeting new friends, or moving to a new and better apartment.

Change. Any time there is change in your normal daily routine, whether good or bad, you will experience stress. The more changes you experience and the more adjustments you must make, the greater the stress effects may be. In 1967, Drs. Thomas Holmes and Richard Rahe analyzed the social readjustments experienced by over 5000 patients, noting which events seemed to occur just prior to disease onset.[9] They determined that certain events (both positive and negative) were predictive of increased risk for illness. They called their scale for predicting stress overload and the likelihood of illness the Social Readjustment Rating Scale (SRRS) and this scale has been used extensively.[10] The SRRS has since been modified for certain groups, including university-aged students. Although many other factors must be considered, it is generally believed that the more stressors you have, the more you need to change your behaviours or situation before problems occur. (See the Rate Yourself box.)

Hassles. While Holmes and Rahe focussed on such major sources of stress as a death in the family, psychologists such as Richard Lazarus have more recently focussed on petty annoyances, irritations, and frustrations—collectively referred to as hassles—as sources of stress.[11] Minor hassles—losing your keys, having the grocery bag rip on the way to the door, slipping and falling in front of everyone as you walk to your seat in a new class, finding that you went through a whole afternoon with a big chunk of spinach stuck in your front teeth—may seem unimportant, but the cumulative effects of these minor hassles may be harmful in the long run.

Pressure. Pressure occurs when we feel forced to speed up, intensify, or shift the direction of our behaviour to meet a higher standard of performance.[12] Pressures can be based on our personal goals and expectations or on a concern about what others may think of us. Pressure can also come from outside influences. Among the most significant and consistent of these are seemingly relentless demands from society that we compete and that we be all that we can be. The forces that push us to compete for the best grades, the nicest cars, the most attractive significant others, and the highest paying jobs create significant pressure to be the personification of success.[13] When we are pressured into doing something we don't want to do (for example, studying when everyone else is going to a movie), significant frustration can occur.

Inconsistent Goals and Behaviours. For many of us, negative stress effects are magnified when there is a conflict between our goals (what we value or hope to obtain in life) and our behaviours (actions or activities that may or may not lead us to achieving these goals). For instance, you may want good grades, and your family may expect them. But if you party and procrastinate throughout the term, your behaviours are inconsistent with your goals, and significant stress in the form of guilt, last-minute frenzy before exams, and disappointing grades may result. On the other hand, if you want to dig in and work, and are committed to getting good grades, much of your negative stress may be eliminated or reduced. Thwarted goals may lead to frustration, and frustration has been shown to be a significant disrupter of homeostasis (see Figure 3.2).

Determining whether our behaviours are consistent with goal attainment is an essential component of our efforts to maintain a balance in our lives. If we consciously strive to attain our goals in a very direct manner, our chances of success are greatly improved. If we deviate from the plan, or if we act in a manner that is inconsistent with

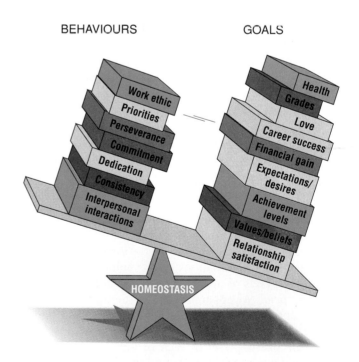

FIGURE 3.2

Stress Affects Homeostatic Balance

How Stressed Are You?

Each of us reacts differently to life's little challenges. Faced with a long line at the bank, most of us will get heated up for a few seconds before we shrug and move on. But for others—the one in five of us whom researchers call hot reactors—such incidents are an assault on good health. That's why rating your stress requires you both to tally your life's stressors (Part One) and to figure out whether you are particularly susceptible to stress (Part Two).

PART ONE

The Stress in Your Life

How often are the following stressful situations a part of your daily life?

1 Never
2 Rarely
3 Sometimes
4 Often
5 All the time

I work long hours	1	2	3	4	5
There are signs my job isn't secure	1	2	3	4	5
Doing a good job goes unnoticed	1	2	3	4	5
It takes all my energy just to make it through the day	1	2	3	4	5
There are severe arguments at home	1	2	3	4	5
A family member is seriously ill	1	2	3	4	5
I'm having problems with child care	1	2	3	4	5
I don't have enough time for fun	1	2	3	4	5
I'm on a diet	1	2	3	4	5
My family and friends count on me to solve their problems	1	2	3	4	5
I'm expected to keep up a certain standard of living	1	2	3	4	5
My neighbourhood is crowded or dangerous	1	2	3	4	5
My home is a mess	1	2	3	4	5
I can't pay my bills on time	1	2	3	4	5
I'm not saving money	1	2	3	4	5

Your Total Score _____

Below 38:   You have a *Lower-Stress Life.*

38 & Above: You have a *High-Stress Life.*

PART TWO

Your Stress Susceptibility

Try to imagine how you would react in these hypothetical situations.

You've been waiting 20 minutes for a table in a crowded restaurant, and the host seats a party that arrived after you.

You feel your anger rise as your face gets hot and your heart beats faster.

True or False

. . . .

Your sister calls out of the blue and starts to tell you how much you mean to her. Uncomfortable, you change the subject without expressing what you feel.

True or False

. . . .

You come home to find the kitchen looking like a disaster area and your spouse lounging in front of the TV. You tense up and can't seem to shake your anger.

True or False

. . . .

Faced with a public speaking event, you get keyed up and lose sleep for a day or more, worrying about how you'll do.

True or False

. . . .

On Thursday your repair shop promises to fix your car in time for a weekend trip. As the hours go by, you become increasingly worried that something will go wrong and your trip will be ruined.

True or False

Two or Fewer True: You're a *Cool Reactor,* someone who tends to roll with the punches when a situation is out of your control.

Three or More True: Sorry, you're a *Hot Reactor,* someone who responds to mildly stressful situations with a "fight-or-flight" adrenaline rush that drives up blood pressure and can lead to heart rhythm disturbances, accelerated clotting, and damaged blood vessel linings. Some hot reactors can seem cool as a cucumber on the outside, but inside their bodies are silently killing them.

WHAT YOUR SCORES MEAN

Combine the results from Parts One and Two to get your total stress rating.

Lower-Stress Life   Cool Reactor

Whatever your problems, stress isn't one of them. Even when stressful events do occur—and they will—your health probably won't suffer.

Lower-Stress Life   Hot Reactor

You're not under stress—at least for now. Though you tend to overreact to problems, you've wisely managed your life to avoid the big stressors. Before you honk at the guy who cuts you off in rush-hour traffic, remember that getting angry can destroy thousands of heart muscle cells within minutes.

(continued)

Robert S. Eliot, author of *From Stress to Strength*, says hot reactors have no choice but to calm themselves down with rational thought. Ponder the fact that the only thing you'll hasten by reacting is a decline in health. "You have to stop trying to change the world," Eliot advises, "and learn to change your response to it."

High-Stress Life   Cool Reactor

You're under stress, but only you know if it's hurting. Even if you normally thrive with a full plate of challenges, now you might be biting off more than you can chew. Note any increase in headaches, backaches, or insomnia; that's your body telling you to lighten your load. If your job is the main source of stress, think about reducing your hours. If that's not possible, find a way to make your job more enjoyable, and stress will become manageable.

High-Stress Life   Hot Reactor

You're in the danger zone. Make an extra effort to exercise, get enough sleep, and keep your family and friends close. Unfortunately, even being physically fit does little to protect you if your body is in perpetual stress mode. To survive, you may need to make major changes—walking away from a life-destroying job or relationship, perhaps—as well as to develop a whole new approach to life's hourly obstacles. Such effort will be rewarded, too. In one experiment, 77 percent of hot reactors were able to cool down—lower their blood pressure and cholesterol levels—by training themselves to stay calm.

Source: Reprinted by permission of the Health Publishing Group, a division of Time Publishing Ventures, Inc., from "How Stressed Are You?" *Health*, October 1994, 47. Researched by Lora Elise Ma. © 1994.

our goals, significant stress may result that makes our goals impossible, and they may become negative sources of stress.

Conflict.   Of all life's troubles, conflict is probably one of the most common. **Conflict** occurs when we are forced to make difficult decisions concerning two or more competing motives, behaviours, or impulses or when we are forced to face two incompatible demands, opportunities, needs, or goals.[14] What if your best friends all choose to smoke marijuana and you don't want to smoke but fear rejection? Such conflicts occur every day for most of us. Worrying about the alternatives, fretting, stewing, and becoming overly anxious are common stress responses when conflict occurs.

Overload.   **Overload** occurs when you suffer from excessive time pressure, excessive responsibility, lack of support, or excessive expectations of yourself and those around you. Have you ever felt that you had so many responsibilities that you couldn't possibly begin to fulfill them all? Have you longed for a weekend when you could just curl up and read a good book or take time out with friends and not feel guilty? These feelings typically occur when a person has been under continued stress for a period of time and is suffering from overload. Students suffering from overload may experience anxiety about tests, poor self-concept, a desire to drop classes or to drop out of school, and other problems. In severe cases, in which they are unable to see any solutions to their problems, students may suffer from depression or turn to substance abuse.

Burnout.   People who regularly suffer from overload, frustration, and disappointment may eventually begin to experience **burnout,** a state of physical and mental exhaustion caused by excessive stress. People involved in the helping professions, such as teaching, social work, drug counselling, nursing, and psychology, appear to experience high levels of burnout, as do people such as police officers and air-traffic controllers who work in high-pressure, dangerous jobs.

Other Forms of Psychosocial Stress.   Other forms of psychosocial stress include problems with adaptation, difficulty in adapting to life's changes; frustration, the thwarting or inhibiting of natural or desired behaviours or goals; overcrowding, the presence of too many people in a space; discrimination, the unfavourable actions taken against people based on prejudices concerning race, religion, social status, gender, lifestyle, national origin, or physical characteristics; and such socioeconomic events as inflation, unemployment, or poverty. People of different ethnic backgrounds may face disproportionately heavy impact from these sources of stress.

Environmental Stress

Environmental stress is stress that results from events occurring in our physical environment as opposed to our social environment. Environmental stressors include natural disasters, such as floods, earthquakes, hurricanes, and forest fires, and industrial disasters, such as chemical spills, accidents at nuclear power plants, and explosions. Often as damaging as one-time disasters are **background**

distressors, such as noise, air, and water pollution, although we may be unaware of them and their effects may not become apparent for decades. As with other distressors, our bodies respond to environmental distressors with the general adaptation syndrome. People who cannot escape background distressors may exist in a constant resistance phase, which may contribute to the development of stress-related disorders.

Self-Imposed Stress

Self-Concept and Stress. How we feel about ourselves, our attitudes toward others, and our perceptions and interpretations of the stressors in our lives are all part of the psychological component of stress. Also included are the defence or coping mechanisms we have learned to use in various stressful situations.

The psychological system that governs our responses to stressors is called the **cognitive stress system.**[15] Our cognitive stress system serves to recognize stressors; evaluate them on the basis of self-concept, past experiences, and emotions; and make decisions regarding how to cope with them.

Our sensory organs serve as input channels for any information reaching the brain. From that point on, attention to the problem, memory, reasoning processes, and problem solving are organized in various parts of the brain before we act on the stressor. Because learning and memory involve the changing of various proteins in brain neurons, the emotions experienced during the stress response also "tickle" the memory storage neurons and contribute to our responses. Behaviourally, we will respond to the stressor in ways consistent with our memories of similar situations.

Self-esteem is closely related to the emotions engendered by past experiences. People with low self-esteem are more likely to become victims of helpless anger, an emotion experienced by people who have not learned to express anger in appropriate ways. People suffering helpless anger have usually learned that they are wrong to feel anger; therefore, instead of learning to express their anger in healthy ways, they turn it inward. They may "swallow" their anger in food, alcohol, or other drugs, or may act in other self-destructive ways.

Research indicates that self-esteem significantly affects various disease processes. People with low self-esteem create a self-imposed distressor that can impair the immune system's ability to combat disease. Some researchers believe that chronic distress can depress the immune system and thus increase the symptoms of such diseases as acquired immune deficiency syndrome (AIDS), herpes, multiple sclerosis, and Epstein-Barr syndrome.

Personality Types and Hardiness. A person's personality may contribute to the kind and degree of self-imposed stress he or she experiences. The coronary-disease-prone personality was first described in 1974 by physicians

Meyer Friedman and Ray Rosenman in their book *Type A Behavior and Your Heart*.[16] Although their work is now considered controversial, it is the basis for much current research.

Friedman and Rosenman identified two stress-related personality types: Type A and Type B. Type A personalities are hard-driving, competitive, anxious, time-driven, impatient, angry, and perfectionistic. Type B personalities are relaxed and noncompetitive. According to Rosenman and Friedman, people with Type A characteristics are more prone to heart attacks than are their Type B counterparts.

Researchers today believe that more needs to be discovered about Type A and Type B personalities before we can say that all Type As will have greater risks for heart disease than will Type Bs. First of all, most people are not one personality type or the other all of the time. Second, there are many other unexplained variables that must be explored, such as why some Type A personalities seem to thrive in stress-filled environments. Now labelled Type C personalities, these individuals appear to succeed more often than Type B personalities and have good health even while displaying Type A patterns of behaviour.

Critics of these categories for stress risk argue that attempts to explain ill health by means of personal behavioural patterns have so far been crude. For example, researchers at Duke University contend that the Type A personality may be more complex than previously described. They have identified a "toxic core" in some Type A personalities. People who have this toxic core are angry, distrustful of others, and have above-average levels of cynicism. People who are angry and hostile often have below-average levels of social support and other increased risks for ill health. It may be this toxic core rather than the hard-driving nature of the Type A personality that makes people more prone to self-imposed stress and its consequences.[17]

Psychologist Susanne Kobasa has identified **psychological hardiness** as a characteristic that has helped some people negate self-imposed stress associated with Type A behaviour. Psychologically hardy people are characterized

---

Conflict: Simultaneous existence of incompatible demands, opportunities, needs, or goals.

Overload: A condition in which we feel overly pressured by demands made on us.

Burnout: Physical and mental exhaustion caused by excessive stress.

Background distressors: Environmental stressors that we may be unaware of.

Cognitive stress system: The psychological system that governs our emotional responses to stress.

Psychological hardiness: A personality characteristic characterized by control, commitment, and challenge.

by control, commitment, and challenge.[18] People with a sense of control are able to accept responsibility for their behaviours and to make changes in behaviours that they discover to be debilitating. People with a sense of commitment have good self-esteem and understand their purpose in life. People with a sense of challenge see changes in life as stimulating opportunities for personal growth.

Modification of Type A behaviour is possible because some of this behaviour is "learned." Some Type A people are able to reduce their hurried behaviour and become more tolerant, more patient, and better-humoured. Unfortunately, many people do not decide to modify their Type A habits until after they have become ill or suffered a heart attack or other circulatory system distress. Prevention of heart and circulatory disorders resulting from stress entails recognizing and changing dangerous behaviours before damage is done.

Self-Efficacy and Control. Whether people are able to cope successfully with stressful situations often depends on their level of self-efficacy, or belief in their skills and performance abilities.[19] If people have been successful in mastering similar problems in the past, they will be more likely to believe in their own effectiveness in future situations. Similarly, people who have repeatedly tried and failed may lack confidence in their abilities to deal with life's problems. In some cases, this insecurity may prevent them from trying to cope.

In addition, people who believe they lack control in a situation may become easily frustrated and give up. Those who feel they have no personal control over anything tend to have an external locus of control and a low level of self-efficacy. People who are confident their behaviour will influence the ultimate outcome of events tend to have an internal locus of control. People who feel that they have limited control over their lives tend to have higher levels of stress. For some suggestions on how to gain more control in angry situations, see the Building Communication Skills box.

STRESS AND THE UNIVERSITY STUDENT

Stress related to university life is not caused only by pressure to excel academically. University students experience numerous distressors, including changes related to being away from home for the first time, climatic differences between home and school, pressure to make friends in a new and sometimes intimidating setting, the feeling of anonymity imposed by large classes, test-taking anxiety, and pressures related to time management.

Some students are stressed by athletic team requirements, dormitory food, roommate habits, peers' expecta-

tions, new questions about personal values and beliefs, relationship problems, fraternity or sorority demands, or financial worries. For older students, worries about competing with 18-year-olds may also be distressful. Most colleges offer stress management workshops through their health centres or student counselling departments.

You should not ignore the following symptoms of stress overload. If you experience one or more of these symptoms, you should act promptly to reduce their impact.

- difficulty keeping up with classes or difficulty concentrating on and finishing tasks
- frequent clashes with close friends, family, or intimate partners about trivial issues such as housekeeping
- frequent mood changes or overreaction to minor problems.
- lethargy caused by lack of sleep or excessive frustration.
- lack of interest in social activities or tendency to avoid others
- avoidance of stressors through use of drugs or alcohol or through other extreme behaviours
- sleep disturbances, TV addiction, free-floating anxiety, or an exaggerated sense of self
- difficulty in maintaining an intimate relationship
- lack of interest in sexual relationships or inability to participate in satisfactory sexual relationships
- tendency to be intolerant of minor differences of opinion
- hunger and cravings or tendency to overeat or to eat while thinking of other things
- lack of awareness of sensory cues
- inability to listen or tendency to jump from subject to subject in conversation
- stuttering or other speech difficulties
- accident-proneness

WHAT DO YOU THINK?

How many of these psychological and emotional reactions have you experienced? Which reactions do you think are the most damaging to you and to your relationships with others? Which ones would be the easiest to change? What actions could you take immediately to cope with these problems? What could you do to cope with these problems in the long run?

Overcoming Test-Taking Anxiety

Doing well on a test is an ability needed far beyond your college days. Many careers require special exams. Tests are a fact of life in government, insurance, medicine, and other fields. And stress is a fact of tests!

But there are things you can do to get the upper hand on your anxiety. Here are some helpful hints that you will find useful now and in the future. Give them a try on your next exam.

Before the exam:

1. *Manage your time.* Effective management will help you find the time to study before the test. Plan to study beginning a week before your test (longer if a career exam). The more advance studying, the less anxiety you will feel. Do not wait to study until the night before the test. The final night should be limited to review. Arrive at the test a half-hour early for a final run-through. You will find that this will ease your anxiety and increase your confidence.

2. *Build your test-taking self-esteem.* Try two things. First, take a three-by-five-inch card and write down the three reasons you will pass the exam. Carry the card with you and look at it whenever you study. Second, when you get the test, write your three reasons on the test or on a piece of scrap paper. Positive affirmations such as this will help you succeed.

3. *Get adequate sleep.* You need to be alert, so try to get a little extra sleep for a few nights before your exam.

4. *Eat well before the exam.* As you'll learn in Chapter 8, sugar doesn't give you energy. In fact, it tires you. Avoid all sugary foods the day before the test and also those foods that might upset your stomach. You want to be feeling your best.

5. *Take caffeine about an hour before the test.* Research shows that caffeine promotes alertness, motor performance, and the capacity for work, as well as a decrease in fatigue. A cup or two of coffee, tea, or a cola drink is sufficient. Some people shouldn't use caffeine. Avoid it if you are one of the small percentage that it leaves feeling shaky and on edge for hours or if you regularly do not use caffeinated products. Test day is not the day to find out how your body reacts to caffeine.

During the test:

1. *Use time management during the test.* If you have 60 minutes to answer 30 multiple-choice questions, you might decide to spend the first 45 minutes taking the test (1 1/2 minutes per question) and 15 minutes reviewing your answers (30 seconds per question). Hold yourself to this schedule. After 15 minutes, you should have completed the first 10 questions, etc. If you don't know an answer, or the question is taking too long, skip it and move on. Since you allotted yourself time at the end to review, you will have the time to go back.

   Test-makers usually allow sufficient time to complete and review a test. However, if you feel that you are a slow reader and may need more time, talk to your teacher or the test administrator *before* the exam.

2. *Slow down.* When you open your test book, always write RTFQ (Read the Full Question) at the top. Make sure you understand the question.

3. *If you begin to get anxious, reread your three reasons for success.* Stay on track.

STRESS MANAGEMENT

Stress can be challenging or defeating depending upon how we learn to view it. The most effective way to avoid defeat is to learn a number of skills known collectively as stress management. Stress management consists primarily of finding balance in our lives. We balance rest, relaxation, exercise, nutrition, work, school, family, finances, and social activities. As we balance our lives, we make the choice to react constructively to our stressors. Robert Eliot, a cardiologist and stress researcher, offers two rules for people trying to cope with life's challenges: (1) "Don't sweat the small stuff," and (2) Remember that "it's all small stuff."[20]

Dealing with Stress

The first step of stress management is to examine thoroughly any problem involving stress. Figure 3.3 shows a decision-making model for stress reduction. As the model shows, dealing with stress involves assessing all aspects of a stressor, examining how you are currently responding to the stressor and how you may be able to change your response, and evaluating various methods of coping with stress. Often we cannot change the requirements at our university, unexpected distressors, or accidents. Inevitably, we will be stuck in classes that bore us and for which we find no application in real life. We feel powerless when a loved one has died. The facts themselves cannot be changed; only our reactions to the distressors in our lives can be changed.

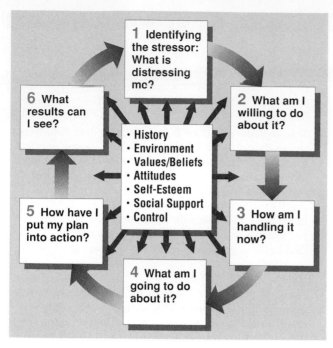

FIGURE 3.3

A Decision-Making Model for Stress Reduction

Source: Adapted from Lester A. Lefton, *Psychology,* 5th ed., 485 (Figure 13.5). © 1994 by Allyn & Bacon. Reprinted by permission.

Assessing Your Stressors.   After recognizing a stressor, you need to assess it. Can you alter the circumstances in any way to reduce the amount of distress you are experiencing, or must you change your behaviour and reactions to the stressor to reduce your stress levels? For example, if five term papers for five different courses are due during the semester, you will probably quickly assess that you cannot alter the circumstances: your professors are unlikely to drop their requirements. You can, however, change your behaviour by beginning the papers early and spacing them over time to avoid last-minute stress. If your boss is vague about directions for assignments, you cannot change the boss. You can, however, ask the boss to clarify in writing the things that are expected of you.

Changing Your Responses.   Changing your responses requires practice and emotional control. If your roommate is habitually messy and this causes you stress, you can choose among several responses. You can express your anger by yelling, you can pick up the mess and leave a nasty note, or you can defuse the situation with humour. The first response that comes to mind is not always the best response. Stop before reacting to gain the time you need to find an appropriate response. Ask yourself, "What is to be gained from my response?"

Many people change their responses to potentially stressful events through *cognitive coping strategies.* These strategies help them prepare for stressors through gradual exposure to increasingly higher stress levels.

Learning to Cope.   Everyone copes with stress in different ways. For some people, drinking and taking drugs helps them to cope. Others choose to get help from counsellors. Still others try to keep their minds off stress or to engage in positive activities such as exercise or relaxation techniques. *Stress inoculation* is one of the newer techniques for helping people prepare for stressful events. Through stress inoculation, people are given warnings, recommendations, and reassurances that may help them to cope with impending dangers or losses. Some health experts compare stress inoculation to a vaccine given to protect against a disease. Essentially, stress inoculation

- increases the predictability of stressful events
- fosters coping skills
- generates self-talking
- encourages confidence about successful outcomes
- builds a commitment to personal action and responsibility for an adaptive course of action

Regardless of how you cope with a given situation, your conscious effort to deal with this situation is an important step in stress management.

Managing Emotional Responses

Have you ever gotten all worked up about something you thought was happening only to find that your perceptions were totally wrong or that a communication problem had caused a misinterpretation of events? If you're like most of us, this has probably happened to you. We often get upset not by realities but by our faulty perceptions.

Stress management requires that you examine your self-talk and your emotional responses to interactions with others. With any emotional response to a distressor, you are responsible for the emotion and the behaviours elicited by the emotion. Learning to tell the difference between normal emotions and those based on irrational beliefs can help you either to stop the emotion or to express it in a healthy and appropriate way. Admitting your feelings and allowing them to be expressed through either communication or action is a stress management technique that can help you get through many difficult situations.

Learning to Laugh and Cry.   For some people, learning to express emotions freely is a difficult task. However, it is a task worth learning. Have you ever noticed that you feel better after a good laugh or cry? It wasn't your imagination. Laughter and crying stimulate the heart and temporarily rev up many body systems. Heart rate and blood pressure then decrease significantly, allowing the body to relax.

Taking Mental Action

Stress management calls for mental action in two areas. First, positive self-esteem, which can help you cope with

Expressing Anger Effectively

Expressing anger constructively is an important skill involved in learning to cope with intimate relationships, family interactions, and other stressful situations. Here are some suggestions for constructive expression of anger.

1. *Determine the real reason behind your anger.* Is it due to a real event (for example, someone you trusted is spreading malicious gossip) or to a perception you have about a situation (friends are avoiding you, so you think someone may be gossiping)?

2. *Don't let your anger build.* When you become angry, take control, and decide what actions you need to take. Try not to act rashly, but don't stew for a long time. If you choose to write a letter expressing your anger, sit down and write it, but don't mail the letter immediately. Put it away, wait a few days, and then reread it. You may choose not to send the letter, but sitting down to write may help you cool off.

3. *If you decide to confront a person, select an appropriate time and place for the meeting.* Try not to attack your target unexpectedly or in the presence of others: the person may become defensive. Give the person a general idea of what you want to discuss ahead of time.

4. *Stick to the major or most recent reason for your anger.* Bringing up a whole list of things that have made you angry over the last year will just complicate the issue and make the other person want to create his or her own list of wrongs that you have committed. Plan in advance which issue you want to discuss.

5. *Attack the problem rather than the person.* Don't get into a battle over personal characteristics. Use "I" statements to communicate resentment or disappointment ("I feel angry that we had to leave the party so early"). "You" statements often put people on the defensive.

6. *Listen carefully to what the other person has to say.* If the other person starts wandering from the issue, gently try to bring him or her back to the point. If the other person attacks you personally, stay in control and don't allow yourself to fight back.

7. *Treat the other person with respect.* Even though you may say the right things, your gestures and body language can reveal that you don't value what the other person has to say, that you are hostile, or that you are losing patience. Drumming your fingers, sighing, or rolling your eyes while the other person is talking can often increase friction.

8. *Recognize when to quit.* Sometimes even the best-laid plans go awry. No matter what you do, the problem may appear impossible to resolve. In such situations, knowing when to quit, either temporarily or permanently, is a key factor in controlling stressful anger levels.

9. *When it's over, let it be over.* After you have done all that you can do, learn to let go of your anger. Don't dwell in the past. Acknowledge your right to be angry, recognize it for what it was, and move on.

---

stressful situations, comes from learned habits. Successful stress management involves mentally developing and practising self-esteem skills.

Second, because you can't always anticipate what the next distressor will be, you need to develop the mental skills necessary to manage your reactions to stresses after they have occurred. The ability to think about and react quickly to stress comes with time, practice, experience with a variety of stressful situations, and patience. Most of all, you must strive to become more aware of potential threats to your stress levels and act quickly to avoid or to deal with potential stressors. Rather than seeing stressors as adversaries, learn to view them as exercises in life.

Changing the Way You Think. Once you realize that some of your thoughts may be irrational or overreactive, making a conscious effort to reframe or change the way you've been thinking and focus on more positive ways of thinking is a key element of stress management. Here are some specific actions you can take to develop these mental skills.

- *Worry constructively.* Don't waste time and energy worrying about things you can't change or things that may never happen.

- *Look at life as being fluid.* If you accept that change is a natural part of living and growing, the jolt of changes may hold much less stress for you.

- *Consider alternatives.* Remember that there is seldom only one appropriate action. Anticipating options will help you plan for change and adjust more rapidly.

- *Moderate expectations.* Aim high, but be realistic about your circumstances and motivation.

- *Weed out trivia.* Don't sweat the small stuff, and remember that most of it is small stuff.

- *Don't rush into action.* Think before you act.

Taking Physical Action

Adopting the attitudes necessary for effective stress management may seem to have little effect. However, developing

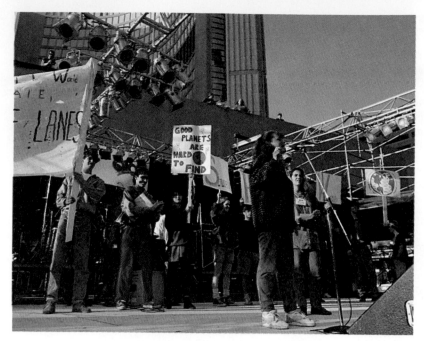

Evaluating stressors and finding a constructive way to react to them can help you cope with stressful situations and events that appear to be beyond your control.

successful emotional and mental coping skills is actually a satisfying accomplishment that can help you gain confidence in yourself. Learning to use physical activity to alleviate stress helps support and complement the emotional and mental strategies you employ in stress management.

Exercise. Exercise is a significant contributor to stress management. Exercise reduces stress by raising levels of endorphins (mood-elevating, pain-killing hormones) in the bloodstream. As a result, exercise often increases energy, reduces hostility, and improves mental alertness.

Relaxation. Like exercise, relaxation can help you to cope with stressful feelings, to preserve adaptation energy stores, and to dissipate the excess hormones associated with the GAS. Relaxation also helps you to refocus your energies and should be practised daily until it becomes a habit. You may find that you even actually enjoy it. When you begin to feel your body respond to distress, make time to relax, both to give yourself added strength and to help alleviate the negative physical effects of stress. As your body relaxes, your heart rate slows, your blood pressure and metabolic rate decrease, and many other body-calming effects occur, allowing you to channel energy appropriately.

Eating Right. Whether foods can calm us and nourish our psyches is a controversial question. Much of what has been published about hyperactivity and its relation to the consumption of candy and other sweets has been shown to be scientifically invalid. High-potency stress-tabs that are supposed to provide you with resistance against stress-related ailments are nothing more than gimmicks. But what is clear is that eating a balanced, healthful diet will help provide you with the stamina needed to get through problems and may stress-proof you in ways that are not fully understood. It is also known that undereating, overeating, and eating the wrong kinds of foods can create distress in the body. For more information about the benefits of sound nutrition in overall health and wellness, see Chapter 7.

Time Management

Time. Everybody needs more of it, especially students trying to balance the demands of classes, social life, earning money for school, family obligations, and time needed for relaxation. The following tips regarding time management should become a part of your stress management program:

- *Clean off your desk.* According to Jeffrey Mayer, author of *Winning the Fight Between You and Your Desk*, most of us spend many stressful minutes each day looking for things that are lost on our desks or in our homes. Go through the things on your desk, toss the unnecessary papers, and put papers for tasks that you must do in folders.

- *Never handle papers more than once.* When bills and other papers come in, take care of them immediately. Write out a cheque and hold it for mailing. Get rid of the envelopes. Read your mail and file it or toss it. If you haven't looked at something in over a year, toss it.

- *Prioritize your tasks.* Make a daily "to do" list and try to stick to it. Categorize the things you must do today, the things that you have to do but not immediately, and the things that it would be nice to do. Prioritize the Must Do Now and Have to Do Later items and put deadlines next to each. Only consider the Nice to Do items if you finish the others or if the Nice to Do list includes something fun for you. Give yourself a reward as you finish each task.

- *Avoid interruptions.* When you've got a project that requires your total concentration, schedule uninterrupted time. Unplug the phone or let your answering machine get it. Close your door and post a Do Not Disturb sign. Go to a quiet room in the library or student union where no one will find you. Guard your time and don't weaken.

- *Reward yourself for being efficient.* If you've planned to take a certain amount of time to finish a task and you finish early, take some time for yourself. Have a cup of coffee or hot chocolate. Go for a walk. Start reading something you've wanted to read but haven't had time for. Differentiate between rest breaks and work breaks. Work breaks simply mean that you switch tasks for awhile. Rest breaks get you away for yourself.

- *Reduce your awareness of time.* Rather than being a slave to the clock, try to ignore it. Get rid of your watch, and try to listen more to your body when deciding whether you need to eat, sleep, and so on. When you feel awake, do something productive. When you are too tired to work, take time out to sleep or to relax to try to energize yourself.

- *Remember that time is precious.* Many people learn to value their time only when they face a terminal illness. Try to value each day. Time spent not enjoying life is a tremendous waste of potential.

- *Become aware of your own time patterns.* For many of us, minutes and hours drift by without us even noticing them. Chart your daily schedule, hour by hour, for one week. Note the time that was wasted and the time spent in productive work or restorative pleasure. Assess how you could be more productive and make more time for yourself.

Making the Most of Support Groups

Support groups are an important part of stress management. Friends, family members, and co-workers can provide us with emotional and physical support. Although the ideal support group differs for each of us, you should have one or two close friends in whom you are able to confide and neighbours with whom you can trade favours. You should take the opportunity to participate in community activities at least once a week. A healthy, committed relationship can also provide vital support.

If you do not have a close support group, you should know where to turn when the pressures of life seem overwhelming. Family members are often a steady base of support on which you can rely. But if friends or family are unavailable, most colleges and universities have counselling services available at no cost for short-term crises. Clergy members, instructors, and dorm supervisors may also be excellent resources. If university services are unavailable or if you are concerned about confidentiality, most communities offer low-cost counselling through mental health clinics.

Alternative Stress Management Techniques

The popularity of stress management as a media topic has increased the amount of advertising for various "stress fighters." We have been made aware of consumer products and services designed to fight stress: hypnosis, massage therapies, meditation, and biofeedback. Some of these services may be provided through extended health coverage at universities.

Hypnosis. **Hypnosis** is a process that requires a person to focus on one thought, object, or voice, thereby freeing the right hemisphere of the person's brain to become more active. The person is then unusually responsive to suggestions. Whether self-induced or induced by another person, hypnosis can reduce certain types of stress.

Massage. If you have ever had someone massage your stiff neck or aching feet, you know that massage is an excellent means of relaxation and thereby stress management. Massage therapists use techniques that vary from the more aggressive methods typical of Swedish massage to the more gentle methods associated with acupressure and Esalen massage. Before selecting a massage therapist, check his or her credentials carefully. He or she should have training from a reputable program that teaches scientific principles for anatomic manipulation.

Meditation. Another way to relax and to manage stress is through meditation. **Meditation** generally focusses on deep breathing, allowing tension to leave the body with each exhalation. There is no "right" way to meditate. Although there are several common forms of meditation, most involve sitting quietly for 15 to 20 minutes, focussing on a particular word or symbol, controlling breathing, and getting in touch with your inner self.

Biofeedback. **Biofeedback** involves self-monitoring by machine of physical responses to stress and attempts to subsequently control these responses. Perspiration, heart rate, respiration, blood pressure, surface body temperature, muscle tension, and other stress responses are monitored. Then, by trial and error, the person using biofeedback techniques learns to lower his or her stress responses through conscious effort. Eventually, the person develops the ability to lower his or her stress responses at will without using the machines.

> **Hypnosis:** A process that allows people to become unusually responsive to suggestion.
> **Meditation:** A relaxation technique that involves deep breathing and concentration.
> **Biofeedback:** A technique involving self-monitoring by machine of physical responses to stress.

Managing Stress Behaviours

Stress is not something that you can run from or wish into nonexistence. To control stress, you must meet it head-on and use as many resources as you can to ensure that your coping skills are fine-tuned and ready to help you. In planning your personal strategy for stress success, you should consider the following:

Making Decisions for You

Following a few simple guidelines may help you not only to enjoy more guilt-free time but also to become more productive during work hours.

- **Plan life, not time.** Determining what you want from life rather than what you can get done may help change the way you use time. Evaluate all your activities, even the most trivial, to determine whether they add to your life. If they don't, get rid of them.

- **Decelerate.** Rushing is part of the Canadian work ethic and mindset that says "Busy is better." It can be addictive. When rushed, ask yourself if you really need to be. What's the worst that could happen if you slow down? Tell yourself at least once a day that failure seldom results from doing a job slowly or too well. Failures happen when rushing causes a lack of attention to detail.

- **Learn to delegate and share.** The need to feel in control is powerful. If you are unusually busy, leave details to someone else. Don't be afraid to ask others to help or to share the work load and responsibilities.

- **Learn to say no.** Give priority to what is most critical to your life, your job, or your current situation. Decide what things you can do, what things you must do, and what things you want to do, and delegate the rest to someone else either permanently or until you complete some of your priority tasks. Before you take on a new responsibility, finish or drop an old one.

- **Schedule time alone.** Find time each day for quiet thinking, reading, exercising, or other enjoyable activities.

Checklist for Change: Assessing Your Life Stressors

✓ Have you assessed the major stressors in your life? Are they people, events, or specific activities?

✓ Have you thought about what you may be doing to worsen your stress levels? Do you often worry about things that never happen? Are you often anxious about nothing?

✓ Have you thought about what you could change to reduce your stress levels?

✓ Do you have a network of friends and family members who can help you reduce your stress levels? Do you know where you could go to get professional advice about how to start reducing them?

✓ Have you thought about what changes you'd like to work on first? Have you developed a plan of action? When do you want to start?

Checklist for Change: Assessing Community Stressors

✓ Have you considered what in your environment may cause stress for you and the people around you?

✓ Could these stressors be changed? How could they be changed? Why would changing them make a difference?

✓ What on your campus or in your living situations causes undue stress for you or your friends? What could you do to change these stressors?

✓ What advice might you give to your school administrators to help them reduce unnecessary stress among students?

Critical Thinking

You just scraped by to pay your tuition bill in January; then your university announces a large tuition hike for next year. You already work a part-time job, and seem to spend all your "free time" studying. The stress you've got now is beginning to get to you, and you realize that you will have to work another five to ten hours per week just to pay your bills next year. And tuition is likely to go up your final year as well. How can you manage your time and finances so that you can complete your degree?

Use the DECIDE model described in Chapter 1 to decide what you should do. Begin with your own current situation: How can you make better use of your time? Could you prioritize your week in a way that you could find the extra time to work? Finally, even if you make enough money, you need to deal with the increased stress. What will you do to keep the stress in check?

Work and Stress Worldwide

Representatives of more than forty collaborating centres of the World Health Organization (WHO) active in occupational health adopted a global strategy on Health at Work, as well as a declaration encouraging WHO and its member states to further develop their occupational health programs on the basis of this new strategy.

Specialists from about thirty countries met in Beijing, China, in 1994 to attend the Second Meeting of the WHO Collaborating Centres in Occupational Health. They reviewed the various aspects of health at work in the light of data showing that depending on the country and the region, 20 to 90 percent of the workers have no access to occupational health services. The need for occupational health services is particularly acute in the developing and newly industrialized countries, where approximately 80 percent of the global working population live.

Globally, about 100 000 chemicals, some 50 physical factors, 200 biological factors and some 20 adverse ergonomic conditions, and an identical number of physical work loads associated with incalculable numbers and types of psychological and social problems have been identified as hazardous conditions of work, which contribute to the risk of occupational injuries, diseases and stress reactions, job dissatisfaction, and absence of well-being. Most of such problems are in principle preventable and should be prevented in the interests of the workers'

health, but also from the economy and productivity point of view.

Approximately 30 to 50 percent of the workers in industrialized countries complain about psychic stress and overload, which has been associated with the occurrence of sleep disturbances and depression, as well as with elevated risks of cardiovascular diseases, particularly hypertension.

In view of all these problems, the World Health Organization's collaborating centres urged a global strategy to promote the improvement of conditions at work based on the following key principles: primary prevention; safe technology; optimization of working conditions; continuous follow-up and development of occupational health and safety; government responsibility, authority, and leadership in the development and control of working conditions; primary responsibility of the employer and economic sectors on health and safety at the workplace; recognition of employees' own interests in occupational health and safety; cooperation and collaboration on an equal basis by employers and workers; right to know and principle of transparency; right to participate in decisions concerning one's own work.

Source: Adapted from World Health Organization, "WHO Collaborating Centres Launch a Global Strategy Towards Health at Work," Press Release WHO/80, October 20, 1994.

Summary

◆ Stress is an inevitable part of our lives. Eustress refers to stress associated with positive events, distress to negative events. Psychoneuroimmunology is the science that attempts to analyze the relationship between the mind's reaction to stress and the function of the immune system. While some evidence links disease susceptibility to stress, it is not conclusive.

◆ The alarm, resistance, and exhaustion phases of the general adaptation syndrome involve physiological responses to both real and imagined stressors.

◆ Multiple factors contribute to stress and to the stress response. Psychosocial factors include change, hassles, pressure, inconsistent goals and behaviours, conflict,

overload, and burnout. Other factors are environmental stressors, and self-imposed stress.

◆ University can be an especially stressful time. Recognition of the signs of stress is the first step in helping yourself toward better health.

◆ Managing stress begins with learning simple coping mechanisms: assessing your stressors, changing your responses, and learning to cope. Finding out what works best for you—probably some combination of managing emotional responses, taking mental or physical action, learning time management, or using alternative stress management techniques—will help you better cope with stress in the long run.

Discussion Questions

1. Compare and contrast distress and eustress. Are both types of stress potentially harmful?

2. Describe the alarm, resistance, and exhaustion phases of the general adaptation syndrome. During which of these phases do your perceptions and feelings about a situation often turn out to be wrong? Discuss the physiological responses that take place if you find you were wrong.

3. What are the major factors that seem to influence the nature and extent of a person's stress susceptibility?

Explain how social support, self-esteem, and personality may make you more or less susceptible to stress.

4. Why are university students often susceptible to excessive stress? What services are available on your campus to help you deal with excessive stress?

5. What can university students do to inoculate themselves against negative stress effects? What actions can you take to manage your stressors? How can you help others to manage their stressors more effectively?

Application Exercise

Reread the What Do You Think? scenario at the beginning of the chapter and answer the following questions:

1. What could Erica have done to help inoculate herself against or prevent negative reactions to the stressful events in her life? What services on your campus could have helped her through the troubles?

2. Why do some people have little social support? Why is social support so important to reducing stress reactions?

3. What direct and indirect health effects of stress may Erica experience? What symptoms of stress should particularly concern her?

4. Do you think that Erica and other university students like her are just suddenly stressed by situations like this? Or do you think that something led them to such reactions for many years? Explain your answer.

Health on the Net

Canadian Institute for Health Information
www.cihi.ca/

Internet Mental Health
www.mentalhealth.com/

Statscan
www.statcan.ca/english/Pgdb/people.htm

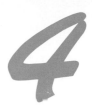

Violence and Abuse

Societal Challenges

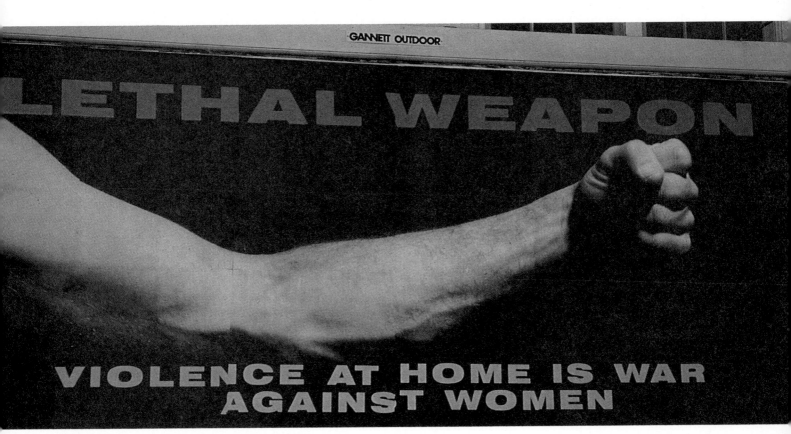

CHAPTER OBJECTIVES

◆ Discuss violence in Canada, including homicide, bias and hate crimes, gang violence, and campus violence.

◆ Discuss domestic violence (abuse against men, women, children, and the elderly committed by their family members) and its causes.

◆ Describe sexual victimization, including sexual assault, rape, date rape, and sexual harassment, and why it happens.

◆ Identify the steps you can take to prevent personal assaults at home, on the street, or in your car.

Freddy is wakened by the sound of loud voices. His parents are fighting again. His father is calling his mother awful names. She is shouting back. Freddy creeps to the top of the stairs. They are just below him. He hears a sickening "whack" as his father hits his mother. Then his father kicks her. There is a knock at the door. The police have been called by the neighbours. They take his father away and talk to his mother. Freddy goes back to his room, but he cannot sleep.

■ What factors in Canadian society have contributed to our growing awareness of violence in the family? What attitudes and beliefs do you encounter as you reflect on family violence? Do you feel violence in the home is increasing, or are we facing up to a problem that has existed for a long time?

Chances are that if you go home from class today and flip on the TV, you will see graphic footage of violent acts and their outcomes. We live in a world caught in an epidemic of violence. The term **violence** is used to indicate a set of behaviours that produce injuries, as well as the outcomes of these behaviours (the injuries themselves). In this chapter, we will focus on those violent acts that have particular relevance to you.

VIOLENCE IN CANADA

Violence is not new in Canada. It is also not as common as in some other countries. Of 15 countries surveyed in 1988, Canada tied with Germany for fifth spot in victimization rates involving the use of force. Australia led, followed by the United States, Finland, and Holland.[1] We have had riots after sporting events and the occasional political confrontation, the melee at the Ontario provincial legislature and the 1995 standoff at Gustafson Lake in British Columbia being recent examples. But we have also had police strikes with no change in the crime rate, and most cities are relatively safe to walk and live in. Canadians are less likely to take precautions against crime when going out than people in other industrialized countries.[2] Yet violence exists here, both in overt forms such as assault or homicide and in more subtle but nonetheless intimidating forms such as stalking. Violence

Violence: Refers to a set of behaviours that produce injuries, as well as the outcomes of these behaviours (the injuries themselves).

can flare up between groups—as it did at Oka between First Nations peoples and the town of Oka over disputed land—or in families, as in child abuse, wife abuse, husband abuse, and elder abuse. In fact, the most violent group in society is the family.

The General Social Survey in 1987 estimated that only 31 percent of violent crimes were reported to police. Why do victims not report violence? Stated reasons were that they felt the incident was minor, believed the police could do nothing about it, were fearful, or had dealt with it informally.[3]

The Department of Justice Canada noted in a 1995 report that there is a long history of violence towards racial or ethnic minorities that can flare up at times. In Vancouver in 1907 a mob of whites attacked the Chinese and Japanese communities, causing damage to stores and several fatalities.[4] The internment of Japanese Canadians during World War II and the confiscation of their property is another example.[5] Compensation and an apology was recently offered to the Japanese-Canadian community by the federal government. A task force has been established to study a wave of attacks against South Asian people in Toronto.[6]

Vulnerable groups such as women and children witnessing or experiencing violence in families are of special concern. The issue of violence by men toward women and children is now accepted as a major social problem in Canadian society. The opening of sexual assault centres and battered women's shelters in the 1970s made this a more visible issue for the public.

Violence relates to health through injuries and deaths that result directly from violence, as well as the subtler forms of damage caused by actual or threatened violence, such as stress, poor mental health, conduct disorders, and lack of social and emotional responsiveness. As well as these social costs, there are indications that the economic costs are very high.[7]

Violence in the form of drive-by shootings, fatal stabbings, domestic beatings, brutalizations of the elderly, and mass bombings are not only a major cause of death and disability in Canada, but also a source of fear and anxiety for all who watch the nightly news or read the morning headlines.

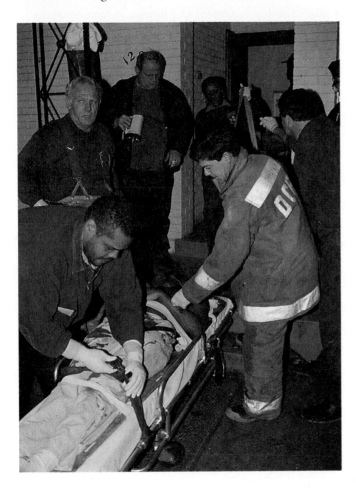

Although the underlying causes of violence and abuse are as varied as the individual crimes and people involved, several social, cultural, and individual factors seem to increase the likelihood of violent acts. Poverty, unemployment, hopelessness, lack of education, inadequate housing, poor parental role models, cultural beliefs that objectify women and empower men to act as aggressors, lack of social support systems, discrimination, ignorance about people who are different, religious self-righteousness, breakdowns in the criminal justice system, stress, economic uncertainty, and a host of other factors may precipitate violent acts.

By learning more about the etiology of homicide, suicide, and other violent acts, you will reduce your own risk of becoming a victim and help ensure your own level of health. By taking steps to help prevent violence against others, you will help safeguard the health of society.

WHAT DO YOU THINK?

Why do you think there is so much violent behaviour in Canada today? What actions can you personally take to prevent violent events from occurring? What actions could be taken on your college campus? In your community?

Homicide

There were 586 homicides in Canada in 1995, a rate of 1.98 per 100 000 population. There has been a steady decrease since the peak in 1975. This rate compares favourably with that of the United States, which is four times higher, but less favourably with that of Europe. For example, the homicide rate in England and Wales is 30 percent lower. The Canadian homicide rate for youth has remained stable. Despite popular fears of the violent stranger, in fact a homicide is likely to be committed by someone known to the victim (47 percent by an acquaintance, 36 percent by a spouse). Males represented 67 percent of the victims of homicide and 87 percent of the accused perpetrators.[8]

Handguns were present in 29 percent of U.S. households and Switzerland was second with 14 percent (about half of these were identified as army guns), in contrast to 6 percent of Canadian households. The United States also had the highest percentage of households with any sort of gun.

Homicide: Death that results from intent to injure or kill.

Suicide

When anger, rage, and hopelessness turn inward rather than outward, violence against the self can result; suicide is the most extreme form of this violence. Suicide attempts may spring from different causes. A suicide attempt can be "a cry for help," a signal of extreme distress and emotional pain. The physical pain of self-injury distracts the person from never-ending emotional pain. A suicide attempt may be an explosive outburst of rage at self; such attempts are usually fatal. Or the suicide may be motivated by a balance of sadness, resignation, and a desire for dignity, in the case of a terminally ill person. Why some people choose suicide while others don't is unclear. Studies indicate that a combination of neurobiological,[9] psychological,[10] and social[11] factors combine to enable suicide (see Chapter 2).

What is the extent of this behaviour? In 1987 Canada ranked eleventh in suicides, at 18 per 100 000 population. Greece, at four per 100 000, was lowest, while Finland (37.6 per 100 000) was highest.[12] In 1992 in Canada, 2923

Overcoming Learned Violence: The Olweus Norwegian Anti-bullying Program

In Norway a nationwide, school-based program seeks to prevent violence by strengthening sanctions against bullying and supporting social norms for inclusive, prosocial behaviour.

This program is based on an analysis of research on bully and victim characteristics. Bullies were found to be generally confident and, among boys, to be physically stronger than others their age; they were not found to have underlying self-esteem or anxiety problems. Bullies tended to come from families where violence was condoned or modelled and where there were low levels of parental supervision. Victims were found to be anxious, socially isolated, and lacking in confidence in their abilities and tended not to respond assertively to aggression.

Major program activities include

- developing awareness of bullying

- involving adults in activities

- surveying bully/victim problems

- holding school conference days and class meetings about bullying

- providing better supervision during recess and lunch hour

- setting specific rules against bullying

- implementing consistent and immediate consequences for aggressive behaviours

- praising prosocial and helpful behaviours

- conducting serious talks with bullies, victims, and parents

- initiating parent-teacher meetings on the topic

Teachers found the program realistic and beneficial. An extensive, large-scale evaluation showed a 50 percent reduction of self-reported victimization over a three-year period, a reduction in antisocial behaviours such as vandalism, and an improvement in the social climate in schools.

Yet the most important effect may appear in future years, when the students in the program form households of their own. It is within the family and intimate relationships that most violence occurs. Studies of violent offenders clearly illustrate a link with a childhood history of violence. Any intervention that can stop a child from becoming a bully—or the victim of a bully—may go a long way toward preventing future domestic violence.

Source: Marlies Sudermann and Peter G. Jaffe, *Preventing Violence: School- and Community-Based Strategies* (National Forum on Health, 1996), 1.

---

men and 786 women (3709 total) committed suicide. This means one death by suicide every two hours.[13]

Suicide is the leading cause of death for men between 30 and 34 years. The rate drops gradually among men over 34 and then more sharply beyond age 45.

Between 1960 and 1991, the rate of suicide for young men increased fourfold: from 5.3 to 23.0 per 100 000. This was six times the rate for young women.

The suicide rate among Indian youth was five times that of the total Canadian population.

The Canadian Institute of Child Health[14] interprets these statistics as a warning that children and youth need more support, recognition, respect, and hope for the future, and that society as a whole must rethink the way we work with and serve youth.

Youth Violence

In 1991 22 percent of federal statute charges were against youths. A higher proportion of youths than of adults were criminally charged. Thirteen percent of the charges against young people related to violence, while 58 percent were property-related. Minor assaults accounted for about half of the violent charges against youth. Total charges against youths were double the number of charges in 1986. But does this statistic truly represent an increase in youth crime? Some of the increase reflects, rather, society's increased sensitivity toward youth violence. Because of school policies of "zero tolerance" for violence, incidents that would previously have been dealt with at a school level now result in police charges and are counted in the statistics.

The youth involved are generally in their late teens (16-to-17-year-olds account for 53 percent of offenders), and the victims are generally youths between 12 and 17 years (50 percent of minor assaults), usually male (76 percent of aggravated assaults). Assaults most commonly occur in dwellings (27 percent) or on the streets (24 percent).[15]

Canada jails a high proportion of young offenders—higher even than the United States—because our justice system makes comparatively little use of alternative approaches. Unlike in the adult system, there is no parole for youth.

Aboriginal youth, youth from certain racial and cultural groups, and young people from lower-income families are over-represented in our justice system. Marginalization fosters resentment and anger, which may be vented on society's symbols such as property.

Yet it should be remembered that most young people in Canada are never in trouble with the law.

The Violence of Hate

Canada historically has welcomed people from other cultures—while marginalizing First Nations people. The degree of acceptance, however, decreases with the immigrants' physical and cultural differences from Northern European peoples. Much as we may wish otherwise, prejudice and racism have always been a part of Canadian society.

Historically, established leaders in Canadian society (both individual and institutional) have made key contributions to interracial violence, for example, to the anti-Chinese riot of 1887 and the anti-Chinese/Japanese riot of 1907 in Vancouver. In both cases, the local newspapers, respectable individuals (businessmen, clergymen, politicians) and organizations played a very prominent role in at least preparing the groundwork and instigating the violence, which claimed "scores" of Chinese lives. The timing of the riots seems to have been related to white workers' alleged fears of economic competition, especially at a time of recession.[16]

Preventing Hate and Bias Crimes.   Although the causes of intolerance remain in question, it is believed that much of it stems from a fear of change and a desire to blame others when forces such as the economy and crime seem to be out of control. What can you do to be part of the solution to the problem rather than part of the problem?

- Support educational programs designed to foster understanding and appreciation for differences in people. Many colleges now require diversity classes as part of their academic curriculum.

- Examine your own attitudes and behaviours. Are you intolerant of others? Do you engage in behaviours that demean any group of individuals? Have you thought about the reasons why you have problems with a particular group?

- Discourage racist jokes and other forms of social or ethnic bigotry? Do not participate in such behaviours and express your dissatisfaction with others who do.

- Vote for community leaders who respect the rights of others, who value diversity, and who do not have racially or ethnically motivated hidden agendas. Vote against intolerant candidates who are attempting to control our school boards and local government through planned infiltration.

- Educate yourself. Read, interact with, and attempt to understand people who may appear to be different from you. Remember that you do not have to like everything about another person or group. Other people may not like everything about you, either. However, respecting people's right to be different is a part of being a healthy, integrated individual.

- Examine your own values in determining the relative worth of your friends and the others in your life. Are you judgemental? Are you somewhat intolerant of others' differences? How do you resolve your own tendencies to be judgemental and bigoted? Do you judge people on appearances? Do you take time to get to know who they are as individuals?

*W*HAT DO YOU THINK?

Think about the bias or hate crimes that you have heard about in the last six months. Who were the victims? Did you know any of the victims? Why do you think people are motivated to initiate such crimes against people they do not know? What can you do to reduce the risk of such crimes in your area? What should be done nationally?

*V*IOLENCE AGAINST WOMEN

The first major empirical study on violence toward women was done by L. MacLeod.[17] She suggested that one in ten women living with a man would be abused each year. This figure, initially ridiculed, is now accepted as an underestimate: more recent figures indicate that more than one woman in four (29 percent) experience some form of domestic violence from their partner.[18] Assaults are eight times as likely in a relationship of less than two years' duration than in partnerships lasting more than twenty years.[19]

The shelter movement lobbied for zero tolerance of abuse and mandatory charging of abusers. This policy has been adopted in virtually all jurisdictions since 1982, when Canada's Attorney General urged police chiefs to lay charges in all cases of suspected wife abuse. The Royal Canadian Mounted Police introduced formal policy in 1984 specifically instructing its members to lay charges in all cases where there are "reasonable and probable grounds" to believe that assault occurred. The assaultive partner may be charged under the assault sections of the Criminal Code of Canada. Not only does a police charge highlight the criminal nature of the act, it relieves the victim of the burden of laying charges.[20]

Canadians were shocked out of denying the existence of violence toward women by the "Montreal Massacre" at Concordia University in Montreal in 1989. Marc Lepine

Justice in China

The emphasis . . . throughout the [Chinese] justice system is a "change in attitude." This orientation manifests itself at every stage of the legal process. In the courts, the first change of attitude is expected to take place prior to a trial; it is a confession of guilt. While the confession does confirm the findings of the investigative panel, it is required for "deeper reasons." As in the past, the confession serves to reestablish the "harmony of the social order . . . after the discord created by the crime. From the accused's point of view the process of confession signals his or her capacity to see the facts from society's standpoint and to engage in self-criticism, and thus in time to be changed in order to fit once more into society". . . . Those who do confess tend to receive lighter sentences, while those who resist this resocialization are labeled as having "bad attitudes" and commonly are given much harsher punishments for the same offense.

The lawyer plays an interesting role in the courtroom process. The profession of lawyer was reestablished only in 1979 and its character is still evolving in today's changing Chinese society. In general, though, in criminal proceedings, rather than taking the adversarial position with which we are familiar, the Chinese lawyer, a governmental official, is an active agent in the resocialization process, assisting the accused in making the right choices. This is not to say that the attorney does not try to defend the client, but rather that the lawyer conducts the defense with the interest of society in mind.

Like the Chinese legal system, the correctional system also stresses change. At the juvenile level, the "gong du" or work study schools attempt to reintegrate youthful offenders into the mainstream of Chinese society. The most distinctive feature of the juvenile system is that the gong du operations are administered by the educational branch of local government and only the most severe juvenile offenders are placed in more traditional correctional facilities. At the gong du school, students are constantly reminded of their responsibility to society both in the classroom and on the job that they are required to have. The adult prisons also place considerable emphasis on changing attitudes. Slogans are displayed throughout the prisons urging the offender to "Get to the bottom of your crimes," "Remold yourself quickly," "Make a start towards a new life," or "Criticize your crimes."

Thus, while crime is considered a violation of the social order as it is in numerous other countries, in China it is also viewed as a break that can be mended.

Source: Excerpted from Daniel J. Curran and Claire M. Renzetti, *Social Problems,* 3rd ed., 546. © 1993 by Allyn & Bacon. Reprinted by permission.

---

shot and killed 14 women at the École Polytechnique, simply because they were women.

Domestic violence and discrimination toward women is a global issue we are slowly trying to face. On the urging of Canada, among other nations, the United Nations Convention on the Elimination of All Forms of Discrimination Against Women adopted a resolution in 1992 accepting that states are responsible for acts of domestic violence between individuals. In December 1993, the UN passed a Declaration Against Violence Against Women.

The extent of wife assault has only recently begun to be well documented. Statistics Canada conducted its first Violence Against Women Survey in 1993. It found that 29 percent of Canadian women have experienced violence at the hands of a current or past marital partner. Between 1974 and 1992, 1435 women were killed by their husbands and 451 men were killed by their wives.[21] While men are sometimes assaulted by women (6 percent of assaults), such assaults are much rarer than assaults by men against women (47 percent of assaults).[22] Over the 18-year period, there were 2.8 million partnerships involving violence against women. In only 24 percent of these cases did either partner use a social service (transition home, crisis centre, community/family service centre, other counsellor); three-quarters of the women had no such help from society.[23] Indeed, answers to an anonymous survey showed that 22 percent of assaulted women had never told *anyone*—not family, friends, police, or community support agencies. Fear and embarrassment were the most common reasons given for this silence.[24]

How many times have you heard of a woman who is repeatedly beaten by her partner or spouse and asked, "Why doesn't she just leave him?" There are many reasons why some women find it difficult, if not impossible, to break their ties with their abusers. Many women, particularly those having small children, are financially dependent on their partners. Others fear retaliation against themselves or their children. There are women who hope that the situation will change with time (it rarely does), and others who stay because their cultural or religious beliefs forbid

Many battered and abused women become trapped in a cycle of violence that also puts their children at risk for physical and psychological abuse.

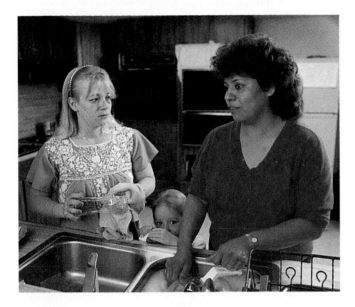

divorce. Finally, there are women who still love the abusive partner and are concerned about what will happen to him if they leave.[25]

Cycle of Violence Theory. Psychologist Lenore Walker has developed a theory known as the "cycle of violence" to explain how women can get caught in a downward spiral without knowing what is happening to them.[26] The cycle has several phases:

- *Phase One: Tension Building.* In this phase, minor battering occurs, and the woman may become more nurturant, more pleasing, and more intent on anticipating the spouse's needs in order to forestall another violent scene. She assumes guilt for doing something to provoke him and tries hard to avoid doing it again.

- *Phase Two: Acute Battering.* At this stage, pleasing her man doesn't help and she can no longer control or predict the abuse. Usually, the spouse is trying to "teach her a lesson," and when he feels he has inflicted enough pain, he'll stop. When the acute attack is over, he may respond with shock and denial about his own behaviour. Both batterer and victim may soft-pedal the seriousness of the attacks.

- *Phase Three: Remorse/Reconciliation.* During this "honeymoon" period, the batterer may be kind, loving, and apologetic, swearing he will never act violently toward the woman again. He may "behave" for several weeks or months, and the woman may come to question whether she overrated the seriousness of past abuse.

Then the kind of tension that precipitated abusive incidents in the past resurfaces, he loses control again, and he once more beats the woman. Unless some form of intervention breaks this downward cycle of abuse, contrition, further abuse, denial, and contrition, it will repeat again and again—perhaps ending only in the woman's or, rarely, the man's death.

It is very hard for most women who get caught in this cycle of violence (which may include forced sexual relations and psychological and economic abuse as well as beatings) to summon up the courage and resolution to extricate themselves. Most need effective outside intervention.

*W*HAT DO YOU THINK?

Can you think of a woman whom you consider a likely victim of domestic violence? What about her has contributed to her current situation? Can you think of a man whom you consider a likely victimizer? What about him has contributed to his current situation?

Causes of Domestic Violence

There is no single explanation for why people tend to be abusive in relationships. Although alcohol abuse is often associated with **domestic violence**, marital dissatisfaction seems to predict physical abuse better than does any other variable.[27] Numerous studies also point to differences in the communication patterns between abusive relationships and nonabusive relationships.[28] While some argue that the hormone testosterone is the cause of male aggression, recent studies have failed to show a strong association between physical abuse in relationships and this hormone.[29] Many experts believe that men who engage in severe violence are more likely than other men to suffer from personality disorders.[30]

The dynamics that both people bring to a relationship can result in violence and allow it to continue. Obtaining help from community support and counselling services may help determine the underlying basis of the problem and may help the victim and the batterer come to a better understanding of the actions necessary to stop the cycle of abuse. The Rate Yourself box may help you determine if you are a victim of abuse.

Domestic violence: The use of force to control and maintain power over another person in the home environment; it includes both actual harm and the threat of harm.

Violence Against Children

Child abuse is found in all societies and is almost always a highly guarded secret, wherever it takes place. In countries with reliable mortality reporting, WHO estimates that as many as one in 5000 to one in 10 000 children under the age of five dies each year from physical violence, although much lower rates are also noted. In the same countries, from one in 1000 to one in 180 children are either brought to a health care facility or are reported to child welfare services as a consequence of abuse every year. According to interviews of children or young adults in Finland, the Republic of Korea, and the United States, from 5 to 10 percent of all children experience physical violence during childhood.[31]

Physical violence often originates in the lack of parenting skills. Typically, abusive parents are unable to respond to a young child's needs and have unrealistic expectations for the stage of a child's development. Another factor is the cultural acceptance of corporal punishment and violence within a society.

Other stresses contributing to child abuse and neglect may include an unwanted child, an unsupported single-parent household, the absence of social support, financial pressures, and/or unemployment.

Child abuse can be aggravated by substance abuse on the part of the parent or guardian. In substance-abusing families there is a strong association between physical violence, sexual abuse, and domestic violence directed at members of the family, particularly women and young children.

The perpetrators of violence or sexual abuse of children are often trusted individuals in a position of authority, usually males, and often family members.[32] (See Table 4.1.)

Children who are victims of violence or **sexual abuse** have a high risk of becoming perpetrators of similar forms of abuse toward younger children. In later years, they may be physically violent to children in their care or to their own children. The normal reactions to harm are the expression of anger and pain. The abused child is forbidden to express anger and cannot bear to endure the pain alone. To survive, the child must repress the feelings and even the memory. The repressed emotions will gain expression in destructive acts—against others, as in criminal behaviour and even mass murder, or against the former victim, as in drug and alcohol abuse.[33]

Child abuse: The systematic harming of a child by a caregiver, generally a parent.

Sexual abuse of children: Sexually suggestive conversations; inappropriate kissing; touching; petting; oral, anal, or vaginal intercourse; and/or other kinds of sexual interaction between a child and an adult or an older child.

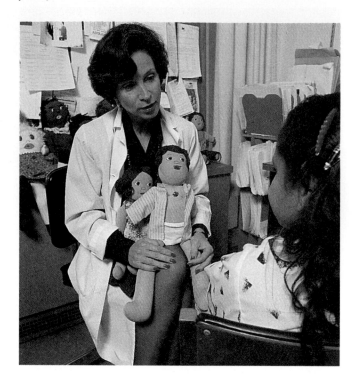

Sympathetic and sensitive therapy can help abused children cope with the mental and physical pain inflicted on them, most commonly by parents or other family members.

Physical violence and sexual abuse in the home is a factor contributing to the phenomenon of street children in both developed and developing countries. Further abuse on the street is an everyday reality.[34]

The use of threat and power by an adult in child abuse breaks the deep trust of the child toward his or her protectors. That they would turn against the child is unthinkable, and so the child divorces awareness of the abuse from everyday thoughts and manages to forget the trauma. But the fear continues to influence the child's behaviour and interactions with others, often in destructive ways. Later in life, when it is safer, the memory may resurface and the person can begin to heal the trauma.

Child welfare statistics are collected at the provincial level, thus complicating the creation of a national picture. The most extensive study on child sexual abuse in Canada was published by the Committee on Sexual Offenses Against Children and Youths in 1984. The study found that 53 percent of females and 31 percent of males had been victims of unwanted sexual acts and that 80 percent of the time these incidents had occurred when they were children or youths.[35]

Not all child violence is physical. Your health can be severely affected by psychological violence—assaults on your personality, character, competence, independence, or general dignity as a human being. The negative conse-

Are You a Victim of Abuse?

Although we often think of abuse as physical, much of the abuse that takes place in intimate relationships is more psychological in nature. If you feel constantly put down or controlled by your partner, ask yourself the following questions.

	Never	Sometimes	Usually	Always
1. Are you blamed by your partner whenever things go wrong?				
2. Does your partner yell at you, curse you, or call you names?				
3. Is your partner a "nasty" drunk or drug user?				
4. Does your partner control your money?				
5. Are you discouraged from enjoying outside friendships?				
6. Is your free time restricted by your partner?				
7. Do you "cover" or make excuses for your partner's behaviour?				
8. Do you do more than your fair share of work around the house?				
9. Are you forced or coerced into having unwanted sex after you've said no?				
10. Do you feel you must ask permission to do things?				
11. Are you sometimes "punished" overtly or more subtly for misbehaving?				
12. Was your mother or your partner's mother abused or was your partner abused in the past?				
13. If you express opinions opposed to those of your partner, does it cause a scene?				
14. Are you afraid of your partner?				
15. Does your partner repeatedly point out things that are wrong with you?				

Scoring

If you answered Usually or Always to

1 or 2 items	Take notice. Work together to improve troubled areas in the relationship.
3 or 4 items	Seriously examine the relationship. Seek joint counselling from a qualified professional.
5 to 7 items	Abuse is definitely a problem. Counselling is necessary (joint counselling may be appropriate).
8 to 15 items	Crisis intervention is needed. Joint therapy is not appropriate.

quences of this kind of victimization in close relationships can be harder to discern and therefore harder to combat. They include depression, lowered self-esteem, and a pervasive fear of doing something that will offend the abuser.

𝒲 HAT DO YOU THINK?

What factors in society lead to child abuse and neglect? What are common characteristics of children's abusers? Why are family members often the perpetrators of child abuse and child sexual abuse? What actions can be taken to prevent such behaviours?

Violence Against Men

While women are most often the targets of violence by men, men are also violent toward other men. Of the nearly 48 000 assaults in 1995, men were the perpetrators *and* the victim in 39 percent of the cases. Men under 34 years are more likely to be perpetrators in major assaults (65 percent). In only 6 percent of reported cases did a woman commit a violent act on a man.[36] Thus, the task of overcoming violence in our society is largely a male issue. The principal reason seems to be that boys are taught—overtly or subtly—that competitiveness, power, and control are valued male attributes. Violence can be seen as an expression of frustration and stress.

TABLE 4.1 ■ Child Abuse: The Victims and the Abusers

Percentage distribution of child victims of family-related physical and sexual assault recorded by the police, by gender of victim and relationship of accused to victim, 1992

Relationship of Accused to Victim	Gender of Victim		
	Total[1] %	Female %	Male[2] %
Physical Assault			
Parent	63	57	73
Parent's spouse	13	20	2
Other immediate family	19	18	20
Extended family	5	5	6
Sexual Assault			
Parent	45	47	34
Parent's spouse	1	2	—
Other immediate family	27	26	31
Extended family	26	25	35

[1] Based on incidents reported by 51 police agencies to the Uniform Crime Reporting database, which represents 30 percent of all reported crime in Canada.

[2] Numbers may not add up to 100 percent because of rounding.

Source: Revised Uniform Crime Reporting Survey, Canadian Centre for Justice Statistics, 1992; *Family Violence in Canada,* Statistics Canada, 1994, 64.

TABLE 4.2 ■ Senior Abuse: The Victims and the Abusers

Percentage distribution of family-related incidents of assault against seniors recorded by the police, by gender of victim and relationship of accused to victim, 1992

Relationship of Accused to Victim	Gender of Victim					
	Total[1] No.	%	Female No.	%	Male No.	%
Spouse	82	31	65	38	17	19
Son or daughter	94	36	54	32	40	45
Parent	29	11	17	11	12	13
Other immediate family	31	12	19	11	12	13
Extended family	24	9	16	9	8	9
Total	**260**	**100[2]**	**171**	**100[2]**	**89**	**100[2]**

[1] Based on incidents reported by 51 police agencies to the Uniform Crime Reporting database, which represents 30 percent of all reported crime in Canada.

[2] Numbers do not add up to 100 percent because of rounding.

Source: Revised Uniform Crime Reporting Survey, Canadian Centre for Justice Statistics, 1992; *Family Violence in Canada,* Statistics Canada, 1994, 89.

Violence Against Seniors

Violence toward seniors, as with other forms of violence in the family, has only recently been getting attention. The first national survey of abuse toward the elderly was done in 1989 by Ryerson University. The survey looked at physical abuse, neglect, chronic verbal aggression, and material abuse (such as forcing seniors to hand over money or valuable goods). They found that 4 percent of Canadians over 65 living in private dwellings (or 98 000 seniors) reported experiencing at least one of these types of abuse in the last 12 months. The victim was more often female (67 percent) and the abuser was most frequently either a spouse or a child of the victim. (See also Table 4.2.)

That 13 percent of seniors refused to lay a charge against the perpetrator indicates how vulnerable this group feels.

SEXUAL VICTIMIZATION

Sexual Assault

Sexual assault can be understood in terms of power imbalance in society. Of the nearly 5000 sexual assaults in 1995, men assaulted women in 83 percent of the incidents. Gunn and Minch describe the power imbalance between men and women "in which violence is implicit" as the base upon which sexual exploitation is built.[37] A survey of more than 6000 university students found that 84 percent of women who had been sexually assaulted knew their attacker and that 57 percent of the rapes had happened on a date.[38] Of male offenders, 32 percent were between 25 and 34 years of age, 23 percent between 35 and 44 years, and 19 percent between 18 and 24 years.

On university campuses, Foot Patrol programs offer safety at night in walking to residence. Women's self-defence courses such as Wendo or karate can provide some protection against attackers as well as improving self-confidence.

Why Some Males Sexually Assault Women

Over the years, psychologists and others have proposed many theories to explain why so many males sexually victimize women. In a recent U.S. study, almost two-thirds of the male respondents had engaged in intercourse unwanted by the woman, primarily because of male peer pressure.[39] Peer pressure is certainly a strong factor in such behaviour, but a growing body of research suggests that sexual assault is encouraged by the normal socialization processes that males experience daily.[40]

The Skills for Behaviour Change box discusses prevention of sexual assault.

WHAT DO YOU THINK?

What factors make men likely to commit sexual assault? What might be effective in preventing such behaviours?

Social Assumptions

According to many experts, certain common assumptions in our society prevent the recognition by both the perpetrator and the wider public of the true nature of sexual assault.[41] The most important of these assumptions are the following.[42]

- *Minimization:* It is often assumed that sexual assault of women is rare because official crime statistics show relatively few offences; however, sexual assault is the most underreported of all serious crimes.

- *Trivialization:* Incredibly enough, sexual assault of women is still often viewed as a jocular matter.

- *Blaming the victim:* Many discussions of sexual violence against women display a sometimes unconscious assumption that the woman did something to provoke the attack—that she dressed too revealingly or flirted too outrageously.

- *"Boys will be boys":* This is the assumption that men just can't control themselves once they become aroused. It has been neatly deflated by one commentator:

  [The] myth that men can't stop once they start is millennia old and typically is stated as "males are slaves to their sexual organs," or "great physical harm can befall the unfortunate male who is denied completion of sexual activity." During my presentations to college-aged audiences, I counter these two statements by pointing out: (a) If a woman's parents walked into the room, it's a sure bet that the male could stop; and (b) there is not a single case reported of a male dying of coitus interruptus.

WHAT DO YOU THINK?

Why do you think women are often reluctant to report sexual harassment cases? Why do you think so many men report that they were unaware of their own sexually harassing behaviours? What can be done to increase awareness in this area?

PREVENTING PERSONAL ASSAULTS

After a violent act is committed against someone we know, we acknowledge the horror of the event, express sympathy for the victim, and then go on with our lives. But the person who has been brutalized often takes a long time to recover—and sometimes complete recovery from the assault is not possible (see Table 4.3 for a summary of the most common consequences of victimization). In this section we discuss prevention of violence and abuse rather extensively because it is far better to stop a violent act than to recover from it.

Self-Defence Against Sexual Assault

Sexual assault can occur no matter what preventive actions you take, but there are some commonsense self-defence

> **Sexual assault:** Any act in which one person is sexually intimate with another person without that other person's consent.

TABLE 4.3 ■ Common Consequences of Victimization

Psychological	Medical
Recurrent and intrusive recollections, dreams, or flashbacks involving traumatic incidents	Death
Generalized anxiety, mistrust, and/or social isolation	Sexual/reproductive symptoms/consequences: Chronic pelvic pain, HIV infection, Urinary tract infections, Premenstrual pain, Fertility problems, Trauma-specific pain, Orgasmic difficulty
Difficulty in forming or maintaining nonexploitive intimate relationships	Battering-related symptoms: Bruises, Black eyes, Fractured ribs/broken teeth, Subdural hematomas, Detached retinas, Other head injuries
Chronic depression	Stress-mediated symptoms: Headaches, Backaches, TMJ symptoms, High blood pressure, Hyperalertness, Sleep disorders, Gastrointestinal disorders
Dissociative reactions: Phobic avoidance, often generalized to apparently unrelated situations Feelings of "badness," stigma, and guilt Impulsive or self-defeating behaviour	Eating disorders Self-mutilation

Source: From Marjorie Whittaker Leidig, "The Continuum of Violence Against Women: Psychological and Physical Consequences," *Journal of American College Health* 40 (1992): 151. Reprinted with permission of the Helen Dwight Reid Educational Foundation. Published by Heldref Publications, 1319 Eighteenth Street NW, Washington, D.C. 20036-1802. © 1992.

tactics that should lower your risk. Self-defence is a process that includes increased awareness, learning self-defence techniques, taking reasonable precautions, and developing the self-confidence and judgement needed to determine appropriate responses to different situations.[43]

Taking Control. Most sexual assaults by assailants unknown to the victim are planned in advance. They are frequently preceded by a casual, friendly conversation. Although many women have said that they started to feel uneasy during such a conversation, they denied the possibility of an attack to themselves until it was too late. Listen to your feelings and trust your intuition. Be assertive and direct to someone who is getting out of line or threatening—this may convince the would-be rapist to back off. Stifle your tendency to be "nice" and don't fear making a scene. Let him know that you mean what you say and are prepared to defend yourself:

- *Speak in a strong voice and use statements like "Leave me alone" rather than questions like "Will you please leave me alone?"* Avoid apologies and excuses.

- *Maintain eye contact with the would-be attacker.*

- *Sound as if you mean what you say.*

- *Stand up straight, act confident, and remain alert.* Walk as if you own the sidewalk.[44]

Many rapists use certain ploys to initiate their attacks. Among the most common are:

- *Request for help.* This allows him to get close—to enter your house to use the phone, for instance.

- *Offer of help.* This can also help him gain entrance to your home: "Let me help you carry that package."

- *Guilt trip.* "Gee, no one is friendly nowadays. . . . I can't believe you won't talk with me for just a little while."

- *Authority.* Many women fall for the old "policeman at the door" ruse. If anyone comes to your door dressed in policeman's garb, ask him to show you his ID before you unlock the door. You can also call the police department to get a confirmation on his ID.

If you are attacked, act immediately:

- *Don't worry about causing a scene.* Draw attention to yourself and your assailant. Scream for help.

- *Report the attack* to the appropriate authorities at once.

To prevent an attack from occurring:

- *Always be vigilant.* Even the safest cities and towns have sexual assaults. Don't be fooled by a sleepy-little-town atmosphere.

- *Use campus escort services whenever possible.*

- *Be assertive in demanding a well-lit campus.*

- *Don't use the same routes all the time.* Think about your movement patterns and vary them accordingly.

Preventing Date Rape

Most date rapes can be prevented by following several general guidelines. To keep yourself from getting into a potentially harmful situation, consider the following:

Women

- Think ahead of time and try to avoid getting into "compromising" situations. If you haven't decided to have sex, stay out of your date's bedroom, the back seat of the car, or other quiet spots that are away from the rest of the crowd.

- Communicate directly. Don't be wishy-washy in your remarks. If things start to go farther than you would like them to go, say NO loudly and with conviction. Do not worry about hurting feelings or seeming too aggressive. Be firm and stick to your words.

- Be aware that some men, in some situations, will interpret a low-cut, sexy dress or other clothing as a come-on. Although this is obviously wrong on their part, it is important that you do not naively assume that everyone is enlightened. Be direct and firm with anyone who seems to be assuming too much from your interactions.

- Avoid any substances, alcohol included, that may cause you not to think as clearly as you normally do.

- Pay attention to the nonverbal and verbal cues that your date is giving you. If he is starting to indicate that he is interested in more, make sure you are not caught unawares. Move to stay close to others and quickly let your date know your intentions.

- Decide ahead of time how far you are interested in going. Remember that it is your game, your rules, and no one should be able to pressure or force you into going beyond the line you have drawn.

- Be concerned about any of the following behaviours or expressions exhibited by your date:
  - Continued suggestive or dirty language indicating a disrespect for you and others.
  - Failure to listen to or to value your opinions about where to go, whom to spend time with, etc.
  - Unusual displays of jealousy/rage concerning your interactions with others.
  - Unusual roughness and forceful pushing or shoving to get you to comply with his wishes.

- Wild anger and violent acts toward others.
- Inability to control drinking and to display appropriate behaviours.
- Lack of concern for your feelings; laughter or derisive comments when you say no.

Men

- Take stock of your past behaviour in potentially sexual situations. How have you behaved, what have been the outcomes of the encounters, etc.? Have you felt uncomfortable about pushing too hard to have sex with your dates in the past?

- Know your sexual limits. If you feel that you are beginning to lose control in an intimate situation, communicate your feelings and indicate why it is time that you stop.

- Understand that NO means NO—and that it is not a sign of rejection. Respect the woman's right to say no, regardless of how far you've gone or what you thought she might have wanted. Stop NOW and quit trying "another line." Think about how you'd want your sister or close female friend to be treated by another guy in a similar situation.

- Just because you may have been intimate with the woman before, don't assume that it's okay now. When you hear the word NO, or if the woman struggles in any way, STOP.

- Avoid alcohol and other drugs that may cause you to think unclearly.

- Avoid situations likely to get you into trouble. Until you are sure of your intentions and your date's intentions, stay out of bedrooms and avoid dark roads and the back seats of cars. Remember, a sexual assault charge is serious business and could ruin your university and future career aspirations, not to mention the damage you may cause the woman.

- If you encounter a particularly aggressive woman, it is not unmanly to tell her you do not want to have sex and are not interested in being intimate in any way. Say NO and avoid situations that may cause you to be caught in a compromising position. Forget about what she may say or what your friends will say. Remember that sexual activity should be a part of a larger relationship.

- *Don't leave a bar alone with a friendly stranger.* Stay with your friends, and let the friendly stranger come along. Don't give your address to anyone you don't know.

- *Let friends/family know where you are going, what route you'll take, and when to expect your return.*

- *Stay close to others.* Avoid shortcuts through dark or unlit paths. Don't be the last one to leave the lab or library late at night.

- *Keep your windows and doors locked.* Don't answer the door to strangers.

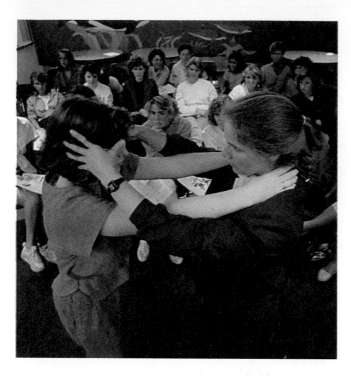

Women who learn self-defence techniques and always remember to take reasonable safety precautions lower their risk for assault.

What to Do When a Sexual Assault Occurs. If you are a sexual assault victim, it should be you who reports the attack. This gives you a sense of control. Calling 911 (if available) is probably the best rule of thumb. Do not bathe, shower, douche, clean up, or touch anything the attacker may have touched. Do not throw away or launder the clothes you were wearing. They will be needed as evidence. Bring a clean change of clothes to the clinic or hospital. Contact the Rape Crisis Centre in your area and ask for advice on therapists or counselling if you need additional advice or help.

If you want to help a sexual assault victim, the best thing you can do is to believe her. Don't ask questions that may appear to implicate her in the assault. Your hindsight may find some questionable judgement on her behalf, but that doesn't mean she's to blame. Sexual assault is a violent act against someone; the victim was certainly not looking for a violent act. Encourage her to talk, and when she does, listen. Hold back on advice.

Encourage her to see a doctor immediately, as she may have medical needs but be too embarrassed to seek help on her own. Be supportive of her reporting of the crime. And stay her friend. It may take six months to a year for emotional recovery, and you should be understanding during this time. Encourage her to seek counselling if any problems persist.

Preventing Assaults at Home

When at home, there are several precautions you can take to avoid being assaulted:[45]

- *Get deadbolts and peepholes and make sure the entryway to your house is lighted and free of shrubs.*

- *Consider putting a lock, solid-core door, and extension phone with a lighted dial in your bedroom.*

- *Get to know your neighbours and organize a neighbourhood watch.*

- *Don't hide your keys under a fake rock or other device.* These are dead giveaways to experienced criminals.

- *Don't open your door to anyone you don't know.*

- *Ask for identification from repairmen and/or call the company to verify that they've sent someone out.*

- *Keep lights on in at least one room other than the one you're in to make it look as if you aren't alone.*

- *Don't put your full name on your mailbox or in the phone book;* use your initials instead.

- *A "Beware of Dog" sign may help deter assailants.* Be careful of "doggy doors." Many an assailant has entered a house through a pet door.

Preventing Assaults on the Street

- *Walk/jog at a steady pace.* Look confident and stay alert to your surroundings.

- *Walk/jog with others.* There is safety in numbers.

- *At night, avoid dark parking lots, wooded areas, and all other good hiding places for assailants.*

- *Listen for footsteps and voices.* Change the pace of your walk if you think you're being followed to see if the person behind you does likewise. If he does, walk down the middle of the street, staying near the streetlights. Run and yell if you feel threatened.

- *Be aware of cars that keep driving around in your area.*

- *Vary your running/walking routes.*[46]

Preventing Assaults in Your Car

Recent carjackings and murders of individuals driving expensive cars, rental cars, and other vehicles point out the necessity for personal actions to help protect yourself and avoid high-risk situations. By taking the following actions, you may avoid a serious assault:

- *Always keep your doors locked and your windows rolled up.*

- *Don't stop for vehicles in distress.* Drive on and call for help.

Confronting Violence in Canadian Society

According to the social causes approach, sexual violence is a learned behaviour created and perpetuated by an intricate set of ideas, values, customs, and institutions, all of which depend on the subjugation of women by men.

Below are some examples of the growing commitment to recognize and confront violence in society.

1965 Ontario becomes the first province to require reporting of child abuse

1970 First Royal Commission report on the Status of Women (no mention of violence)

1970 First women's studies course offered (University of Toronto)

1972 Canada's first shelter for abused women opened in Vancouver

1973 Canadian Advisory Council on Status of Women (CACSW) established

1973 Newfoundland's Neglected Adults Welfare Act becomes the first North American legislation to protect adults with physical or mental limitations from abuse or neglect

1976 House Standing Committee holds hearings and issues a report on child abuse and neglect

1980 National Advisory Council on Aging established

1980 CACSW releases report, *Wife Battering in Canada: The Vicious Circle*

1981 Media reports of laughter in House of Commons over report on prevalence of wife abuse prompt public outcry

1982 National Clearinghouse on Family Violence established

1982 Canada's Solicitor General urges police to lay charges in cases of wife battering when there are reasonable grounds to believe that an assault has taken place

1983 Broad amendments made to Canadian sexual assault legislation including making sexual assault in marriage a crime

1984 Speech from the Throne includes wife battering as a priority concern

1984 The Committee on Sexual Offenses Against Children and Youth (Badgley Committee) releases report

1986 Health and Welfare Canada creates Family Violence Division

1987 CACSW releases report, *Battered, But Not Beaten: Preventing Wife Battering in Canada*

1989 Fourteen women killed in Montreal in what becomes known as the "Montreal Massacre"

1989 First major Canadian survey on the extent and nature of elder abuse

1990 Special Advisor on Child Sexual Abuse to the Minister of National Health and Welfare releases report, *Reaching for Solutions*

1993 Canadian Panel on Violence Against Women releases report, *Changing the Landscape: Ending Violence, Achieving Equality*

1993 Statistics Canada conducts Violence Against Women Survey

Source: Planned Parenthood of Toronto, "Sex and Violence—What's the Connection?" *Sex Wise* (Summer 1993); with acknowledgement to Ron Thorne-Finch, *Enduring the Silence: The Origins and Treatment of Male Violence Against Women.*

- *If your car breaks down, lock the doors and wait for help from the police.* Do not accept assistance from strangers, particularly from individuals on isolated roads.

- *If you think someone is following you, do something to attract attention.* Stay in your car with locked windows and doors and drive to a fire station, police station, all-night grocery, restaurant, or other place where there are people. If you are forced to stop on a deserted road, leave your engine running and in gear. Wait until your pursuer gets out of his car, then drive away as fast as you can.

- *Stick to well-travelled routes.* Avoid dark, isolated shortcuts.

- *Fill your car with gas and keep it in good running order.*

- *Don't put your name and address on your key ring.*

Sexual Harassment

Sexual harassment is a form of sex discrimination, and a violation of the human rights law of most provinces. Sexual harassment is sex discrimination. Most victims of sexual harassment are women, but sometimes men are victims of sexual harassment.

Everyone wants the right to be able to use public services, housing, and most importantly, to work, without being sexually harassed. Sexual harassment is unwelcome conduct of a sexual nature that has an adverse impact on the person harassed. Here are some examples.

Sexual harassment is any sexually oriented conduct that interferes with your ability to do your job, or creates a hostile, intimidating, or offensive environment.

Sexual harassment can also include any sexually oriented behaviour that you feel that you have to put up with in order to keep your job or to get a promotion.

Sexual harassment can also involve the displaying of pictures that are sexual in nature, such as pinups, that are offensive to you.

Sexual harassment can involve unwanted touching, patting, or grabbing. If you feel uncomfortable when a co-worker or supervisor touches you, you should tell that person that you do not like to be touched. Touching or grabbing genitals or breasts is never appropriate behaviour.

An invitation to dinner or a movie from a co-worker or even a supervisor is not necessarily sexual harassment. Invitations can be made, accepted, or rejected innocently. When a supervisor implies that an invitation must be accepted or there will be employment consequences, however, that may be sexual harassment.

What to Do

If you believe that you are being sexually harassed, your response should be immediate and direct. In some cases, it works to tell the harasser that his or her behaviour is unwelcome and unacceptable, and that if it happens again, you will report it.

It sometimes works to discuss the problem with your supervisor, a member of your personnel or human resources department, or a union steward.

If the harassment is repeated over a period of time, it is a good idea to keep a diary of the incidents as they occur. The diary is a written record. It is also important that you tell someone that you are being harassed. This could be a trusted co-worker, friend, or family member. The diary and the fact that you told someone may be important as evidence if you choose to file a complaint.

If you believe that you are being sexually harassed, you should first advise your employer and your union. See if they will do something to deal with the problem. You can also file a complaint under the Human Rights Code of your province. If you believe that you are being sexually harassed, but are not certain if you wish to file a complaint, you may call and discuss your concerns with the staff of your provincial Human Rights Commission. Your call will be kept confidential.

How to Make a Complaint

To file a complaint, phone the Human Rights Commission and tell them that you wish to file a complaint. What happens next will depend on the procedures that are being followed at that time. You should ask the person you speak with what is the normal procedure. Usually in these situations, the staff will investigate your complaint to decide if it should be referred for a hearing. Information is gathered from all the people involved in the complaint, including any witnesses identified by either side.

Source: BC Branch, Canadian Bar Association © 1996 (http://www.acjnet.org/dialalaw/bc/bc271.html).

- *Before getting into your car, walk around it and check the back seat, floor, and undercarriage.*

- *On long trips, don't make it obvious you're travelling alone.* Never take a map into a restaurant.

- *Don't sleep in your car along the highway.* This is no longer safe in many areas.

- *When you stop for a traffic light, leave a car's length so that if you are approached you'll have room to pull out.* If someone does approach, blow your horn and attract attention.

- *Never get out of the car if someone bumps into you until a police officer arrives.* A recent rash of murders and carjackings have involved assailants ramming victims'

cars from behind and then shooting or attacking victims who got out to investigate.[47]

Violence and Health

If the health sector is to adequately understand and respond to violence, greater emphasis is needed on a Population Health model—the model now adopted by the federal government, which sees health as embracing not only medical services and personal health practices, but also the physical, social, and economic environment (see Chapter 1). Prevention of violence must be based on creation of life conditions that would reduce the occurrence of violence and lessen its effects.

Managing Campus Safety

College campuses today may be healthy places for student interactions, or they may be settings for violent and aggressive interactions between students. Most campuses have initiated programs, services, and policies designed to protect students from possible violations of their personal health and safety. Answering the following questions may help you determine your college administrators' degree of interest in and commitment to a violence-free setting.

Making Decisions for You

Setting limits on where you go, at what time, and with whom seem to be running themes of this chapter. What types of limits do you set yourself? Think for a moment about your next night out with friends or with your lover. What limits will you set yourself? Will you decide ahead of time to limit your drinking? What time do you want to be home? How far you will go sexually? Will you use condoms? Decide how you will achieve your goals.

Choices for Change: Making Personal Choices

✓ Do you decide before a date to limit your sexual behaviour?

✓ Do you travel in groups whenever possible?

✓ Do you avoid being out alone at night?

✓ Do you avoid high-crime areas?

Choices for Change: Making Community Choices

✓ Does your campus have a student health centre with a trained staff of health educators?

✓ Does your health centre offer workshops on prevention of sexual assault?

✓ Does your campus offer courses focussing on understanding human diversity?

✓ Does your campus offer workshops and/or seminars for men to help them understand their sexuality and refrain from rape and other kinds of assault against women?

✓ Does your campus offer workshops/information for students to help them avoid situations that put them at risk for violent sexual or other interactions?

✓ Does your campus offer confidential counselling and/or assistance to victims of sexual assault?

✓ Does your campus offer workshops/educational sessions dealing with suicide?

✓ Does your campus offer information/workshops/services dealing with partner/domestic violence?

✓ Does your campus offer information/workshops/services dealing with child abuse and/or sexual abuse?

✓ Does your campus offer workshops/seminars that help males learn how to confront peers who express attitudes supportive of "overcoming" women sexually?

✓ Does your campus have strict substance abuse policies designed to reduce the likelihood of possible sexual assaults?

✓ Are sessions designed to negate myths and to increase understanding between the sexes offered in "safe" environments where discussions are open and positive role models encourage positive actions?

✓ Are services such as rides and escort services available to students after hours to prevent assaults? Do security guards patrol the campus?

✓ Is your campus well-lighted and open in the evenings?

✓ Are campus health educators, counsellors, and other professionals trained to spot victimization in clients and recommend appropriate services?

✓ Does your campus have a code of conduct that mandates swift and prudent punishment for alcohol and other drug abuse and acts of campus violence?

Critical Thinking

Your best friend and roommate has been accused of date rape; if the charge is substantiated, he could be dismissed from university. The way your friend tells it, they had a few drinks, started making out, and eventually had intercourse. He claims that she did not try to stop him. Your friend asks you to talk to the girl; after all, she's a friend of yours from high school and you introduced them. He wants you to "find holes in her story" and see if you can get her to "forget about the whole thing." It's hard to believe your best friend is a rapist. But then it's also hard to believe she is lying.

Using the DECIDE model described in Chapter 1, decide what you will do. Reconsider the information about rape in the chapter. Would it make a difference if she came to you to talk?

Clearly, a violence-free environment is a prerequisite for health.[48] Violence is both a barrier to health and a consequence of an unhealthy environment. In fact, the Ottawa Charter for Health Promotion (an international statement on health promotion) states:

… the fundamental conditions and resources for health are peace, shelter, education, food, income, a stable ecosystem, sustainable resources, social justice and equity. Improvement in health requires a secure foundation in these basic prerequisites.[49]

Summary

◆ Violence affects everyone in society—from the direct victims, to those who live in fear, to those who pay higher taxes and insurance premiums. Over half of homicides are committed by people who knew their victims. Bias and hate crimes divide people, but teaching tolerance can reduce risks. Gang violence can be combatted by programs aimed at reducing the problems that lead to gang membership.

◆ Sexual victimization refers to sexual assault, date rape, and sexual harassment. The possible reasons accounting for why males sexually assault females include male socialization, attitudes, sexual history and hostility, misperceptions, and situational factors. Sexual assault is not a sexual act, but a violent act.

◆ Prevention of violent acts begins with keeping yourself out of situations in which harm may occur.

Discussion Questions

1. What are common ways that violence is expressed in Canada?

2. What are the health care issues of violence in society?

3. Compare spousal abuse against men and against women: What are the differences? What are the similarities? What are the causes of domestic violence?

4. What puts a child at risk for abuse? Is there anything that can be done to prevent or to decrease the amount of child abuse?

5. What is sexual harassment and what factors contribute to it in the workplace?

6. List the actions you can take to protect yourself from personal assault in your home, in your car, or on the streets.

7. If your friend were to tell you that she was sexually assaulted last night, what would you do? What would you suggest she do?

Application Exercise

Reread the What Do You Think? scenario at the beginning of the chapter and answer the following questions:

1. What do you think are the major reasons that this situation occurred? What actions could we take as a society to reduce violence?

2. Do you believe that violence is really much worse than it was back in the "good old days"? Or are we just made more aware of it due to increased media coverage?

Health on the Net

Access to Justice Network
www.acjnet.org/acjeng.html

Forty-Ninth World Health Assembly; Prevention of Violence: A Public Health Priority
www.who.ch/programmes/eha/wha49-25.htm

Stopping Family Violence
www.cfc-efc.ca/docs/00000124.htm

$\mathcal{H}$ealthy Relationships and Sexuality

$\mathcal{M}$aking Commitments

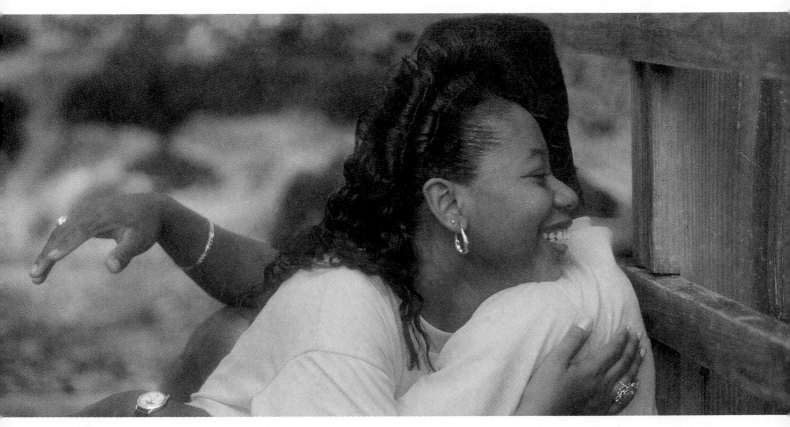

$\mathcal{C}$HAPTER OBJECTIVES

- Explain the characteristics of intimate relationships, the purposes they serve, and the types of intimacy that each of us may be able to have.

- Explain the development of relationships, potential barriers to healthy relationships, and factors that are important in maintaining intimate relationships.

- Discuss what remaining single means for many Canadians.

- Examine child-rearing practices in Canada and the importance of a healthy family environment.

- Discuss the warning signs of relationship decline, where you can go to get help with a relationship crisis,

and factors that ultimately lead to relationship problems.

- Define sexual identity, and discuss the role of gender identity.

- Identify the components of male and female reproductive anatomy and physiology and their functions.

- Discuss the options available for the expression of one's sexuality.

- Classify sexual dysfunctions and describe each disorder.

- Learn to develop your own sexual identity.

Michael and Sara have been dating seriously for over two years and have talked about marriage. Sara has noticed that Michael often seems overly possessive of her and jealous of her time spent with others. They fight regularly about who she does things with, potential threats to their relationship, and the like. Recently, Michael took a weekend to go hunting with the guys while Sara stayed home to get caught up on her work. When Sara's friends called her to ask her to go to a party, she decided to go. She had worked hard all weekend and needed a break. When she talks to Michael on the phone the next day, he asks her what she did the night before. Wanting to avoid a fight, she tells him that she stayed home to work. He responds angrily, "I tried to call you all night and you weren't home."

- ■ What should Sara do in this situation? Why do you think she felt the need to lie? Is dishonesty in a relationship ever justified? Is Michael's jealousy a healthy aspect of their relationship? What factors may have contributed to his jealousy? Can a relationship based on mistrust and half-truths survive?

Friendship, close family bonds, and loving intimate and nonintimate relationships are viewed as significant factors in achieving overall health. The eternal quest to be loved and to love others appears to be one of our most basic human needs.

For many, the motivation to seek and receive love appears to be a natural result of previous life experiences and our development as sexual beings. For others, the struggle to find, develop, and maintain relationships becomes a difficult, often painful and frustrating experience, punctuated by unhappy sexual and nonsexual interactions. What makes one person more successful in his or her relationships than another? What role does friendship and the family environment have on the development of healthy relationships later in life? What effect, if any, does sexual identity have on one's ability to form healthy relationships?

CHARACTERISTICS OF INTIMATE RELATIONSHIPS

There are many possible definitions of **intimate relationships.** One classic definition calls these relationships "close relationships with another person in which you offer, and are offered, validation, understanding, and a sense of being valued intellectually, emotionally, and physically."[1] In this context, friends, family, lovers, partners, and even people you work with or interact with at the grocery store may be included in the sphere of intimate interactions.

For the purposes of this chapter, we define intimate relationships in terms of three characteristics: *behavioural interdependence, need fulfillment,* and *emotional attachment.* Each of these three characteristics may be related to interactions with family, close friends, and romantic relationships.[2]

Behavioural interdependence refers to the mutual impact that people have on each other as their lives and daily activities become intertwined. What one person does may influence what the other person may want to do and can do. Such interdependence may become stronger over time to the point that each person would find a great void in his or her life if the other person was gone.

Another characteristic of intimate relationships is that they serve to fulfill psychological needs and, as such, are a means of *need fulfillment.* These needs may often be met only through relationships with others:

- ■ The need for approval and for a sense of purpose in life—requiring the sense that what we say and do counts.

- ■ The need for intimacy—requiring someone with whom we can share our feelings freely.

- ■ The need for social integration—requiring someone with whom we can share our worries and concerns.

- ■ The need for being nurturant—requiring someone whom we can take care of.

- ■ The need for assistance—requiring someone to help us in times of need.

- ■ The need for reassurance or affirmation of our own worth—requiring someone who will tell us that we matter.

Emotional bonding and other elements of intimate relationships are rooted in a caring, supportive family environment.

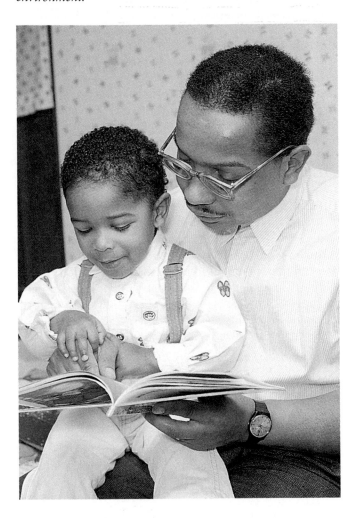

In close, rewarding, intimate relationships, partners or friends meet each other's needs. They disclose feelings, share confidences, and discuss practical concerns, helping each other and providing reassurance. They serve as major sources of social support and reinforce our feelings that we are important and serve a purpose in life.

In addition to behavioural interdependence and need fulfillment, intimate relationships involve strong bonds of *emotional attachment*, or feelings of love and attachment. The intimacy level experienced by any two people cannot easily be judged by those outside the relationship. A relationship may be very intimate and not be sexual, although sex may be an important part of an intimate relationship. Important relationships having high levels of intimacy may be either sexual or nonsexual. Many satisfying and lasting intimate relationships go well beyond the need for sexual contact.

*W*HAT DO YOU THINK?

Do you have at least one person in your life right now who helps fulfill your psychological needs? Who makes you feel loved and important? Who would support you if you really needed help? Are you a source of psychological support for someone else? If you don't have this type of relationship, what could you do to develop one?

Emotional availability, the ability to give to and receive from others emotionally without fear of being hurt or rejected, is another characteristic of intimate relationships. At times, all of us may need to protect ourselves psychologically by making ourselves unavailable emotionally. For example, after the end of a relationship, a young woman may close down emotionally and carefully avoid letting herself feel too much. This gives her time for regrouping and healing before she reaches out to people again. It also reduces the risk of a rebound romance that is often doomed to failure as a result of unresolved personal hurts and issues.

Types of Intimate Relationships

Balanced intimacy involves developing levels of intimacy in several dimensions. *Sexual intimacy* is one possible expression of closeness. Another dimension of intimacy is *intellectual intimacy,* the sharing of ideas. *Emotional intimacy* involves the sharing of significant meanings and feelings. *Aesthetic intimacy* refers to the sharing of experiences with one another. *Recreational intimacy* is the freedom to let the child within us come out when we are with others. *Work intimacy* is the sharing of common tasks such as housework, family responsibilities, employment, and community undertakings. *Crisis intimacy* implies the successful coping with either internal or external threats. *Commitment intimacy* involves the mutual concern for issues and philosophies that go beyond the immediate relationship (for example, a political cause). *Spiritual intimacy* is the sharing of ultimate concerns regarding the meanings of

Intimate relationships: "[C]lose relationships with another person in which you offer, and are offered, validation, understanding, and a sense of being valued intellectually, emotionally, and physically."

Emotional availability: The ability to give to and receive from other people emotionally without being inhibited by fears of being hurt.

life. By achieving balanced levels in mutually selected areas of intimacy, two people contribute to *creative intimacy,* or the sharing of emotional and social factors that help each other grow and learn.

Balanced intimacy is a goal most people pursue either directly or indirectly. The chances for balanced intimacy are greater for people who were raised in an environment where close relationships were valued, where there were positive role models for friendships, close family bonds, and romantic attachments.

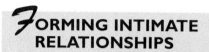

FORMING INTIMATE RELATIONSHIPS

Throughout our lives, we go through predictable patterns of relationships. In our early years, our families are our most significant relationships. Gradually, our relationships widen to include circles of friends, co-workers, and acquaintances. Ultimately, most of us develop romantic or sexual relationships with significant others. Each of these relationships plays a significant role in psychological, social, spiritual, and physical health. Each has the potential either to serve as a growth experience or to "bring us down" as a result of unhealthy interactions.

Families: The Ties That Bind

Although many people consider the family the foundation of Canadian society and talk about a return to "family values" as a desirable objective, it is clear that the modern Canadian family may look quite different from families of previous generations. The *Leave It to Beaver* family type encouraged during the 1950s, composed of Mom with her apron, staying at home and content with her role as mother and spouse; Dad with his briefcase, trying to move up the corporate ladder; and two or three happy, well-adjusted children, is often not the norm. Over half of today's moms work outside the home and large numbers of children are raised by single parents, grandparents, relatives, stepparents, nannies, day-care centres, and other "parents."

Regardless of the form or structure of each family, all families have in common one unique characteristic: the special caring, regard, and bonding that a group of people having shared interests have for each other. Whether the family is related by birth, a high level of love and regard, living arrangement, or some other factor, the family network often provides the sense of security that humans need to develop into healthy adults. The definition of *family* changes dramatically from culture to culture and from place to place over time.

The Vanier Institute on the Family defines family as "any combination of two or more persons who are bound together over time by ties of mutual consent, birth and/or adoption/placement and who, together, assume responsibilities for variant combinations of the following: Physical maintenance and care of family members; Addition of new members, Socialization of children; Social control of members; Production, consumption and distribution of goods and services; Love and affective nurturance."[3]

Families are not inherently good or bad based on the structure or roles that people bring to the family setting. Those that result in the most positive health outcomes for all members appear to be those that offer a sense of security, safety, and love, and that provide the opportunity for members to grow as a result of positive interactions.

Today's Family Unit

The United Nations defines seven basic types of families, including single-parent families, communal families (unrelated people living together for ideological, economic, or other reasons), extended families, and others. But most of us think of family in terms of the "family of origin" or the "nuclear family." The *family of origin* includes the people present in the household during a child's first years of life—usually parents and siblings. However, the family of origin may also include a stepparent, parents' lovers, or significant others such as grandparents, aunts, or uncles. The family of origin has a tremendous impact on the child's psychological and social development. The *nuclear family* consists of parents (usually married, but not necessarily) and their offspring.

If parents are not afraid to share feelings, affection, or love with each other and their offspring, their children are more likely to become emotionally connected adults. If the home environment provides stability and seems a safe place to be, it is likely that the children will learn to express feelings and develop intimacy skills. Sibling interactions provide a way to learn and practise interpersonal skills.[4] The family of origin and the nuclear family have the potential for encouraging significant positive interactions and growth. People can practise positive behaviours and learn the rights and wrongs of negative behaviours in a safe and nonjudgemental environment when the family itself is healthy. However, if the family is psychologically or physically unhealthy, it may pose significant barriers to later relationships.

Friendships: Finding the Right Ingredients

A Friend is one who knows you as you are
understands where you've been
accepts who you've become, and
still gently invites you to grow.

—Author Unknown

Although most of us have a fairly clear idea of the distinction between a friend and a lover, this difference is not always easy to verbalize. Some people believe that the major difference is that there is no intimate physical involvement between friends. Others have suggested that intimacy levels are much lower between friends than between lovers. But as we have stated, people can be intimate with each other without being sexually involved. Confused? You are probably not alone. Surprisingly, there has not been a great deal of research to clarify these terms. Psychologists Jeffrey Turner and Laurna Rubinson provide a basic overview of what friendship actually entails.[5] Beyond the fact that two people participate in a relationship as equals, friendships include the following characteristics:

- *Enjoyment.* Friends enjoy each other's company most of the time, although there may be temporary states of anger, disappointment, or mutual annoyance.

- *Acceptance.* Friends accept each other as they are, without trying to change or make the other into a different person.

- *Trust.* Friends have mutual trust in the sense that each assumes that the other will act in his or her friend's best interests.

- *Respect.* Friends respect each other in the sense that each assumes that the other exercises good judgement in making life choices.

- *Mutual assistance.* Friends are inclined to assist and support one another. Specifically, they can count on each other in times of need, trouble, or personal distress.

- *Confiding.* Friends share experiences and feelings with each other that they don't share with other people.

- *Understanding.* Friends have a sense of what is important to each and why each behaves as he or she does. Friends are not puzzled or mystified by each other's actions.

- *Spontaneity.* Friends feel free to be themselves in the relationship rather than required to play a role, wear a mask, or inhibit revealing personal traits.

Significant Others, Partners, Couples

Although family and friends are necessary intimate relationships, most people choose at some point whether or not to enter into an intimate sexual relationship with another person. Numerous studies have analyzed the ways in which couples form significant partnering relationships. Most couples fit into one of four categories of significant sexual or committed relationships: married heterosexual couples, cohabiting heterosexual couples,

lesbian couples, and gay male couples. These groups are discussed in greater detail later in this chapter.

Love relationships in each of these four groups typically include all the characteristics of friendship as well as other characteristics related to passion and caring:[6]

- *Fascination.* Lovers tend to pay attention to the other person even when they should be involved in other activities. They are preoccupied with the other and want to think about, look at, talk to, or merely be with the other.

- *Exclusiveness.* Lovers have a special relationship that usually precludes having the same relationship with a third party. The love relationship takes priority over all others.

- *Sexual desire.* Lovers want physical intimacy with the partner, desiring to touch, hold, and engage in sexual activities with the other. They may choose not to act on these feelings because of religious, moral, or practical considerations.

- *Giving the utmost.* Lovers care enough to give the utmost when the other is in need, sometimes to the point of extreme sacrifice.

- *Being a champion/advocate.* The depth of lovers' caring may show up as an active, unselfish championing of each other's interests and a positive attempt to ensure that the other succeeds.

For obvious reasons, the best love relationships share friendships, and the best friendships include several love components. Both relationships share common bonds of nurturance, enhancement of personal well-being, and a genuine sense of mutual regard, trust, and security.

This Thing Called Love

What is love? Finding a definition of love may be more difficult than listing characteristics of a loving relationship. The term *love* has more entries in *Bartlett's Familiar Quotations* than does any other word except *man*.[7] This four-letter word has been written about and engraved on walls; it has been the theme of countless novels, movies, and plays. There is no one definition of *love,* and the word may mean different things to people depending on cultural values, age, gender, and situation.

Many social scientists maintain that love may be of two kinds: *companionate* and *passionate.* Companionate love is a secure, trusting attachment, similar to what we may feel for family members or close friends. In companionate love, two people are attracted, have much in common, care about each other's well-being, and express reciprocal liking and respect. Passionate love is, in contrast, a state of high arousal, filled with the ecstasy of being loved by the partner and the agony of being rejected.[8] The person experiencing passionate love tends to be preoccupied with his or her partner and to perceive the love object as being perfect.[9] According to Hatfield and Walster, passionate love will not occur unless three conditions are met.[10] First, the person must live in a culture in which the concept of "falling in love" is idealized. Second, a "suitable" love object must be present. If the person has been taught by parents, movies, books, and peers to seek partners having certain levels of attractiveness or belonging to certain racial groups or having certain socioeconomic status and none is available, the person may find it difficult to allow him- or herself to become involved. Finally, for passionate love to occur, there must be some type of physiological arousal that occurs when a person is in the presence of the object of desire. Sexual excitement is often the way in which such arousal is expressed.

In his article "The Triangular Theory of Love," researcher Robert Sternberg attempts to clarify further what love is by isolating three key ingredients:

- *Intimacy.* The emotional component, which involves feelings of closeness.
- *Passion.* The motivational component, which reflects romantic, sexual attraction.
- *Decision/commitment.* The cognitive component, which includes the decisions you make about being in love and the degree of commitment to your partner.

According to Sternberg's model, the higher the levels of intimacy, passion, and commitment, the more likely a person is to be involved in a healthy, positive love relationship (see Table 5.1).

Anthropologist Helen Fisher, a research associate at the American Museum of Natural History and author of *Anatomy of Love: The Natural History of Monogamy, Adultery, and Divorce,* has attempted to shed new light on the process of falling in love.[11] According to Fisher (and others), attraction and falling in love follow a fairly predictable pattern based on (1) *imprinting,* in which our evolutionary patterns, genetic predispositions, and past experiences trigger romantic reaction; (2) *attraction,* in which neurochemicals produce feelings of euphoria and elation; (3) *attachment,* in which endorphins—natural opiates—cause lovers to feel peaceful, secure, and calm; and (4) *production of a cuddle chemical,* in which the brain secretes the chemical oxytocin, thereby stimulating sensations during lovemaking and eliciting feelings of satisfaction and attachment.[12]

Lovers who claim that they are swept away by passion may not, therefore, be far from the truth.

A meeting of the eyes, a touch of the hands or a whiff of scent may set off a flood that starts in the brain and races along the nerves and through the blood. The familiar results—flushed skin, sweaty palms, heavy breathing—are identical to those experienced when under stress. Why? Because the love-smitten person is secreting chemical substances such as dopamine, norepinephrine, and phenylethylamine (PEA) that are chemical cousins of amphetamines.[13]

Although attraction may in fact be a "natural high," with PEA levels soaring, this hit of passion loses effectiveness over time as the body builds up a tolerance. Needing a continual fix of passion, many people may become attraction junkies, seeking the intoxication of love much as the drug user seeks a chemical high.[14]

Fisher speculates that PEA levels drop significantly over a three-to-four-year period, leading to the "four-year itch" that shows up in the peaking fourth-year divorce rates present in over 60 cultures. Those romances that last beyond the four-year decline of PEA are influenced by another set of chemicals, known as endorphins, soothing substances that give lovers a sense of security, peace, and calm.[15]

TABLE 5.1 ■ The Triangular Theory of Love: Types of Relationships

	Intimacy	Passion	Decision and Commitment
Nonlove	Low	Low	Low
Liking	High	Low	Low
Infatuated love	Low	High	Low
Romantic love	High	High	Low
Empty love	Low	Low	High
Companionate love	High	Low	High
Fatuous love	Low	High	High
Consummate love	High	High	High

Source: R. J. Sternberg, "The Triangular Theory of Love," *Psychological Review* 93 (1986): 119–135. Copyright 1986 by the American Psychological Association. Reprinted by permission.

Is It Love or Infatuation?

In the early stages, love and infatuation can be very similar emotions. They both produce a characteristic rush of excitement as well as a strong desire to have more of the loved one's time, energy, and contact. The primary difference is that with love, the feelings often grow deeper as you get to know the person better and come to appreciate him or her more. With infatuation or a crush, you begin to realize that Ms. or Mr. Right wasn't all you had thought. Taking the following test may help you determine whether it's the real thing or merely a case of infatuation. Respond YES or NO to the following statements:

1. I knew I was in love with the person almost immediately.

2. Even though I've known the person for a while, I still really love his/her personality.

3. I wonder sometimes if the person has changed a lot since I've known him/her because he/she acts differently around me now.

4. The more I'm with the person, the more I want to be around him/her.

5. I am less interested in the person sexually than I was in the beginning.

6. The more I know about the person, the more I want to know.

7. The more I know about the person, the less interested I am in him/her.

8. I feel really good associating with this person and being regarded as a couple.

9. I have begun to notice more things wrong with this person and spend a lot of time trying to get him/her to change.

10. Even though I have been with this person for a while, I am still just as sexually interested as I was in the beginning.

11. I find that I'd just as soon do things with other people as with this person because I'd probably have more fun.

12. I am able to share my feelings with this person and trust him/her completely.

13. I really love this person but don't feel good about sharing intimate feelings with him/her yet.

14. This person brings out the best in me and genuinely seems to care about me.

15. I love this person, but I don't respect him/her the way I respect others.

Scoring

There are no right or wrong responses to these statements. However, answering YES to the even-numbered statements may indicate that your feelings are more likely to be love-directed. In contrast, answering YES to the odd-numbered statements may indicate a tendency toward infatuation rather than love. Count the number of YESes to the even-numbered statements and the number of YESes to the odd-numbered statements. Look carefully at each statement. Are these things that you feel important enough to work on? Or are your responses telling you that another person may be a better choice?

Oxytocin is also being studied for its role in the love formula. Produced by the brain, it sensitizes nerves and stimulates muscle contractions, the production of breast milk, and the desire for physical closeness between mother and infant. Scientists speculate that oxytocin may encourage similar cuddling between men and women. Oxytocin levels have also been shown to increase dramatically during orgasm for both men and women.[16]

In addition to such possible chemical influences, our past experiences may significantly affect our attractions for others. Our parents' modelling of traits we believe are desirable or undesirable may play a role in drawing us to people with similar traits. Many researchers have investigated the possible link between males seeking their own mothers in partners and females seeking their fathers in partners. To date, research on chemical attractions and parent-seeking tendencies is inconclusive and should be viewed only as preliminary findings. Much more research is needed to confirm these provocative new attraction theories.

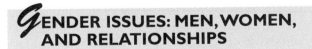

GENDER ISSUES: MEN, WOMEN, AND RELATIONSHIPS

In any relationship, understanding and communication are important ingredients for success. Sometimes it may seem that the relating styles of men and women are so different that obtaining true understanding and open communication may be next to impossible. Deborah Tannen summarized the frustration often felt between men and women who are trying to relate to one another in her best-selling book *You Just Don't Understand: Women and Men in Conversation*.[17] According to Tannen, men's and women's social conditioning is so different that it is almost as if they are raised in two different cultures. Women are brought up to feel comfortable and to share freely in their intimate relationships. They tend to be more nurturing and less afraid to share their fears, anxieties, and emotions. It's okay if they cry, scream, or express wide emotional swings. Big boys, however, are not supposed to cry—at least according to popular beliefs. Unlike their female counterparts, they are not supposed to show emotions, and they are brought up to believe that being strong is often more important than having close friendships. As a result, according to research, only one male in ten has a close male friend to whom he divulges his innermost thoughts.[18]

Why the Differences?

Although there are various theories about why males and females relate in the way they do, Lillian Rubin has provided the most comprehensive analysis. Rubin sees a serious barrier to intimacy in what she considers a basic difference in the development patterns of men and women.[19] In her view, men are less able to express emotions and achieve intimacy than are women owing to the process of identity development in infancy, which she sees as more difficult for males than for females. Males initially achieve intimacy with a female caregiver, usually a mother, at a preverbal stage. By the time they have developed verbal skills, boys have physically separated from the caregiver. Thus, for males, intimacy may consist of physical proximity rather than verbal sharing. Because females do not need to separate themselves from a female caregiver, they do not separate their feelings of intimacy from their verbal constructs. Consequently, women often are able to express intimacy verbally, whereas men often are not. This male/female disparity in the ability to express emotions is both the single greatest difference between the sexes and the greatest threat to intimacy in many relationships. Rubin's theories have received widespread acceptance among sociologists and psychologists today. The disparity in the ability to express emotions may account for common female complaints about male attitudes toward sex. Rubin feels that emotion generates sexual feelings in women, whereas sexual feelings generate emotion in men. Sex, it seems, is one area in which men are allowed to contact deeper emotional states. In fact, sexual activity carries the major burden of emotional expression for many males and may explain the urgency with which some men approach sex.

*W*HAT DO YOU THINK?

Who are the people with whom you feel most comfortable talking about very personal issues? Do you talk with both males and females about these issues, or do you tend to gravitate toward just one sex? Why do you think you do this?

Picking Partners: Similarities and Differences Between Genders

Just as males and females may find different ways to express themselves, the process of partner selection also shows distinctly different patterns. In both males and females, more than just chemical and psychological processes influence the choice of partners.[20] One of these factors is *proximity*, or being in the same place at the same time. The more you see a person in your hometown, at social gatherings, or at work, the more likely that an interaction will occur. Thus, if you live in Winnipeg, you'll probably end up with another Winnipeger. If you live in Prince Edward Island, you'll probably end up with another Islander.

You also pick a partner on the basis of *similarities* (attitudes, values, intellect, interests); the adage that "opposites attract" usually isn't true. Even though you may initially be attracted to someone who is extremely different from you, first flames usually die quickly and there is a subliminal hunt for common ground.

If your potential partner expresses interest or liking, you may react with mutual regard known as *reciprocity*. The more you express interest, the safer it is for someone else to return the regard, and the cycle spirals onward.

Another factor that apparently plays a significant role in selecting a partner is *physical attraction*. Whether such attraction is caused by a chemical reaction or a socially learned behaviour, males and females appear to have different attraction criteria. Men tend to select their mates primarily on the basis of youth and physical attractiveness. Although physical attractiveness is an important criterion for women in mate selection, they tend to place greater emphasis on partners who are somewhat older, have good financial prospects, and are dependable and industrious. Good grooming is an almost universally desirable trait for both men and women. If you smell or appear less than squeaky clean, you may have problems in the partner arena regardless of your sex.

*B*ARRIERS TO INTIMACY

Obstacles to intimacy include lack of personal identity, emotional immaturity, and a poorly developed sense of responsibility. The fear of being hurt, low self-esteem, mishandled hostility, chronic "busyness" (and its attendant lack of emotional presence), a tendency to "parentify" loved ones, and a conflict of role expectations may be equally detrimental. In addition, individual insecurities and difficulties in recognizing and expressing emotional needs can lead to an intimacy barrier. These barriers to intimacy may have many causes, including the different emotional development of men and women or an upbringing in a dysfunctional family.

Dysfunctional Families

As noted earlier, the ability to sustain genuine intimacy is largely developed in the family of origin. Unfortunately, sharing, trust, and openness do not always occur in the family. In fact, the assumption that such intimacy existed in the family of origin may actually be unrealistic. As adults, we may discover that although we thought our family encouraged emotional intimacy, it was actually judgemental, full of expectations, controlling, and, in many ways, dysfunctional. A **dysfunctional family** is one in which the interaction between family members inhibits psychological growth rather than encouraging self-love, emotional expression, and individual growth. If you were to examine even the most pristine family under a microscope, you would likely find some type of dysfunction. No group of people who live together day in and day out can interact perfectly all the time. However, many people have begun to overuse the term *dysfunctional* to refer to even the smallest problems in the family unit. As such, the term becomes relatively meaningless. True dysfunctionality refers to settings where negative interactions are the norm rather than the exception. Children raised in these settings tend to face tremendous obstacles to growing up healthy. Coming to terms with past hurts may take years. However, with careful planning and introspection, support from loved ones, and counselling when needed, children from even the worst homes have proved to be remarkably resilient. Many are able to forget the past and to focus on the future, developing into healthy, well-adjusted adults.[21] It is important to note that dysfunctional families are found in every social, ethnic, religious, economic, and racial group.

Recently, social scientists have been studying the impact of the alcoholic home environment on the sexual and intimate behaviour of adult children of alcoholics (ACOAs). Therapist Mary Ann Klausner has identified a number of intimacy problems as typical of ACOAs. Many ACOAs claim that they become involved in unhealthy relationships, have difficulty trusting others, have problems in communicating with partners, and have difficulty defining a healthy relationship.[22]

Another tragically large group of people struggling with intimacy problems originating in the family of origin are survivors of childhood emotional, physical, and sexual abuse. Experiencing or witnessing physical and emotional abuse as a child can have an impact on a person's intimate relations as an adult. Domestic violence, whether directed at a child or at another family member, can affect a child's ability to trust others and to maintain an intimate relationship later in life. Physical abuse may vary from the use of spanking to discipline a child to violent beatings. Emotional abuse includes name-calling and other tactics that damage a child's self-esteem.

Jealousy: The Green-Eyed Monster of Relationships

Jealousy has been described as an aversive reaction evoked by a real or imagined relationship involving your partner and a third person.

Contrary to what many of us may believe, jealousy is not a sign of intense devotion or of passionate love for the person who is the target of it. Instead, jealousy is often a sign of underlying problems that may prove to be a significant barrier to a healthy intimate relationship. The roots of jealous feelings and behaviours may run deep. Causes of jealousy typically include the following:

- *Overdependence on the relationship.* People who have few social ties and who rely exclusively on their significant others tend to be fearful of losing them.

- *High value on sexual exclusivity.* People who believe that sexual exclusiveness is a crucial indicator of a love relationship are more likely to become jealous. As the expectation of sexual exclusivity increases, the likelihood of becoming jealous also increases.

- *Severity of the threat.* People may feel uneasy if a person with a fantastic body, stunning good looks, and a great personality appears interested in their partners. But they may brush off the threat if they appraise the person as "unworthy" in terms of appearance or other characteristics.

- *Low self-esteem.* People who feel good about themselves are less likely to feel unworthy and to fear that someone else is going to snatch their partners away from them. The underlying question that torments people with low self-esteem is, "Why would anyone want me?" Thus, everyone other than the "beloved" becomes a threat.

- *Fear of losing control.* Some people need to feel in control of the situation. Feeling that they may be losing the attachment of or control over a partner can cause jealousy.

COMMITTED RELATIONSHIPS

Feelings of love or sexual attraction are not always equated with commitment in a relationship. There can be love without commitment and there can be sex without commitment. Commitment in a relationship with another person means that there is an intent to act over time

---

Dysfunctional family: A family in which the interaction between family members inhibits rather than enhances psychological growth.

Jealousy: An aversive reaction evoked by a real or imagined relationship involving a person's partner and a third person.

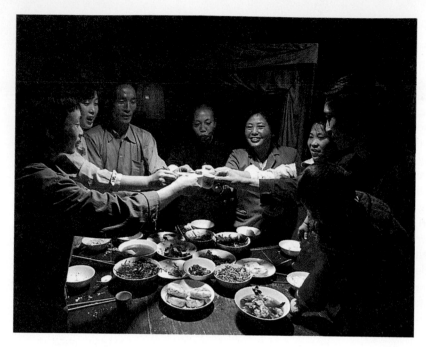

The negative interactions in dysfunctional families that damage self-esteem and deter psychosocial growth do not exist in healthy families that encourage emotional intimacy for all members throughout their lives.

in a way that perpetuates the well-being of the other person, yourself, and the relationship. A committed relationship involves tremendous diligence on the part of both partners. Over the years, partners learn about one another and constantly adjust the direction of their relationship. The Building Communication Skills box may help you evaluate your relationship's present state and may point to positive changes you can make. What separates committed from uncommitted relationships is the willingness of committed partners to dedicate themselves to acquiring and using the skills that will ensure a lasting relationship.

Marriage

Marriage is the traditional committed relationship in many societies around the world. For many people, marriage is the ultimate expression of an intimate relationship. When two people marry in Canada, they enter into a legal agreement that includes shared financial plans, property, and responsibility in raising children. For religious people, marriage is also a sacrament that stresses the spirituality, rights, and obligations of each person.

In 1991, 83 percent of the population lived in a family; 17 percent did not. Of families, 77 percent involved married couples, with or without children; 10 percent involved a common-law couple, and 13 percent were lone-parent families. Marriage is somewhat less prevalent in Quebec, where 69 percent of families included a married couple, than in the rest of the country, where the proportion is 80 percent.[23]

Most people believe that marriage involves **monogamy,** or exclusive sexual involvement with one partner.

The lifetime pattern for many Canadians appears to be **serial monogamy,** which means that a person has a monogamous sexual relationship with one partner for the duration of a relationship before moving on to another monogamous relationship. Some people prefer to have an **open relationship,** or open marriage, in which the partners agree that there may be sexual involvement for each person outside their relationship.

Humans are not naturally monogamous; that is, most of us are capable of being sexually and/or emotionally involved with more than one person at a time. Yet, Canadian society frowns on involvement with an outsider when we are involved in a relationship and profess to be committed. Many people find themselves being attracted to others while in a relationship and consciously try to stop any subsequent interactions. Others find themselves involved unintentionally. Still others actively seek out extra-relationship affairs. Whether by choice or chance, sexual infidelity is a common factor in divorces and breakups. Perhaps only those having strong self-images and a dedication to the principles of open relationships are able to maintain nonmonogamy over a period of time.

As with all relationships, there are marriages that work well and bring much satisfaction to the partners, and there are marriages that are unhealthy for the people involved. A good marriage can yield much support and stability, not only for the couple, but also for those involved in the couple's life. Considerable research also indicates that married people live longer, are happier, remain mentally alert longer, and suffer fewer bouts with physical and mental ailments. In the late 1980s, however, Wood and Glenn found that modern married women may not be as happy as their parents were and that the happiness of never-married men had increased.[24] Regardless, behavioural scientists agree that couples who make some type of formal commitment are more likely to stay together and develop the fulfilling relationship they initially sought than are those who do not commit.

Cohabitation

For various reasons, many people prefer to live together without the bonds of matrimony. Commonly called **cohabitation,** this type of relationship is defined as two people who have an intimate connection with each other who live together in the same household. The relationship can be very stable with a high level of commitment between the partners.

Among people born prior to World War II (1939–1945), common-law marriage was very much the exception to the rule. The 1990 General Social Survey (GSS) found that, of people aged between 45 and 54, only 5 percent of men and 2 percent of women had lived common-law before marriage or before age 30. In contrast, among those born between 1954 and 1960 (who ranged in age from 29 to 35 at the time of the survey) 40 percent of men and 36 percent of women had lived common-law before marriage or before age 30. Slightly more than half of these relationships resulted in marriage to the same partner.[25]

This dramatic increase may be partly attributed to youth's inclination to question traditional values and to the expanding recognition that marriage may not be the only legitimate basis for sexual relations. Cheaper, more effective birth control has probably been another factor. Many couples also believe that living together simply because they want to may be more important than being bound by a legal document.

Although cohabitation is a viable alternative for some, many cohabitors eventually marry because of pressures from parents and friends, difficulties in obtaining insurance and tax benefits, legal issues over property, and a host of other reasons.

The disadvantage of cohabitation lies in the lack of societal validation for the relationship and, in some cases, in the societal disapproval of living together without being married. Cohabiting partners do not usually experience the social incentives to stay together that they would if they were married. If they decide to separate, however, they do not experience the legal problems involved in going through a divorce. In most provinces, cohabitation that lasts more than three years is viewed as a **common-law marriage** in the eyes of the court on issues of child care and spousal support. It is not the same, however, as becoming legally married. Some laws treat common-law spouses the same as married spouses. For example, responsibilities of parents to their children are the same whether the parents are married to each other or not. On the other hand, some laws apply to married people and not to common-law couples, such as the one that divides matrimonial property. In still other situations, how the law treats a common-law couple depends on how long they lived together. For example, Employment Canada considers moving to be with a spouse a valid reason to quit a job, and, for this purpose, considers a couple who have been living together for at least one year to be spouses.[26]

Gay and Lesbian Partnerships

Most people seek intimate, committed relationships during their adult years. This is no different for gay and lesbian (homosexual) couples. Lesbians and gay men are socialized like other people in our culture and tend to place a high value on relationships. They seek the same things in their primary relationships as do heterosexual partners: friendship, communication, validation, companionship, and a sense of stability. Studies of lesbian couples indicate high levels of attachment and satisfaction and a tendency toward monogamous, long-term relationships. Gay men, too, tend to form committed, long-term relationships, especially as they age.[27]

Challenges to successful lesbian and gay male relationships often stem from the discrimination they face as homosexuals and to difficulties dealing with social, legal, and religious doctrines.

SUCCESS IN COMMITTED RELATIONSHIPS

Because the traditional marriage ceremony includes the vow "till death do us part," the definition of success in a relationship tends to be based on whether a couple stays together over the years. Marriage has become the model that relationships must conform to in order to be considered stable or healthy. One reason for the increase in cohabitation and other alternative relationships is the need

Monogamy: Exclusive sexual involvement with one partner.

Serial monogamy: Monogamous sexual relationship with one partner before moving on to another.

Open relationship: A relationship in which partners agree that there can be sexual involvement outside the relationship.

Cohabitation: Living together without being married.

Common-law marriage: Cohabitation lasting a designated period of time (usually three years) treated as equivalent to marriage for some, but not all, legal purposes.

Communicating with Your Partner

How well do you and your partner know each other? Do you communicate your feelings, fears, frustrations, and hopes to one another? Completing this exercise may help you evaluate areas that you may need to work on.

1. Do you feel that your partner often does not seem to understand you? _____

2. Do you think your partner is pleased with your overall appearance? _____

3. Are you able to give constructive criticism to each other? _____

4. In appropriate places, do you openly show your affection? _____

5. When you disagree, does the same person usually give in? _____

6. Are you able to discuss money matters with each other? _____

7. Are you able to discuss religion and politics without arguing? _____

8. Do you often know what your partner is going to say before he/she says it? _____

9. Are you afraid of your partner's reactions to things that you do or say? _____

10. Do you know where your partner wants to be in five years? _____

11. Is your sense of humour basically the same as your partner's? _____

12. Do you have the persistent feeling you do not really know each other or have never really talked about important issues? _____

13. Would you be able to give an accurate biography of your partner? Do you know about his/her past experiences? _____

14. Do you know your partner's secret fantasy? _____

15. Do you feel you have to avoid discussion of many topics with your partner? _____

16. Does your partner know your biggest flaw? _____

17. Does your partner know what you are most afraid of? _____

18. Do you take a genuine interest in each other's work? _____

19. Can you judge your partner's mood accurately by watching his/her body language? _____

20. Do you know who your partner's favourite relatives are and why? _____

21. Do you know what things you may say that could hurt your partner's feelings? _____

22. Do you know the number of children your partner would like to have? _____

Scoring

Look over your responses and give yourself one point for each YES response to numbers 2, 3, 4, 6, 7, 8, 10, 11, 13, 14, and 16 to 22 and one point for each NO response to numbers 1, 5, 9, 12, and 15.

1–5: This may indicate a low level of communication/interaction between you and your partner. However, you are together, so you must be fulfilling some need through your relationship. Perhaps the two of you simply need to develop better communication.

6–9: This may indicate that your communication/interaction level is rather low, but perhaps you are trying to improve your interactions. What actions might you take?

10–14: This may indicate a moderate communication/interaction level with some room for improvement. Just keep working on the development of open and honest communication.

15–18: You seem to have a strong communication/interaction level, but you do have your differences. With open communication, you are learning to deal with your differences, which will strengthen the relationship.

19–22: You seem to have a great understanding of each other and what it takes to make a successful relationship. Keep being honest, talking, and sharing your feelings.

After rating yourself, what areas do you need to work on? What steps can you take to improve your overall level of communication and intimacy levels?

_____

Source: Adapted by permission of McGraw-Hill, Inc., from Robert F. Valois and Sandra Kammermann, *Your Sexuality: A Personal Inventory* (New York: Random House, 1984), 128–129.

for new forms in which people can express their love and commitment to one another and still have individual needs met more adequately. Success in relating to another human being may have more to do with the quality of the interaction between two people than with the number of years they continue to live together. Many social scientists agree that the ideal in relating to another person is to develop a committed bond, the boundaries and form of which can change to allow the maximum degree of growth over time.

Partnering Scripts

Most parents love their children and want them to be happy. They often believe that their children will achieve happiness by living much as they have. They chose to marry and raise a family, and they expect their children to follow a similar pattern. These expectations usually come from wanting the best for their children rather than from an overt desire to control their lives. Accordingly, children are reared with a very strong script for what is expected of them as adults. This "scripting" is part of what maintains stability within a society. By individuals partnering with someone similar to their families of origin, groups within society remain discernible; children of upper-class parents usually remain in the upper class, children of white partners usually marry a white partner, and so forth. Each group in society has its own partnering script that includes similarities of sex, age, social class, race, religion, physical attributes, and personality types of the prospective partner. By adolescence, people generally know exactly what type of person they are expected to befriend or to date.

As Canadian society becomes increasingly multicultural, in-group partnering is giving way to more frequent mixing of cultures and backgrounds. A relationship between people of different cultural backgrounds can bring with it increased tension. Yet tension is not always a bad thing: it provides an opportunity for individuals to create more flexible behaviour patterns.

For people who select a potential mate on the basis of the script with which they were raised, an elaboration of the concept may seem unnecessary. Yet there are two reasons why it is important to consider the concept of partnering scripts: (1) you may be among the group that has not chosen an "appropriate" partner or (2) social approval of your mate selection may bring with it other subtle expectations of your behaviour as a couple.

People who have not chosen an "appropriate" partner are subject to a great deal of external stress. Recognizing that this stress is external to the relationship can help alleviate criticism and distancing between the partners.

Society provides constant reinforcement for traditional couples. People who choose an "appropriate" partner usually have plenty of validation for the relationship. The love and support they feel from friends and family is genuine. It also comes with expectations of what will occur within the relationship. Decisions that the couple feel should be exclusively theirs may provoke unsolicited advice from friends and family.

Most people who try to influence a couple's relationship do so out of love and respect for the people involved. It is important to remember, especially when relating to parents, that their concern usually comes from a desire for the couple's well-being. They associate well-being with living the way they lived or, in some cases, with living better than they lived. In either case, it is possible to appreci-ate parents' viewpoints but choose to live in a different manner if that is what the couple wants.

WHAT DO YOU THINK?

What characteristics are most important to you in a potential partner? Which of these would be important to your parents or friends? If your parents or friends didn't like a potential partner, how important would their opinion be?

The Importance of Self-Nurturance

It is often stated that you must love yourself before you can love someone else. What does this mean? Learning how you function emotionally and how to nurture yourself through all life's situations is a lifelong task. There seems to be a certain level of individual maturity that needs to be reached before a successful intimate relationship becomes possible. Over half of marriages between teenagers end in divorce. The divorce rate drops to 37 percent among people over 25 years of age at marriage.

Two concepts that are especially important to knowing yourself and maintaining a good relationship are "accountability" and "self-nurturance." **Accountability** means that both partners see themselves as responsible for their own decisions and actions. The other person is not held responsible for the positive or negative experiences in life. Each and every choice is one's own responsibility. A partner can no longer leave a relationship saying, "She ruined my life," or, "He made me do it!" When two people are accountable for their own emotional states, partners can be angry, sad, or frustrated without the other person taking it personally. Accountable people may even say something like, "This has nothing to do with you; I just happen to be angry right now."

Self-nurturance goes hand-in-hand with accountability. In order to make good choices in life, a person needs to maintain a balance of sleeping, eating, exercising, working, relaxing, and socializing. When the balance is disrupted, as it will inevitably be, self-nurturing people are patient with themselves and try to put things back on course. When they make bad choices, as all people do, self-nurturing people learn from the experience. It is a lifelong

Accountability: Accepting responsibility for personal decisions, choices, and actions.

Self-nurturance: Developing individual potential through a balanced and realistic appreciation of self-worth and ability.

process to learn to live in a balanced and healthy way. Two people who are on a path of accountability and self-nurturance together have a much better chance of maintaining satisfying relationships.

Elements of Good Relationships

Relationships that are satisfying and stable share certain elements. Some of these are achieved through conscious efforts and communication; others evolve over time. People in healthy, committed relationships trust one another. Without trust, intimacy will not develop and the relationship will experience trouble and possible failure. **Trust** can be defined as the degree of confidence felt in a relationship. Trust includes three fundamental elements: predictability, dependability, and faith.

- *Predictability* means that you can predict your partner's behaviour. This sense of predictability is based on the knowledge that your partner acts in consistently positive ways.

- *Dependability* means that you can rely on your partner to give support in all situations, particularly in those in which you feel threatened with hurt or rejection.

- *Faith* means that you feel absolutely certain about your partner's intentions and behaviour.

Trust and intimacy are the foundation of healthy committed relationships. Spouses who like and enjoy one another as people and find each other interesting frequently are happier than those who don't. Many spouses describe their partners as their best friends. Although most marriages have their share of ups and downs, members of successful couples are able to talk to, listen to, and touch one another in an atmosphere of caring. They value a good sense of humour and exhibit communication, cooperation, and the ability to resolve conflicts constructively.

Sexual intimacy is also a major part of healthy relationships, but sex is not a major reason for the existence of the relationship. Some couples admit to sexual dissatisfaction within their relationships but feel the relationship is more important than sexual satisfaction. Rather than seek an outlet in an extramarital affair, those who are dissatisfied with their sex lives adjust and spend little energy worrying about it because the relationship is satisfying in other, more important ways. Many couples report that as communication and trust increase in a long-term, committed relationship, the entire sexual relationship also improves.

Trust: The degree of confidence felt in a relationship.

Autonomy: The ability to care for oneself emotionally, socially, and physically.

STAYING SINGLE

While many people choose to marry, have children, and follow in the footsteps of their ancestors, increasing numbers of young and older adults have elected to remain single. Of the 17 percent of people who did not live in a family in 1994, half lived alone. Many of these were women over 65, 34 percent of whom lived alone, in contrast to 14 percent of men in the same age group and 8 percent of the general population aged 15 to 64. Of the remainder not living in a family, 6 percent lived with non-relatives, 2 percent were in institutions, and 1 percent lived with a relative other than a parent, spouse, or never-married child.[28]

Today, large numbers of people choose to or are forced by circumstances to remain single. While many of these people seek or have sought committed relationships, in the absence of a suitable partner, they find singlehood preferable. Singles clubs, social outings arranged by communities and churches, extended-family environments, and a large number of social services support the single lifestyle. Although some research indicates that single people live shorter lives, are more unhappy, are more likely to be financially distressed, and are more prone to illnesses than their married counterparts, other studies contradict these conclusions.[29]

HAVING CHILDREN

When a couple decides to raise children, their relationship changes. Resources of time, energy, and money are split many ways, and the partners no longer have each other's undivided attention. Babies and young children do not time their requests for food, sleep, and care to the convenience of adults. Therefore, individuals or couples whose own basic needs for security, love, and purpose are already met make better parents. Any stresses that already exist in a relationship are further accentuated when parenting is added to the list of responsibilities. Having a child does not save a bad relationship and, in fact, only seems to compound the problems that already exist. A child cannot and should not be expected to provide the parents with self-esteem and security.

Changing patterns in family life affect the way children are raised. In modern society, it is not always clear which partner will adjust his or her work schedule to provide the primary care of children. Remarriage creates a new family of stepparents and stepsiblings. In addition, an increasing number of individuals are choosing to have children in a family structure other than a heterosexual marriage. Single women can choose adoption or alternative (formerly "artificial") insemination as a way to create a family. Single men can choose to adopt or can obtain the services of a surrogate mother. Regardless of the structure of the family, certain factors remain important to the well-being of the unit: consistency, communication, affection, and mutual respect.

Some people become parents without a lot of forethought. Some children are born into a relationship that was supposed to last and didn't. This does not mean it is too late to do a good job of parenting. Attention, consistency, and caring can be provided by other adults if a parent cannot be physically or emotionally present for a period of time. Children are amazingly resilient and forgiving if parents show respect to them and communicate about household activities that affect their lives. Even children who grew up in a household of conflict can feel loved and respected if the parents treat them fairly. This means that parents take responsibility for any of their own conflicts and make it clear to the children that they are not the reason for the conflict.

Changes in the traditional family structure have forced society to examine alternative means of raising children. Day-care centres, extended families, and live-in babysitters will all become important alternatives to the traditional parental unit.

*W*HAT DO YOU THINK?

What are the essential characteristics of a healthy "family" environment? Why is having such an environment so important to the future development of our children? Do you think that day-care centres, extended family units, and full-time babysitters have equal chances of providing a positive environment for personal growth? Why or why not?

*E*NDING A RELATIONSHIP

The Warning Signs

The symptoms of a troubled relationship are relatively easy to recognize. Many couples choose to ignore them, however, until the situation erupts into some type of emotional confrontation. By then, the relationship may be beyond salvaging.

Breakdowns in relationships usually begin with a change in communication, however subtle. Either partner may stop listening, ceasing to be emotionally present for the other. In turn, the other feels ignored, unappreciated, or unwanted. Unresolved conflicts may increase, and unresolved anger can cause problems in sexual relations, with one partner not wanting sex and perhaps giving in and subsequently feeling used.

When a couple who previously enjoyed spending time alone together find themselves continually in the company of others or spending time apart, it may be a sign that the relationship is in trouble. Of course, individual privacy and **autonomy** (the ability to care for oneself emotionally, socially, and physically) are important. If, however, a partner decides to make a change in the amount and quality of time spent together without the input or understanding of the other, it may be a sign of hidden problems.

Honesty and verbal affection are usually very positive aspects of a relationship. In a troubled relationship, however, they can be used to cover up irresponsible or hurtful behaviour. "At least I was honest" is not an acceptable substitute for acting in a trustworthy way. The words "But I really do love you" should not be used as a licence to be inconsiderate, rude, or hurtful to a partner.

Seeking Help: Where to Look

The first place some people look for help when there are problems in a relationship is a trusted friend. Although friends can offer needed support during trying times, few have the training and detachment necessary to resolve problems. Others find that they do not have the type of friendships that lend themselves to divulging deep secrets or problems.

Most communities have private practitioners trained to counsel married or committed couples. Community mental health centres usually have trained counsellors as well. These practitioners may be psychiatrists, licensed psychologists, social workers, or counsellors having advanced degrees. These counsellors are often specially equipped to deal with the unique needs of young adults having relationship, sexual, emotional, financial, or other concerns. Most student health centres and/or counselling centres on campus have reduced student fees for students who need help. If you are unaware of such services, talk with your instructor and ask for his or her advice about where someone with your type of problem may get help.

Trial Separations

Sometimes a relationship becomes so dysfunctional that even counselling cannot bring about significant change. Moving apart for a period of time may allow some preliminary healing and give both parties an opportunity to reassess themselves and their commitment to the relationship. Trial separations do not guarantee that the situation will improve, nor do they mean the relationship is ending. If both people are involved in counselling or have other support systems and mutually agree on the need for a trial separation, it may be a way to regroup and save a failing relationship.

Why Relationships End

In 1995, 77 636 couples in Canada ended their marriages. Many others end relationships of all types. The reasons for relationship breakdown are numerous. Tragedies such as the death of a child, serious illness of one partner, severe financial reverses, and career failures certainly contribute to divorces and relationship endings. Somehow, communication and cooperation between partners break down under the additional stress of these burdens.

What about breakups between people who have never experienced these tragedies? These breakups arise from unmet expectations regarding marriage or relationships in general or personal roles within the relationship. Many people enter marriage with expectations about what marriage will be like and how they and their partner will behave. Many people enter relationships looking for someone to fill the empty spots in their lives. Failure to communicate such expectations to your partner can lead to resentment and disappointment. Because many premarital expectations may be unreasonable, early exploration of these expectations is important. This exploration may take place together or within a support program.

Differences in sexual needs may also contribute to the demise of a relationship. Many partners find that their spouses desire sex at different times or in different styles and frequencies than they do. Unless sexual differences are resolved, one or both partners may begin to feel used and resent sexual activity.

The bottom line is that if couples do not grow together, they often grow apart. Without a commitment to working on their differences, many find it easier to move on, and this decision may be best for all concerned.

Deciding to Break Up

At some point, troubled couples may feel that their relationship is not worth saving. The decision to end the relationship is usually difficult, even for couples whose relationship was over long before the decision.

For married couples, wading through divorce or dissolution proceedings may be painful as they decide child-custody issues, alimony questions, and division of property. Finding legal assistance may be difficult, because painful emotions usually affect judgement. Friends or counsellors may be able to recommend lawyers who understand the emotions that follow the ending of a relationship.

Cohabiting couples also experience difficulty in separating. Legal problems involving property, children, and alimony are often more ambiguous than in a marriage. Some couples expend much time, money, and energy working out settlements with lawyers who specialize in problems following the breakup of a nonmarried committed relationship.

Aside from legal worries, many newly separated or divorced people experience painful emotions of anger, guilt, rejection, and unworthiness. No matter how miserable the relationship, feelings of failure are not uncommon or abnormal following a divorce or breakup, and the emo-

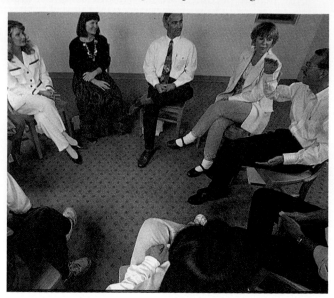

Unresolved conflicts and frequent emotional confrontations are signs of a troubled relationship, but if the partners are committed to staying together, counselling can often bring about positive change.

tional wounds take varying amounts of time to heal. Counsellors familiar with loss and grieving estimate that it takes at least a year and often longer to recover from the loss of a major relationship, whether by death or separation. With time, support from others, and community or professional help, most people do recover and establish new relationships.

Coping with Loneliness

Some people find establishing and maintaining relationships difficult. Others find that through death, illness, or distance, their relationships disappear or grow dim with time. Loneliness, or the unfulfilled desire to engage in a close personal relationship, is a difficult emotion to experience, even for the most determined person.

The loss of an important committed relationship is usually too painful for a person ever to want to repeat. Reflecting on the beginning, the course, and the ending of the relationship can help you avoid the same mistakes in the future. Concentrating on the negative aspects of past behaviour of an ex-partner is a natural tendency but is only helpful in getting in touch with emotions or in learning from the situation. It is equally important to spend time remembering what was loved in the other person and what is lovable about oneself. Intimacy, love, and commitment between people always change the lives of those involved. It is through relationships that we both give and receive our greatest support and validation as worthwhile human beings. When we accept the risk and

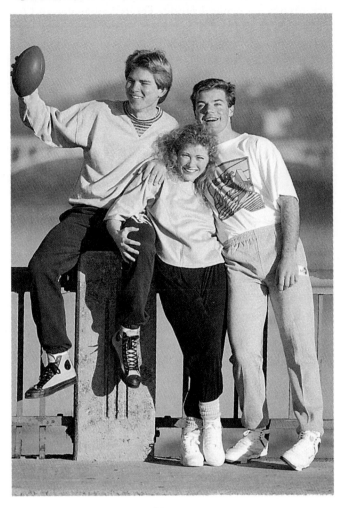

Sexual identity includes not only the physical features that determine one's sex, but also the healthy attitudes expressed in femininity or masculinity.

challenge of close relationships, we accept one of the greatest gifts life has to offer.

DEFINING YOUR SEXUAL IDENTITY

You are a sexual being from birth, but, ironically, you are not born knowing all about your sexuality. Learning about and becoming comfortable with your sexual self is a lifelong process. Taboos, mores, laws, and sexual myths abound. In addition, family members, friends, the media, popular music, your religion, and the educational institutions you have attended all provide you with information about your sexuality and how you should or should not express it. In the end, it is up to you to blend all this information with your personal experience and values to create your own sexual identity.

Your **sexual identity** is determined by a complex interaction of genetic, physiological, and environmental factors. The beginning of your sexual identity occurs at conception with the combining of chromosomes that determine your sex. Actually, it is your biological father who determines whether you will be a boy or a girl. Here's how it works. All eggs (ova) carry an X sex chromosome; sperm may carry either an X or a Y chromosome. If a sperm carrying an X chromosome fertilizes an egg, the resulting combination of sex chromosomes (XX) provides the blueprint to produce a female. If a sperm carrying a Y chromosome fertilizes an egg, the XY combination produces a male (see Figure 5.1).

The genetic instructions included in the sex chromosomes lead to the differential development of male and female **gonads** at about the eighth week of foetal life. Once the male gonads (testes) and the female gonads (ovaries) are developed, they play a key role in all future sexual development because the gonads are responsible for the production of sex hormones. The primary sex hormones produced by females are estrogen and progesterone. In males, the hormone of primary importance is testosterone. The release of testosterone in a maturing foetus signals the development of a penis and other male genitals. If no testosterone is produced, female genitals form.

At the time of **puberty,** sex hormones again play major roles in development. Hormones released by the **pituitary gland,** called gonadotropins, stimulate the gonads (testes and ovaries) to make appropriate sex hormones. The increase of estrogen production in females and testosterone production in males leads to the development of **secondary sex characteristics.** The development of secondary sex characteristics in males includes deepening of the voice, development of facial and body hair, and growth of the skeleton and musculature. In females, the development of secondary sex characteristics includes growth of the breasts, widening of the hips, and the development of pubic and underarm hair.

Sexual identity: Our recognition of ourselves as sexual creatures; a composite of gender, gender roles, sexual preference, body image, and sexual scripts.

Gonads: The reproductive organs in a male (testes) or female (ovaries).

Puberty: The period of sexual maturation.

Pituitary gland: The endocrine gland controlling the release of hormones from the gonads.

Secondary sex characteristics: Characteristics associated with gender but not directly related to reproduction, such as vocal pitch, degree of body hair, and location of fat deposits.

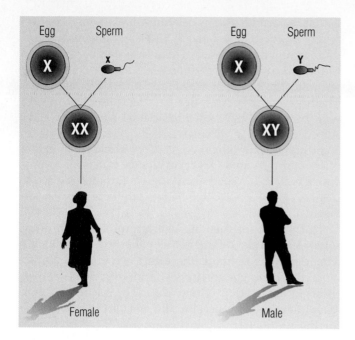

Egg   Sperm   Egg   Sperm

X   x   X   Y

XX   XY

Female   Male

FIGURE 5.1

How Sex Is Determined

Gender Identity and Roles

Thus far, we have described sexual identity only in terms of a person's sex. Sex simply refers to the biological condition of being male or female based on physiological and hormonal differences. **Gender,** on the other hand, refers to your sense of masculinity or femininity as defined by the society in which you live. Each of us expresses our maleness or femaleness to others on a daily basis by the **gender roles** we play. **Gender identity** refers to your per-sonal sense or awareness of being masculine or feminine, a male or a female. It may sometimes be difficult for you to express your true sexual identity because you feel bound by existing gender-role stereotypes. **Gender-role stereotypes** are generalizations about how males and females should express themselves and the characteristics each possesses. Our traditional sex roles are an example of gender-role stereotyping. Men are thought to be independent, aggressive, better in math and science, logical, and always in control of their emotions. Women, on the other hand, are traditionally expected to be passive, nurturing, intuitive, sensitive, and emotional. **Androgyny** is the combination of traditional masculine and feminine traits in a single person. Androgynous people do not always follow traditional sex roles but, rather, try to act appropriately according to the given situation. The process by which a society transmits behavioural expectations to its individual members is called **socialization.** Gender roles are shaped or socialized by our parents, peers, schools, textbooks, advertisements, and many forms of media including television, music, and movies. Think about the current television shows you watch. Do the characters play out traditional gender roles?

By now you can see that defining your sexual identity is not a simple matter. It is a lifelong process of growing and learning. The Skills for Behaviour Change box identifies the characteristics that make up a sexually healthy adult. Your sexual identity is made up of the unique combination of your sex, gender identity, chosen gender roles, sexual preference, and personal experiences. No other person on this earth is exactly like you, and it is up to you to take every opportunity to get to know and like yourself so that you may enjoy your life to the fullest. As the saying goes, sex is what you are born with, but sexuality is who you are.

Gender: Your sense of masculinity or femininity as defined by the society in which you live.

Gender roles: Expression of maleness or femaleness exhibited on a daily basis.

Gender identity: Your personal sense or awareness of being masculine or feminine, a male or female.

Gender-role stereotypes: Generalizations concerning how males and females should express themselves and the characteristics each possesses.

Androgyny: Combination of traditional masculine and feminine traits in a single person.

Socialization: Process by which a society identifies behavioural expectations to its individual members.

External female genitals: The mons pubis, labia majora and minora, clitoris, urethral and vaginal openings, and vestibule of the vagina and its glands.

ℛEPRODUCTIVE ANATOMY AND PHYSIOLOGY

Sexual activity is physical in nature and depends on anatomical and physiological characteristics and conditions. An understanding of the functions of the male and female reproductive systems will help you derive pleasure and satisfaction from your sexual relationships, be sensitive to your partner's wants and needs, and be more responsible in your choices regarding your own sexual health.

Characteristics of Sexually Healthy Adults

Do you have the resources and skills needed to accomplish the tasks listed below? These items have been identified as important aspects of sexual health. If you feel that one or more is beyond your current reach, make a list of the resources and skills you would need to reach this objective.

- Appreciate your own body.
- Interact with both genders in appropriate and respectful ways.
- Express love and intimacy in appropriate ways.
- Avoid exploitative relationships.
- Identify your values.
- Take responsibility for your own behaviour.
- Communicate effectively with family and friends.
- Ask questions of parents and other adults about sexual issues.
- Enjoy sexual feelings without necessarily acting upon them.
- Be able to communicate and negotiate sexual limits.
- Decide what is personally "right" and act on these values.

- Understand the consequences of sexual activity.
- Talk with a partner about sexual activity before it occurs, including limits, contraceptive and condom use, and meaning in the relationship.
- Communicate desires not to have sex and accept refusals to sex.
- If sexually active, use contraception effectively to avoid pregnancy and use condoms and safer sex to avoid contracting or transmitting a sexually transmitted disease.
- Practice health-promoting behaviours, such as regular checkups, and breast or testicular self-exams.
- Demonstrate tolerance for people with different values.
- Understand the impact of media messages on thoughts, feelings, values, and behaviours related to sexuality.
- Seek further information about sexuality as needed.

Source: Reproduced with permission from D. W. Haffner, "Toward a New Paradigm on Sexual Health," *SIECUS Report*, 21, No. 2 (December 1992/January 1993). Copyright Sexuality Information and Education Council of the United States, 130 West 42nd Street, Suite 350, New York, NY 10036.

Female Reproductive Anatomy and Physiology

The female reproductive system includes two major groups of structures, the external genitals and the internal genitals (see Figure 5.2). The **external female genitals** include all structures that are outwardly visible and are often referred to as the vulva. Specifically, the **vulva**, or external genitalia, includes the mons pubis, the labia minora and majora, the clitoris, the urethral and vaginal openings, and the vestibule of the vagina. The **mons pubis** is a pad of fatty tissue covering the pubic bone. The mons serves to protect the pubic bone, and after puberty it becomes covered with coarse hair. The **labia minora** are folds of mucous membrane and the **labia majora** are folds of skin and erectile tissue that enclose the urethral and vaginal openings. The labia minora are found just inside the labia majora.

The female sexual organ whose only known function is sexual pleasure is called the **clitoris.** It is located at the upper end of the labia minora and beneath the mons pubis. Directly below the clitoris is the **urethral opening** through which urine leaves the body. Below the urethral opening is the vaginal opening, or opening to the **vagina.** In some women, the vaginal opening is covered by a thin membrane called the **hymen.** It is a myth that an intact hymen is proof of virginity. The **perineum** is the area between the vulva and the anus. Although not technically part of the external genitalia, the tissue in this area has many nerve endings and is sensitive to touch; it can play a part in sexual excitement.

Vulva: The female's external genitalia.

Mons pubis: Fatty tissue covering the pubic bone in females; in physically mature women, the mons is covered with coarse hair.

Labia minora: "Inner lips" or folds of tissue just inside the labia majora.

Labia majora: "Outer lips" or folds of tissue covering the female sexual organs.

Clitoris: A pea-sized nodule of tissue located at the top of the labia minora.

Urethral opening: The opening through which urine is expelled.

Vagina: The passage in females leading from the vulva to the uterus.

Hymen: Thin tissue covering the vaginal opening.

Perineum: Tissue extending from the vulva to the anus.

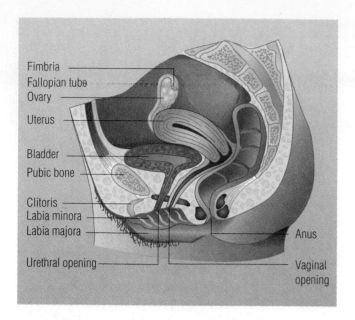

FIGURE 5.2

Side View of the Female Reproductive Organs

Source: From Jeffrey S. Turner and Laurna Rubinson, *Contemporary Human Sexuality,* © 1993, 64. Reprinted by permission of Prentice-Hall, Englewood Cliffs, NJ.

The **internal female genitals** of the reproductive system include the vagina, uterus, fallopian tubes, and ovaries. The vagina is a tubular organ that serves as a passageway from the uterus to the outside of a female's body. This passageway allows menstrual flow to exit from the uterus during a female's monthly cycle and serves as the birth canal during childbirth. The vagina also receives the penis during intercourse. The **uterus,** also known as the womb, is a hollow,

muscular, pear-shaped organ. Hormones acting on the inner lining of the uterus, called the **endometrium,** either prepare the uterus for implantation and development of a fertilized egg or signal that no fertilization has taken place, in which case the endometrium deteriorates and becomes menstrual flow.

The lower end of the uterus is called the **cervix** and extends down into the vagina. The **ovaries** are almond-sized structures suspended on either side of the uterus. The ovaries produce the hormones estrogen and progesterone and are also the reservoir for immature eggs. All the eggs a female will ever have are present in the ovaries at birth. Eggs mature and are released from the ovaries in response to hormone levels. Extending from the upper end of the uterus are two thin, flexible tubes called the **fallopian tubes.** The fallopian tubes are where sperm and egg meet and fertilization takes place. Following fertilization, the fallopian tubes serve as the passageway to the uterus, where the fertilized egg implants and development continues (see Figure 5.3).

The Onset of Puberty and the Menstrual Cycle. With the onset of **puberty,** the female reproductive system matures, and the development of secondary sex characteristics transforms young girls into young women. Under the direction of the endocrine system, the **pituitary gland,** the **hypothalamus,** and the ovaries all secrete hormones that act as the chemical messengers among them. Working in a feedback system, hormonal levels in the bloodstream act as the trigger mechanism for release of more or different hormones (see Figure 5.4).

At around the age of 11 or 12 in females, the hypothalamus receives the message to begin secreting **gonadotropin-releasing hormone (GnRH).** The release of GnRH in turn signals the pituitary gland to release hormones called gonadotropins. **Follicle-stimulating hormone (FSH)** and

---

Internal female genitals: The vagina, uterus, fallopian tubes, and ovaries.

Uterus (womb): Hollow, pear-shaped muscular organ whose function is to contain the developing foetus.

Endometrium: Soft, spongy matter that makes up the uterine lining.

Cervix: Lower end of the uterus that opens into the vagina.

Ovaries: Almond-sized organs that house developing eggs and produce hormones.

Fallopian tubes: Tubes that extend from the ovaries to the uterus.

Puberty: The maturation of the female or male reproduction system.

Pituitary gland: A gland located deep within the brain; controls reproductive functions.

Hypothalamus: An area of the brain located near the pituitary gland. The hypothalamus works in conjunction with the pituitary gland to control reproductive functions.

Gonadotropin-releasing hormone (GnRH): Hormone that signals the pituitary gland to release gonadotropins.

Follicle-stimulating hormone (FSH): Hormone that signals the ovaries to prepare to release eggs and to begin producing estrogens.

Luteinizing hormone (LH): Hormone that signals the ovaries to release an egg and to begin producing progesterone.

Estrogens: Hormones that control the menstrual cycle.

Progesterone: Hormone secreted by the ovaries; helps keep the endometrium developing in order to nourish a fertilized egg; also helps maintain pregnancy.

Menarche: The first menstrual period.

luteinizing hormone (LH) are two gonadotropins, and their role is to signal the gonads, in this case the ovaries, to start producing **estrogens** and **progesterone.** Increased estrogen levels assist in the development of female secondary sex characteristics. In addition, estrogens are responsible for regulating the reproductive cycle. The normal age range for the onset of the first menstrual period, termed the **menarche,** is 10 to 16 years, with the average age being 13 or 14 years.

The average menstrual cycle is 28 days long and divided into three phases, the proliferatory phase, the secretory phase, and the menstrual phase. During the proliferatory phase, the pituitary gland releases FSH and LH. The FSH acts on the ovaries to stimulate the maturation process of several **ovarian follicles (egg sacs).** These follicles secrete estrogens and, in response to this estrogen stimulation, the lining of the uterus, the endometrium, begins to grow and develop. The inner walls of the uterus become coated with a thick, spongy lining composed of blood and mucus. In the event of fertilization, the endometrial tissue will become a nesting place for the developing embryo. The increased estrogen level also signals the pituitary to slow down FSH production but to increase LH secretion. Of the several follicles developing in the ovaries, only one each month normally reaches complete maturity. Under the influence of LH, this one ovarian follicle rapidly matures, and on or about the fourteenth day of the proliferatory phase, it releases an ovum into the fallopian tube—a process referred to as **ovulation.** Just prior to ovulation, the mature egg's follicle begins to increase secretion of progesterone, the first function of which is to spur the addition of further nutrients to the developing endometrium.

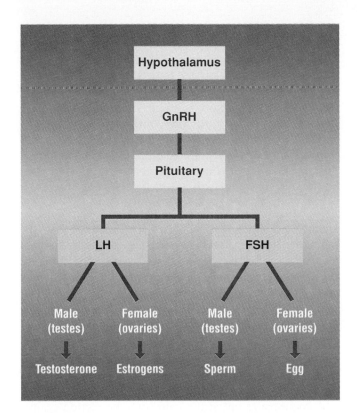

FIGURE 5.4

Hormonal Direction of the Human Reproductive System

After ovulation, the ovarian follicle is converted into the *corpus luteum,* or yellow body, which continues to secrete estrogen and progesterone but in decreasing amounts. In addition, FSH also falls back to its preproliferatory levels. Essentially, the woman's body is "waiting" to see whether fertilization will occur. During this time after ovulation, LH declines, and progesterone levels begin to rise, causing additional tissue growth in the endometrium. This phase of the cycle is called the secretory phase.

If fertilization takes place, cells surrounding the developing embryo release a hormone called **human chorionic gonadotropin (HCG).** This hormone leads to increased levels of estrogen and progesterone secretion, which maintains the endometrium while signalling the pituitary gland not to start a new menstrual cycle.

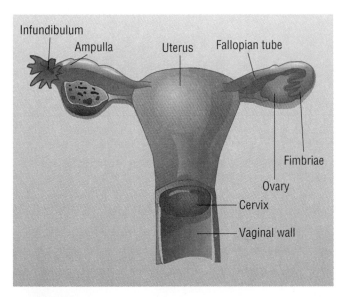

FIGURE 5.3

The Ovaries and Fallopian Tubes

Ovarian follicles (egg sacs): Areas within the ovary in which individual eggs develop.

Ovulation: The point of the menstrual cycle at which a mature egg ruptures through the ovarian wall.

Human chorionic gonadotropin (HCG): Hormone that calls for increased levels of estrogen and progesterone secretion if fertilization has taken place.

When fertilization does not occur, the egg gradually disintegrates within approximately 72 hours. The corpus luteum gradually becomes nonfunctional, causing levels of progesterone and estrogen to decline. As hormonal levels decline, the endometrial lining of the uterus loses its nourishment, dies, and is sloughed off as menstrual flow. Menstruation is the third phase of the menstrual cycle.

Some issues associated with menstruation that you may be interested in reading about are premenstrual syndrome (PMS), toxic shock syndrome (TSS), and dysmenorrhea, or painful menstruation.

Menopause.   Just as menarche signals the beginning of a female's potential reproductive years, **menopause**—the permanent cessation of menstruation—signals the end. Generally occurring between the ages of 50 and 55, menopause results in decreased estrogen levels, which may produce troublesome symptoms in some women. Decrease in vaginal lubrication, hot flashes, headaches, dizziness, and joint pains have all been associated with the onset of menopause. Since estrogen plays a protective role in women by guarding against heart disease and osteoporosis (loss of bone mineral density), postmenopausal women may not only reduce some of the symptoms associated with menopause but also regain some protection against heart disease and osteoporosis by going on hormone-replacement therapy (HRT), or estrogen-replacement therapy (ERT), as it is sometimes called.[30] Unfortunately, HRT/ERT is not without potential risks. Increased risk of gall bladder disease and breast cancer has been reported in some women. But overall, for most women, the benefits of hormone therapy outweigh the risks. Certainly lifestyle changes such as regular exercise and a diet low in fat and adequate in calcium can also help protect postmenopausal women from heart disease and osteoporosis.

WHAT DO YOU THINK?

Why is it so important that we understand the function of our sexual anatomy? Do men need to understand how the menstrual cycle works? Why? Some people are not comfortable using the medical terms for parts of the sexual anatomy. Why do you think this is so?

Male Reproductive Anatomy and Physiology

The structures of the male reproductive system may be divided into external and internal genitals (see Figure 5.5). The penis and the scrotum make up the **external male genitals.** The **internal male genitals** include the testes, epididymides, vasa deferentia, and urethra, and three other structures—the seminal vesicles, the prostate gland, and the Cowper's glands—that secrete components that, with sperm, make up semen. These three structures are sometimes referred to as the **accessory glands.**

The **penis** serves as the organ that deposits sperm in the vagina during intercourse. The urethra, which passes through the center of the penis, acts as the passageway for both semen and urine to exit the body. During sexual arousal, the spongy tissue in the penis becomes filled with blood, making the organ stiff, or erect. Further sexual excitement leads to **ejaculation,** a series of rapid spasmodic contractions that propel semen out of the penis.

Situated behind the penis and also outside the body is a sac called the **scrotum.** The scrotum serves to protect the testes and also helps control the temperature within the testes, which is vital to proper sperm production. The **testes** (singular: *testis*) are egg-shaped structures in which

Menopause: The permanent cessation of menstruation.

External male genitals: The penis and scrotum.

Internal male genitals: The testes, epididymides, vasa deferentia, ejaculatory ducts, urethra, and accessory glands.

Accessory glands: The seminal vesicles, prostate gland, and Cowper's glands.

Penis: Male sexual organ designed for releasing sperm into the vagina.

Ejaculation: The propulsion of semen from the penis.

Scrotum: Sac of tissue that encloses the testes.

Testes: Two organs, located in the scrotum, that manufacture sperm and produce hormones.

Testosterone: The male sex hormone manufactured in the testes.

Spermatogenesis: The development of sperm.

Epididymis: A comma-shaped structure atop the testis where sperm mature.

Vas deferens: A tube that transports sperm toward the penis.

Seminal vesicles: Storage areas for sperm where nutrient fluids are added to them.

Semen: Fluid containing sperm and nutrient fluids that increase sperm viability and neutralize vaginal acid.

Prostate gland: Gland that secretes nutrients and neutralizing fluids into the semen.

Foreskin: Flap of skin covering the end of the penis; it is removed during circumcision.

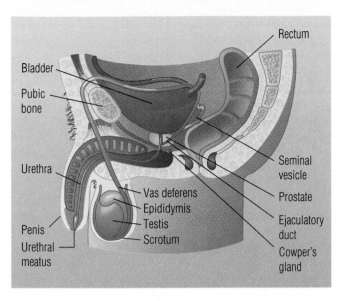

FIGURE 5.5

Side View of the Male Reproductive Organs

Source: From Jeffrey S. Turner and Laurna Rubinson, *Contemporary Human Sexuality,* © 1993, 67. Reprinted by permission of Prentice-Hall, Englewood Cliffs, NJ.

sperm are manufactured. The testes also contain cells that manufacture **testosterone,** the hormone responsible for the development of male secondary sex characteristics.

Spermatogenesis is the term used to describe the development of sperm. Like the maturation of eggs in the female, this process is governed by the pituitary gland. Follicle-stimulating hormone (FSH) is secreted into the bloodstream to stimulate the testes to manufacture sperm. Immature sperm are released into a comma-shaped structure on the back of the testis called the **epididymis** (plural: *epididymides*), where they ripen and reach full maturity.

The epididymis contains coiled tubules that gradually "unwind" and straighten out to become the **vas deferens.** The two vasa deferentia, as they are called in the plural, make up the tubular transportation system whose sole function is to store and move sperm. Along the way, the **seminal vesicles** provide sperm with nutrients and other fluids that compose **semen.**

The vasa deferentia eventually connect each epididymis to the ejaculatory ducts, which pass through the prostate gland and empty into the urethra. The **prostate gland** contributes more fluids to the semen, including chemicals to aid the sperm in fertilization of an ovum, and, more importantly, a chemical that neutralizes the acid in the vagina to make its environment more conducive to sperm motility (ability to move) and potency (potential for fertilizing an ovum).

Just below the prostate gland are two pea-shaped nodules called the Cowper's glands. Their primary function is to secrete a fluid that lubricates the urethra and neutralizes any acid that may remain in the urethra after urination. Urine and semen do not come into contact with each other. During ejaculation of semen, the tube to the urinary bladder is closed off by a small valve.

Circumcision: Risk Versus Benefit. Many new parents must decide whether their male infant will be circumcised. Circumcision involves the surgical removal of the **foreskin,** a flap of skin covering the tip of the penis. Most circumcisions have traditionally been performed for religious/cultural reasons or because of concerns about hygiene. In the uncircumcised male, oily secretions and sloughed-off dead cells (smegma) can collect under the foreskin and create an irritation or set up a breeding ground for infection. Removing the foreskin makes cleansing of the penis easier. Recent studies have shown that about one in ten uncircumcised male babies develops urinary tract infections. Other studies have suggested that uncircumcised males may be at slightly greater risk for penile cancer or HIV infection. These studies are not conclusive, and more research is clearly needed.

Today, infants can be given a local anesthetic, and circumcisions can be performed with little or no pain. This does not mean, however, that the procedure itself is without risk. All surgery involves some risk. If circumcision is performed later in life under a general anesthetic, the risk of complications is greater.

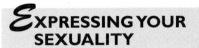

EXPRESSING YOUR SEXUALITY

Finding healthy ways to express your sexuality is an important part of developing sexual maturity. With the many avenues of sexual expression open to you, discovering one that will bring you satisfaction can be very difficult.

Human Sexual Response

Sexual response is a physiological process that involves different stages. The biological goal of the response process is the reproduction of the species. Human psychological traits greatly influence sexual response and sexual desire. Thus, we may find relationships with one partner vastly different from those we might experience with other partners.

Sexual response generally follows a pattern. Laboratory research has delineated four or five stages within the response cycle, and researchers agree that each individual has a personal response pattern that may or may not conform to the stages observed in experimental research. Both males and females exhibit four common stages: excitement/arousal, plateau, orgasm, and resolution. In addition, some males experience a fifth stage, the refractory period. Identification of these stages was achieved in laboratory situations in which genital response was carefully measured using specially designed instruments. Regardless of the type of sexual activity (stimulation by a partner or self-stimulation), the response stages are the same.

During the first stage, *excitement/arousal,* male and female genital responses are caused by **vasocongestion,** or increased blood flow in the genital region. Increased blood flow to these organs causes them to swell. The vagina begins to lubricate in preparation for penile penetration and the penis becomes partially erect. Both sexes may exhibit a "sex flush," or light blush all over their bodies. Excitement/arousal can be generated by touching other parts of the body, by kissing, through fantasy, by viewing films or videos, or by reading erotic literature.

The *plateau phase* is characterized by an intensification of the initial responses. Voluntary and involuntary muscle tensions increase. The female's nipples and the male's penis become erect. A few drops of semen, which may contain sperm, are secreted from the penis at this time.

During the *orgasmic phase,* vasocongestion and muscle tensions reach their peak, and rhythmic contractions occur through the genital regions. In females, these contractions are centered in the uterus, the outer vagina, and the anal sphincter. In males, the contractions occur in two stages. First, contractions within the prostate gland begin propelling semen through the urethra. In the second stage, the muscles of the pelvic floor, the urethra, and the anal sphincter contract. Semen usually, but not always, is ejaculated from the penis. In both sexes, spasms in other major muscle groups also occur, particularly in the buttocks and abdomen. Feet and hands may also contract, and facial features often contort.

Muscle tension and congested blood subside in the *resolution phase,* as the genital organs return to their prearousal states. Both sexes usually experience deep feelings of well-being and profound relaxation. In some

males, a fifth, or *refractory phase,* occurs. Males experience a period of time in which their systems are incapable of subsequent arousal. This refractory period may last from a few minutes to several hours. The length of the refractory period increases with age.

Following orgasm and resolution, many females are capable of being aroused and brought to orgasm again. Males and females experience the same stages in the sexual response cycle; however, the length of time spent in any one stage is variable. Thus, one partner may be in the plateau phase while the other is in the excitement or orgasmic phase. Such variations in response rates are entirely normal. Some couples believe that simultaneous orgasm is desirable for sexual satisfaction. Although simultaneous orgasm is pleasant, so are orgasms achieved at different times.

Sexual pleasure and satisfaction are possible without orgasm or intercourse. Achieving sexual maturity includes learning that sex is not a contest with a real or imaginary opponent. The sexually mature person enjoys sexual activity whether or not orgasm occurs. Expressing love and sexual feelings for another person involves many pleasurable activities, of which intercourse and orgasm may only be a part.

*W*HAT DO YOU THINK?

Why do North Americans place so much importance on the orgasmic phase of sexual response? Do you think there should be a "psychological phase" added to descriptions of the sexual response cycle?

Sexual Orientation

An essential part of your sexual identity is your sexual orientation. **Sexual orientation** refers to a person's potential to respond with sexual excitement to other persons.[31] You may be primarily attracted to members of the other sex (**heterosexual**), your same sex (**homosexual**), or both sexes (**bisexual**).

Homosexuality refers to emotional and sexual attachment to persons of your same sex. Many homosexuals prefer the use of the terms *gay* and *lesbian* to describe their sexual orientations, as these terms go beyond the exclusively sexual connotation of the term *homosexual.* The term *gay* can be applied to both men and women, but the term *lesbian* is applied only to women. Contrary to popular belief, most gays and lesbians are well adjusted and emotionally stable.[32] Some clinicians propose that when maladaptive behaviour does occur in gays and lesbians, it is triggered by the social stigma our society attaches to being gay rather than by something inherently pathological in the homosexual person.[33] **Homophobia,** as defined by Martin Weinberg, is the irrational fear of homosexuality in others, the fear of homosexual feelings within one-

Vasocongestion: The engorgement of the genital organs with blood.

Sexual orientation: Attraction to and interest in members of the opposite sex, the same sex, or both sexes in emotional, social, and sexual situations.

Heterosexual: Refers to attraction to and preference for sexual activity with people of the opposite sex.

Homosexual: Refers to attraction to and preference for sexual activity with people of the same sex.

Bisexual: Refers to attraction to and preference for sexual activity with people of both sexes.

Homophobia: Irrational hatred or fear of homosexuals or homosexuality.

Sexuality and Aging

In our society, we often make the assumption that older adults are sexless. Here are six simple facts about sexuality and aging we should all know.

- *All older people are sexual.* They may not all be having sex, but they all do have sexual beliefs, values, memories, and feelings. To deny this sexuality is to exclude a significant part of the lives of older people.

- *Many older people have a need for a good sexual relationship.* The warmth, intimacy, and security of a good sexual relationship is as important to a 70-year-old as it is to a 20-, 30-, or 40-year-old.

- *Sexual physiology changes with age.* Older men may find that erections occur less frequently, take longer to achieve, are less firm, and are more easily lost. After menopause, older women may find decreased vaginal lubrication a problem. Estrogen replacement or certain over-the-counter lubricants can alleviate this problem in most women.

- *Social attitudes are often frustrating.* Society tends to deny the sexuality of the aged, and in doing so creates complications in their sometimes already difficult lives. A good example is the many rules, customs, and lack of privacy which severely inhibit the establishment of intimate relationships in our retirement facilities and nursing homes.

- *Use it or lose it.* Sexual activity is a physiologic function that tends to deteriorate if not exercised. It is particularly fragile in the elderly.

- *Older folks do it better.* Older people often enjoy sex more because they are experienced, they take their time, they're not goal- (orgasm-) oriented, and they tend to be more leisurely and relaxed.

Do you make the assumption that older people are no longer sexual? Do you treat the older people in your life as sexual beings? What can be done to change our social attitudes toward sexuality and aging?

Source: Adapted with permission from Richard J. Cross, "What Doctors Need to Know: Six Facts on Human Sexuality and Aging," *SIECUS Report,* 21, No. 5 (June/July 1993): 7–9. Copyright Sexuality Information and Education Council of the United States, 130 West 42nd Street, Suite 350, New York, NY 10036.

---

self, or self-loathing because of one's homosexuality.[34] Homophobia in our society is expressed in many ways subtle and not so subtle. Homophobic behaviour can range from avoiding hugging same-sex friends to "gay bashing" (physical and verbal attacks on gays). The emergence of AIDS (acquired immune deficiency syndrome) seems to have magnified antihomosexual prejudice, as many people have erroneously assumed that homosexuality rather than high-risk behaviours is responsible for the epidemic.

Bisexuality refers to emotional attachment and sexual attraction to members of both sexes. Bisexuals may face great social stigma, as they are often ostracized by homosexuals as well as by heterosexuals. Little research has been done on this segment of the population, and many bisexuals remain hidden or closeted. This fear of revealing one's bisexuality to others has been increased during the current AIDS epidemic.

Origins of Sexual Orientation. A variety of theories, both biological and psychosocial, have been proposed to explain why some people are gay or lesbian. One of the most comprehensive and well-done studies on the psychosocial origins of sexual orientation was by Bell, Weinberg, and Hammersmith. They found that (1) sexual preference appears to be largely determined before adolescence; (2) individuals seem to experience homosexual feelings for about three years prior to any open displays of homosexual activity, and these feelings play a larger role in the subject's sexual orientation than does any particular activity; (3) homosexuals tend to have a history of heterosexual experiences during childhood and adolescence but report these experiences as unsatisfying; and (4) identification with a parent of either sex appears to play no significant role in determining one's sexual orientation.[35]

The major biological theories are based upon prenatal hormone levels, structural differences in the brain, and genetic factors. In 1991, Simon LeVay[36] found that in homosexual men, one part of the hypothalamus that influences sexual behaviour was smaller than that same region of the hypothalamus in heterosexual men. Also in 1991, Bailey and Pillard[37] conducted research on the role of genetic factors in the development of sexual orientation. They studied identical twins, fraternal twins, and adoptive brothers of gay men. The researchers wanted to know the percentage of cases in which a gay orientation was present in both siblings when it was present in one sibling. They found that 52 percent of the identical twin brothers of gay men were also gay. In fraternal twins, 22 percent of the brothers were also gay. For genetically unrelated (adopted) brothers, however, it was only 11 percent. These two studies don't prove being gay or lesbian is determined strictly by biological factors, but biology may play a part.

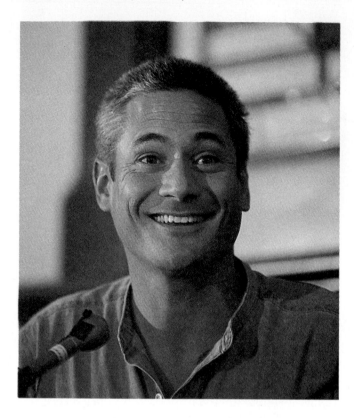

In a society where anti-homosexual attitudes prevail, a gay person's decision to make his or her sexual preference known to the public involves courage and a strong belief in himself or herself.

The cause or causes of sexual orientation are complex. At present there is no single, conclusive explanation for how sexual orientation develops.[38] Most probably the determinants are a combination of various biological and environmental factors that are unique to each person.

*W*HAT DO YOU THINK?

Why is sexual orientation such a controversial subject for some people? Do you think the origin of homosexuality is primarily biological or environmental?

Developing Sexual Relationships

Perhaps the most important part of developing mature sexuality is learning to develop rewarding sexual relationships. Like all skills, developing relationships takes time, patience, and practice. Your sexual education begins with your family. You watch the significant adults in your life and pattern your behaviours after theirs. At puberty, when extrafamilial elements, peers, and the media become more

important, you adapt some of their standards to your behaviours. Your shyness, aggressiveness or assertiveness, passiveness, and levels of comfort with your sexuality come from your own personality and from what you have learned from others.

Not only do you bring your history to your sexual relationships, but you also bring your peculiar chemistry. The human potential for passionate sexual love has been defined as **limerence**. The word *limerence* is derived from the name of the portion of the brain that controls sexual response, the limbic cortex. Limerence is what makes us feel sexually "turned on" by a person. This powerful feeling can overshadow common sense. Sexual relationships based on limerence may or may not develop into long-lasting or committed relationships. Limerence is thought to last only two years at most. Relationships based upon a love that has taken time to mature are much more likely to last. Following are some of the "symptoms" of limerence:

- Intrusive thoughts about the object of desire.

- Dependence of mood on love object's actions.

- Fear of rejection, along with almost incapacitating shyness.

- Sharp sensitivity to interpret desired person's actions favourably and ability to interpret any signs from the other as hidden passion.

- Buoyant, walking-on-air feeling when reciprocation is evident.

- Intensity of feelings that leaves other concerns in the background.

- Ability to emphasize what is admirable in the love object and to avoid dwelling on the negative or even ability to reconceptualize the negative into a positive attribute.[39]

Sexual Expression: What Are Your Options?

The range of human sexual expression is virtually infinite. What you find personally satisfying and enjoyable may not be an option for someone else. The ways you choose to meet your sexual needs today may be very different two weeks or two years from now. Knowing and accepting yourself as a sexual person with individual desires and preferences is the first step in achieving sexual satisfaction.

Celibacy. **Celibacy** is avoidance of or abstention from sexual activities with others. A completely celibate person also does not engage in masturbation (self-stimulation), whereas a partially celibate person avoids sexual activities with others but may enjoy autoerotic behaviors such as masturbation. Some individuals choose to be celibate for religious or moral reasons. Others may be celibate for a period of time due to illness, the breakup of a long-term relationship, or lack of an acceptable partner. For some, celibacy is a lonely, agonizing state, but others find that it can be a time for introspection, value assessment, and personal growth.

Autoerotic Behaviours. The goal of **autoerotic behaviours** is sexual self-stimulation. Sexual fantasy and masturbation are the two most common autoerotic behaviours. **Sexual fantasies** are sexually arousing thoughts and dreams. Fantasies may reflect real-life experiences or forbidden desires or may provide the opportunity for practice of new or anticipated sexual experiences. The fact that you may fantasize about a particular sexual experience does not mean that you want to, or have to, act that experience out. Sexual fantasies are just that—fantasy. Another common autoerotic behaviour is **masturbation**. Masturbation is self-stimulation of the genitals. Although many people feel uncomfortable discussing masturbation, it is a common sexual practice across the life span. Masturbation is a natural, pleasure-seeking behaviour in infants and children. It is a valuable and important means for adolescent males and females, as well as adults, to explore their sexual feelings and responsiveness. In addition, masturbation is an important means of sexual expression for older adults who have lost a lifelong companion or whose companion has a prolonged illness.

Kissing and Erotic Touching. Kissing and erotic touching are two very common forms of nonverbal sexual communication or expression. Both males and females have **erogenous zones,** or areas of the body that when touched lead to sexual arousal. Erogenous zones may include genital as well as nongenital areas, such as the earlobes, mouth, breasts, and inner thighs. Almost any area of the body can be conditioned to respond erotically to touch. Spending time with your partner exploring and learning about his or her erogenous areas is another pleasurable, safe, and satisfying means of sexual expression.

Oral-Genital Stimulation. **Cunnilingus** is the term used for oral stimulation of a female's genitals, and **fellatio** is the term used for oral stimulation of a male's genitals. Many partners find oral-genital stimulation an intensely pleasurable means of sexual expression. For some people, oral sex is not an option because of moral or religious beliefs. It is necessary to remember that HIV and other sexually transmitted diseases (STDs) can be transmitted via unprotected oral-genital sex. Use of an appropriate barrier device is strongly recommended if either partner's disease status is in question or unknown.

Anal Intercourse. The anal area is highly sensitive to touch, and some couples find pleasure in the stimulation

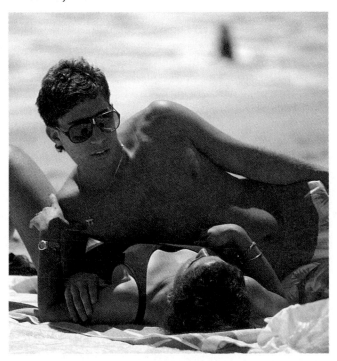

As couples become more comfortable together, each partner learns what pleases the other sexually and emotionally.

of this area. **Anal intercourse** is insertion of the penis into the anus. Stimulation of the anus by mouth or with the fingers is also practiced. As with all forms of sexual expression, anal stimulation or intercourse is not for everyone. If you do enjoy this form of sexual expression, remember to use condoms to prevent disease transmission. Also,

Limerence: The quality of sexual attraction based on chemistry and gratification of sexual desire.

Celibacy: State of not being involved in a sexual relationship.

Autoerotic behaviours: Sexual self-stimulation.

Sexual fantasies: Sexually arousing thoughts and dreams.

Masturbation: Self-stimulation of genitals.

Erogenous zones: Areas in the body of both males and females that, when touched, lead to sexual arousal.

Cunnilingus: Oral stimulation of a female's genitals.

Fellatio: Oral stimulation of a male's genitals.

Anal intercourse: The insertion of the penis into the anus.

anything inserted into the anus should not be directly inserted into the vagina, as bacteria commonly found in the anus can cause infections when introduced into the vagina.

Vaginal Intercourse. The term *intercourse* is generally used to refer to **vaginal intercourse,** or insertion of the penis into the vagina. *Coitus* is another term for vaginal intercourse, which is the most often practised form of sexual expression for most couples. A great variety of positions can be used during coitus. Examples include the missionary position (man on top facing the woman), woman on top, side by side, or man behind (rear entry). Many partners enjoy changing and experimenting with different positions. Sexual intercourse can take on different meanings under different circumstances. It can be a hurried, unplanned event involving little communication in the back seat of a car or an erotic, sensual experience including the exchange of love and mutual emotions in a private setting. Knowledge of yourself and your body, along with your ability to communicate effectively with others, will play a large part in determining the enjoyment or meaning of intercourse for you and your partner. Whatever your circumstance, you should practise safe sex to avoid disease transmission or unwanted pregnancy.

What Is Right for Me?

Invariably, whenever people talk about the spectrum of sexual behaviours, someone in the group will bring up the issue of normality. In *The Joy of Sex,* Alex Comfort summarizes "normality" succinctly:

> Accordingly, if you must talk about "normality," any sex behavior is normal which (1) you both enjoy, (2) hurts nobody, (3) isn't associated with anxiety, (4) doesn't cut down your scope. . . . "Normal" implies there is something which sex ought to be. That is, it ought to be a wholly satisfying link between two affectionate people, from which both emerge unanxious, rewarded, and ready for more.[40]

Many couples worry that they don't have sex often enough. Popular magazines frequently give the "average" number of times couples engage in sex every week. Such numbers are meaningless. Rather than compare yourself to these statistics, you would be wise simply to follow your own feelings. The bottom line is that you must decide what is right or "normal" for you.

Variant Sexual Behaviour

Although attitudes toward sexuality have changed radically since the Victorian era, some people believe that any sexual behaviour other than heterosexual intercourse is abnormal, deviant, or perverted. Rather than using these negative terms, people who study sexuality prefer to use the nonjudgemental term **variant sexual behaviour** to describe sexual behaviours that are not engaged in by most people. The following list of variant sexual behaviours includes behaviours that are illegal in some states and some behaviours that could be harmful to others:

- *Group sex.* Sexual activity involving more than two people. Participants in group sex run a high risk of exposure to HIV infection and other sexually transmitted diseases.

- *Transvestitism.* The wearing of clothing of the opposite sex. Most transvestites are male, heterosexual, and married.

- *Transsexualism.* Strong identification with the opposite sex in which men or women feel that they are "trapped in the wrong body." In some cases, transsexuals undergo sex-change operations.

- *Fetishism.* Describes sexual arousal achieved by looking at or touching inanimate objects, such as underclothing or shoes.

- *Exhibitionism.* The exposure of one's genitals to strangers in public places. Most exhibitionists are seeking a reaction of shock or fear from their victims.

Vaginal intercourse: The insertion of the penis into the vagina.

Variant sexual behaviour: A sexual behaviour that is not engaged in by most people.

Sexual dysfunction: Problems associated with achieving sexual satisfaction.

Inhibited sexual desire (ISD): Lack of sexual appetite or simply a lack of interest and pleasure in sexual activity.

Sexual aversion disorder: Type of desire dysfunction characterized by sexual phobias and anxiety about sexual contact.

Erectile dysfunction: Also known as impotence; difficulty in achieving or maintaining a penile erection sufficient for intercourse.

Impotence: Inability to attain or maintain an erection sufficient for intercourse.

Premature ejaculation: Ejaculation that occurs prior to or almost immediately following penile penetration of the vagina.

Retarded ejaculation: The inability to ejaculate once the penis is erect.

- *Voyeurism.* Observing other people for sexual gratification. Most voyeurs are men who attempt to watch women undressing or bathing. Voyeurism is an invasion of privacy and is illegal.

- *Sadomasochism.* Sexual activities in which gratification is received by inflicting pain (verbal or physical abuse) on a partner or by being the object of such infliction. A sadist is a person who receives gratification from inflicting pain, and a masochist is a person who receives gratification from experiencing pain.

- *Pedophilia.* Sexual activity or attraction between an adult and a child. Any sexual activity involving a minor, including possession of child pornography, is illegal.

*W*HAT DO YOU THINK?

How does our society decide what sexual behaviours are normal and which are variant? Are some sexual behaviours that we consider normal looked upon as abnormal or perverse in other countries or cultures? Why are some individuals very willing to try various sexual behaviours while others are not?

*D*IFFICULTIES THAT CAN HINDER SEXUAL FUNCTIONING

Research indicates that problems that can hinder sexual functioning are quite common in this country. The label given to the various problems that can interfere with sexual pleasure is **sexual dysfunction.** You should not be embarrassed if you experience a sexual dysfunction at some point in your life. The sexual part of yourself does not come with a lifetime warranty. You can have breakdowns involving your sexual function just as you can have breakdowns in any of your other body systems. Sexual dysfunctions can be divided into four major classes: sexual desire disorders, sexual arousal disorders, orgasm disorders, and sexual pain disorders. We will look briefly at each of these categories. In most cases, sexual dysfunctions can be treated successfully if both partners are willing to work together to solve the problem.

Sexual Desire Disorders

The most frequent problem that causes people to seek out a sex therapist is **ISD,** or **inhibited sexual desire.**[41] ISD is the lack of a sexual appetite or simply a lack of interest and pleasure in sexual activity. In some instances, it can result from stress or boredom with sex. **Sexual aversion disorder** is another type of desire dysfunction, characterized by sexual phobias (unreasonable fears) and anxiety about sexual contact. The psychological stress of a punitive upbringing, rigid religious background, or a history of physical or sexual abuse may be one source of these desire disorders.

Sexual Arousal Disorders

The most common disorder in this category is erectile dysfunction. **Erectile dysfunction,** or **impotence,** is difficulty in achieving or maintaining a penile erection sufficient for intercourse. At some time in his life, every man experiences impotence. Causes are varied and include underlying diseases, such as diabetes or prostate problems; reactions to some medications (for example, medication for high blood pressure); depression; fatigue; stress; alcohol; performance anxiety; and guilt over real or imaginary problems (such as when a man compares himself to his partner's past lovers).

Impotence generally becomes more of a problem as men age. Statistics indicate that 2 percent of men at age 40 and 25 percent of men over age 65 experience the problem occasionally.[42]

Chronic impotence (impotence lasting more than three months) should be treated by a physician. A complete medical examination and history are necessary to rule out physical causes. For impotence related to physical causes, new treatments are being explored. These include hormone therapy, treatment with vasoactive drugs (drugs that work on the circulatory system), and vascular surgery to correct abnormalities in the blood vessels that supply the penis.

Impotence due to psychological factors can be treated with psychotherapy. Such treatment is effective in 90 percent of cases.

Orgasm Disorders

Up to 50 percent of the male population are affected by premature ejaculation at some time in their lives. **Premature ejaculation** is ejaculation that occurs prior to or very soon after the insertion of the penis into the vagina. Another orgasm disorder in males is **retarded ejaculation,** or the inability to ejaculate once the penis is erect. Treatment for premature ejaculation involves a physical examination to rule out organic causes. If the cause of the problem is not physiological, therapy is available to help a man learn how to control the timing of his ejaculation. Fatigue, stress, performance pressure, and alcohol use can all be contributing factors to orgasmic disorders in men.

When a woman is unable to achieve orgasm with her partner, she often blames herself and learns to fake orgasm in order to preserve her partner's ego. Research has reported

Building Better Relationships

After reading this chapter, it should be apparent that relationships involve complex interactions between individuals. To build strong relationships, you must carefully assess the values that you put on friendships, significant others, and other forms of interpersonal interactions. Healthy relationships involve developing intimacy in several dimensions. It may be helpful for you to take a personal inventory of your relationships to assess how healthy they are.

Making Decisions for You

Think about the most important relationship in your life. Why is this relationship important to your overall health and well-being? Are there any behaviours that you could change to strengthen this relationship? To make such a change, begin by listing the reasons that the change is important. Who will benefit from this change? What steps will you take to make this change occur? What will you do to make sure that you stay with this behaviour change?

Checklist for Change: Making Personal Choices

✓ What relationships are most important to you right now?

✓ How have these relationships affected your relationships with others? Are you giving enough time to your other relationships?

✓ Have you thought about how good your relationships are from an emotional perspective? A psychological perspective? A physical perspective? Which of these factors is the most important to you? Why?

✓ What would an ideal set of relationships look like for you? How many close interactions would you want to make time for? What would the nature and extent of these relationships be?

✓ Do you feel comfortable with yourself sexually? Are you satisfied with your current choice(s) of sexual expression?

✓ What do you expect in a long-term, committed relationship? What would you be willing to accept in terms of behaviours from your committed partner?

✓ What do you think are the three most important attributes of a friend? Have you displayed these attributes when dealing with your friends?

✓ Do you feel limited or bound by any gender-role stereotypes?

✓ Have you considered your own values/beliefs about what is most important to you in a prospective lifelong partner? Are you asking for the same attributes that you would be able to give to a partner?

Checklist for Change: Making Community Choices

✓ Do you make a habit of putting yourself in the other person's shoes when discussing how your actions may have made that person feel or how that person may be feeling in general?

✓ Do you take time to listen to your friends? Your parents? Your acquaintances? Do you find yourself thinking about your own problems, thoughts, or issues when someone is trying to tell you about their problems?

✓ Do you reach out to friends who are having problems in their relationships?

✓ Are you supportive of couples who are having problems without being judgemental or taking sides?

✓ Do you try to work through your problems with others, or do you run from, avoid, or get angry about rather than try to talk through your difficulties?

✓ Are you supportive of counselling services and other campus/community services that offer help for people who have troubled relationships?

✓ Do you listen carefully to what your legislators propose in the way of family and individual policies and programs that may unfairly harm others?

Critical Thinking

After leading what you consider a normal sexual life, which included several intimate sexual relationships, you meet that special person. When you first started dating, you learned that this person was a practising member of an Eastern religion, but you never really gave much thought to what that meant to your relationship. Now, several months later, as you want to become intimate, you realize that this religion does not accept intercourse before marriage.

You feel sexually frustrated. But at the same time, you are sincerely in love and believe that this relationship could lead to marriage. Using the DECIDE model in Chapter 1, think about what the two of you could do to satisfy both physical and emotional feelings.

that up to 66 percent of women have faked an orgasm at one time or another.[43] Until recently, our society dictated that women were not supposed to enjoy sex but were to engage in it only to fulfill the "marital duty." The Kinsey reports in the 1950s and Masters and Johnson's findings in the 1960s and 1970s raised questions about these female sexual myths.

We recognize today that women enjoy sexual pleasure as much as men do. In the past, women who did not experience orgasm were called frigid. This term is no longer used because it implies that the woman is at fault. Instead, the term **preorgasmic** has been substituted, since most women can be taught to become orgasmic.

For women whose sexual pleasure is hampered, therapy is available. A physical examination to rule out organic causes is generally the first step. Masturbation is usually a primary focus in teaching a woman to become orgasmic. Through masturbation, a woman can learn how her body responds sexually to various types of touch. Once a woman has become orgasmic through masturbation, she learns to communicate her needs to her partner. The investment of time and caring by both partners is usually worth the effort, for 70 percent of preorgasmic women can be helped.

Sexual Pain Disorders

Two common disorders in this category are dyspareunia and vaginismus. **Dyspareunia** is pain experienced by a female during intercourse. This pain may be caused by diseases such as endometriosis, uterine tumours, chlamydia, gonorrhea, or urinary tract infections. Damage to tissues during childbirth and insufficient lubrication during intercourse may also cause pain or discomfort. Dyspareunia can also be psychological in origin. As with other problems, dyspareunia can be treated with good results. The first step in treatment is a thorough pelvic examination to rule out physical disease. Diseases or disorders can usually be cured with medication or surgery. Vaginal lubricants can be purchased to help with inadequate lubrication. Psychologically caused dyspareunia is much more difficult to treat.

Vaginismus is the involuntary contraction of vaginal muscles, making penile insertion painful or impossible. Most cases of vaginismus are related to fear of intercourse or to unresolved sexual conflicts. Treatment of vaginismus involves teaching a woman to achieve orgasm through nonvaginal stimulation. Becoming orgasmic is important because research has indicated that treatment for vaginismus is more successful in orgasmic women. The woman and her partner are then taught methods for dilating the vagina, either with fingers or a vibrator. As dilation is achieved, the woman is taught to relax in order to effect penetration. Cure rates are close to 100 percent.

Drugs and Sex

Because psychoactive drugs affect our entire physiology, it is only logical that they affect our sexual behaviour. Promises of increased pleasure make drugs very tempting to those seeking greater sexual satisfaction. Too often, however, drugs become central to sexual activities and damage the relationship.

Alcohol is notorious for reducing inhibitions and giving increased feelings of well-being and desirability. At the same time, alcohol inhibits sexual response; thus, the mind may be willing, but not the body.

Perhaps the greatest danger associated with use of drugs during sex is the tendency to blame the drug for negative behaviour. "I can't help what I did last night because I was stoned" is a response that demonstrates sexual immaturity. A sexually mature person carefully examines risks and benefits and makes decisions accordingly. If drugs are necessary to increase erotic feelings, it is likely that the partners are being dishonest about their feelings for each other. Good sex should not be dependent on chemical substances.

Preorgasmic: In women, the state of never having experienced an orgasm.

Dyspareunia: Pain experienced by women during intercourse.

Vaginismus: A state in which the vaginal muscles contract so forcefully that penetration cannot be accomplished.

---

*W*HAT DO YOU THINK?

Why do we find it so difficult to discuss sexual dysfunction in our society? Do you think it is more difficult for men than for women to talk about dysfunction? Have you ever used alcohol or some other drug to enhance your sexual performance? Why did you feel the need to rely on something outside yourself?

Summary

◆ Intimate relationships have several different characteristics that play significant roles in determining how happy, healthy, and well adjusted you are as you interact with others.

◆ Men and women often relate very differently in intimate relationships. Understanding these differences and learning how to deal with them is an important aspect of healthy relationships.

◆ Success in committed relationships requires understanding the roles that partnering scripts play, the importance of self-nurturance, the elements of a good relationship, and the ability to confront couple issues.

◆ Today's family structure may look different from that of previous generations, but love, trust, and commitment to a child's welfare continue to be the cornerstones of successful child rearing.

◆ Sexual identity is determined by a complex interaction of genetic, physiological, and environmental factors. Gender, gender roles, and gender-role stereotypes are all blended into our sexual identity.

◆ The major components of the female sexual anatomy include the mons pubis, labia minora and majora, clitoris, urethral and vaginal openings, vagina, cervix, fallopian tubes, and ovaries. The major components of the male sexual anatomy are the penis, scrotum, testes, epididymides, vasa deferentia, ejaculatory ducts, and urethra.

◆ Sexuality can be expressed in many ways. Physiologically, males and females experience four phases of sexual response: excitement/arousal, plateau, orgasm, and resolu-

tion. In addition, men experience a fifth phase known as the refractory period. Sexual orientation refers to a person's preference for emotional, social, and sexual attractions. Sexual activities include celibacy, autoerotic behaviours, kissing and erotic touch, oral-genital stimulation, anal intercourse, and vaginal intercourse. Numerous variant sexual behaviours also exist in our society.

◆ There are many strategies for building better relationships. Taking a careful look at your own behaviours, those things you may need to change, and those things that you are willing to do to help develop a relationship are all important ingredients of success.

Discussion Questions

1. What are behavioural interdependence, need fulfillment, and emotional attachment, and why are each of these important in subsequent relationship development?

2. What are the common types of intimate relationships? Which of these do you think is most important to you right now? Why?

3. Why are your relationships with your family important? Explain how your family unit was similar to or different from the family unit of the early 1900s. Who made up your family of origin? Your nuclear family?

4. How can you tell the difference between a love relationship and one that is based primarily on attraction? What common characteristics do love relationships share?

5. What can serve as barriers to intimacy? Are there actions that you can take to reduce or remove these barriers?

6. What are common elements of good relationships?

7. What actions can you take to improve your own interpersonal relationships?

8. What are the functions of the various hormones during puberty? What physical changes are brought about by menopause?

9. What is "normal" sexual behaviour? Is sexual orientation primarily determined by biological or environmental factors? Do men and women differ in sexual response?

10. Do drugs and alcohol enhance sexual performance? What risks are involved in such experimentation?

Application Exercise

Reread the What Do You Think? scenario at the beginning of the chapter and answer the following question.

From what you have read in this chapter, what problems do Michael and Sara have in their relationship? Why do you think people are often forced to tell lies or half-truths

in their relationships with others? Are there times when it is okay to be dishonest or to not tell the truth, or should you always be totally honest and truthful about your actions? Do you believe that you should tell your partner about all of your sexual interactions? Why or why not?

Health on the Net

Vanier Institute of the Family
www.familyforum.com/vanier/family.htm

Sexual and reproductive health rights in Canada
**www.hc-sc.gc.ca/main/hc/web/datapcb/datawhb/
conference/papers/canada/english/reprod.htm**

6

Birth Control, Pregnancy, and Childbirth

Managing Your Fertility

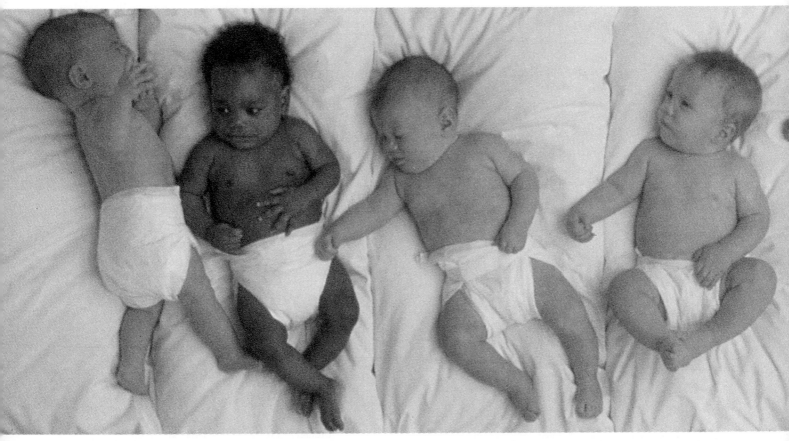

Chapter Objectives

- List permanent and reversible contraceptive methods, discuss their effectiveness in preventing pregnancy and sexually transmitted infections, and describe how these methods are used.

- Summarize the legal decisions surrounding abortion and the various types of abortion procedures used today.

- Discuss emotional health, maternal health, financial evaluation, and contingency planning in terms of your own life's goals as aspects that you should consider before becoming parents.

- Explain the importance of prenatal care and the process of pregnancy.

- Describe the basic stages of childbirth as well as some of the complications that can arise during labour and delivery.

- Review some of the primary causes of and possible solutions to infertility.

Kari and Dave have been dating for several months. After a romantic evening, they go back to Dave's room in the residence hall with the intention of having sex. When they arrive at Dave's, Kari discovers that Dave does not have any condoms. He thought that Kari either would have a diaphragm or was taking the pill. Rather than spoil the evening, Kari and Dave have unprotected sex. The next day, they have an argument over who exactly was responsible for the birth control.

- ■ What mistakes were made in this relationship? Who is responsible for providing birth control? What were the risks involved in having unprotected sex? What were the alternatives?

Fertility is a mixed blessing for some women. The ability to participate in the miracle of birth is an overwhelming experience for many. Yet the responsibility to control one's fertility can also seem overwhelming. Today, we not only understand the intimate details of reproduction but also possess technologies designed to control or enhance our fertility. Along with information and technological advance comes choice, and choice goes hand-in-hand with responsibility. Choosing if and when to have children is one of our greatest responsibilities. A woman and her partner have much to consider before planning or risking a pregnancy. Children, whether planned or unplanned, change people's lives. They require a lifelong personal commitment of love and nurturing.

For couples who want to avoid pregnancy, a wide variety of contraceptives are available, including male and female condoms, IUDs, cervical caps, diaphragms, and different types of pills.

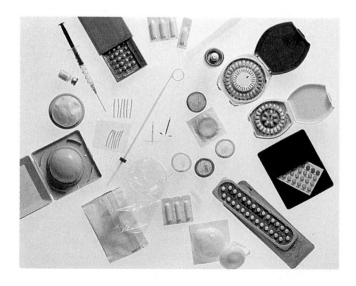

Before you plan or risk a pregnancy, you have the responsibility to make certain you are physically, emotionally, and financially prepared to care for another human being. One measure of maturity is the ability to discuss reproduction and birth control with one's sexual partner before succumbing to sexual urges. Men often assume that their partners are taking care of birth control. Women often feel that if they bring up the subject, it implies that they are "easy" or "loose." You will find embarrassment-free discussion a lot easier if you understand human reproduction and contraception and honestly consider your attitudes toward these matters before you get into compromising situations.

METHODS OF FERTILITY CONTROL

Conception refers to the fertilization of an ovum by a sperm. The sperm enters the ovum. Its tail breaks off, and a protective chemical barrier secreted by the ovum surrounds the sperm and prevents other sperm from entering. The following conditions are necessary for conception:

1. a viable egg

2. a viable sperm

3. possible access to the egg by the sperm

Contraception refers to methods of preventing conception. Ever since people first associated sexual activity with pregnancy, society has searched for a simple, infallible, and risk-free method of preventing pregnancy. We have not yet succeeded in finding one.

Our present methods of contraception fall into two categories: *reversible methods,* such as the pill, condoms, and abstinence; and *permanent methods,* such as vasectomy (for men) and tubal ligation (for women). Let's discuss some of the methods in each category in detail so you

Which Contraceptive Method Is Right for You and Your Partner?

If you are sexually active, you need to use the contraceptive method that will work best for you. A number of factors may be involved in your decision. The following questions will help you sort out these factors and choose an appropriate method. Answer yes (Y) or no (N) for each statement as it applies to you and, if appropriate, your partner.

1. I like sexual spontaneity and don't want to be bothered with contraception at the time of sexual intercourse.
2. I need a contraceptive immediately.
3. It is very important that I do not become pregnant now.
4. I want a contraceptive method that will protect me and my partner against sexually transmissible infections.
5. I prefer a contraceptive method that requires the co-operation and involvement of both partners.
6. I have sexual intercourse frequently.
7. I have sexual intercourse infrequently.
8. I am forgetful or have a variable daily routine.
9. I have more than one sexual partner.
10. I have heavy periods with cramps.
11. I prefer a method that requires little or no action or bother on my part.
12. I am a nursing mother.
13. I want the option of conceiving immediately after discontinuing contraception.
14. I want a contraceptive method with few or no side-effects.

If you answered yes to the statements listed on the left, the method on the right may be a good choice for you.

1, 3, 6, 10, 11	Oral contraceptives
1, 3, 6, 8, 10, 11	Norplant
1, 3, 6, 8, 10, 11, 12	Depo-Provera
1, 3, 6, 8, 11, 12, 13	IUD
2, 4, 5, 7, 8, 9, 12, 13, 14	Condoms (male and female)
5, 7, 12, 13, 14	Diaphragm and spermicide
5, 7, 12, 13, 14	Cervical cap
2, 5, 7, 8, 12, 13, 14	Vaginal spermicides
5, 7, 13, 14	FAM

Your answers may indicate that more than one method would be appropriate for you. To help narrow your choices, circle the numbers of the statements that are *most* important for you. Before you make a final choice, talk with your partner(s) and your physician. Consider your own lifestyle and preferences as well as characteristics of each method (effectiveness, side-effects, costs, and so on). For maximum protection against pregnancy and STDs, you might want to consider combining two methods.

Source: Reprinted by permission from Bryan Strong and Christine DeVault, *Human Sexuality,* © 1994 Mayfield Publishing Company.

---

will have the information you need to make an informed choice (also see the Rate Yourself box).

Reversible Contraception

Abstinence and "Outercourse." Strictly defined, abstinence means deliberately shunning intercourse. This strict definition would allow one to engage in such forms of sexual intimacy as massage, kissing, and solitary masturbation. But many people today have broadened the definition of abstinence to include all forms of sexual contact, even those that do not culminate in sexual intercourse.

Couples who go a step farther than massage and kissing and engage in such activities as oral-genital sex and mutual masturbation are sometimes said to be engaging in "outercourse." Like abstinence, outercourse can be 100 percent effective for birth control as long as the male does not ejaculate near the vaginal opening. Unlike abstinence, however, outercourse is not 100 percent effective against

sexually transmitted infections (STIs). Oral-genital contact can result in transmission of an STI, although the practice can be made safer by using a condom on the penis or a dental dam on the vaginal opening.

The Condom. The **condom** is a strong sheath of latex rubber or other material designed to fit over an erect penis.

Fertility: A person's ability to reproduce.

Conception: The fertilization of an ovum by a sperm.

Contraception: Methods of preventing conception.

Condom: A sheath of thin latex or other material designed to fit over an erect penis and to catch semen upon ejaculation.

The condom catches the ejaculate, thereby preventing sperm migration toward the egg. The condom is the only temporary means of birth control available for men and the only barrier that effectively prevents the spread of STIs and HIV infection. Regardless of your preferred method of birth control, you should always use a condom. Condoms come in a wide variety of styles: coloured, ribbed for "extra sensation," lubricated, nonlubricated, and with or without reservoirs at the tip. All may be purchased with or without spermicide in pharmacies, in some schools, and in some public washrooms. Some health clinics provide condoms free of charge. A new condom must be used for each act of intercourse or oral sex.

Condoms help prevent the spread of some sexually transmitted infections, including genital herpes and HIV infection. They may also slow or reduce the development of cervical abnormalities in women that can lead to cancer. The theoretical **contraceptive effectiveness rate** for condoms is 98 percent, meaning that *when they are used correctly,* 2 women out of 100 using condoms will become pregnant in one year. In actuality, however, their effectiveness rate is only 88 percent because they are so often used incorrectly. The failure rates of contraceptives are shown in Table 6.1. Condoms should be used during every act of intercourse or oral sex. They must be rolled on the erect penis before the penis touches the vagina, leaving about a 1 centimetre space at the tip to collect ejaculated semen. The condom should be held at the base when the penis is

removed from the vagina after ejaculation to avoid spilling any semen. For greatest efficacy, they should be used with a spermicide containing nonoxynol-9.

Another reason that condoms are not as effective in real life as in theory is that they can break during intercourse, especially if they are old or poorly stored. They must be stored in a cool place (not in a wallet or hip pocket) and should be inspected before use for small tears.

Some people claim that a condom ruins the spontaneity of sex. Stopping to put it on breaks the mood for them. Others report that the condom decreases sensation. These perceived inconveniences contribute to improper use of the device. Couples who learn to put the condom on together as part of foreplay are generally more successful with this form of birth control.[1]

Oral Contraceptives. **Oral contraceptive** pills were first marketed in Canada in 1961 though they were theoretically illegal at that time. In 1960, a Toronto pharmacist was put in jail for selling condoms. The use of contraception became legal in Canada in 1969. The convenience of oral contraceptives quickly made them the most widely used reversible method of fertility control.

Most oral contraceptives work through the combined effects of synthetic estrogen and progesterone. Because the levels of estrogen in the pill are higher than those produced by the body, the pituitary gland is never signalled to produce follicle-stimulating hormone (FSH), without which

---

TABLE 6.1 ■ Available Methods of Contraception and Failure Rates

Nearly half of unplanned pregnancies occur to women who were using contraception, mainly because of inconsistent and incorrect use. Listed below are methods of contraception and their ranges of failure rates. While these data are taken from U.S. studies, Canadian patterns are probably similar.

	Percentage of Sexually Active Couples Who Use It	Failure Rate	
		Perfect Use	Average Use
For women			
• Pill	25	0.1%	6.0%
• Diaphragm/cervical cap	5.7	6%	18%
• Sponge	1.1	8%	24%
• IUD	1.0	0.8%	4.0%
• Spermicides (foams, creams, gels)	6.0	3.0%	30%
For men and women			
• Condoms	19	2.0%	16%
• Sterilization			
Tubal ligation	27	0.2%	0.5%
Vasectomy	NA	0.1%	0.2%
• Withdrawal/rhythm	7.0	4.0%	24%

Source: Adapted with permission of Ortho-McNeil Pharmaceutical and the Alan Guttmacher Institute from Robin Herman, "Whatever Happened to the Contraceptive Revolution?" *Washington Post,* Health Section, December 13, 1994, 12–16. Contraceptive usage data from the 1993 Ortho Annual Birth Control Study; failure rate data from the Alan Guttmacher Institute.

Talking with Your Partner About Using Condoms

Knowing what's best for our health and doing something about it can be two different things. Even bringing up the subject of condoms can be hard. Here are some suggestions:

- Think about what you want to say ahead of time. Sort out your own feelings about using condoms before you talk with your partner.

- Choose a time to talk before that first intimate moment. Getting things straight before you make love means you'll both be prepared and relaxed.

- Decide how you want to start the conversation. You might say, "I need to talk with you about something that's important to both of us," or, "I've been hearing a lot lately about safer sex. Have you ever tried condoms?" or, "I feel kind of embarrassed, but I care too much about you not to talk about this."

- Remember, starting to talk is the hardest part. Don't be surprised if your partner responds with, "I'm glad you brought it up. I was worried too," or, "I like sharing the responsibility of sex. I appreciate a woman who's willing to let me."

- Once you've both agreed to use condoms, do something positive and fun. Go to the store together. Buy lots of different brands and colors. Plan a special day when you can experiment. Just talking about how you'll use all those condoms can be a turn on.

Source: Reprinted with permission from *Condoms: Talking with Your Partner,* ETR Associates, Santa Cruz, CA. For more information about this and other related materials, call 1-800-321-4407.

---

ova will not develop in the ovaries. Progesterone in the pill prevents proper growth of the uterine lining and thickens the cervical mucus, forming a barrier against sperm.

Pills are meant to be taken in a cycle. At the end of each three-week cycle, the user discontinues the drug or takes a placebo pill for one week. The resultant drop in hormones causes the uterine lining to disintegrate, and the user will have a menstrual period, usually within one to three days. The same cycle is repeated every 28 days. Menstrual flow is generally lighter than in a non-pill-user because the hormones in the pill prevent thick endometrial buildup.

Today's pill is different from the one introduced more than three decades ago. The original pill contained large amounts of estrogen, which caused certain risks for the user, whereas the current pill contains the minimal amount of estrogen necessary to prevent pregnancy.

Because the chemicals in oral contraceptives change the way the body metabolizes certain nutrients, all women using the pill should check with their prescribing practitioners regarding dietary supplements. The nutrients of concern include vitamin C and the B-complex vitamins—B_2, B_6, and B_{12}. A nutritious diet that includes whole grains, fresh fruits and vegetables, lean meats, fish and poultry, and nonfat dairy products is advised.

Oral contraceptives can interact negatively with other drugs. Some antibiotics diminish the pill's effectiveness, as can the 24-hour flu or diarrhea. A backup contraceptive should be used for the rest of the pill pack if these circumstances occur. Women in doubt should check with their prescribing practitioners, their pharmacists, or other knowledgeable health professionals. You can learn more about health methods and contraceptive choice in the Skills for Behaviour Change box.

Return of fertility may be delayed after discontinuing the pill, but the pill is not known to cause infertility. Women who had irregular menstrual cycles before going on the pill are more likely to have problems conceiving, regardless of pill use.

The effectiveness rate of oral contraceptives is 97 percent, making them one of the most effective reversible methods of fertility control. Use of the pill is convenient and does not interfere with lovemaking. It may lessen menstrual difficulties, such as cramps and premenstrual syndrome (PMS). Women using oral contraceptives have lower risks for developing endometrial and ovarian cancers. They are also less likely than nonusers to develop fibrocystic breast disease. In addition, pill users have lower incidences of ectopic pregnancies, ovarian cysts, pelvic inflammatory disease, and iron deficiency anemia.[2] But possible serious health problems associated with the pill include the tendency for pill users' blood to form clots and an increased risk for high blood pressure in a few women. Clotting can lead to strokes or heart attacks. The risk is low for most healthy women under 35 who do not smoke; it increases with age and, especially, with cigarette smoking.

Contraceptive effectiveness rate: The percentage rate of women who will become pregnant in one year when the contraceptive method is used correctly.

Oral contraceptive pills: Pills taken daily for three weeks of the menstrual cycle which prevent ovulation by regulating hormones.

Outside these risk factors and certain side-effects associated with the pill, its greatest disadvantage is that it must be taken every day. If a woman misses taking one pill, she is advised to use an alternative form of contraception for the remainder of that cycle. The cost of the pill may also be a problem for some women. Finally, some younger teenagers report that the requirement to have a complete gynecological examination in order to get a prescription for the pill is a huge obstacle. Fully 69 percent of female teenagers think that this requirement frightens their peers away from use of the pill.[3] Educating young women about what goes on in a gynecological exam would certainly help ease their anxiety.

Progestin-Only Pills.

Progestin-only pills (or minipills) contain small doses of progesterone. Women who feel uncertain about using estrogen pills, who suffer from side-effects related to estrogen, or who are nursing may want to take these pills rather than combination pills. There is still some question about the specific ways progestin-only pills work. Current thought is that they change the composition of the cervical mucus, thus impeding sperm travel. They may also inhibit ovulation in some women. The effectiveness rate of progestin-only pills is 96 percent, which is slightly lower than that of estrogen-containing pills. Also, their use usually leads to irregular menstrual bleeding.

The Morning-After Pill.

The term **morning-after pill** refers to drugs that can be taken up to three days after unprotected intercourse to prevent fertilization or implantation. The most common drug prescribed is a combination of estrogen and progesterone. Other preparations include large doses of progesterone or a large dose of estrogen called **diethylstilbestrol (DES).** Of all the drugs available to prevent pregnancy, DES is the most risky. Between 1941 and 1970, DES was given to pregnant women to prevent miscarriage. Babies born to these women are today at increased risk for developing a rare vaginal cancer (in women) or genital abnormalities (in men). Nausea or vomiting is the most likely side-effect of these drugs. Other risks are the same as those associated with combination pills.

The morning-after pill is for a one-time emergency use only. It is not a method to be used regularly. No serious side-effects have been observed when women take these drugs under medical supervision.

Foams, Suppositories, Jellies, and Creams.

Like condoms, these contraceptive preparations are available without a prescription. Chemically, they are referred to as **spermicides**—substances designed to kill sperm.

Jellies and creams are packaged in tubes, and foams are available in aerosol cans. They must be inserted far enough into the vagina to cover the cervix, providing both a chemical barrier that kills sperm and a physical barrier that stops sperm from continuing toward an egg.

Suppositories are waxy capsules that are placed deep in the vagina and melt once they are inside. They must be inserted 10 to 20 minutes before intercourse to have time to melt but no longer than one hour prior to intercourse or they lose their effectiveness. Additional contraceptive chemicals must be applied for each subsequent act of intercourse (see Figure 6.1).

Jellies, creams, suppositories, and foam do not require a prescription. When used in conjunction with a condom, their effectiveness rate is nearly 98 percent. They help prevent the spread of certain sexually transmitted infections.

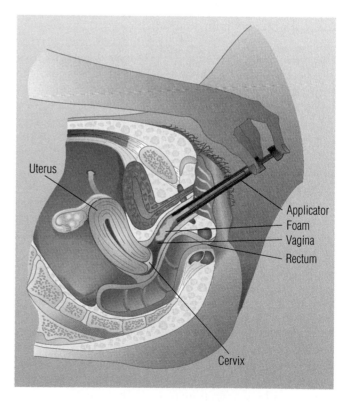

FIGURE 6.1

The Proper Method of Applying Spermicide Within the Vagina

Morning-after pill: Drugs taken within three days after intercourse to prevent fertilization or implantation.

Diethylstilbestrol (DES): Type of morning-after pill containing large amounts of estrogen.

Spermicides: Substances designed to kill sperm.

Female condom: A single-use polyurethane sheath for internal use by women.

Diaphragm: A latex, saucer-shaped device designed to cover the cervix and block access to the uterus; should always be used with spermicide.

Toxic shock syndrome (TSS): A potentially life-threatening disease that occurs when specific bacterial toxins are allowed to multiply unchecked in wounds or through improper use of tampons or diaphragms.

Jellies and creams are designed to be used with a diaphragm. Used alone, their effectiveness rate is only 79 percent. Foam, which is designed to be used alone, also has an effectiveness rate of 79 percent.

Contraceptive Film. This is available in Canada but is not widely distributed. It is a translucent square that is inserted to cover the cervix, like jellies or foams, close to the time of intercourse. Some women prefer it as it is less messy than jellies or foam. It does not have to be removed, as it dissolves.

The Female Condom. This new contraceptive device for internal use by women has now been approved by the Health Protection Branch of Health Canada. The **female condom** is a single-use, soft, loose-fitting polyurethane sheath. It is designed as one unit with two diaphragm-like rings. One ring, which lies inside the sheath, serves as an insertion mechanism and internal anchor. The other ring, which remains outside the vagina once the device is inserted, protects the labia and the base of the penis from infection. Tests conducted by the company that manufactures the female condom found that it was 87.6 percent effective among women in the United States. Many women like the female condom because it gives them more control over their reproduction than does the male condom.

The Diaphragm with Spermicidal Jelly or Cream. Invented in the mid-nineteenth century, the **diaphragm** was the first widely used birth control method for women. Prior to that time, most women had to rely on their male partners to use a condom or to withdraw the penis before ejaculation.

The diaphragm is a soft, shallow cup made of thin latex rubber. Its flexible, rubber-coated ring is designed to fit snugly behind the pubic bone in front of the cervix and over the back of the cervix on the other side. Diaphragms are manufactured in different sizes and must be fitted to the woman by a trained practitioner. The practitioner should also be certain that the user knows how to insert her diaphragm correctly before she leaves the practitioner's office.

Diaphragms must be used with spermicidal cream or jelly. The spermicide is applied to the inside of the diaphragm before insertion. The jelly or cream is held in place by the diaphragm, creating a physical and chemical barrier against sperm. Additional spermicide must be applied before each subsequent act of intercourse, and the diaphragm must be left in place for six to eight hours after intercourse to allow the chemical to kill any sperm remaining in the vagina (see Figure 6.2).

The effectiveness rate of the diaphragm is only 82 percent. Using the diaphragm during the menstrual period or leaving the diaphragm in place beyond the recommended time slightly increases the user's risk of developing **toxic shock syndrome (TSS).** This condition results from the multiplication of a type of bacteria that spreads to the bloodstream and causes sudden high fever, rash, nausea, vomiting, diarrhea, and a sudden drop in blood pressure. If not treated, TSS can be fatal. The diaphragm (as well as tampons left too long in place) creates conditions conducive to the growth of these bacteria. To reduce the risk of TSS, women should wash their hands carefully with soap and water before inserting or removing the diaphragm.

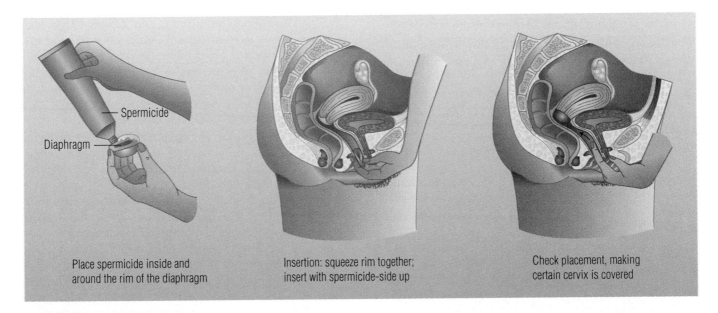

Place spermicide inside and around the rim of the diaphragm

Insertion: squeeze rim together; insert with spermicide-side up

Check placement, making certain cervix is covered

FIGURE 6.2

The Proper Use and Placement of a Diaphragm

Choosing a Contraceptive

Part of sexual maturity is taking responsibility for your personal health regarding contraceptives. Aside from simply worrying about contraceptive effectiveness and convenience, you need to consider the effects that your birth control method may have on your health now and in the future. Here are some things to keep in mind when you decide on your contraceptive method:

1. Talk to your medical professional about your and your family's medical history. Is there anything that would discourage use of one method or another? For example, contraceptive methods may have serious side-effects according to your medical history. Someone with diabetes would not be a good candidate for Norplant.

2. Learn about the potential side-effects. If you find yourself experiencing the side-effects of a contraceptive, you should talk to your doctor immediately. Your doctor may suggest switching to a different contraceptive or may simply assure you that the "side-effects" don't appear related to contraceptive use.

3. Devise a method to ensure that you can't miss using it. If you take the pill, take it at the same time every day. Associating it with a certain time or event (for instance,

taking a morning shower) will reinforce your memory. If you use condoms, you might keep some in your sport coat jacket so that they will be there when you need them. Or you might keep your diaphragm packed in your overnight bag.

4. Learn how to talk to your partner about your choice of contraception. Decisions about contraceptives should be made as a couple, taking each person's health and desires into account.

5. Learn about drug interactions with your birth control method. While we will discuss this in more detail in Chapter 10, it is important to know what medications may interact with your method of birth control. For example, reactions may occur between alcohol and contraceptive pills or between antibiotics and contraceptive pills. In other words, alcohol and antibiotics may diminish the effectiveness of birth control pills in some women. Ask your doctor about drug interactions if you receive a prescription drug. If there is a potential for diminished effectiveness of your contraceptive, ask when can you resume normal sexual relations without taking added precautions.

Another problem with the diaphragm is that it can put undue pressure on the urethra, blocking urinary flow and predisposing the user to bladder infections. A further disadvantage is that inserting the device can be awkward, especially if the woman is rushed. When inserted incorrectly, the effectiveness rate of the diaphragm decreases.

The Contraceptive Sponge. First manufactured in 1983, the contraceptive sponge gained in popularity among young women during the 1980s and early 1990s. Plagued by problems with reliability, allergic reactions, and other serious concerns, the original sponge was discontinued. In Canada, a new sponge is available called Protectaid.

Cervical Cap. Cervical caps are one of the oldest methods used to prevent pregnancy. Early caps were made from beeswax, silver, or copper. The modern cervical cap has been available in Europe for several years and has been approved for use in Canada by the Health Protection Branch since 1982.

The cervical cap is a small cup made of latex that is designed to fit snugly over the entire cervix. It must be fitted by a practitioner and is designed for use with contraceptive jelly or cream. It is somewhat more difficult to insert than a diaphragm because of its smaller size.

The cap keeps sperm out of the uterus. It is held in place by suction created during application. Insertion

may take place anywhere up to two days prior to intercourse, and the device must be left in place for six to eight hours after intercourse. The maximum length of time the cap can be left on the cervix is 48 hours. If removed and cleaned, it can be reinserted immediately.

The effectiveness rate of the cap is only 82 percent. Some women report unpleasant vaginal odours after use. Because the device can become dislodged during intercourse, placement must be checked frequently. It cannot be used during the menstrual period or for longer than 48 hours because of the risk of toxic shock syndrome.

Intrauterine Devices. Widespread use of **intrauterine devices (IUDs)** for contraception began in the mid-1960s, when these devices were advertised as less risky and more convenient than the pill.

The devices began to fall out of favour in the mid-1970s following negative publicity about the Dalkon Shield, a device associated with pelvic inflammatory disease and sterility. The manufacturer stopped making Dalkon shields in 1975.

We are not certain how IUDs work, despite the fact that women have been using them since 1909. Although it was once thought that IUDs act by preventing implantation of a fertilized egg, most experts now believe that they interfere with the sperm's fertilization of the egg.

Two IUDs are currently available. The first is Nova-T, and the second is Gyne-T.

A physician must fit and insert the IUD. For insertion, the device is folded and placed into a long, thin plastic applicator. The practitioner measures the depth of the uterus with a special instrument and then uses these measurements to place the IUD accurately. When in place, the arms of the T open out across the top of the uterus. One or two strings extend from the IUD into the vagina so the user can check to make sure that her IUD is in place. The device is removed by a practitioner when desired.

IUDs are 95 percent effective. But the discomfort and cost of insertion may be a disadvantage for some. When in place, the device can cause heavy menstrual flow and severe cramps. There is a risk of uterine perforation. Women using IUDs have a higher risk of ectopic pregnancy, pelvic inflammatory disease, infertility, and tubal infections. If a pregnancy occurs while the IUD is in place, the chance of miscarriage is 25 to 50 percent. Removal of the device as soon as the pregnancy is known is advised. Doctors often offer therapeutic abortion to women who become pregnant while using an IUD because of the serious risks (including premature delivery, infection, and congenital abnormalities) associated with continuing the pregnancy.

Withdrawal. This not very effective method of birth control is most commonly used by people who have not taken the time to consider alternatives. The **withdrawal** method involves withdrawing the penis from the vagina just prior to ejaculation. Because there can be up to half a million sperm in the drop of fluid at the tip of the penis before ejaculation, this method is unreliable. Timing withdrawal is also difficult; males concentrating on accurate timing may not be able to relax and enjoy intercourse. The effectiveness rate for the withdrawal method is 82 percent.

New Methods of Birth Control

Depo-Provera. **Depo-Provera** is a long-acting synthetic progesterone that is injected intramuscularly every three months. Although used in other countries for years, the Health Protection Branch did not approve it for use in Canada until 1997. Researchers believe that the drug prevents ovulation.

Depo-Provera encourages sexual spontaneity because the user does not have to remember to take a pill or to insert a device. Its effectiveness in preventing pregnancy is higher than 99 percent, which is better than the pill's effectiveness. There are fewer health problems associated with Depo-Provera than with estrogen-containing pills. The main disadvantage is irregular bleeding, which can be troublesome at first, but within a year, most women are amenorrheic (have no menstrual periods). Weight gain (an average of five pounds in the first year) is common. Other possible side-effects include dizziness, nervousness,

and headache. Unlike other methods of contraception, this method cannot be stopped immediately if problems arise. Fertility may not occur immediately after Depo-Provera is discontinued.

Norplant. One of the newest forms of hormonal contraception is **Norplant**. It has been tested by more than 1 million women in 45 countries and is now approved for use in 14 countries.

Six silicon capsules that contain progestin are surgically inserted under the skin of a woman's upper arm. For five years, small amounts of progestin are continuously released. The progestin in Norplant works the same way as oral contraceptives do; it suppresses ovulation, prevents growth of uterine lining, and thickens the cervical mucus.

Norplant is one of the most effective methods of birth control ever developed. With a greater than 99 percent success rate in preventing pregnancy, its effectiveness approaches that of sterilization.[4]

Norplant can be inserted by a specially trained doctor, nurse, or nurse practitioner in 10 to 15 minutes. A local anesthetic is administered to the upper arm, a small injection is made, and, with a special needle, the six capsules are placed just under the skin in a fan shape. The capsules are similarly removed after five years or, if necessary, at any point after their insertion. Another type of Norplant is being developed that lasts for three years.

The capsules usually cannot be seen, nor does insertion leave a scar in most women. At this time, no serious side-effects are known. Less serious side-effects include irregular bleeding and irregular menstrual periods, acne, weight gain, breast tenderness, headaches, nervousness, and nausea.

An effectiveness rate greater than 99 percent makes Norplant one of the most effective reversible methods of fertility control. In addition to being very convenient, the implant is easy for a trained practitioner to do, so there is little chance of error, and costs less than the contraceptive pill.[5]

Cervical cap: A small cup made of latex that is designed to fit snugly over the entire cervix.

Intrauterine device (IUD): A T-shaped device that is implanted in the uterus to prevent pregnancy.

Withdrawal: A method of contraception that involves withdrawing the penis from the vagina before ejaculation. Also called "coitus interruptus."

Depo-Provera: An injectable method of birth control that lasts for three months.

Norplant: A long-lasting contraceptive that consists of six silicon capsules surgically inserted under the skin in a woman's upper arm.

Infant Mortality Among First Nations

Although there have been significant changes in infant mortality rates between registered Indians and other Canadians in the years 1976–1991, there are still differences that favour non-Indians. Risks that increase infant mortality include lack of prenatal medical care, poor nutrition due to lack of income, lack of availability of necessary nutrients, and alcohol abuse.

Infant Mortality—Registered Indians* and Canada

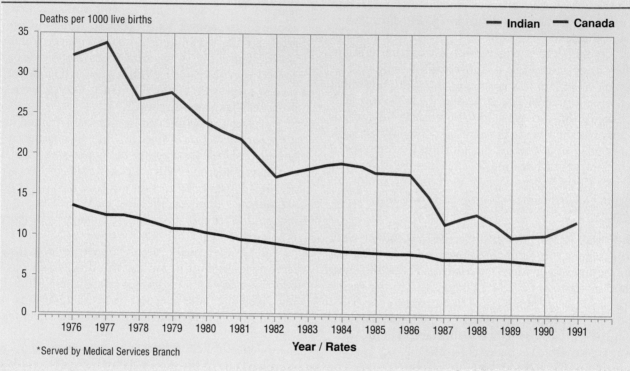

*Served by Medical Services Branch

Oral Contraceptives for Men? The development of an oral contraceptive for men has been slow. Evidently, the mechanisms involved in the manufacture and release of sperm are not as easy to manipulate as are the ovulatory and uterine cycles of the female. Some oral contraceptives for men have been tested, but they produced unpleasant side-effects such as diminished sex drive and impotence.

At the present time, research into the development of new male contraceptives is being carried on in various countries. Many researchers expect to develop a new male contraceptive by the end of the present decade.

One compound being researched is *gossypol,* a substance derived from the cotton plant. Chinese and Canadian researchers have found that gossypol inhibits sperm production, causing infertility. Difficulties in reversing the effects of the drug are presenting problems, as are concerns over long-term health consequences and possible genetic effects.

Scientists in Sweden have pioneered research into a nasal spray containing hormones designed to inhibit sperm production. As with gossypol, questions regarding side-effects and long-term health hazards remain unanswered.

Other researchers are investigating the possibility of using ultrasound as a male contraceptive. In this method, a high-frequency sound machine is placed in contact with the scrotum. The device emits sound waves that slow sperm production, thereby lowering sperm counts. In some cases, sperm counts have remained lowered for up to two years after the procedure. Reduced sperm count, as opposed to total destruction of sperm, may suffice as a contraceptive measure because a minimum number of sperm are needed for fertilization. Before this method can be made available, the risks for testicular cancer and genetic damage must be thoroughly explored.

Fertility Awareness Methods (FAM)

Methods of fertility control that rely upon the alteration of sexual behaviour are called **fertility awareness methods (FAM).** These methods include observing female "fertile periods" by examining cervical mucus and/or keeping track of internal temperature and then abstaining from sexual intercourse (penis-vagina contact) during these fertile times.

Two decades ago, the "rhythm method" was the object of much ridicule because of its low effectiveness rates. However, it was the only method of birth control available to women belonging to religious denominations that forbid the use of oral contraceptives, barrier methods, and sterilization. Our present reproductive knowledge enables women and their partners to use natural methods of birth control with fewer risks of pregnancy, although these methods remain far less effective than others.

Fertility awareness methods of birth control rely upon basic physiology. A released ovum can survive for up to 48 hours after ovulation. Sperm can live for as long as five days in the vagina. Natural methods of birth control teach women to recognize their fertile times. Changes in cervical mucus prior to and during ovulation and a rise in basal body temperature are two indicators frequently used in natural contraceptive techniques. Another method involves charting a woman's menstrual cycle and ovulation times on a calendar. Any combination of these methods may be used to determine fertile times more accurately.

Cervical Mucus Method. The **cervical mucus method** requires women to examine the consistency and colour of their normal vaginal secretions. Prior to ovulation, vaginal mucus becomes gelatinous and stringy in consistency, and normal vaginal secretions may increase. Sexual activity involving penis-vagina contact must be avoided while this "fertile mucus" is present and for several days following the mucus changes.

Body Temperature Method. The **body temperature method** relies on the fact that the female's basal body temperature rises between 0.4 and 0.8 degrees after ovulation has occurred. For this method to be effective, the woman must chart her temperature for several months to learn to recognize her body's temperature fluctuations. Abstinence from penis-vagina contact must be observed preceding the temperature rise until several days after the temperature rise was first noted.

The Calendar Method. The **calendar method** requires the woman to record the exact number of days in her menstrual cycle. Since few women menstruate with complete regularity, a record of the menstrual cycle must be kept for 12 months, during which time some other method of birth control must be used. The first day of a woman's period is counted as day 1. To determine the first fertile unsafe day of the cycle, she subtracts 18 from the number of days in the shortest cycle. To determine the last unsafe day of the cycle, she subtracts 11 from the number of days in the longest cycle. This method assumes that ovulation occurs during the midpoint of the cycle (see Figure 6.3). The couple must abstain from penis-vagina contact during the fertile time.

Women interested in fertility awareness methods of birth control are advised to take supervised classes in their use. The risks of an unwanted pregnancy are great for the untrained woman. Reading a book or watching a film on the subject or talking to the proprietor of the local health food store will not provide the necessary training to ensure maximum effectiveness. Incidentally, information on these methods can be helpful to couples who are trying to conceive.

Permanent Contraception

Sterilization has become increasingly common among married couples in Canada. Since the 1970s, perfection of sterilization procedures has made this method popular. Although some of the newer surgical techniques make reversal of sterilization theoretically possible, anyone considering sterilization should assume that the operation is *not* reversible. Before becoming sterilized, people should think through such possibilities as divorce and remarriage or a future improvement in their financial status that may make them want a larger family.

Fertility awareness methods (FAM): Include several types of birth control that require alteration of sexual behaviour rather than chemical or physical intervention into the reproductive process.

Cervical mucus method: A birth control method that relies upon observation of changes in cervical mucus to determine when the woman is fertile so the couple can abstain from intercourse during those times.

Body temperature method: A birth control method that requires a woman to monitor her body temperature for the rise that signals ovulation and to abstain from intercourse around this time.

Calendar method: A birth control method that requires mapping the woman's menstrual cycle on a calendar to determine presumed fertile times and abstaining from penis-vagina contact during those times.

Sterilization: Permanent fertility control achieved through surgical procedures.

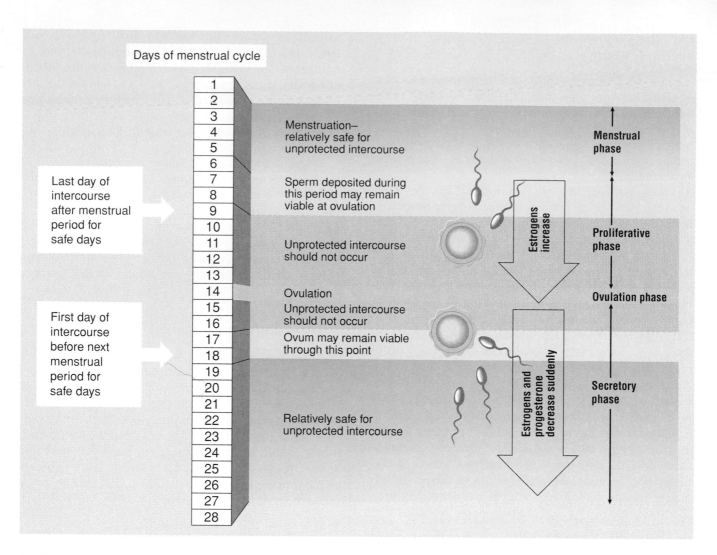

FIGURE 6.3

The Fertility Cycle

Female Sterilization.   One method of sterilization in females is called **tubal ligation.** It is achieved through a surgical procedure that involves tying the fallopian tubes closed or cutting them and cauterizing (burning) the edges to seal the tubes so that access by sperm to released eggs is blocked. The operation is usually done in a hospital on an outpatient basis. First, the abdomen is inflated with carbon dioxide gas through a small incision in the navel. The surgeon then inserts a *laparoscope* into another incision just above the pubic bone. This specially designed instrument has a fibre-optic light source that enables the physician to see the fallopian tubes clearly. Once located, the tubes are cut and tied or cauterized (see Figure 6.4).

Ovarian and uterine functions are not affected by a tubal ligation. The woman's menstrual cycle continues, and released eggs simply disintegrate and are absorbed by the lymphatic system. As soon as her incision is healed,

the woman may resume sexual intercourse with no fear of pregnancy.

As with any kind of surgery, there are risks. Some patients are given general anesthesia, which presents a small risk; others receive local anesthesia. The procedure itself usually takes less than an hour, and the patient is generally allowed to return home within a short time after waking up. Women considering a tubal ligation should thoroughly discuss all the risks with their physician before the operation.

The **hysterectomy,** or removal of the uterus, is a method of sterilization requiring major surgery. It is usually done only when the patient has a disease of or damage to the uterus.

Male Sterilization.   Sterilization in men is less complicated than in women. The procedure, called a **vasectomy,**

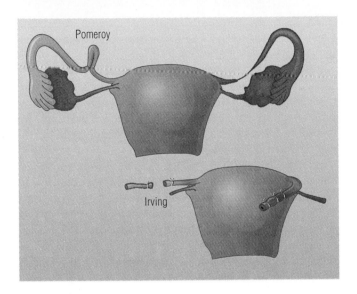

FIGURE 6.4

Two Methods of Tubal Ligation

Although a vasectomy should be considered a permanent procedure, surgical reversal is sometimes successful in restoring fertility. Recent improvements in microsurgery techniques have resulted in annual pregnancy rates of between 40 and 60 percent for women whose partners have had reversals. The two major factors influencing the success rate of reversal are the doctor's expertise and the time elapsed since the vasectomy.

is usually done on an outpatient basis using a local anesthetic. The surgeon (generally a urologist) makes an incision on each side of the scrotum. The vas deferens on each side is then located, and a piece is removed from each. The ends are usually tied or sewn shut (see Figure 6.5).

The man usually experiences some discomfort, local pain, swelling, and discolouration for about a week. In a small percentage of cases, more serious complications occur: formation of a blood clot in the scrotum (which usually disappears without medical treatment), infection, and inflammatory reactions. Because sperm are stored in other areas of the reproductive system besides the vas deferens, couples must use alternative methods of birth control for at least one month after the vasectomy. The man must check with his physician (who will do a semen analysis) to determine when unprotected intercourse can take place. The pregnancy rate in women whose partners have had vasectomies is about 15 in 10 000.

Many men are reluctant to consider sterilization because they fear the operation will affect their sexual performance. Such fears are unfounded (although not abnormal) and can be alleviated by talking to men who have already had a vasectomy.

A vasectomy in no way affects sexual response. Because sperm constitute only a small percentage of the semen, the amount of ejaculate is not changed significantly. The testes continue to produce sperm, but the sperm are prevented from entering the ejaculatory duct because of the surgery. After a time, sperm production may diminish. Any sperm that are manufactured disintegrate and are absorbed into the lymphatic system.

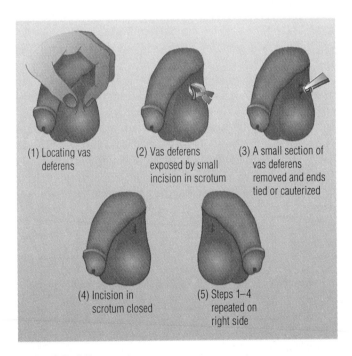

(1) Locating vas deferens

(2) Vas deferens exposed by small incision in scrotum

(3) A small section of vas deferens removed and ends tied or cauterized

(4) Incision in scrotum closed

(5) Steps 1–4 repeated on right side

FIGURE 6.5

Vasectomy

Tubal ligation: Sterilization of the female that involves the cutting and tying off of the fallopian tubes.

Hysterectomy: The removal of the uterus.

Vasectomy: Sterilization of the male that involves the cutting and tying of both vasa deferentia.

ABORTION

The law on **abortion** has seen a number of changes in Canada and much activity both federally and provincially. In 1869, two years after Confederation, a law was enacted that prohibited abortion and the penalty for someone found guilty of such an offence was life imprisonment. Those who oppose abortion believe that the embryo or foetus is a human being with rights that must be protected. Others have worked to get easier access to abortion for women.

In 1967, the Federal Standing Committee on Health and Welfare began consideration of proposed amendments to the Criminal Code relating to abortion. Dr. Henry Morgentaler, an abortion activist and physician, appeared "on behalf of the Humanist Fellowship of Montreal, urging the repeal of the abortion law and freedom of choice on abortion."[6] In 1969, Dr. Morgentaler closed his general practice and opened a clinic in Montreal to specialize in abortion using the vacuum aspiration method. In 1970, 1971, and 1973, 13 charges of illegal abortion were brought against Dr. Morgentaler. On November 13, 1973, a jury acquitted Dr. Morgentaler. The next year, however, the Quebec Court of Appeal convicted him.

Dr. Morgentaler appealed to the Supreme Court but in 1975 the appeal was dismissed and he served ten months in jail. In 1976, the newly elected Parti Québécois government declared that there would be no prosecution of Dr. Morgentaler for the outstanding charges against him. In 1983, Dr. Morgentaler opened clinics in Toronto and Winnipeg and was again charged, along with other clinic doctors and the head nurse. Appeal procedures and renewed charges continued through 1986.

Abortion: The medical means of terminating a pregnancy.

Vacuum aspiration: The use of gentle suction to remove foetal tissue from the uterus.

Dilation and evacuation (D&E): An abortion technique that combines vacuum aspiration with dilation and curettage; foetal tissue is both sucked and scraped out of the uterus.

Dilation and curettage (D&C): An abortion technique in which the cervix is dilated with laminaria for one to two days and the uterine walls are scraped clean.

Hysterotomy: The surgical removal of the foetus from the uterus.

Induction abortion: A type of abortion in which chemicals are injected into the uterus through the uterine wall; labour begins and the woman delivers a dead foetus.

In 1988 the Supreme Court of Canada ruled that Canada's abortion law was unconstitutional because it violated Canada's Charter of Rights and Freedoms and a woman's right to "life, liberty and security of the person."[7] In an attempt to recriminalize abortion, Bill C-43 was introduced in Parliament. This bill, which sought to prohibit abortion unless a physician deemed it necessary for the mother's physical, mental, or psychological health, was defeated by the Senate in 1991.

Along with the legal battle, abortion doctors, clinics, and patients have been harassed by anti-abortion protesters in Canada. Harassment and threats of violence have caused some physicians to stop performing abortions. On May 8, 1992, a firebomb destroyed the Morgentaler clinic in Toronto. On November 8 in British Columbia, abortion provider Dr. Garson Romalis was shot and seriously wounded at his home in Vancouver.

Another focus of debate is who will pay for abortions. Most medical procedures in Canada are covered under public health insurance plans. Abortions conducted in hospitals are covered by public health insurance. Clinics, though, may be fully covered, partly covered, or not covered at all.[8] In 1995, the federal government ruled that if the provinces accept that abortion is medically necessary, they must pay the full cost of abortions or lose money from federal transfer payments under the Canada Health Act.[9]

Only a few Canadian hospitals perform abortions. Yet, in 1994, 106 255 abortions were performed, up 1.8 percent over the previous year. The growth came from the number of abortions performed in clinics. The national abortion rate was 27.6 abortions per 100 live births.[10]

In 1994, half of all women obtaining therapeutic abortions were between the ages of 20 and 29, and a third were over 30. One in five was under 20. Over the ten-year period 1984–1994, women aged 40 and over accounted for 2 to 3 percent of the annual number of abortions.[11]

The best birth control methods can fail. Women may be raped. Pregnancies can occur despite every possible precaution. When an unwanted pregnancy does occur, the decision whether to terminate, to carry to term and keep the baby, or to carry to term and give the baby away must be made. This is a personal decision to be made by each woman according to her personal beliefs, values, and resources after careful consideration of all alternatives.

Methods of Abortion

The type of abortion procedure used is determined by how many weeks pregnant the woman is. Pregnancy length is calculated from the first day of a woman's last menstrual period.

If performed during the first trimester of pregnancy, abortion presents a relatively low risk to the mother. The most commonly used method of first-trimester abortion is **vacuum aspiration.** The procedure is usually per-

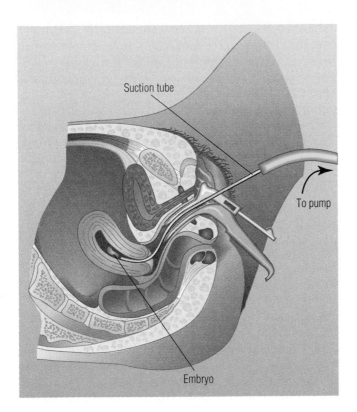

Suction tube

To pump

Embryo

FIGURE 6.6

Vacuum Aspiration Abortion

formed with local anesthetic. The cervix is dilated with instruments or by placing *laminaria,* a sterile scaweed product, in the cervical canal. The laminaria is left in place for a few hours or overnight and slowly dilates the cervix. After it is removed, a long tube is inserted into the uterus through the cervix. Gentle suction is then used to remove the foetal tissue from the uterine walls.

Pregnancies that progress into the second trimester can be terminated through **dilation and evacuation (D&E),** a procedure that combines vacuum aspiration with a technique called **dilation and curettage (D&C).** For this procedure, the cervix is dilated with laminaria for one to two days and a combination of instruments and vacuum aspiration is used to empty the uterus (see Figure 6.6). Second-trimester abortions are frequently done under general anesthetic. Both procedures can be performed on an outpatient basis (usually in the physician's office) with or without pain medication. Generally, however, the woman is given a mild tranquillizer to help her relax. Both procedures may cause moderate to severe uterine cramping and blood loss.

The **hysterotomy,** or surgical removal of the foetus from the uterus, may be used during emergencies or when the mother's life may be in danger and when other types of abortions are deemed too dangerous.

The risks associated with abortions include infection, incomplete abortion (when parts of the placenta remain in the uterus), missed abortion (when the foetus is not ac-

tually removed), excessive bleeding, and cervical and uterine trauma. Follow-up and attention to dangerous signs decrease the chances of any long-term problems.

The mortality rate for first-trimester abortions averages out to 0.8 per 100 000. The rate for second-trimester abortions is higher, 4.3 per 100 000. This higher rate is due to the increased risk of uterine perforation, bleeding, infection, and incomplete abortion due to the fact that the uterine wall becomes thinner as the pregnancy progresses.

Two other methods used in second-trimester abortions, though less commonly than the D&E method, are prostaglandin or saline **induction abortions.** In these methods, prostaglandin hormones or a saline solution is injected into the uterus. The injected solution kills the foetus and causes labour contractions to begin. After 24 to 48 hours the foetus and placenta are expelled from the uterus.

---

*W*HAT DO YOU THINK?

If you or your partner unexpectedly became pregnant, would you choose to terminate the pregnancy? How might an abortion affect your relationship? If you were married, would your decision be different? Why?

---

*P*LANNING A PREGNANCY

The technological ability to control your fertility gives you choices not available when your parents were born. The loosening of social restrictions in the areas of marriage and parenting also affords single men and women the opportunity to become parents. Regardless of whether you are married or single, the preparation to become a parent involves similar considerations and decisions. If you are in the process of deciding whether to have children, you need to take the time to evaluate your emotions, finances, and health.

Emotional Health

The first and foremost evaluation you should make is why you want to have a child: To fulfill an inner need to carry on the family? Out of loneliness? Any other reasons? Can you care for this new human being in a loving and nurturing manner? Are you ready to make all the sacrifices necessary to bear and raise a child? You can prepare yourself for this change in your life in several ways. Reading about parenthood, taking classes, talking to parents of children of all ages, and joining a support group are all helpful forms of preparation. If you choose to adopt, you will find many support groups available to you as well. If you and your partner agree you are ready to have a child, then consider the following as well.

Maternal Health

Before becoming pregnant, a woman should have a thorough medical examination. **Preconception care** should include assessment of possible pregnancy complications. Medical problems such as diabetes and high blood pressure should be discussed, as should any genetic disorders that run in either family.

Paternal Health

It is common wisdom that mothers-to-be should steer clear of toxic chemicals that can cause birth defects. Even women who are trying to conceive are cautioned to avoid toxic environments and to eat a nourishing diet, to stop smoking and drinking alcohol, and to avoid most medications.

Now similar precautions are being urged for fathers-to-be. New research suggests that a man's exposure to chemicals influences not only his ability to father a child but also the future health of his child. Fathers-to-be have been overlooked in the past for several reasons. Researchers assumed that the genetic damage leading to birth defects and other health problems always occurred while a child was in the mother's womb. After all, they reasoned, that's where embryonic and foetal development take place. Conventional medical wisdom also held that defective-looking sperm (those with misshapen heads, crooked tails, or retarded swimming ability) were incapable of fertilizing an egg.

Scientists have recently discovered that how sperm look has little to do with how they act. Misshapen sperm can penetrate an egg, and they do not necessarily carry defective genetic goods. Moreover, sperm that look healthy and swim well can be the true genetic culprits. DNA fluorescent markers have identified normal-looking, yet genetically flawed, sperm that carry too many or too few chromosomes. Fathers contribute the extra chromosome 21 in about 6 percent of children with Down's syndrome, which causes mental retardation; the extra X chromosome in 50 percent of boys with Klinefelter's syndrome, which causes abnormal sexual development; and the shortened chromosome 15 in about 85 percent of children with Prader-Willi syndrome, a disorder characterized by retardation and obesity.

Although some birth defects are caused by the random errors of nature, it now appears that some disorders can be traced to sperm damaged by chemicals. Sperm are naturally vulnerable to toxic assault and genetic damage.

Preconception care: Medical care received prior to becoming pregnant that helps a woman assess and address potential maternal health.

Many drugs and ingested chemicals can readily invade the testes from the bloodstream; others ambush sperm after they leave the testes and pass through the epididymides, where they mature and are stored. By one route or another, half of 100 chemicals studied so far (including by-products of cigarette smoke) apparently harm sperm.

Some researchers believe that vitamin C is nature's way of protecting sex cells from damage. Bad diets, exposure to toxic chemicals, cigarette smoking, and not enough foods rich in vitamin C are probably the biggest culprits in sperm damage.[12]

Financial Evaluation

You also need to evaluate your finances. Both partners should find out about their employers' policies concerning parental leave, including length of leave available and conditions for returning to work.

Raising a child exacts a tremendous strain on most family's finances. Expenses during the first year of life averages $9500. The expense of raising a child from birth to 21 years of age is presently estimated to be over $155 000—not including the cost of a college education!

The cost and availability of quality child care should also be considered. Prospective parents should realistically assess how much family assistance they can expect with a new baby as well as the availability of nonfamily child care.

Contingency Planning

A final consideration is how to provide for the child should something happen to you and your partner. If both of you were to die while the child is young, do you have relatives or close friends who would raise the child? If you have more than one child, would they have to be split up or could they be kept together? Unpleasant though it may be to think about, this sort of contingency planning is highly important.

---

*W*HAT DO YOU THINK?

Do you think most parents plan when they will have their children? At what point in your life do you think you will be ready to take on the responsibilities of becoming a parent? What are your biggest concerns about parenthood?

---

*P*REGNANCY

Prenatal Care

A successful pregnancy requires the mother's ability to take good care of herself and her unborn child. It is essential to have regular medical checkups, beginning as soon as possible (certainly within the first three months). Early detection of foetal abnormalities and identification of high-risk mothers and infants are the major purposes of prenatal care. On the first visit, the practitioner should obtain a complete medical history of the mother and her family and note any hereditary conditions that could put a woman or her foetus at risk.

Regular checkups to measure weight gain and blood pressure and monitor the size and position of the foetus should continue throughout the pregnancy. This early care reduces infant mortality and low birthweight. Experts recommend obstetrical visits once a month to 28 weeks, biweekly to 36 weeks, and weekly to 40 weeks.

Additional concerns include the mother's physical condition, her level of nutrition, her confidence in her ability to give birth, her use of drugs and medications, and the availability of a skilled practitioner who can oversee the pregnancy and delivery. A woman planning a pregnancy also needs a support system (spouse or partner, family, friends, community groups) willing to give her and her child the love and emotional support needed during and after her pregnancy. In some areas prenatal classes are available for pregnant teens.

Choosing a Practitioner. A woman should carefully choose a practitioner to attend her pregnancy and delivery. If possible, this choice should be made before she becomes pregnant. Recommendations from friends who were satisfied with the care they received during pregnancy may be a good starting point in the search for a practitioner. The woman's family physician may also be able to recommend a specialist. The pregnant woman needs to find a practitioner she can trust with both her own life and that of the baby and with whom she can communicate freely.

When choosing a practitioner, parents should ask a number of questions concerning credentials and professional qualifications. Besides this information, a pregnant woman must ask questions specific to her condition. Prospective parents should also inquire about the practitioner's experience in handling various complications, commitment to being at the mother's side during delivery, and beliefs and practices concerning the use of anesthesia, foetal monitoring, induced labour, and forceps delivery. What are the practitioner's attitudes toward birth control, abortion, and alternative birthing procedures? The practitioner's approach to nutrition and medication during pregnancy should be similar to the woman's own. Finally, the parents must learn under what circumstances the practitioner would perform a caesarean section.

Two types of physicians can attend pregnancies and deliveries. The *obstetrician-gynecologist* (ob-gyn) is an M.D. who specializes in obstetrics (pregnancy and birth) and gynecology (care of women's reproductive organs). These practitioners are trained to handle all types of pregnancy- and delivery-related emergencies.

A *family practitioner* is a licensed M.D. who provides comprehensive care for people of all ages. The majority of family practitioners have obstetrical experience but will refer a patient to a specialist if necessary. Unlike the ob-gyn, the family practitioner can serve as the baby's physician after attending the birth.

Midwives are also experienced practitioners who can attend both pregnancies and deliveries. Most midwives work in private practice or in conjunction with physicians. Those who work with physicians have access to traditional medical facilities to which they can turn in an emergency.

Alcohol and Drugs. A woman should avoid all types of drugs during pregnancy unless prescribed by a doctor—and then she should ask whether the medication is really necessary and whether there are safer alternatives. Always tell a physician, dentist, or other practitioner if you are pregnant. Even common over-the-counter medications such as aspirin and beverages such as coffee and tea can damage a developing foetus.

During the first three months of pregnancy, the foetus is especially subject to the **teratogenic** (birth-defect-causing) effects of some chemical substances. The foetus

TABLE 6.2 ▪ Teratogenic Effects of Drugs

Drug	Effect
Alcohol	Mental retardation; growth retardation; increased spontaneous abortion rate
Amphetamines	Suspected nervous system damage
Aspirin	Newborn bleeding
Cocaine	Uncontrolled jerking motions; paralysis; depressed interactive behaviour; poor organizational response to environmental stimuli
Opioids	Immediate withdrawal in newborns; permanent learning disabilities
Tetracycline	Tooth discolouration
Sulfa drugs	Facial and skeletal abnormalities
Barbiturates	Congenital malformations
Streptomycin	Deafness
Accutane	Small or absent ears; small jaw; heart defects
Valium	Possible congenital anomalies

Source: Mike Samuels, M.D., and Nancy Samuels, *The Well Pregnancy Book* (New York: Summit Books, 1986), 131. Copyright 1986. Reprinted by permission of the Elaine Markson Literary Agency and Mike Samuels, M.D., and Nancy Samuels.

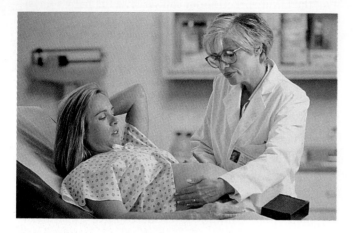

Good prenatal care involves regular medical checkups by a practitioner with whom the mother feels she can communicate freely.

can also develop an addiction to or tolerance for drugs that the mother is using.

Of particular concern to medical professionals is the use of tobacco and alcohol during pregnancy. Women who are heavy drinkers may have normal first babies but subsequently deliver children having foetal alcohol syndrome. The symptoms of **foetal alcohol syndrome (FAS)** include mental retardation, slowed nerve reflexes, and small head size. The exact amount of alcohol necessary to cause FAS is not known, but researchers doubt that any level of alcohol consumption is safe. Therefore, total abstinence from alcohol during pregnancy is recommended. Table 6.2 provides a list of teratogenic effects of alcohol and other drugs ingested by the mother.

Cigarette smoking during pregnancy has more predictable effects than alcohol. Studies have shown a 25 to 50 percent higher rate of foetal and infant deaths among women who smoke during pregnancy than among those who do not.[13] Women who smoke more than 10 to 15 cigarettes a day during pregnancy have higher rates of miscarriage, stillbirth, premature births, and low-birthweight babies than do nonsmokers. Foetal research on the effects

---

Teratogenic: Causing birth defects; may refer to drugs, environmental chemicals, X-rays, or diseases.

Foetal alcohol syndrome (FAS): A collection of symptoms, including mental retardation, that can appear in infants of women who drink too much alcohol during pregnancy.

Down's syndrome: A condition characterized by mental retardation and a variety of physical abnormalities.

---

of "secondhand" or sidestream smoke (inhaling smoke produced by others) is inconclusive, but babies whose parents smoke can be twice as susceptible to pneumonia, bronchitis, and related illnesses as other babies.

X-rays. X-rays present a clear danger to the foetus. Although most diagnostic tests produce minimal amounts of radiation, even low levels may cause birth defects or other problems, particularly if several low-dose X-rays are taken over a short time period. Pregnant women are advised to avoid X-rays unless absolutely necessary.

Nutrition and Exercise. Pregnant women have additional needs for protein, calories, and certain vitamins and minerals, so their diets should be carefully monitored by a qualified practitioner. Special attention should be paid to getting enough folic acid (found in dark leafy greens), iron (dried fruits, meats, legumes, liver, egg yolks), calcium (nonfat or lowfat dairy products, some canned fish), and fluids. Vitamin supplements can correct some deficiencies, but there is no true substitute for a well-balanced diet. Babies born to mothers whose nutrition has been poor run high risks of substandard mental and physical development (see Table 6.3).

Weight gain during pregnancy helps nourish a growing baby. For a woman of normal weight before pregnancy, the acceptable weight gain during pregnancy ranges from 11–16 kilograms (25–35 pounds); a woman carrying twins needs to gain about 16–20 kilograms (35–45 pounds). Usually the mother can expect to gain about 5 kilograms (ten pounds)

TABLE 6.3 ■ Nutrient Deficiency Effects

Nutrient	Deficiency Effect
Overall caloric intake	Low infant birthweight
Protein	Reduced infant head circumference
Folic acid	Miscarriage and neural tube defects
Vitamin D	Low infant birthweight
Calcium	Decreased infant bone density
Iron	Low infant birthweight and premature birth
Iodine	Varying degrees of mental and physical retardation in the infant
Zinc	Congenital malformations

Source: Reprinted by permission from Linda Kelly Debruyne and Sharon Rady Rolfes, *Life Cycle Nutrition: Conception Through Adolescence.* Copyright 1989 by West Publishing Company. All rights reserved.

during the first 20 weeks and about 0.5 kilograms (one pound) per week during the rest of the pregnancy.

Of the total number of kilograms gained during pregnancy, about 3–4 are the baby's weight. The baby's birth weight is important, since low weight can mean health problems during labour and the baby's first few months. Eating right and gaining enough weight helps reduce the chances of having a low-birthweight baby. If a woman gains an appropriate amount of weight while pregnant, chances are that her baby will gain weight properly, too. Pregnancy is not a time to think about losing weight—doing so may endanger the baby.[14]

As in all other stages of life, exercise is an important factor in weight control during pregnancy as well as in overall maternal health. A balanced 45-minute exercise session three days per week has been associated in one study with heavier-birthweight babies, fewer surgical births, and shorter hospital stays after birth.[15] Pregnant women should consult with their physicians before starting any exercise program.

Other Factors. A pregnant woman should avoid exposure to toxic chemicals, heavy metals, pesticides, gases, and other hazardous compounds. She should not clean cat-litter boxes because cat faeces can contain organisms that cause a disease called toxoplasmosis. If a pregnant woman contracts this disease, her baby may be stillborn or suffer mental retardation or other birth defects.

Before becoming pregnant, a woman should be tested to determine if she has had rubella (German measles). If she has not had the disease, she should get an immunization for it and wait the recommended length of time before becoming pregnant. A rubella infection can kill the foetus or cause blindness or hearing disorders in the infant. If the woman has ever had genital herpes, she should inform her physician. The physician may want to deliver the baby by caesarean section, especially if the woman has active lesions. Contact with an active herpes infection during birth can be fatal to the infant.

A Woman's Reproductive Years

More than half of the average Canadian woman's expected life span is spent between menarche (first menses) and menopause (last menses), a period of approximately 40 years. During this 40-year period, she must make many decisions regarding her reproductive health. Deciding if and when to have children, as well as how to prevent pregnancy when necessary, are long-term concerns.[16]

Today, a woman over 35 who is pregnant has plenty of company. While births to women in their 20s are declining, the rate of first births to women between the ages of 30 and 39 has doubled in the past decade, and births to women over 39 have increased by more than 50 percent. Many women who wait until their 30s to consider having

A doctor-approved exercise program during pregnancy not only helps the mother control her weight, but also contributes to easier deliveries and healthier babies.

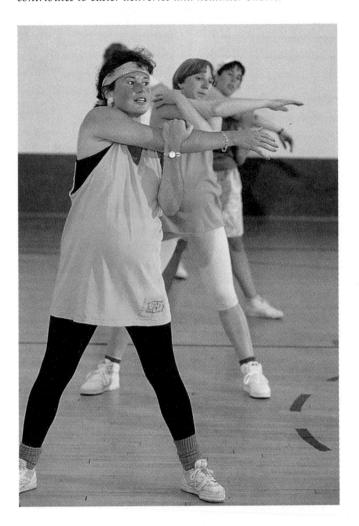

a child find themselves wondering, "Am I too old to have a baby?" Researchers believe that there is a decline in both the quality and viability of eggs produced after age 35. Statistically, the chances of having a baby with birth defects do rise after the age of 35. **Down's syndrome,** a condition characterized by mild to severe mental retardation and a variety of physical abnormalities, is the most common birth defect found in babies born to older mothers. The incidence of Down's syndrome in babies born to mothers aged 20 is 1 in 10 000 births; it rises to 1 in 365 births when the mother is 35, to 1 in 109 when she is 40, and to 1 in 32 when she is 45.

Women who choose to delay motherhood until their late 30s also worry about their physical ability to carry and deliver their babies. For these women, a comprehensive exercise program will assist in maintaining good posture and promoting a successful delivery.

Pregnancy Testing

A woman may suspect she is pregnant before she has any type of pregnancy tests. A typical sign is a missed menstrual period, yet this is not always an accurate indicator. A woman can miss her period for a variety of reasons: stress, exercise, emotional upset. Confirmation of a pregnancy can be obtained from a pregnancy test scheduled in a medical office or birth control clinic.

Women who wish to know immediately whether or not they are pregnant can purchase home pregnancy test kits. These kits, sold over the counter in drugstores, are about 85 to 95 percent reliable. A positive test is based on the secretion of **human chorionic gonadotropin (HCG)** found in the woman's urine. Home test kits come equipped with a small sample of red blood cells coated with HCG antibodies, to which the user adds a small amount of urine. If the concentration of HCG is great enough, it will clump together with the HCG antibodies, indicating that the user is pregnant.

There are some problems with the accuracy of these home tests. If taken too early in the pregnancy, they may show a false negative. Other causes of false negatives are unclean test tubes, ingestion of certain drugs, and vaginal or urinary infections. Accuracy also depends on the quality of the test itself and the user's ability to perform it and interpret the results. Blood tests administered and analyzed by a medical laboratory give more accurate results.

The Process of Pregnancy

Pregnancy begins the moment a sperm fertilizes an ovum in the fallopian tubes (see Figure 6.7). From there, the single cell multiplies, becoming a sphere-shaped cluster of cells as it travels toward the uterus, a journey that may last three to four days. Upon arrival, the embryo burrows into the thick, spongy endometrium and is nourished from this carefully prepared lining.

Early Signs of Pregnancy. The first sign of pregnancy is usually a missed menstrual period (although some women "spot" in early pregnancy, and such spotting may be mistaken for a period). Other signs of pregnancy include:

- Breast tenderness
- Extreme fatigue
- Sleeplessness
- Emotional upset
- Nausea
- Vomiting (especially in the morning)

Pregnancy typically lasts 40 weeks. The due date is calculated from the expectant mother's last menstrual period. Pregnancy is typically divided into three phases, or **trimesters,** of approximately three months each.

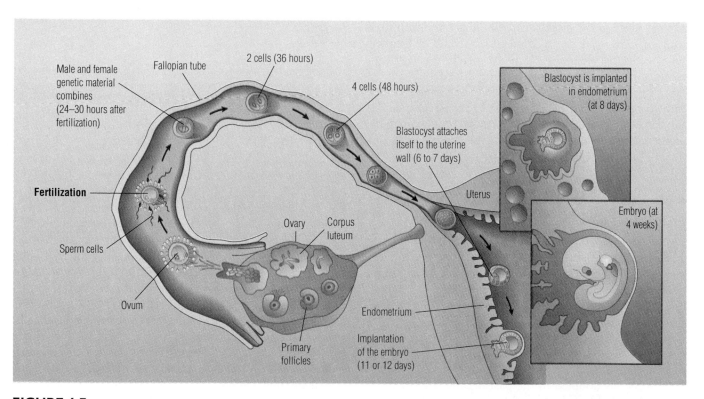

FIGURE 6.7

Fertilization

The First Trimester. During the first trimester, there are few noticeable changes in the maternal body. The expectant mother may urinate more frequently and experience morning sickness, swollen breasts, or undue fatigue. But these symptoms may not be frequent or severe, so she may not realize she is pregnant at this time unless she has a pregnancy test.

During the first two months after conception, the **embryo** differentiates and develops its various organ systems, beginning with the nervous and circulatory systems. At the start of the third month, the embryo is called a **foetus,** indicating that all organ systems are in place. For the rest of the pregnancy, growth and refinement occur in each major body system so that they can function independently, yet in coordination, at birth.

The Second Trimester. At the beginning of the second trimester, physical changes in the mother become more visible. Her breasts swell and her waistline thickens. During this time, the foetus makes greater demands upon the mother's body. In particular, the **placenta,** the network of blood vessels that carry nutrients and oxygen to the foetus and foetal waste products to the mother, becomes well established.

The Third Trimester. From the end of the sixth month through the ninth is considered the third trimester. This is the period of greatest foetal growth. The foetus gains most of its weight during these last three months. During the third trimester, the foetus must get large amounts of calcium, iron, and nitrogen from the food the mother eats. Approximately 85 percent of the calcium and iron the mother digests goes into the foetal bloodstream.

Although the foetus may live if it is born during the seventh month, it needs the layer of fat it acquires during the eighth month and time for the organs (especially the respiratory and digestive organs) to develop to their full potential. Babies born prematurely thus usually require intensive medical care.

Prenatal Testing and Screening

Modern technology has enabled medical practitioners to detect health defects in a foetus as early as the 14th to 18th weeks of pregnancy. One common testing procedure, **amniocentesis,** which is strongly recommended for women over the age of 35, involves inserting a long needle through the mother's abdominal and uterine walls into the **amniotic sac,** the protective pouch surrounding the baby (see Figure 6.8). The needle draws out 3 to 4 teaspoons of fluid, which is analyzed for genetic information about the baby. This test can reveal the presence of 40 genetic abnormalities, including Down's syndrome, Tay-Sachs disease (a fatal disorder of the nervous system common among Jewish people of Eastern European

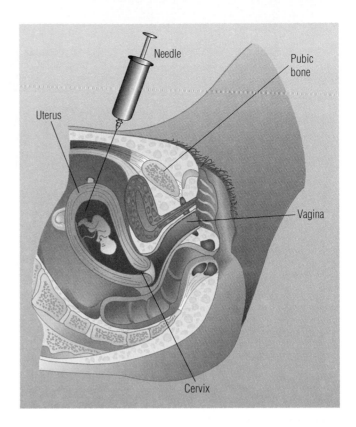

FIGURE 6.8

The process of amniocentesis can detect certain congenital problems as well as the sex of the foetus.

Human chorionic gonadotropin (HCG): Hormone detectable in blood or urine samples of a mother within the first few weeks of pregnancy.

Trimester: A three-month segment of pregnancy; used to describe specific developmental changes that occur in the embryo or foetus.

Embryo: The fertilized egg from conception until the end of two months' development.

Foetus: The name given the developing baby from the third month of pregnancy until birth.

Placenta: The network of blood vessels that carries nutrients to the developing infant and carries wastes away; it connects to the umbilical cord.

Amniocentesis: A medical test in which a small amount of fluid is drawn from the amniotic sac; it tests for Down's syndrome and genetic diseases.

Amniotic sac: The protective pouch surrounding the baby.

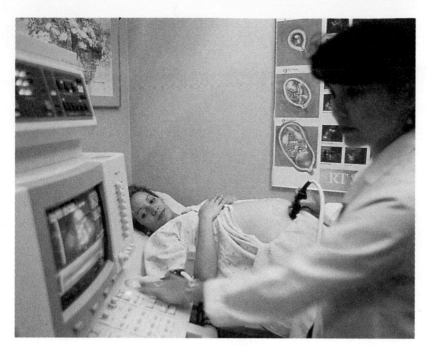

Ultrasound testing can reveal defects in the developing foetus, and, as the time of delivery nears, it can provide useful information about the size and position of the unborn child.

descent), and sickle-cell anemia (a debilitating blood disorder found primarily among blacks). Amniocentesis can also reveal the sex of the child, a fact many parents choose not to know until the birth. Although widely used, amniocentesis is not without risk. Chances of foetal damage and miscarriage as a result of testing are 1 in 400.

Another procedure, *ultrasound* or *sonography*, uses high-frequency sound waves to determine the size and position of the foetus. Ultrasound can also detect defects in the central nervous system and digestive system of the foetus. Knowing the position of the foetus assists practitioners in performing amniocentesis and in delivering the child.

A third procedure, *foetoscopy*, involves making a small incision in the abdominal and uterine walls and then inserting an optical viewer into the uterus to view the foetus directly. This method is still experimental and involves some risk. It causes miscarriage in approximately 5 percent of cases.

A fourth procedure, *chorionic villus sampling (CVS)*, involves snipping tissue from the developing foetal sac. CVS can be used at 10 to 12 weeks of pregnancy, and the test results are available in 12 to 48 hours. This test is an attractive option for couples who are at high risk for having a baby with Down's syndrome or a debilitating hereditary disease.

If any of these tests reveals a serious birth defect, parents are advised to undergo genetic counselling. In the case of a chromosomal abnormality such as Down's syndrome, the parents are usually offered counselling regarding their options.

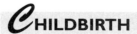

*W*HAT DO YOU THINK?

What are the most important concerns you have considering your choice of a health practitioner for your or your partner's pregnancy? What behaviours might you have to change if you found out that you or your partner were pregnant? In what ways would your life change if you had a child who was born with a birth defect? What type of prenatal tests would you consider before the birth of your child?

*C*HILDBIRTH

Choosing Where to Have Your Baby

Today's prospective mothers have many delivery options. These range from the traditional hospital birth to home birth. When considering birthing alternatives, parental values are important. Many couples, for instance, feel that the modern medical establishment has dehumanized the birth process; thus they choose to deliver at home or at a *birthing centre*, a homelike setting outside a hospital where women can give birth and receive postdelivery care by a team of professional practitioners, including physicians and registered nurses.

Birth Attendants

Over the years, the World Health Assembly has adopted a number of resolutions drawing attention to the facts that most of the populations in various developing countries around the world depend for primary health care on ways of protecting and restoring health that existed before the arrival of modern medicine; that the work force represented by practitioners of traditional medicine is a potentially important resource for the delivery of health care; and that medicinal plants are of great importance to the health of individuals and communities.

The reasons for the inclusion of traditional healers in primary health care are manifold: the healers' knowing the sociocultural background of the people; their being highly respected and experienced in their work; economic consider- ations; the distances to be covered in some countries; the strength of traditional beliefs; and the shortage of health professionals, particularly in rural areas—to name just a few.

A large proportion of the population in a number of developing countries still relies on traditional practitioners, including traditional birth attendants. WHO estimates that traditional birth attendants assist in up to 95 percent of all rural births and 70 percent of urban births in developing countries.

Source: Adapted from World Health Organization, *Fact Sheet N134, September 1996: Traditional Medicine.* See web site: http://www.who.ch/programmes/;nf/facts/fact134.htm.

Labour and Delivery

The birth process has three stages. The exact mechanisms that signal the mother's body that the baby is ready to be born are unknown. During the few weeks preceding delivery, the baby normally shifts and turns to a head-down position, and the cervix begins to dilate (open up). The junction of the pubic bones also loosens to permit expansion of the pelvic girdle during birth (see Figure 6.9).

In the first stage of labour, the amniotic sac breaks, causing a rush of fluid from the vagina (commonly referred to as "breaking of the waters"). Contractions in the abdomen and lower back also signal the beginning of labour. Early contractions push the baby downward, putting pressure on the cervix and thereby causing it to dilate further. The first stage of labour may last from a couple of hours to more than a day for a first birth, but is usually much shorter during subsequent births.

The end of the first stage of labour, called **transition,** is the part of the process when the cervix becomes fully dilated and the baby's head begins to move into the vagina, or the birth canal. Contractions usually come quickly during transition. Transition usually lasts 30 minutes or less.

The second stage of labour follows transition when the cervix has become fully dilated. Contractions become rhythmic, stronger, and more painful as the uterus works to push the baby through the birth canal. The second stage of labour (called the *expulsion stage*) may last between one and four hours and concludes when the infant is finally pushed out of the mother's body. In some cases, the attending practitioner will do an **episiotomy,** a straight incision in the mother's **perineum,** to prevent the baby's head from causing tearing of vaginal tissues and to speed the baby's exit from the vagina. Sometimes women can avoid the need for an episiotomy by exercising and getting good nutrition throughout pregnancy, by trying different birth positions, or by having an attendant massage the perineal tissue. However, the skin's natural elasticity and the baby's size are limiting factors.

After delivery, the attending practitioner cleans the baby's mucus-filled breathing passages, and the baby takes its first breath, generally accompanied by a loud wail. (The traditional "slap" on the baby's buttocks, often romanticized in old movies, is no longer a common practice because of the trauma associated with it.)

In the meantime, the mother continues into the third stage of labour, during which the placenta, or **afterbirth,** is expelled from the womb. This stage is usually completed within 30 minutes after delivery. The umbilical cord is then tied and severed. The stump of cord attached to the baby's navel dries up and drops off within a few days.

Transition: The process during which the cervix becomes nearly fully dilated and the head of the foetus begins to move into the birth canal.

Episiotomy: A straight incision in the mother's perineum.

Perineum: The area between the vulva and the anus.

Afterbirth: The expelled placenta.

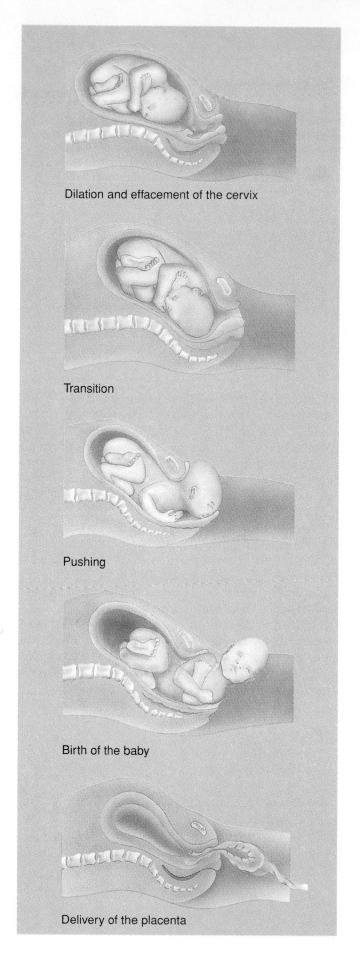

Dilation and effacement of the cervix

Transition

Pushing

Birth of the baby

Delivery of the placenta

Prenatal Education

Expectant parents in Canada can receive a variety of services for prenatal education depending upon the resources in terms of facilities and professionals in the community where they live. Most prenatal programs include instruction in a range of comfort measures as well as preparation in breathing.

Drugs in the Delivery Room

Because painkilling drugs given to the mother during labour can cause sluggish responses in the newborn, many women choose drug-free labours and deliveries. Drug-free labour involves the use of exercise, massage, and controlled rhythmic breathing to control pain. Many women who choose "natural" childbirth mistakenly believe that the exercises they are taught in their classes will make their labour and delivery painless. When their time comes to give birth, they may feel inadequate because they experience the normal pain associated with childbirth. Pain is to be expected, and if it becomes too intense, the mother can be given painkilling medication.

A discussion with the attending physician before the birth of the baby will alert the mother to the practitioner's feelings about the use of painkilling drugs during delivery. Many experts believe that women should be offered the option of drugs during delivery both before and during the event. To refuse to give a mother medicine to take the edge off the pain is considered poor medical practice by some authorities.

Breast-Feeding and the Postpartum Period

Although the new mother's milk will not begin to flow for two or more days, her breasts secrete a thick yellow substance called *colostrum*. Because this fluid contains vital antibodies to help fight infection, the newborn baby should be allowed to suckle.

As a result of recent scientific findings, it is strongly recommended that full-term newborns be breast-fed. This recommendation does not mean that breast milk is the only adequate method of nourishing a baby. Prepared formulas can provide nourishment that allows a baby to grow and thrive.

Still, there are many advantages to breast-feeding. Breast milk is perfectly suited to a baby's nutritional needs. Breast-fed babies have fewer illnesses and a much lower hospitalization rate because breast milk contains maternal antibodies and immunological cells that stimulate the infant's immune system. When breast-fed babies do get sick, they recover more quickly. They are also less likely to be obese than babies fed on formulas, and they have fewer allergies.

FIGURE 6.9 The Birth Process

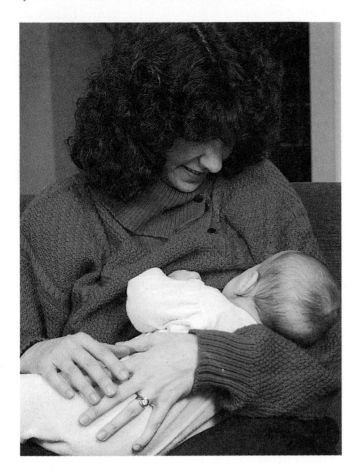

Breast-feeding is one way to enhance the development of intimate bonds between mother and child.

When deciding whether to breast- or bottle-feed, mothers need to consider their own desires and preferences. Both feeding methods can supply the physical and emotional closeness so essential to the parent-child relationship.

The *postpartum period* lasts from four to six weeks after delivery. During this time, the mother's reproductive organs revert to a nonpregnant state. Many women experience energy depletion, anxiety, mood swings, and depression during this period. This experience, known as **postpartum depression,** appears to be a normal end-product of the birth process. For most women, the symptoms gradually disappear as their bodies return to normal. For others, the symptoms, coupled with the stresses of managing a new family, can cause more severe depression that lasts for several months.

Complications

Problems and complications can occur during labour and delivery even following a successful pregnancy. Such possibilities should be discussed with the practitioner prior to labour so the mother understands what medical procedures may be necessary for her safety and for that of her child. Although pregnancy still involves a certain amount of risk, the risk is lower than for many other common activities.

Caesarean Section (C-Section).   If labour lasts too long or if a baby is presenting wrong (about to exit the uterus anything but head first), a **caesarean section (C-section)** may be necessary. This surgical procedure involves making an incision across the mother's abdomen and through the uterus to remove the baby. This operation is also performed in cases in which labour is extremely difficult, maternal blood pressure falls rapidly, the placenta separates from the uterus too soon, the mother has diabetes, or other problems occur.

A caesarean section can be traumatic for the mother if she is not prepared for it. Risks to the mother are the same as for any major abdominal surgery, and recovery from birth takes considerably longer after a C-section. Although a caesarean section may be necessary in certain cases, some physicians and critics feel that the option has been used too frequently in this country. The 1986 National Conference on Aspects of Cesarean Birth recommended guidelines to deal with rising caesarean rates. Overall rates of caesarean section subsequently dropped from 20 percent in 1987 to 15 percent in 1993. The guidelines dealt with three scenarios: breech presentation, prolonged labour, and previous caesarean section. The adage was "Once a caesarean, always a caesarean." Now, however, surgical techniques allow many women who have had a caesarean section to deliver later children vaginally. Repeat caesareans decreased from 39 percent in the mid-1980s to 34 percent in 1993.[17]

Miscarriage.   One in ten pregnancies does not end in delivery. Loss of the foetus before it is viable is called a **miscarriage** (also referred to as spontaneous abortion). An estimated 70 to 90 percent of women who miscarry eventually become pregnant again.

Reasons for miscarriage vary. In some cases, the fertilized egg has failed to divide correctly. In others, genetic abnormalities, maternal illness, or infections are responsible. Maternal hormonal imbalance may also cause a miscarriage, as may a weak cervix or toxic chemicals in the environment. In most cases, the cause is not known.

Postpartum depression: The experience of energy depletion, anxiety, mood swings, and depression that women may feel during the postpartum period.

Caesarean section (C-Section): A surgical procedure in which a baby is removed through an incision made in the mother's abdominal and uterine walls.

Miscarriage: Loss of the foetus before it is viable; also called spontaneous abortion.

A blood incompatibility between mother and father can cause **Rh factor** problems, and sometimes miscarriage. Rh is a blood protein. Rh problems occur when the mother is Rh-negative and the foetus is Rh-positive. During a first birth, some of the baby's blood passes into the mother's bloodstream. An Rh-negative mother may manufacture antibodies to destroy the Rh-positive blood introduced into her bloodstream at the time of birth. Her first baby will be unaffected, but subsequent babies with positive Rh factor will be at risk for a severe anemia called *hemolytic disease* because the mother's Rh antibodies will attack the foetus's red blood cells.

Medical advances now offer both prevention and treatment for this condition. The mother and foetus can be tested, and if Rh incompatibility is found, intrauterine transfusions can be given or an early delivery by caesarean section can be done, depending upon the individual case. Prevention of the problem is preferable to treatment. All women with Rh-negative blood should be injected with a medication called RhoGAM within 72 hours of any birth, miscarriage, or abortion. This injection will prevent them from developing the Rh antibodies.

Another cause of miscarriage is **ectopic pregnancy,** or implantation of a fertilized egg outside the uterus. A fertilized egg may implant itself in the fallopian tube or, occasionally, in the pelvic cavity. Because these structures are not capable of expanding and nourishing a develop-

ing foetus, the pregnancy cannot continue. Such pregnancies are surgically terminated. Most often, the affected fallopian tube is also removed.

Ectopic pregnancy is generally accompanied by pain in the lower abdomen or an aching feeling in the shoulders as the blood flows up toward the diaphragm. If bleeding is significant, blood pressure drops and the woman can go into shock. If an ectopic pregnancy goes undiagnosed and untreated, the fallopian tube ruptures, and the woman is then at great risk of hemorrhage, peritonitis (infection in the abdomen), and even death.

Over the past 12 years, the incidence of ectopic pregnancy has tripled, and no one really understands why. We do know that ectopic pregnancy is a potential side-effect of pelvic inflammatory disease (PID), which has become increasingly common in recent years, because the scarring or blockage of the fallopian tubes characteristic of this disease prevents the fertilized egg from passing to the uterus. About 50 percent of women who have had an ectopic pregnancy conceive again. But women who have had one ectopic pregnancy run a higher risk of having another.

Stillbirth is one of the most traumatic events a couple can face. A stillborn baby is one that is born dead, often for no apparent reason. The grief experienced following a stillbirth is usually devastating and can last for years. In many cases, no amount of reassurance from the attending physician, relatives, or friends can assuage the grief or guilt.

Sudden Infant Death Syndrome. The sudden death of an infant under one year of age, for no apparent reason, is called sudden infant death syndrome (SIDS). While SIDS is the leading cause of death for children aged one month to one year, affecting about 1 in 1000 infants in the United States each year, it is not a disease. Rather, it is ruled the cause of death after all other possibilities are ruled out. A SIDS death is sudden and silent; the death occurs quickly, often associated with sleep and no signs of suffering.

Because SIDS is a diagnosis of exclusion, doctors do not know what causes SIDS. However, research done in countries including England, New Zealand, Australia, and Norway has shown that by placing children on their backs or sides to sleep, the rate of SIDS was cut by as much as half. Prenatal classes instruct parents in SIDS prevention in Canada. Additional precautions against SIDS include having a firm surface for the infant's bed, not allowing the infant to become too warm, maintaining a smoke-free environment, having regular paediatric visits, breast-feeding, and seeking prenatal care.

Because the death of an infant is a disruption of the natural order, it is traumatic for parents, family, and friends. The lack of a discernible cause, the suddenness of the tragedy, and the involvement of the legal system make

---

Rh factor: A blood protein related to the production of antibodies. If an Rh-negative mother is pregnant with an Rh-positive foetus, the mother will manufacture antibodies that can kill the foetus, causing miscarriage.

Ectopic pregnancy: Implantation of a fertilized egg outside the uterus, usually in a fallopian tube; a medical emergency that can end in death from hemorrhage for the mother.

Stillbirth: The birth of a dead baby.

Infertility: Difficulties in conceiving.

Pelvic inflammatory disease (PID): An infection that scars the fallopian tubes and consequently blocks sperm migration, causing infertility.

Endometriosis: A disorder in which uterine lining tissue establishes itself outside the uterus; it is the leading cause of infertility in the United States.

Low sperm count: A sperm count below 60 million sperm per millilitre of semen; it is the leading cause of infertility in men.

Fertility drugs: Hormones that stimulate ovulation in women who are not ovulating; often responsible for multiple births.

a SIDS death especially difficult, leaving a great sense of loss and a need for understanding. Some communities have support groups to help parents and other family members through this grieving process.

*W*HAT DO YOU THINK?

Have you talked to your health care provider about a birth plan and arranged for it to be in your chart? What do you think would be the advantages and disadvantages of breast-feeding?

*I*NFERTILITY

An estimated one in six American couples experiences **infertility,** or difficulties in conceiving. The reasons for this phenomenon include the trend toward delaying childbirth (as a woman gets older, she is less likely to conceive), the use of IUDs, and the rise in the incidence of pelvic inflammatory disease.

Causes in Women

One cause of infertility in women is **pelvic inflammatory disease (PID),** a serious infection that scars the fallopian tubes and blocks sperm migration. Women often develop PID as a result of a gonorrhea or chlamydia infection that progresses to the fallopian tubes and the ovaries. The risk of infertility after one bout of PID is 12 percent. After two bouts, it doubles to nearly 25 percent, and following three bouts, it jumps to more than 50 percent.[18]

Endometriosis is a major cause of infertility. In this disorder, parts of the endometrial lining of the uterus implant themselves outside the uterus—in the fallopian tubes, lungs, intestines, outer uterine walls, ovarian walls, and/or on the ligaments that support the uterus. The disorder can be treated surgically or with hormonal preparations. Success rates vary. Approximately 35 percent of women diagnosed with endometriosis are infertile.

Causes in Men

Among men, the single largest fertility problem is **low sperm count.** Although only one viable sperm is needed for fertilization, research has shown that all the other sperm in the ejaculate aid in the fertilization process. There are normally 60 to 80 million sperm per millilitre of semen. When the count drops below 20 million, fertility begins to decline.

Low sperm count may be attributable to environmental factors such as exposure of the scrotum to intense heat or cold, radiation, or altitude, or even to wearing excessively tight underwear or outerwear. The mumps virus damages the cells that make sperm. Varicose veins above one or both testicles can also render men infertile. Male infertility problems account for around 40 percent of infertility cases.

Treatment

For the couple desperately wishing to conceive, the road to parenthood may be frustrating. Fortunately, medical treatment can identify the cause of infertility in about 90 percent of affected couples. The chances of becoming pregnant range from 30 to 70 percent, depending on the specific cause of the infertility. The countless tests and the invasion of privacy that characterize some couples' efforts to conceive can put stress on an otherwise strong, healthy relationship. Before starting fertility tests, the wise couple will reassess their priorities. Some will choose to undergo counselling to help them clarify their feelings about the fertility process. A good physician or fertility team will take the time to ascertain the couple's level of motivation.

Fertility work-ups for men include a sperm count, a test for sperm motility, and analysis of any disease processes present. Women are thoroughly examined by an obstetrician/gynecologist for the composition of cervical mucus, extent of tubal scarring, and evidence of endometriosis.

Complete fertility work-ups may take four to five months and can be unsettling. In some cases, surgery can correct structural problems such as tubal scarring. In others, administering hormones can improve the health of ova and sperm. Sometimes pregnancy can be achieved by collecting the husband's sperm from several ejaculations and inseminating the wife at a later time.

When all surgical and hormonal methods fail, the couple still has some options. **Fertility drugs** such as Clomid and Pergonal stimulate ovulation in women who are not ovulating. Ninety percent of women who use these drugs will begin to ovulate, and half will conceive.

Fertility drugs are associated with a great number of side-effects, including headaches, irritability, restlessness, depression, fatigue, edema (fluid retention), abnormal uterine bleeding, breast tenderness, vasomotor flushes (hot flashes), and visual difficulties. Women using fertility drugs are also at increased risk of multiple ovarian cysts (fluid-filled growths) and liver damage. The drugs sometimes trigger the release of more than one egg. Thus a woman treated with one of these drugs has a 1 in 10 chance of having multiple births. Most such births are twins, but triplets and even quadruplets are not uncommon.

Alternative insemination of a woman with her partner's sperm is another treatment option. If this procedure fails, the couple may choose insemination by an anonymous donor through a "sperm bank." Many men sell their sperm to such banks. The sperm are classified according to the physical characteristics of the donor (for example, blonde hair, blue eyes), and then frozen for future use. Sperm can survive in this frozen state for up to five years. The woman being inseminated usually chooses sperm from a man whose physical characteristics resemble those of her partner or match her own personal preferences.

In the last few years, concern has been expressed about the possibility of transmitting the AIDS virus through alternative insemination. As a result, donors are routinely screened for the disease before they donate.

In vitro fertilization, often referred to as "test tube" fertilization, involves collecting a viable ovum from the prospective mother and transferring it to a nutrient medium in a laboratory, where it is fertilized with sperm from the woman's partner or a donor. After a few days, the embryo is transplanted into the mother's uterus, where, it is hoped, it will develop normally. Until 1984, in vitro fertilization was classified as "experimental." Since then, it has moved into the mainstream of standard infertility treatments.

In **gamete intrafallopian transfer (GIFT),** the egg is "harvested" from the wife's ovary and placed in the fallopian tube with her husband's sperm. Less expensive and time-consuming than in vitro fertilization, GIFT mimics nature by allowing the egg to be fertilized in the fallopian tube and to migrate to the uterus according to the normal timetable. The success rate for this procedure is approximately 20 percent.

In **nonsurgical embryo transfer,** a donor egg is fertilized by the husband's sperm and then implanted in the wife's uterus. This procedure may also be used in cases involving the transfer of an already-fertilized ovum into the uterus of another woman.

Embryo transfer is another treatment for infertility. In this procedure, an ovum from a donor's body is artificially inseminated by the husband's sperm, allowed to stay in the donor's body for a time, and then transplanted into the wife's body.

Some laboratories are experimenting with **embryo freezing,** in which a fertilized embryo is suspended in a solution of liquid nitrogen. When desired, it is gradually thawed and implanted into the prospective mother. The first United States birth of a frozen embryo was reported in June 1986. In the future, this technique may make it possible for young couples to produce an embryo and save it for later implantation when they are ready to have a child, thus reducing the risks of fertilization of older eggs.

Alternative insemination: Fertilization accomplished by depositing a partner's or a donor's semen into a woman's vagina via a thin tube; almost always done in a doctor's office.

In vitro fertilization: Fertilization of an egg in a nutrient medium and subsequent transfer back to the mother's body.

Gamete intrafallopian transfer (GIFT): An egg is harvested from the female partner ovary and placed with the male partner's sperm in her fallopian tube, where it is fertilized and then migrates to the uterus for implantation.

Nonsurgical embryo transfer: In vitro fertilization of a donor egg by the male partner's (or donor's) sperm and subsequent transfer to the female partner's or another woman's uterus.

Embryo transfer: Alternative insemination of a donor with male partner's sperm; after a time, the embryo is transferred from the donor to the female partner's body.

Embryo freezing: The freezing of an embryo for later implantation.

Surrogate Motherhood

Between 60 and 70 percent of infertile couples are able to conceive after treatment. The rest decide to live without children, to adopt, or to attempt surrogate motherhood. In this option, the couple hires a woman to be alternatively inseminated by the husband. The surrogate then carries the baby to term and surrenders it upon birth to the couple. Surrogate mothers are reportedly paid about $10 000 for their services and are reimbursed for medical expenses. Legal and medical expenses can run as high as $30 000 for the infertile couple. Couples considering surrogate motherhood are advised to consult a lawyer regarding contracts between all involved parties.

𝒲HAT DO YOU THINK?

What are the rights of surrogate mothers? What option would you most likely select if you found that you and your spouse had fertility problems? Why? Do you think cloning or embryo freezing is ethical? Why or why not? Do you think men should participate in prenatal counselling?

Managing Your Fertility

After reading this chapter, you should realize that pregnancy, childbirth, and reproductive issues are not to be taken lightly. The choices between different types of birth control and the ethical issues surrounding fertility are complex. As you read through this chapter, we hope you were able to sort through issues and begin to contemplate some of the decisions you may have to face. We hope that you have begun the process of self-exploration and that you will be able to make informed decisions and choices.

Making Decisions for You

It's important to take control of your own fertility and to share this responsibility in your relationships. What kind of birth control do you currently use or would you use in a sexual relationship? Do you know the potential side-effects? Are there any potential drug interactions? If the contraceptive has a low effectiveness rate, what further means of protection can you take? Finally, have you protected yourself from sexually transmitted infections?

Checklist for Change: Making Personal Choices

✓ If you are in a stable relationship and are considering having a child, is it something both you and your partner want?

✓ Do you have a network of family and friends who will help if you decide to have a baby?

✓ Do you know and feel comfortable with your philosophical beliefs about children?

✓ Have you assessed your health to make sure that if you choose to get pregnant you will begin the pregnancy as healthy as possible?

✓ Do you feel comfortable discussing birth control with your partner?

✓ Do you feel comfortable choosing a method of birth control that meets both your own and your partner's needs?

✓ Are you familiar with the resources available if you have trouble conceiving?

✓ Have you discussed alternatives should you become pregnant or get someone pregnant?

Checklist for Change: Making Community Choices

✓ Have you taken the time to become educated about the issues and concerns related to parenting?

✓ Have you decided to become involved in issues that concern children and parenting?

✓ Do you listen with an open mind to issues involving reproduction and sexual health and then make informed decisions?

✓ When you think about having children, do you think of it in terms of long-range planning?

✓ Are you an advocate for people making choices that are in their best interests, regardless of your own personal philosophy or opinions?

✓ Do you believe in providing support for community agencies and social services that assist in meeting the sexual and reproductive health needs of your community?

✓ Do you try to volunteer your time to other people or agencies that may need your assistance?

Critical Thinking

Rebecca and Bryant are the 37-year-old parents of a five-year-old daughter. They had always planned on having several children, but are now facing a difficult decision: should they have another child now, wait a few more years, or perhaps not have any more children at all? Bryant thinks that they should have more children before they get to be too old. As an only child, he remembers being "lonely all the time." But Rebecca is concerned about the additional expense of having another child. With their daughter about to start school, she is considering going back to work. Anyway, she recently read an article about the advantages of being an only child.

Using the DECIDE model described in Chapter 1, decide what you would do if you were Rebecca or Bryant. Is there more than one decision with which you could feel comfortable?

Summary

◆ Only latex condoms, when used correctly for oral sex or intercourse, are effective in preventing sexually transmitted diseases. Other contraceptive methods include abstinence, outercourse, oral contraceptives, foams, jellies, suppositories, creams, the female condom, the diaphragm, the cervical cap, intrauterine devices, withdrawal, Norplant, Depo-Provera, film, and the sponge. Fertility awareness methods rely on altering sexual practices to avoid pregnancy. Sterilization is permanent contraception.

- Abortion is currently legal through the second trimester. Abortion methods include vacuum aspiration, dilation and evacuation (D&E), dilation and curettage (D&C), hysterotomy, and induction abortion.

- Parenting is a demanding job requiring careful planning. Emotional health, maternal health, financial evaluation, and contingency planning all need to be taken into account.

- Prenatal care includes a complete physical exam within the first trimester and avoidance of alcohol, drugs, cigarettes, X-rays, and chemicals having teratogenic effects. Full-term pregnancy covers three trimesters.

- Childbirth occurs in three stages. Parents should jointly make decisions about labour early in the pregnancy to be better prepared for labour when it occurs. Complications of pregnancy and childbirth include miscarriage, ectopic pregnancy, stillbirth, and the necessity for caesarean section.

- Infertility in women may be caused by pelvic inflammatory disease or endometriosis. In men, it may be caused by low sperm count. Treatment may include alternative insemination, in vitro fertilization, gamete intrafallopian transfer, nonsurgical embryo transfer, and embryo transfer. Surrogate motherhood involves hiring a fertile woman to be alternatively inseminated by the male partner.

Discussion Questions

1. Draw up a list of the most effective contraceptive methods. What drawbacks keep everyone from using them? What medical conditions should keep you from using them?

2. Discuss the varied methods of abortion.

3. What are some of the most important decisions that your parents made concerning raising you? Would you raise your child differently from how you were raised?

4. Discuss the growth of the foetus through the three trimesters. What medical checkups or tests should be done during each trimester?

5. List the varied decisions that parents face when thinking about childbirth. Consider where to have the child and whether to use painkilling drugs during delivery. How does the first-time parent decide what to do?

6. If you and your spouse were having difficulty getting pregnant, what would your options be? If you proved infertile, what would your options be then? What would you do?

Application Exercise

Reread the What Do You Think? scenario at the beginning of the chapter and answer the following questions.

1. What concerns you most about Kari and Dave's relationship? Is it realistic that two people can date for several months and never discuss having sex? What would you have done or not done differently from Kari and Dave?

2. If you could tell incoming first-year students three personal rules about using birth control, what would they be?

Health on the Net

Health Canada Health Protection Branch
www.hwc.ca/datahpb/policy/poltab.html

Canadian Pediatric Society
www.cps.ca/english/index.htm

Canadian Association of Family Resource Programs
www.cfc-efc.ca/frpc/htmle/home.htm

7

Nutrition
Eating for Optimum Health

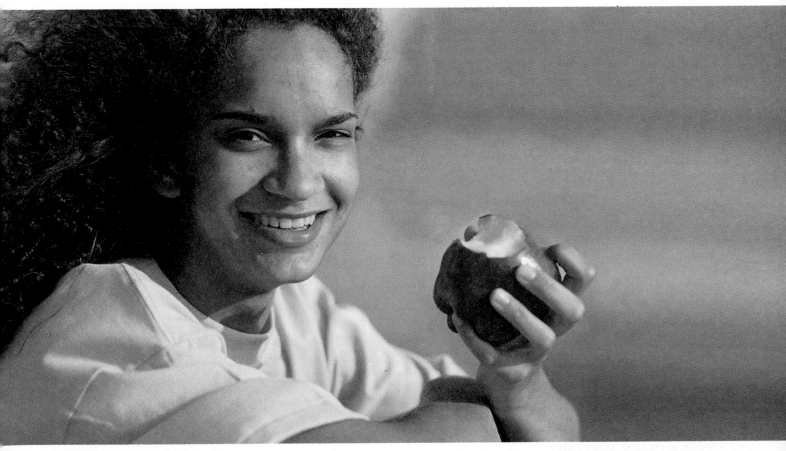

CHAPTER OBJECTIVES

◆ Examine the factors that influence dietary decisions and discuss how *Canada's Food Guide* can be used to help break bad habits.

◆ Explain major essential nutrients (water, proteins, carbohydrates, fibre, fats, vitamins, and minerals) and indicate what purpose they serve in maintaining your overall health.

◆ Define the different types of vegetarianism and discuss possible health benefits and risks.

◆ Describe the unique problems that university students may have when trying to eat healthy foods and the actions they can take to ensure compliance with the food guide.

◆ Explain some of the food safety concerns of which consumers should be aware, including food irradiation, food-borne illnesses, food allergies, and other food health concerns.

Jasper is a first-year student living in the dormitory of a small college. His parents opted for the food service meal plan in the hope that Jasper would eat at least one hot meal per day. This particular food service has few choices for students; foods are overcooked, there are few salads or vegetables, and most entrées tend to be high in fat content. Jasper eats at the food service most of the time, but supplements his diet with fast food and ice cream snacks. He is gaining weight and is worried about some of the recent news stories on TV discussing high-fat diets and diets lacking certain nutrients. He decides he'd better do something about his eating habits, but when he goes to the cafeteria at school, he finds he has few healthy options.

- ■ Why do some people find their dietary choices to be relatively easy, while others have huge problems making dietary changes? What factors may have contributed to their attitudes and behaviours? What would you suggest Jasper do to change his eating habits, if anything? Do you have friends who have similar problems? Where on your campus could they go for help?

Today, we face dietary choices and nutritional challenges that our grandparents never dreamed of—exotic foreign foods; dietary supplements; artificial sweeteners; no-fat, low-fat, and artificial-fat alternatives; cholesterol-free, high-protein, high-carbohydrate, and low-calorie products—thousands of alternatives bombard us daily. Caught in the crossfire of advertised claims by the food industry and advice provided by health and nutrition experts, most of us find it difficult to make wise dietary decisions. The ability to sift through the untruths, half-truths, and scientific realities and select a nutrition plan designed to meet your individual needs is an essential health-promoting skill.

When you are living away from home for the first time, suddenly having to make your own choices about food may be a formidable task. A 1994 study of over 2000 U.S. college students found that they often had considerable difficulty planning their own menus, eating healthfully, and having the resources to prepare meals.[1] Past patterns of eating may be influencing your current behaviours more than you realize. Understanding the reasons behind your nutritional choices may help you change negative dietary patterns and enhance positive behaviours.

HEALTHY EATING

Eating is one activity that most of us take for granted. We assume that we will have sufficient food to get us through the day and rarely are we forced to eat things that we do not like for the sake of staying alive. In fact, although we have all undoubtedly experienced **hunger** before mealtime, few of us have ever experienced the type of hunger that continues for days and threatens our survival.

Many factors influence when we eat, what we eat, and how much we eat. Sensory stimulation, such as smelling, seeing, and tasting foods, can entice us to eat. Social pressures, including family traditions, social events that involve eating, and busy work schedules, can also influence our diets. Although our ancestors typically sat down to three complete meals per day, they also laboured heavily in the fields or at other work and burned off many of those calories. Today, eating three large meals per day combined with an inactive lifestyle is just the right recipe for weight gain.

Cultural factors also play a role in how we eat. People from Middle Eastern cultures tend to eat more rice, fruits, and vegetables than does the typical Canadian. The Japanese eat more fish. Clearly, each culture has both healthy and unhealthy eating habits. The Global Perspectives box suggests ethnic foods to eat and ethnic foods to avoid.

Other factors also influence our dietary choices. Our economic status may determine what types of foods we purchase; those having low incomes probably find some foods or food groups too expensive, while those having high incomes have boundless choices.

If our **appetite** for food is stimulated, we may want to eat something because it looks or smells good, even though we are not actually hungry. Finding the right balance between eating to maintain body functions (eating

Hunger: The feeling associated with the physiological need to eat.

Appetite: The desire to eat; normally accompanies hunger, but is more psychological than physiological.

Changing the way you think about food can mean the difference between choosing healthy foods (eating to live) and foods that satisfy your cravings (living to eat).

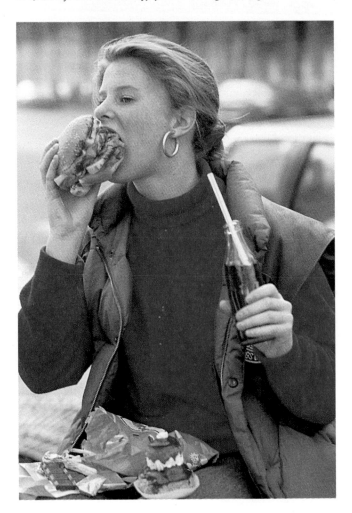

to live) and eating to satisfy our appetites (living to eat) is a problem for many of us.

Nutrition is the science that investigates the relationship between physiological function and the essential elements of the foods we eat. With our overabundance of food, our vast number of choices, and our easy access to almost every **nutrient** (proteins, carbohydrates, fats, vitamins, minerals, and water), Canadians should have few nutritional problems. But nutritionists believe that our "diets of affluence" are responsible for many of our diseases and disabilities. Our history as a land of agricultural abundance accounts for the traditional Canadian diet: high in fats and calories and weighted toward red meats, potatoes, and rich desserts. More recent trends have indicated that Canadians are changing to a white-meat diet having fewer fats and more fruits and vegetables. The Focus on Canada box shows some of these changes.

Despite these dietary improvements, heart disease, certain types of cancer, hypertension (high blood pressure), cirrhosis of the liver, tooth decay, and chronic obesity continue to be major health risks. Why do so many of us have nutritional problems? Much of our preoccupation with food and our tendency to eat the wrong types and amounts of foods stem from our early eating habits. Find out how much you know about nutrition by taking the Rate Yourself test.

𝒲HAT DO YOU THINK?

Think about your own eating habits. Do you eat significant amounts of red meats and dairy products? Are you a vegetarian? Would you be happy with a veggie-laden salad and some wheat bread for your evening meal or do you crave a hot, meat-and-potatoes dining experience? Why do you think you feel the way you do? How did your family eat when you were growing up? Is everyone in your family of origin still eating the same way they did when they were young? Why or why not?

Responsible Eating: Changing Old Habits

Canadians consume more calories per person than do many other peoples in the world. A **calorie** is a unit of measure that indicates the amount of energy we obtain from a particular food. Calories are eaten in the form of *proteins, fats,* and *carbohydrates,* three of the basic nutrients necessary for life. Three other nutrients, *vitamins, minerals,* and *water,* are necessary for bodily function but do not contribute any calories to our diets.

Excess calorie consumption is a major factor in our tendency to be overweight. However, it is not so much the quantity of food we eat that is likely to cause weight problems and resultant diseases as it is the relative proportion of nutrients in our diets and our lack of physical activity. Canadians typically get approximately 38 percent of their calories from fat,[2] 15 percent from proteins, 22 percent from complex carbohydrates, and 24 percent from simple sugars. Dietitians recommend that complex carbohydrates be increased to make up 48 percent of our total calories and that proteins be reduced to 12 percent, simple sugars to 10 percent, and fats to no more than 30 percent of our total diets.

It is the high concentration of fats in the Canadian diet, particularly saturated fats (largely animal fats), that appears to increase our risk for heart disease. High concentrations of highly processed sugars seem to increase the risk for certain other diseases, particularly tooth decay. Over the years, several agencies have worked to modify the average Canadian's diet through a series of dietary goals and guidelines.

Canadian Eating Habits: Changing Patterns

For the past twenty years, Canadians have eaten more poultry and reduced their consumption of beef and eggs. This trend began in the mid-1970s when Canadians were eating almost twice as much beef as poultry per person. By 1987, beef and poultry consumption were at the same level and since then, poultry has surpassed beef as the meat of choice on Canadian tables. Although beef has become a leaner product, economic conditions, cheaper poultry retail prices, and the quest for low-fat protein may have spurred the steady increase in poultry consumption. In 1995, poultry consumption reached 31 kilograms per person, up from 18 kilograms in 1975. Canadians ate 23 kilograms of beef (on a retail weight basis) per person in 1995, down from 35 in 1975.

Egg consumption has also continued its steady downward trend and stood at 14 dozen eggs in 1995, down almost 25% from 19 dozen in 1975. However, processed egg consumption has increased in the form of products such as fresh pasta. Total production of processed eggs has more than doubled over the last 15 years.

Source: Statistics Canada Livestock and Animal Products Section, *Apparent per Capita Food Consumption in Canada Part I, 1995* (1996). Catalogue No. 32-229-XPB.

Consumption of Meat Products and Eggs (Index: 1975=100)

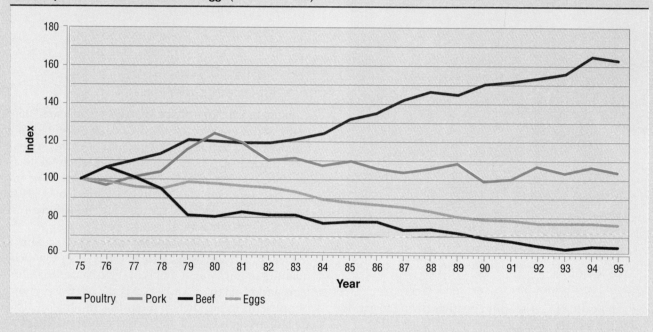

Nutrition: The science that investigates the relationship between physiological function and the essential elements of foods we eat.

Nutrients: The constituents of food that sustain us physiologically: proteins, carbohydrates, fats, vitamins, minerals, and water.

Calorie: A unit of measure that indicates the amount of energy we obtain from a particular food.

Canada's Food Guide

Recent changes in the way we think about food groups and eating were consolidated with the development of *Canada's Food Guide*, promoted by Health and Welfare Canada. The *Guide* was designed to illustrate graphically the importance of grains, cereals, vegetables, and fruits compared to meat, fish, poultry, dairy products, and other foods. Figure 7.1 shows *Canada's Food Guide*, including recommended foods. On the second page of the *Guide* are examples of the equivalent of one serving from each of the major food groups.

Guidelines for Healthy Ethnic Eating

Ethnic Food	Healthy Ideas	Things to Avoid
Italian	▪ Stick to pasta dishes with low-fat sauces; plain red and meatless marinara. Use fresh ingredients such as mushrooms. ▪ Rinse pasta to remove starch. ▪ Choose vegetarian pizzas. ▪ Use skim-milk mozzarella.	▪ Sausages, carbonara sauces, meatballs, garlic/butter breads, cream sauces, heavy-cheese pastas, pepperoni. ▪ Extra cheese.
Mexican	▪ Ask that cheeses and sour cream be provided on the side or left out altogether. ▪ Select white-meat chicken fillings. ▪ Fill up on beans, rice, and vegetables. ▪ Ask what types of oils are used in stir-frying fajitas.	▪ Refried beans fried in fat. ▪ Fried tortillas and burrito and taco shells. ▪ Pork, beef, and sausage fillings. ▪ Thick cheese sauces or toppings.
Chinese	▪ Focus on brown rice as a major part of the meal; if unavailable, ask for steamed (*not* fried) white rice. ▪ Make vegetables the key part of the meal. Stir-frying in vegetable oil is preferable to deep-frying. ▪ Choose a low-fat appetizer such as wonton soup. ▪ Choose chicken or fish and ask if meat content of a dish can be reduced and vegetables increased.	▪ Fried rice, egg rolls, spring rolls, and crispy noodles—are all high in fat. ▪ MSG and high-sodium soy sauces. ▪ Rich lobster or egg dishes.
Japanese	▪ Focus on steamed rice and vegetables. ▪ Substitute tofu for meat; although high in fat, the fat is largely unsaturated. ▪ Eat chicken or fish broiled or steamed.	▪ Soy sauces. ▪ Fried rice dishes. ▪ Miso—it is extremely high in sodium. ▪ Tempura—it is high in fat. ▪ Sashimi and sushi (raw fish) dishes, because of possible bacteria or parasites.
Thai	▪ Choose clear broth soups. ▪ Order steamed seafood in wine sauces, stir-fried chicken, vegetables, or grilled meats.	▪ Coconut milk. ▪ Peanut drippings/sauces. ▪ Deep-fried dishes.
Cajun	▪ Choose tomato-based sauces. ▪ Order vegetable gumbo or jambalaya. ▪ Ask for fish that is grilled. ▪ Hold the salt.	▪ Deep-fried foods. ▪ Andouille and other sausages. ▪ Sauces on sandwiches.

Canada's Food Guide was developed in 1942; the first version was called *Canada's Official Food Rules*. It has since undergone two name changes and three major revisions to make it a better tool for nutrition education. As nutritional knowledge advances, further modifications to the relative numbers of servings recommended are likely.

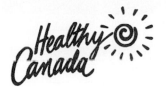

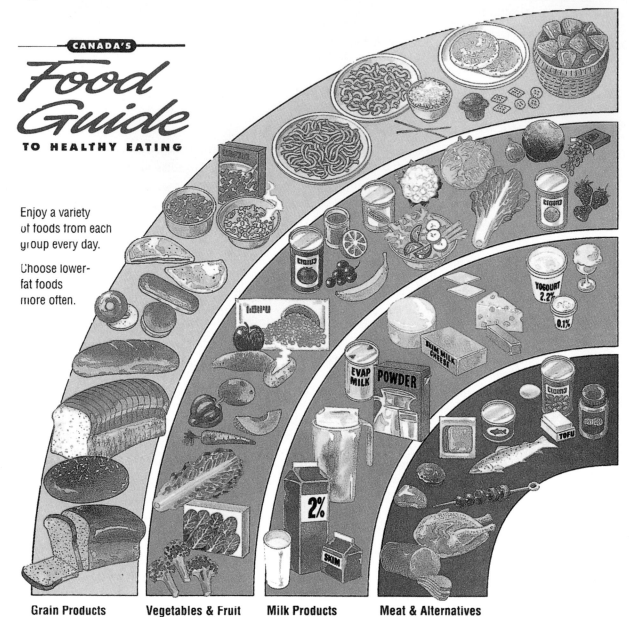

Health and Welfare Canada   Santé et Bien-être social Canada

CANADA'S
Food Guide
TO HEALTHY EATING

Enjoy a variety of foods from each group every day.

Choose lower-fat foods more often.

Grain Products
Choose whole grain and enriched products more often.

Vegetables & Fruit
Choose dark green and orange vegetables and orange fruit more often.

Milk Products
Choose lower-fat milk products more often.

Meat & Alternatives
Choose leaner meats, poultry and fish, as well as dried peas, beans and lentils more often

Canada

FIGURE 7.1

Canada's Food Guide to Healthy Eating

Source: Minister of Supply and Services Canada, 1992. Cat. No. H39-252/1992E.

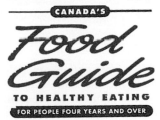

Different People Need Different Amounts of Food

The amount of food you need every day from the 4 food groups and other foods depends on your age, body size, activity level, whether you are male or female and if you are pregnant or breast-feeding. That's why the Food Guide gives a lower and higher number of servings for each food group. For example, young children can choose the lower number of servings, while male teenagers can go to the higher number. Most other people can choose servings somewhere in between.

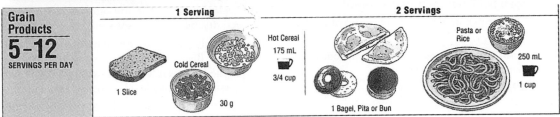

Grain Products
5-12 SERVINGS PER DAY

1 Serving — 1 Slice — Cold Cereal 30 g — Hot Cereal 175 mL 3/4 cup

2 Servings — 1 Bagel, Pita or Bun — Pasta or Rice 250 mL 1 cup

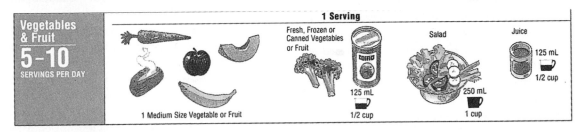

Vegetables & Fruit
5-10 SERVINGS PER DAY

1 Serving — 1 Medium Size Vegetable or Fruit — Fresh, Frozen or Canned Vegetables or Fruit 125 mL 1/2 cup — Salad 250 mL 1 cup — Juice 125 mL 1/2 cup

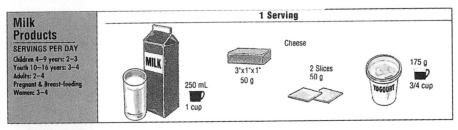

Milk Products
SERVINGS PER DAY
Children 4–9 years: 2–3
Youth 10–16 years: 3–4
Adults: 2–4
Pregnant & Breast-feeding Women: 3–4

1 Serving — MILK 250 mL 1 cup — Cheese 3"x1"x1" 50 g — 2 Slices 50 g — 175 g 3/4 cup

Other Foods

Taste and enjoyment can also come from other foods and beverages that are not part of the 4 food groups. Some of these foods are higher in fat or Calories, so use these foods in moderation.

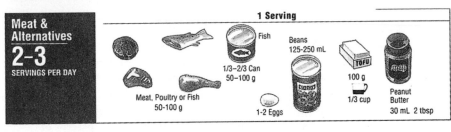

Meat & Alternatives
2-3 SERVINGS PER DAY

1 Serving — Meat, Poultry or Fish 50-100 g — Fish 1/3–2/3 Can 50–100 g — 1-2 Eggs — Beans 125-250 mL — TOFU 100 g 1/3 cup — Peanut Butter 30 mL 2 tbsp

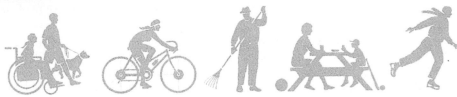

Enjoy eating well, being active and feeling good about yourself. That's VITALITÉ

FIGURE 7.1 *(continued)*

Canada's Food Guide to Healthy Eating

Nutrition Quiz

Which of the following statements are true?

_____ 1. Large amounts of gelatin strengthen finger-nails.

_____ 2. Toast has fewer calories than bread.

_____ 3. Food grown on depleted soils is nutritionally inferior.

_____ 4. Commercially canned and frozen foods are nearly worthless nutritionally.

_____ 5. Athletes need more protein in their diets than does the general population.

_____ 6. Feed a cold and starve a fever.

_____ 7. Taking extra vitamins and minerals will pep you up if you are fatigued.

_____ 8. Eating certain food combinations (such as fish and milk or cucumbers and milk) is dangerous.

_____ 9. Cheese causes constipation.

_____ 10. Celery and fish are brain foods.

_____ 11. Prunes, bran, and fresh fruits are sure cures for constipation.

_____ 12. Yogurt is a nutritionally superior wonder food that will make you healthy.

_____ 13. Vitamin supplements are necessary if you are to be well-nourished.

_____ 14. Oysters and black olives are aphrodisiacs (love potions).

_____ 15. Any food craving indicates that the body needs the nutrients in that food.

_____ 16. Obesity is usually caused by glandular disorders.

_____ 17. "Health foods" are nutritionally superior to regular brands.

_____ 18. Megadoses of vitamin C help to prevent colds.

Answers: All the statements are false.

1. Many factors influence fingernail formation including disease, environment, hormones, and nutrition. Gelatin is not one of them.

2. Toasting browns and dehydrates the exterior of the bread but does not reduce its caloric value.

3. Poor soil produces poor yields. Quantity is affected, not quality. For example, depleted soil produces fewer and smaller beans, but each bean is still nutritionally complete.

4. Some methods of food preparation—including home preparation—reduce the nutrient value of certain foods. But commercial methods of processing foods are designed to preserve their nutrient values.

5. Athletes may need more calories because of increased activity, but they do not need more protein.

6. The only valid guideline with colds and fever is to increase fluid intake. With a fever, more calories are burned as a result of increased metabolic rate, but the person often eats less because of malaise and nausea.

7. Vitamins and minerals are not pep pills. They contain no calories (energy), nor are they stimulants. If fatigue persists, see a physician.

8. There are no known poisonous food combinations providing, of course, that neither food is contaminated or spoiled.

9. Generally, over 90 percent of the carbohydrate, protein, and fat in cheese is absorbed; constipation is not produced.

10. No one particular food builds any one body tissue.

11. There are several causes of constipation. If constipation is atonic, roughage may be helpful, but if it is spastic or obstructive, roughage is undesirable and the person is placed on a low-fibre diet.

12. Yogurt is a cultured milk product. It has the same nutritive value as the milk from which it was made. There are no "wonder foods."

13. A well-balanced diet provides all necessary vitamins. Hypervitaminosis can result from high amounts of ingested fat-soluble vitamins.

14. There are no known aphrodisiacs for humans.

15. Craving is a learned preference for a food rather than an indication that the body "needs" that food.

16. At the present time, it is thought that only 5 percent of obesity cases are caused by metabolic or glandular problems. The remaining 95 percent of cases are regulatory, which means too much food and too little exercise.

17. Foods claiming to be "natural" or "organic" are not superior to general foods available at the supermarket. Foods should be selected for their nutritional value, not their advertising value.

18. Many controlled and double-blind studies have been run. So far there is no statistical evidence that high doses of vitamin C help to prevent the common cold.

Making the *Guide* Work for You

Some people are overwhelmed by their first glance at the *Guide.* But when you consider breakfast, lunch, dinner, and snacks in between, it is really quite easy to get all the servings that you need.

Although everyone is different, it is generally recommended that you try to consume foods from the grain products group throughout the day, starting perhaps with a large bowl of cereal for breakfast or a bowl of cereal and a bagel or English muffis. Keep in mind that with any bread, cereal, or grain product you must consider the amount of fat. Many people are duped into thinking that granola is a health food and that bran muffins are better than bagels or bread. Sometimes these products are loaded with fat, sugar, and calories. Read the labels on packaged products and opt for reduced-fat, whole-grain products when trying to meet *Canada's Food Guide* requirements.

The Digestive Process

Food provides us with the chemicals we need for energy and body maintenance. Because our bodies cannot synthesize or produce certain essential nutrients, we must obtain them from the foods we eat. Even though we may take in adequate amounts of foods and nutrients, if our body systems are not functioning properly, much of the nutrient value in our food may be lost. Before foods can be utilized properly, the digestive system must break the larger food particles down into smaller, more usable forms. The process by which foods are broken down and either absorbed or excreted by the body is known as the **digestive process.**

Even before you take your first bite of pizza, your body has already begun a series of complex digestive responses. Your mouth prepares for the food by increasing production of **saliva.** Saliva contains mostly water, which aids in chewing and swallowing, but it also contains important enzymes that begin the process of food breakdown, including amylase, which begins to break down carbohydrates. From the mouth, the food passes down the **esophagus**, a 23-to-25-centimetre tube that connects the mouth and stomach. A series of contractions and relaxations by the muscles lining the esophagus gently moves food to the next digestive organ, the **stomach.** Here food mixes with enzymes and stomach acids. Hydrochloric acid begins to work in combination with pepsin, an enzyme, to break down proteins. In most people, the stomach secretes enough mucus to protect the stomach lining from these harsh digestive juices. In others, there are problems with the lining that can result in ulcers or other gastric problems.

Further digestive activity takes place in the **small intestine**, an eight-metre-long coiled tube containing three sections: the *duodenum,* the *jejunum,* and the *ileum.* Each of these sections secretes digestive enzymes that, when combined with enzymes from the liver and the pancreas, further contribute to the breakdown of proteins, fats, and carbohydrates. Once broken down, these nutrients are absorbed into the bloodstream to supply body cells with energy. The liver is the major organ that determines whether nutrients are stored, sent to cells or organs, or excreted. Solid wastes consisting of fibre, water, and salts are dumped into the large intestine, where most of the water and salts are reabsorbed into the system and the fibre is passed out through the anus. The entire digestive process takes approximately 24 hours (see Figure 7.2).

*O*BTAINING ESSENTIAL NUTRIENTS

Water

If you were to go on a survival trip, which would you take with you—food or water? You may be surprised to learn that you could survive for much longer periods without food than you could without water. Even in severe conditions, the average person can go for weeks without certain vitamins and minerals before experiencing serious deficiency symptoms. **Dehydration**, however, can cause serious problems within a matter of hours; after a few days without water, death is likely.

Digestive process: The process by which foods are broken down and either absorbed or excreted by the body.

Saliva: Fluid secreted by the salivary glands; enzymes in the fluid aid in the breakdown of certain foods for digestion.

Esophagus: Tube that transports food from the mouth to the stomach.

Stomach: Large muscular organ that temporarily stores, mixes, and digests foods.

Small intestine: Muscular, coiled digestive organ; consists of the duodenum, jejunum, and ileum.

Dehydration: Abnormal depletion of body fluids; a result of lack of water.

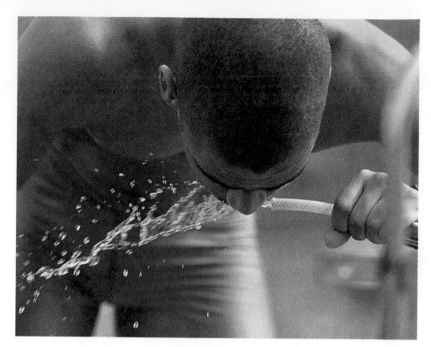

While you may not be conscious of your body's need for water until an unquenchable thirst comes along, water is actually our most necessary nutrient.

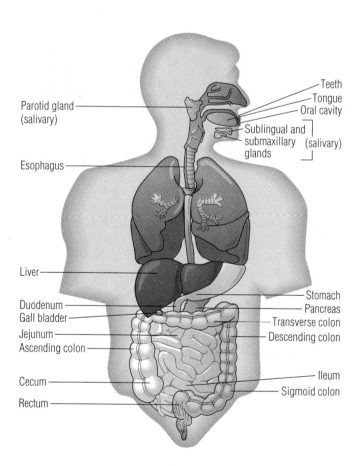

Parotid gland (salivary)

Teeth
Tongue
Oral cavity

Sublingual and submaxillary (salivary) glands

Esophagus

Liver

Duodenum
Gall bladder
Jejunum
Ascending colon

Cecum

Rectum

Stomach
Pancreas
Transverse colon
Descending colon

Ileum
Sigmoid colon

FIGURE 7.2

The Human Digestive System. Digestion occurs throughout this system, from the mouth through the rectum.

Just what function does water serve in the body? Between 50 and 60 percent of our total body weight is water. The water in our system bathes cells, aids in fluid and electrolyte balance, maintains pH balance, and transports molecules and cells throughout the body. Water is the major component of the blood, which carries oxygen and nutrients to the tissues and is responsible for maintaining cells in working order.

How much water do you need? Most experts believe that six to eight glasses of water per day are necessary. Because of high concentrations of water in most of the foods we consume, however, the actual number of glasses needed each day is somewhat less than this for the average person. Individual needs vary drastically according to dietary factors, age, size, environmental temperature and humidity levels, exercise, and the effectiveness of the individual's system.

Proteins

Next to water, **proteins** are the most abundant substances in the human body. Proteins are major components of nearly every cell and have been called the "body builders" because of their role in the development and repair of bone, muscle, skin, and blood cells. Proteins are also the key elements of the antibodies that protect us from disease, of enzymes that control chemical activities in the body, and of hormones that regulate bodily functions. Moreover, proteins aid in the transport of iron, oxygen, and nutrients to all of the body's cells and supply another source of energy to body cells when fats and carbohydrates are not readily available. In short, adequate amounts of protein in the diet are vital to many body functions and to your ultimate survival.

Most Canadians, like their U.S. counterparts, consume more protein than required, and too much of it in the form of high-fat animal flesh and dairy products.[3] The recommended protein intake for the average man is only 63 grams, while the average woman needs only 50 grams under normal circumstances. The excess is stored, like other extra calories, as fat.

Proteins are made up of smaller molecules known as **amino acids**. These acids are composed of chains that link together like beads on a necklace in differing combinations. Over 22 different types of amino acids are found in animal tissue, and humans cannot synthesize all of them. The eight amino acids that the adult body cannot synthesize in adequate amounts are referred to as **essential amino acids**. They must be obtained from foods.

Complete (high-quality) proteins are those proteins that naturally contain all the eight essential amino acids. If we consume a food that contains protein but is deficient in some of the essential amino acids, the total amount of protein that can be synthesized by the other amino acids is decreased. It is important to remember that just because essential amino acids are present in a food does not guarantee that they will be synthesized. Quality of protein depends on the presence of amino acids in digestible form and in amounts proportional to body requirements.

The most common sources of dietary protein in Canada are red meats, poultry, fish, beans, nuts, and dairy products. In addition to providing high-quality proteins, these sources of protein (with the exception of fish, beans, and nuts) also contain high levels of saturated fat and cholesterol. Selecting leaner cuts of meat, removing the fat and skin from chicken, and choosing low-fat dairy products will enable you to get high-quality proteins without the excess calories and fat.

What about plant sources of protein? Proteins from plant sources are often **incomplete proteins** in that they are missing one or two of the essential amino acids. Nevertheless, it is relatively easy for the non-meat eater to combine plant foods effectively and to eat complementary sources of plant protein (see Figure 7.3). An excellent example of this mutual supplementation process is eating peanut butter on whole-grain bread. Although each of these foods is deficient in essential amino acids, eating them together provides high-quality protein.

Plant sources of protein fall into three general categories: legumes (beans, peas, peanuts, and soy products), grains (whole grains, corn, and pasta products), and nuts and seeds. Certain vegetables, such as leafy green vegetables and broccoli, also contribute valuable plant proteins. Mixing two or more foods from each of these categories during the same meal will provide all of the essential amino acids necessary to ensure adequate protein absorption. People who are not interested in obtaining all of their protein from plants can combine incomplete plant proteins with complete low-fat animal proteins such as chicken, fish, turkey, and lean red meat. Low-fat or nonfat cottage cheese, skim milk, egg whites, and nonfat dry milk all provide high-quality proteins and have few calories and little dietary fat.

Carbohydrates

Although the importance of proteins in the body cannot be underestimated, it is **carbohydrates** that supply us with the energy needed to sustain normal daily activity. Long maligned by weight-conscious people, carbohydrates can actually be metabolized more quickly and efficiently than can proteins. Carbohydrates are a quick source of energy for the body, being easily converted to glucose, the fuel for the body's cells. These foods also play an important role in the functioning of the internal organs, the nervous system, and the muscles. They are the best source of energy for endurance athletics because they provide both an immediate and a time-released energy source as they are digested easily and then consistently metabolized in the bloodstream.[4] For many people, a plate of pasta represents an attractive, healthy alternative to a fatty steak.

There are two major types of carbohydrates: **simple sugars**, which are found primarily in fruits, and **complex carbohydrates**, which are found in grains, cereals, dark green leafy vegetables, yellow fruits and vegetables (carrots, yams), *cruciferous* vegetables (such as broccoli, cabbage, and cauliflower), and certain root vegetables, such as potatoes. Most of us do not get enough complex carbohydrates in our daily diets.

Proteins: The essential constituents of nearly all body cells. Proteins are necessary for the development and repair of bone, muscle, skin, and blood, and are the key elements of antibodies, enzymes, and hormones.

Amino acids: The building blocks of protein.

Essential amino acids: Eight of the basic nitrogen-containing building blocks of protein that we must obtain from foods to ensure our personal health.

Complete (high-quality) proteins: Proteins that contain all of the eight essential amino acids.

Incomplete proteins: Proteins that are lacking in one or more of the essential amino acids.

Carbohydrates: Basic nutrients that supply the body with the energy needed to sustain normal activity.

Simple sugars: A major type of carbohydrate that provides short-term energy.

Complex carbohydrates: A major type of carbohydrate that provides sustained energy.

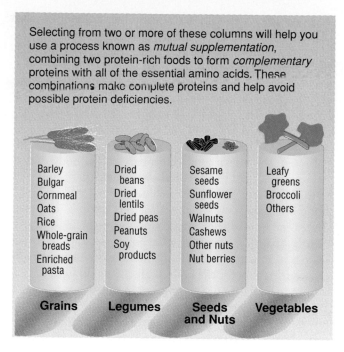

Grains	Legumes	Seeds and Nuts	Vegetables
Barley	Dried beans	Sesame seeds	Leafy greens
Bulgar	Dried lentils	Sunflower seeds	Broccoli
Cornmeal	Dried peas	Walnuts	Others
Oats	Peanuts	Cashews	
Rice	Soy products	Other nuts	
Whole-grain breads		Nut berries	
Enriched pasta			

FIGURE 7.3

Complementary Proteins

Source: Adapted by permission from page 205 of *Nutrition Concepts and Controversies,* 6th ed., by Eva Hamilton, Eleanor Whitney, and Frances Sizer. Copyright 1994 by West Publishing Company. All rights reserved.

A typical diet contains large amounts of simple sugars. The most common form is *glucose.* Eventually, the human body converts all types of simple sugars to glucose to provide energy to cells. In its natural form, glucose is sweet and is obtained from substances such as corn syrup, honey, molasses, vegetables, and fruits. *Fructose* is another simple sugar found in fruits and berries. Glucose and fructose are **monosaccharides** and contain only one molecule of sugar.

Disaccharides are combinations of two monosaccharides. Perhaps the best-known example is common granulated table sugar (known as sucrose), which consists of a molecule of fructose chemically bonded to a molecule of glucose. Lactose, found in milk and milk products, is another form of disaccharide, formed by the combination of glucose and galactose (another simple sugar). Disaccharides must be broken down into simple sugars before they can be used by the body.

Controlling the amount of sugar in your diet can be difficult because sugar, like sodium, is often present in food products in which you might not expect to find it. Such diverse items as ketchup, Russian dressing, Coffee-Mate, and Shake 'n' Bake derive between 30 and 65 percent of their calories from sugar. Reading labels carefully before purchasing food products is a must.

Polysaccharides are complex carbohydrates formed by the combining of long chains of saccharides. Like disac-

charides, they must be broken down into simple sugars before they can be utilized by the body. There are two major forms of complex carbohydrates: *starches* and *fibre,* or **cellulose.**

Starches make up the majority of the complex carbohydrate group. Starches in our diets come from flours, breads, pasta, potatoes, and related foods. They are stored in body muscles and the liver in a polysaccharide form called **glycogen.** When the body requires a sudden burst of energy, it breaks down glycogen into glucose. While we often think of starches as an alternative to fats, starches aren't better for some people, such as those who are insulin-resistant.

Carbohydrates and Athletic Performance. In the last decade, carbohydrates have become the "health foods" of many people involved in athletic competition. Many fitness enthusiasts consume concentrated sugary foods or drinks before or during athletic activity, thinking that the sugars will provide extra energy. However, in some situations, they may actually be counterproductive.[5]

One possible problem involves the gastrointestinal tract. If your intestines react to activity (or the nervousness before competition) by moving material through the small intestine more rapidly than usual, undigested disaccharides and/or unabsorbed monosaccharides will reach the colon, which can result in a very inopportune bout of diarrhea.[6]

Consuming large amounts of sugar during exercise can also have a negative effect on hydration. Concentrations exceeding 24 grams of sugar per 200 grams of fluid can delay stomach emptying and hence absorption of water. Some fruit juices, fruit drinks, and other sugar-sweetened beverages have more than this amount of sugar. If you use these products, you should dilute them with ice cubes or water.

Marathon runners and other people who require reserves of energy for demanding tasks often attempt to increase stores of glycogen in the body by a process known as *carbohydrate loading.* This process involves modifying the nature of both workouts and diet, usually during the week or so before competition. The athlete trains very hard early in the week while eating small amounts of carbohydrates. Right before competition, the athlete dramatically increases intake of carbohydrates to force the body to store increased levels of glycogen, to be used during endurance activities (such as the last kilometres of a marathon).

The Myth of Sugar and Hyperactivity. Contrary to early media reports, extensive research done in the last decade indicates that sugars *do not* cause hyperactivity.[7] In well-controlled dietary challenge studies, consumption of sugar has not been shown to have negative effects on motor activity, spontaneous behaviour, performance in psychological tests, learning, memory, attention span, or problem-solving ability.

Fibre

The role fibre plays in promoting nutrition and health has been a controversial subject in recent years. What exactly is fibre? How effective is it in reducing certain health risks? Are certain types of fibres more effective than others?

Fibre, often referred to as "bulk" or "roughage," is the indigestible portion of plant foods that helps move foods through the digestive system and softens stools by absorbing water. *Insoluble fibre,* which is found in bran, whole-grain breads and cereals, and most fruits and vegetables, is associated with these gastrointestinal benefits and has also been found to reduce the risk for several forms of cancer. *Soluble fibre* appears to be a factor in lowering blood cholesterol levels, thereby reducing risk for cardiovascular disease. Major sources of soluble fibre in the diet include oat bran, dried beans (such as kidney, garbanzo, pinto, and navy beans), and some fruits and vegetables.

Carbo-loading with bread and pasta before an endurance event is a training strategy used by many athletes to build energy reserves for the "last mile."

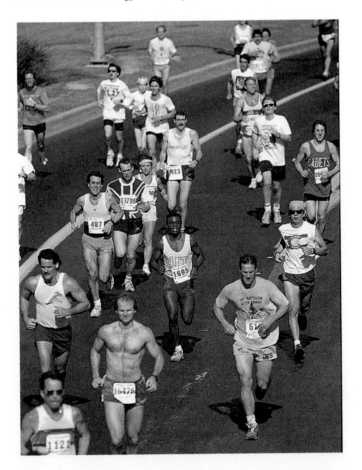

The best way to increase your dietary fibre is to eat more complex carbohydrates, such as whole grains, fruits, vegetables, dried peas and beans, nuts, and seeds. As with most nutritional advice, however, too much of a good thing can pose problems. Sudden increases in dietary fibre may cause flatulence (intestinal gas), cramping, or a bloated feeling. Consuming plenty of water or other liquids may reduce such side-effects.

Fibre and Your Health. A few years ago, fibre was thought by some to be the remedy for just about everything. Much of this hope was exaggerated. However, current research does support many benefits of fibre, including the following:[8]

- *Protection against colon and rectal cancer.* Several studies have supported the theory that fibre-rich diets, particularly those including insoluble fibre, prevent the development of precancerous growths.

- *Protection against breast cancer.* Research into the effects of fibre on breast-cancer risks is very inconclusive. However, some studies have indicated that wheat bran (rich in insoluble fibre) reduces blood-estrogen levels, which may affect the risk for breast cancer. Another theory suggests that people who eat more fibre have proportionally less fat in their diets and that this is what reduces overall risk. The jury is still very much out in this area.

- *Protection against constipation.* Insoluble fibre, consumed with adequate fluids, is the safest, most effective way to prevent or treat constipation. The fibre acts like a sponge, absorbing moisture and producing softer, bulkier stools that are easily passed. Fibre also helps produce gas, which, in turn, may initiate a bowel movement.

- *Protection against diverticulosis.* About half of all Canadians over 60 suffer from *diverticulosis,* a condition in which tiny bulges or pouches form on the large intestinal wall. These bulges become irritated and cause chronic pain if under strain from constipation. Insoluble fibre helps to reduce constipation and added pain. The condition is rare in those under 30.

Monosaccharide: A simple sugar that contains only one molecule of sugar.

Disaccharide: A combination of two monosaccharides.

Polysaccharide: A complex carbohydrate formed by the combination of long chains of saccharides.

Cellulose: Fibre, a major form of complex carbohydrates.

Glycogen: The polysaccharide form in which glucose is stored in the liver.

- *Protection against heart disease.* Many studies have indicated that soluble fibre (as in oat bran, barley, and fruit pectin) helps reduce blood cholesterol, primarily by lowering LDL ("bad") cholesterol. Whether this reduction is a direct effect or occurs instead through the displacement of fat calories by fibre calories in a high-fibre diet remains in question.

- *Protection against diabetes.* Some studies have suggested that soluble fibre improves control of blood sugar and can reduce the need for insulin or medication in people with diabetes. Exactly why isn't clear, but soluble fibre seems to delay the emptying of the stomach and slow the absorption of glucose by the intestine.

- *Protection against obesity.* Because most high-fibre foods are high in carbohydrates and low in fat, they help control caloric intake. Many take longer to chew, which slows you down at the table and makes you feel full sooner.

Most experts believe that Canadians should double their current consumption of dietary fibre—to 20 to 30 grams per day for most people. To do this, the following steps are recommended:

1. Eat a variety of foods.
2. Eat at least five servings of fruits and vegetables and three to six servings of whole-grain breads, cereals, and legumes per day.

3. Eat less processed food.
4. Eat the skins of fruits and vegetables.
5. Get your fibre from foods rather than pills or powders.
6. Spread out your fibre intake.
7. Drink plenty of liquids.

Fats

Fats (or *lipids*), another group of basic nutrients, are perhaps the most misunderstood of the body's required energy sources. Most of us do not realize that fats play a vital role in the maintenance of healthy skin and hair, insulation of the body organs against shock, maintenance of body temperature, and the proper functioning of the cells themselves. Fats make our foods taste better and carry the fat-soluble vitamins A, D, E, and K to the cells. They also provide a concentrated form of energy in the absence of sufficient amounts of carbohydrates. If fats perform all these functions, why are we constantly urged to reduce our intake of them?

Although moderate consumption of fats is essential to health maintenance, overconsumption can be dangerous. The most common form of fat circulating in the blood is the **triglyceride**, which makes up about 95 percent of total body fat. When we consume too many calories, the excess is converted into triglycerides in the liver, which are stored in all-too-obvious places on our bodies.

The remaining 5 percent of body fat is composed of substances such as **cholesterol**, which can accumulate on the inner walls of arteries, causing a narrowing of the channel through which blood flows. This buildup, called **plaque**, is a major cause of *atherosclerosis* (hardening of the arteries). At one time, the amount of circulating cholesterol in the blood was thought to be crucial. Current thinking is that the actual amount of circulating cholesterol itself is not as important as the ratio of total cholesterol to a group of compounds called **high-density lipoproteins (HDLs)**. Lipoproteins are the transport facilitators for cholesterol in the blood. High-density lipoproteins are capable of transporting more cholesterol than are **low-density lipoproteins (LDLs)**. Whereas LDLs transport cholesterol to the body's cells, HDLs apparently transport circulating cholesterol to the liver for metabolism and elimination from the body. People with a high percentage of HDLs therefore appear to be at lower risk for development of cholesterol-clogged arteries. Regular vigorous exercise plays a part in reduction of cholesterol by increasing high-density lipoproteins.

Fat cells consist of chains of carbon and hydrogen atoms. Those that are unable to hold any more hydrogen in their chemical structure are labelled **saturated fats**. They generally come from animal sources, such as meats and dairy products, and are solid at room temperature. **Unsaturated fats**, which come from plants and include

Fats: Basic nutrients composed of carbon and hydrogen atoms; needed for the proper functioning of cells, insulation of body organs against shock, maintenance of body temperature, and healthy skin and hair.

Triglyceride: The most common form of fat in the body; excess calories consumed are converted into triglycerides and stored as body fat.

Cholesterol: A form of fat circulating in the blood that can accumulate on the inner walls of arteries.

Plaque: Cholesterol buildup on the inner walls of arteries, causing a narrowing of the channel through which blood flows; a major cause of atherosclerosis.

High-density lipoproteins (HDLs): Compounds that facilitate the transport of cholesterol in the blood to the liver for metabolism and elimination from the body.

Low-density lipoproteins (LDLs): Compounds that facilitate the transport of cholesterol in the blood to the body's cells.

Saturated fats: Fats that are unable to hold any more hydrogen in their chemical structure; derived mostly from animal sources; solid at room temperature.

Unsaturated fats: Fats that do have room for more hydrogen in their chemical structure; derived mostly from plants; liquid at room temperature.

most vegetable oils, are generally liquid at room temperature and have room for additional hydrogen atoms in their chemical structure. The terms *monounsaturated fat* and *polyunsaturated fat* refer to the relative number of hydrogen atoms that are missing. Peanut and olive oils are high in monounsaturated fats, whereas corn, sunflower, and safflower oils are high in polyunsaturated fats. There is currently a great deal of controversy about which type of unsaturated fat is most beneficial. Although polyunsaturated fats were favoured by nutritional researchers in the early 1980s, today many researchers believe that polyunsaturates may decrease beneficial HDL levels while reducing LDL levels. Monounsaturated fats seem to lower only LDL levels and thus are the "preferred" fats of the 1990s. For a breakdown of the types of fats found in common vegetable oils, see Figure 7.4.

Reducing Fat in Your Diet.   Finding the best ways to cut fat in your diet is largely dependent on you, your lifestyle, and determining what works for you. The following basic guidelines are a good place to start to reduce your fat intake:

- *Know what you are putting in your mouth.* Read food labels. Remember that no more than 10 percent of your total calories should come from saturated fat, and no more than 30 percent should come from all forms of fat.

- *Choose fat-free or low-fat versions of cakes, cookies, crackers, or chips.*

- *Use olive oil for baking and sautéing.* Animal studies have shown that it doesn't raise cholesterol or promote the growth of tumours.

- *Whenever possible, use liquid, diet, or whipped margarine: they have far less trans-fatty acids than solid fat.*

- *Choose lean meats, fish, or poultry.* Remove skin. Broil or bake whenever possible. In general, the more well-done the meat, the fewer the calories. Drain off fat after cooking.

- *Choose fewer cold cuts, bacon, sausage, hot dogs, and organ meats.* Be careful of those products claiming to be "95 percent fat-free" as they may still have high levels of fat.

- *Select nonfat dairy products whenever possible.* Part-skim-milk cheeses such as mozzarella, farmer's, lappi, and ricotta are good choices.

- *When cooking, use substitutes for butter, margarine, oils, sour cream, mayonnaise, and salad dressings.* Chicken broths, wine, vinegar, and low-calorie dressings make good flavourings and/or cooking ingredients.

- *Remember to think of your food intake as an average over a day or a couple of days.* If you have a high-fat breakfast or lunch, have a low-fat dinner to balance it.

For more specific ways to cut fat from your diet, see the Skills for Behaviour Change box.

Trans-Fatty Acids: Still Bad?   Since the mid-1960s, Canadians have shown that they have heeded the dire warnings about cholesterol and saturated fat by decreasing their intake of butter by almost two-thirds and substituting margarine, which became known as the "better butter" after reports labelled unsaturated fats the "heart-healthy" alternative. But a widely publicized study in 1990

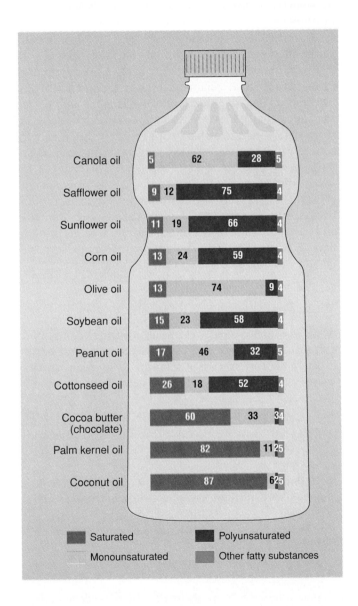

FIGURE 7.4

Percentages of Saturated, Polyunsaturated, and Monounsaturated Fats in Common Vegetable Oils

questioned the benefits of margarine; it indicated that margarine contains fats that raise blood cholesterol at least as much as the saturated fat in butter does.[9] The culprits? **Trans-fatty acids,** fatty acids having unusual shapes that are produced when polyunsaturated oils are *hydrogenated,* a process in which hydrogen is added to unsaturated fats to make them more solid and resistant to chemical change.[10] Besides raising cholesterol levels, trans-fatty acids have been implicated in the development of certain types of cancer.[11]

While the 1990 study pointed an accusing finger at the potential "bad" margarine, researchers Walter Willet and Albert Ascherio of the Harvard School of Public Health recently provided a resounding "wake-up call" for those of us who have faithfully avoided butter in favour of the healthier margarine alternative. According to their analysis of several fat studies, the trans-fatty acids found in margarine may not just be potentially harmful; they may in fact pose an even greater risk for heart disease than does eating saturated fat villains such as butter and lard.[12] But before you dash out and fill your refrigerator with butter, remember that Willet and Ascherio's research is also controversial. Wondering what to do? Probably the best advice is to continue to reduce overall fat in your diet to less than 30 percent of total calories. Whenever possible, opt for other condiments on your bread, such as jams, fat-free cream cheeses, garlic, or other toppings. Some experts advocate using low-fat salad dressings as toppings for bread and pasta, or using olive oil in moderation to add a bit of flavour. If you have high cholesterol, reducing all types of fat and cholesterol in the diet is still sound advice.

Vitamins

Vitamins are potent, essential, organic compounds that promote growth and help maintain life and health. Every minute of every day, vitamins help maintain your nerves and skin, produce blood cells, build bones and teeth, heal wounds, and convert food energy to body energy. And they do all of this without adding any calories to your diet.

Age, heat, and other environmental conditions can destroy vitamins in food. Vitamins can be classified as either *fat-soluble,* meaning that they are absorbed through the intestinal tract with the help of fats, or *water-soluble,* meaning that they are easily dissolved in water. Vitamins A, D, E, and K are fat-soluble; B complex vitamins and vitamin C are water-soluble. Fat-soluble vitamins tend to be stored in the body, and toxic accumulations in the liver may cause cirrhosis-like symptoms. Water-soluble vitamins are generally excreted and cause few toxicity problems (see Table 7.1).

Despite all of the media suggestions to the contrary, few Canadians suffer from true vitamin deficiencies if they eat a diet containing all of the food groups at least part of the time. Nevertheless, Canadians continue to purchase large quantities of vitamin supplements. For the most part, vitamin supplements are unnecessary and, in certain instances, may even be harmful. Overuse of vitamin supplements can lead to a toxic condition known as **hypervitaminosis.**

Recommended Nutrient Intake. A document called the "Recommended Nutrient Intake (RNI)" is the standard guide for nutrient intake in Canada. Health and Welfare Canada revises RNI values periodically. The RNIs reflect the fact that a person's actual level of need for a nutrient can be influenced by age, sex, body size, growth, and reproductive status. Thus, pregnant and lactating women have their own set of RNIs. RNIs given on food packaging are often for adult males, and may be misleading for women, children, the elderly, and other groups who have different nutritional needs.

In Canada, macronutrients, such as protein and carbohydrates, are measured in grams, while micronutrients, such as vitamins, are given as a percentage of RNI.

Trans-fatty acids: Fatty acids that are produced when polyunsaturated oils are hydrogenated to make them more solid.

Vitamins: Essential organic compounds that promote growth and reproduction and help maintain life and health.

Hypervitaminosis: A toxic condition caused by overuse of vitamin supplements.

Minerals: Inorganic, indestructible elements that aid physiological processes.

Macrominerals: Minerals that the body needs in fairly large amounts.

Trace minerals: Minerals that the body needs in only very small amounts.

𝒲HAT DO YOU THINK?

Of all of the nutrients discussed in this section, which one do you worry most about not getting enough in your diet? What is the basis for your worry? Are you planning to take any action to make sure your daily intake is adequate? What steps will you take?

Minerals

Minerals are the inorganic, indestructible elements that aid physiological processes within the body. Without minerals, vitamins could not be absorbed. Minerals are readily excreted and are usually not toxic. **Macrominerals** are those minerals that the body needs in fairly large amounts: sodium, calcium, phosphorus, magnesium, potassium,

How to Cut the Fat from Your Diet

The small choices you make in your daily diet can add up to a tremendous difference in how much fat you consume over time. Trimming just one teaspoon each day can cut over five pounds of fat from your diet in a year's time. It's still possible to eat great-tasting foods and barely notice these small personal choices. Consider the following:

1. "Butter" your toast and muffins with "fruit-only" jams instead of sugary jellies and jams, butter, margarine, or other high-calorie spreads.

15 mL butter	108 calories	12 g fat
15 mL sugarless jam	18 calories	0 g fat
Savings	90 calories	12 g fat

2. Sauté meat and vegetables in chicken broth or wine (most of which burns off during cooking) rather than in oil.

15 mL oil	240 calories	27 g fat
wine or broth	0 calories	0 g fat
Savings	240 calories	27 g fat

3. Remove the skin from chicken before cooking.

100 g breast	193 calories	8 g fat
100 g skinless breast	142 calories	3 g fat
Savings	51 calories	5 g fat

4. Use low-calorie, low-fat salad dressings on your sandwiches instead of mayonnaise.

15 mL mayonnaise	100 calories	11 g fat
15 mL low-cal dressing	7 calories	0 g fat
Savings	93 calories	11 g fat

5. When you crave ice cream, splurge instead on nonfat frozen yoghurt. Today's flavours are so delicious that you may give ice cream the permanent cold shoulder.

125 mL ice cream	400 calories	25 g fat
125 mL nonfat yogurt	120 calories	0 g fat
Savings	280 calories	25 g fat

6. For a skinny version of cream cheese that only tastes fattening, mix three parts blenderized low-fat cottage cheese with one part nonfat yogurt and use as a delicious dip, spread, or topping.

30 mL cream cheese	99 calories	10 g fat
30 mL mock cream cheese	20 calories	0 g fat
Savings	79 calories	10 g fat

7. For a warming meal minus a lot of fat and calories, sip broth-based rather than cream-based soups.

250 mL cream of chicken soup	191 calories	15 g fat
250 mL chicken noodle soup	75 calories	2 g fat
Savings	116 calories	13 g fat

8. Substitute fish for meat at least once a week.

85 g top round beef	162 calories	5 g fat
85 g cod	70 calories	0.5 g fat
Savings	92 calories	4.5 g fat

9. Substitute two egg whites for one whole egg in recipes or omelets.

1 whole egg	79 calories	6 g fat
2 egg whites	32 calories	0 g fat
Savings	47 calories	6 g fat

10. Load up on protein without overdosing on fat by selecting meatless entrées such as lentil soup and vegetarian chili.

270 g beef chili	256 calories	6 g fat
270 g lentil soup	164 calories	1 g fat
Savings	92 calories	5 g fat

General Advice. Become a fat sleuth. Read food labels faithfully and select those products that contain no more than three grams of fat for every 100 calories, which will keep your fat calories to a maximum of 30 percent of total calories.

List the small changes that you can make this week to cut the fat from your diet.

1.

2.

3.

4.

5.

What other things can you do to help reduce your overall fat consumption?

Source: Adapted by permission of the author from Evelyn Tribole, "24 Ways to Trim Fat," *Shape,* July 1990, 92–93.

sulfur, and chloride. **Trace minerals** include iron, zinc, manganese, copper, iodine, and cobalt. Only trace amounts of these minerals are needed, and serious problems may result if excesses or deficiencies occur. Specific types of minerals are listed in Table 7.1.

Although minerals are necessary for body function, there are limits on the amounts of each that we should consume. Canadians tend to overuse or underuse certain minerals.

Sodium. Sodium is necessary for the regulation of blood and body fluids, for the successful transmission of nerve impulses, for heart activity, and for certain metabolic functions. However, we consume much more

TABLE 7.1 ■ Summary of Recommended Nutrient Intakes

Examples of Recommended Nutrient Intake Based on Age and Body Weight, Expressed as Daily Rates

Age	Sex	Weight kg	Protein g	Vit. A RE[a]	Vit. D µg	Vit. E mg	Vit. C mg	Folate µg	Vit. B12 µg	Calcium mg	Phosphorus mg	Magnesium mg	Iron mg	Iodine µg	Zinc mg
Months															
0–4	Both	6.0	12[b]	400	10	3	20	25	0.3	250[c]	150	20	0.3[c]	30	2[c]
5–12	Both	9.0	12	400	10	3	20	40	0.2	400	200	32	7	40	3
Years															
1	Both	11	13	400	10	3	20	40	0.5	500	300	40	6	55	4
2–3	Both	14	16	400	5	4	20	50	0.6	550	350	50	6	65	4
4–6	Both	18	19	500	5	5	25	70	0.8	600	400	65	8	85	5
7–9	M	25	26	700	2.5	7	25	90	1.0	700	500	100	8	110	7
	F	25	26	700	2.5	6	25	90	1.0	700	500	100	8	95	7
10–12	M	34	34	800	2.5	8	25	120	1.0	900	700	130	8	125	9
	F	36	36	800	2.5	7	25	130	1.0	1100	800	135	8	110	9
13–15	M	50	49	900	2.5	9	30	175	1.0	1100	900	185	10	160	12
	F	48	46	800	2.5	7	50	170	1.0	1000	850	180	13	160	9
16–18	M	62	58	1000	2.5	10	40[c]	220	1.0	900	1000	230	10	160	12
	F	53	47	800	2.5	7	30[c]	190	1.0	700	850	200	12	160	9
19–24	M	71	61	1000	2.5	10	40[c]	220	1.0	800	1000	240	9	160	12
	F	58	50	800	2.5	7	30[c]	180	1.0	700	850	200	13	160	9
25–49	M	74	64	1000	2.5	9	40[c]	230	1.0	800	1000	250	9	160	12
	F	59	51	800	2.5	6	30[c]	185	1.0	700	850	200	13	160	9
50–74	M	73	63	1000	5	7	40[c]	230	1.0	800	1000	250	9	160	12
	F	63	54	800	5	6	30[c]	195	1.0	800	850	210	8	160	9
75–	M	69	59	1000	5	6	40[c]	215	1.0	800	1000	230	9	160	12
	F	64	35	800	5	5	30[c]	200	1.0	800	850	210	8	160	9
Pregnancy (additional)															
1st Trimester			5	0	2.5	2	0	200	0.2	500	200	15	0	25	6
2nd Trimester			20	0	2.5	2	10	200	0.2	500	200	45	5	25	6
3rd Trimester			24	0	2.5	2	10	200	0.2	500	200	45	10	25	6
Lactation (additional)			20	400	2.5	3	25	100	0.2	500	200	65	0	50	6

a. Retinol equivalents.

b. Protein is assumed to be from breast milk and must be adjusted for infant formula.

c. Infant formula with high phosphorus should contain 375 mg calcium.

d. Breast milk is assumed to be the source of the mineral.

e. Smokers should increase vitamin C by 50%.

sodium every day than we need. It is estimated that the average adult who does not sweat profusely has a need for only 3 to 5 grams of sodium (about 1/4 teaspoon) per day; yet the average Canadian consumes at least 12 times this amount. Sodium should be restricted to no more than 2400 milligrams per day; less is better. The most common source of sodium in the Canadian diet is table salt. The remainder of dietary sodium comes from the water we drink and from highly processed foods that are infused with sodium to enhance flavour. Pickles, salty snack foods, processed cheeses, many breads and bakery products, and smoked meats and sausages often contain several hundred milligrams of sodium per serving. Many fast-food entrées and convenience entrées have 500 to 1000 milligrams of sodium per serving. Soft drinks are also likely culprits for added sodium.

TABLE 7.1 *(continued)* ▪ Summary of Recommended Nutrient Intakes

Examples of Recommended Nutrients Based on Energy, Expressed as Daily Rates

Age	Sex	Energy kcal	Thiamin mg	Riboflavin mg	Niacin NE[a]
Months					
0–4	Both	600	0.3	0.3	4
5–12	Both	900	0.4	0.5	7
Years					
1	Both	1100	0.5	0.6	8
2–3	Both	1300	0.6	0.7	9
4–6	Both	1800	0.7	0.9	13
7–9	M	2200	0.9	1.1	16
	F	1900	0.8	1.0	14
10–12	M	2500	1.0	1.3	18
	F	2200	0.9	1.1	16
13–15	M	2800	1.1	1.4	20
	F	2200	0.9	1.1	16
16–18	M	3200	1.3	1.6	23
	F	2100	0.8	1.1	15
19–24	M	3000	1.2	1.5	22
	F	2100	0.8	1.1	15
25–49	M	2700	1.1	1.4	19
	F	1900	0.8[b]	1.0[b]	14[b]
50–74	M	2300	0.9	1.2	16
	F	1800	0.8[b]	1.0[b]	14[b]
75–	M	2000	0.8	1.0	14
	F[c]	1700	0.8[b]	1.0[b]	14[b]
Pregnancy (additional)					
1st Trimester		100	0.1	0.1	1
2nd Trimester		300	0.1	0.3	2
3rd Trimester		300	0.1	0.3	2
Lactation (additional)		450	0.2	0.4	3

a. Niacin equivalents.

b. Level below which intake should not fall.

c. Assumes moderate (more than average) physical activity.

Source: Reprinted from Health and Welfare Canada, *Nutrition Recommendations: The Report of the Scientific Review Committee* (Ottawa: Supply and Services Canada, 1990). © Health and Welfare Canada.

Many experts believe that there is a link between excessive sodium intake and hypertension (high blood pressure). Although this theory is controversial, many organizations have recommended that Canadians cut back on sodium consumption to reduce their risk for cardiovascular disorders. Sodium has also been linked to stomach cancer.

Calcium. The issue of calcium consumption has gained national attention with the rising incidence of osteoporosis (see Chapter 14) among elderly women. Although calcium plays a vital role in building strong bones and teeth, muscle contraction, blood clotting, nerve impulse transmission, regulating heart beat, and fluid balance within cells, most Canadians do not consume the 800 milligrams of calcium per day established by Health and Welfare Canada.

Improving Your Calcium Levels. Because calcium intake is so important throughout your life for a strong bone structure, it is critical that you consume the minimum required amounts each day. Over half of our calcium intake

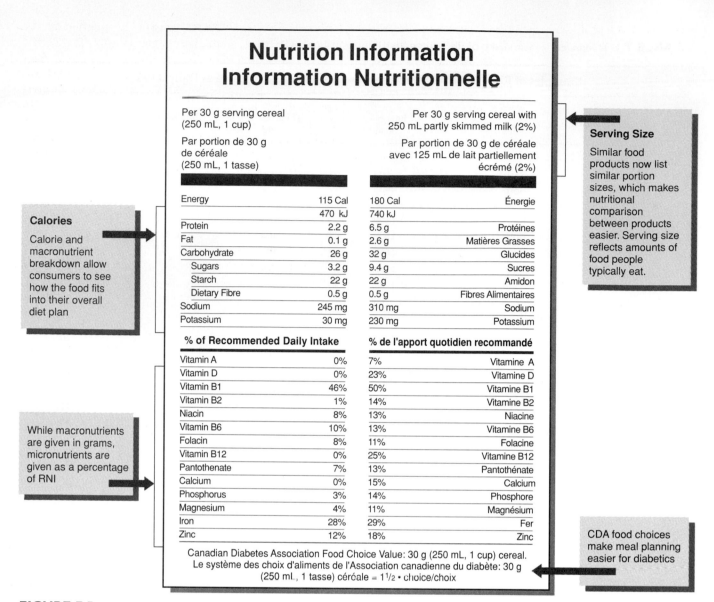

Nutrition Information
Information Nutritionnelle

Per 30 g serving cereal (250 mL, 1 cup) Par portion de 30 g de céréale (250 mL, 1 tasse)		Per 30 g serving cereal with 250 mL partly skimmed milk (2%) Par portion de 30 g de céréale avec 125 mL de lait partiellement écrémé (2%)	
Energy	115 Cal	180 Cal	Énergie
	470 kJ	740 kJ	
Protein	2.2 g	6.5 g	Protéines
Fat	0.1 g	2.6 g	Matières Grasses
Carbohydrate	26 g	32 g	Glucides
Sugars	3.2 g	9.4 g	Sucres
Starch	22 g	22 g	Amidon
Dietary Fibre	0.5 g	0.5 g	Fibres Alimentaires
Sodium	245 mg	310 mg	Sodium
Potassium	30 mg	230 mg	Potassium

% of Recommended Daily Intake		% de l'apport quotidien recommandé	
Vitamin A	0%	7%	Vitamine A
Vitamin D	0%	23%	Vitamine D
Vitamin B1	46%	50%	Vitamine B1
Vitamin B2	1%	14%	Vitamine B2
Niacin	8%	13%	Niacine
Vitamin B6	10%	13%	Vitamine B6
Folacin	8%	11%	Folacine
Vitamin B12	0%	25%	Vitamine B12
Pantothenate	7%	13%	Pantothénate
Calcium	0%	15%	Calcium
Phosphorus	3%	14%	Phosphore
Magnesium	4%	11%	Magnésium
Iron	28%	29%	Fer
Zinc	12%	18%	Zinc

Canadian Diabetes Association Food Choice Value: 30 g (250 mL, 1 cup) cereal. Le système des choix d'aliments de l'Association canadienne du diabète: 30 g (250 mL, 1 tasse) céréale = 1½ • choice/choix

Serving Size

Similar food products now list similar portion sizes, which makes nutritional comparison between products easier. Serving size reflects amounts of food people typically eat.

Calories

Calorie and macronutrient breakdown allow consumers to see how the food fits into their overall diet plan

While macronutrients are given in grams, micronutrients are given as a percentage of RNI

CDA food choices make meal planning easier for diabetics

FIGURE 7.5

The New Food Label

usually comes from milk, one of the highest sources of dietary calcium. Many green, leafy vegetables are good sources of calcium, but some contain oxalic acid, which makes their calcium harder to absorb. Spinach, chard, and beet greens are not particularly good sources of calcium, whereas broccoli, cauliflower, and many peas and beans offer good supplies (pinto beans and soybeans are among the best). Many nuts, particularly almonds, brazil nuts, and hazelnuts, and seeds such as sunflower and sesame contain good amounts of calcium. Molasses is fairly high in calcium. Some fruits—such as citrus fruits, figs, raisins, and dried apricots—have moderate amounts.

Of interest to those who drink carbonated soft drinks is the fact that the added phosphoric acid (phosphate) in these drinks can cause you to excrete extra calcium, which may result in calcium being pulled out of your bones. Cal-

cium/phosphorus imbalances may lead to kidney stones and other calcification problems as well as to increased atherosclerotic plaque.[13]

We also know that sunlight increases the manufacture of vitamin D in the body, and is therefore like having an extra calcium source because vitamin D improves absorption of calcium. Stress, on the other hand, tends to contribute to calcium depletion. It is generally best to take calcium throughout the day, consuming foods containing protein, vitamin D, and vitamin C with it for optimum absorption. Experts differ on which type of supplemental calcium is most readily and efficiently absorbed, although bone meal, aspartate, or citrate salts of calcium are among those most often recommended. The best way to obtain calcium, like all the other nutrients, is to consume it as part of a balanced diet.

Iron. Iron is a problem mineral for millions of people. Although it is found in every cell of all living things, many humans have difficulty getting enough iron in their daily diets. Females aged 19 to 50 need about 18 milligrams per day, and males aged 19 to 50 need about 10 milligrams. Iron deficiencies can lead to **anemia**, a problem resulting from the body's inability to produce hemoglobin, the bright red, oxygen-carrying component of the blood. When this occurs, body cells receive less oxygen, and carbon dioxide wastes are removed less efficiently. These problems cause a person to feel tired and run down. Anemia can be caused by accidents, cancers, ulcers, and other conditions, but iron deficiency is a common cause. Generally, women are more likely than men to suffer from iron deficiency problems, partly because they typically eat less than men, and their diets therefore contain less iron. Also, because blood loss is the major reason for iron depletion, women having heavy menstrual flows may be prone to iron deficiency. Another problem with iron deficiency is that the immune system becomes less effective, which can lead to increased risk of illness.

Recently, researchers have speculated that too much iron in the body may increase the risk for heart disease. They point to the low risk for heart disease in premenopausal women and the striking rise in risk in postmenopausal women as a possible indicator of such an association. Men who consume high-iron diets also appear to be at increased risk. But this research is preliminary; nutrition scientists are planning further studies of this possible connection.[14] Blood donors and pregnant women may need to increase iron intake. A less common problem, iron toxicity, is caused by too much iron in the blood.

Package labelling can assist you in making food choices. The labels indicate nutrient content. (See Figure 7.5.)

> **Anemia:** Iron-deficiency disease that results from the body's inability to produce hemoglobin.

Sex Differences in Nutritional Needs

Men and women differ in body size, body composition, and overall metabolic rates. They therefore have differing needs for most nutrients throughout the life cycle (see tables on vitamin and mineral requirements) and face unique difficulties in keeping on track with their dietary goals. Some of these differences have already been discussed. However, there are some diet/nutrition factors that need further consideration. One factor is that women have a lower ratio of lean body mass to adipose (fatty) tissue at all ages and stages of life. Also, after sexual maturation, metabolism is higher in men, meaning that they will burn more calories than women doing the same things.

Different Cycles, Different Needs. In addition to the above differences, women have many more "landmark" times in their lives when their nutritional needs vary significantly from what they are at other times in their lives. From menarche to menopause, women undergo cyclical physiological changes that can have dramatic effects on metabolism, nutritional needs, and efforts to stick to a nutritional plan. For example, during pregnancy and lactation, nutritional requirements increase substantially for women. Those who are unable to follow the strict dietary recommendations of their doctors may find themselves gaining much more weight during pregnancy and retaining it afterwards. During the menstrual cycle, many women report significant food cravings that may cause them to overconsume. Later in women's lives, with the advent of menopause, nutritional needs again change rather dramatically. With depletion of the hormone estrogen, the body's need for calcium to ward off bone deterioration becomes pronounced. Women must pay closer attention to their exercise patterns and to getting enough calcium through diet or dietary supplements or run the risk of severe osteoporosis.

Changing the Meat and Potatoes Man. Although men do not have the same cyclical patterns and dietary needs as women, they do suffer from a heritage of dietary excesses that are difficult to change. Consider the following:

- Men who eat red meat as a main dish five or more times a week have four times the risk of colon cancer of men who eat red meat less than once a month.

- Heavy-red-meat-eaters are more than twice as likely to get prostate cancer and nearly five times as likely to get colon cancer.

- For every three servings of fruits or vegetables per day men can expect a 22 percent lower risk of stroke.

- High fruit and vegetable diets may lower the risk of lung cancer in smokers from 20 times the risk of nonsmokers to "only" 10 times the risk. They may also protect against oral, throat, pancreas, and bladder cancers, all of which are more common in smokers.

- While obesity seems to be a factor in cancer of the esophagus, an increasingly common malignancy among men, fruits and vegetables are the protectors.

*W*HAT DO YOU THINK?

Think about the women that you know who seem to have weight problems. What are their ages? What factors may have influenced them to have more problems keeping weight off than you may have? What advantages, if any, do men have in controlling their eating behaviours and managing their weight?

VEGETARIANISM: EATING FOR HEALTH

For aesthetic, animal rights, economic, personal, health, cultural, or religious reasons, some people choose specialized diets. Between 3 and 7 percent of all Canadians today claim to be some form of vegetarian, and numbers are rising among 15-to-25-year-olds.[15] Normally, vegetarianism provides a superb alternative to our high-fat, high-calorie, meat-based cuisine, but, without proper information, vegetarians can also have dietary problems.

The term **vegetarian** means different things to different people. Strict vegetarians, or *vegans,* avoid all foods of animal origin, including dairy products and eggs. The few people who fall into this category must work hard to ensure that they get all of the necessary nutrients. Far more common are *lacto-vegetarians,* who eat dairy products but avoid flesh foods. Their diet can be low in fat and cholesterol, but only if they consume skim milk and other low-fat or nonfat products. *Ovo-vegetarians* add eggs to their diet, while *lacto-ovo-vegetarians* eat both dairy products and eggs. *Pesco-vegetarians* eat fish, dairy products, and eggs, while *semivegetarians* eat chicken, fish, dairy products, and eggs. Some people in the semivegetarian category prefer to call themselves "non-red-meat-eaters."

Generally, people who follow a balanced vegetarian diet have lower weights, better cholesterol levels, fewer problems with irregular bowel movements (constipation and diarrhea), and a lower risk of heart disease than non-vegetarians. Some preliminary evidence suggests that vegetarians may also have a reduced risk for colon and breast cancer. Whether these lower risks are due to the vegetarian diet per se or to some combination of lifestyle variables remains unclear.

Although in the past vegetarians often suffered from vitamin deficiencies, the vegetarian of the 1990s is usually extremely adept at combining the right types of foods to ensure proper nutrient intake. People who eat dairy products and small amounts of chicken or fish are seldom nutrient-deficient; in fact, while vegans typically get 50 to 60 grams of protein per day, lacto-ovo vegetarians normally consume between 70 and 90 grams per day, well

---

Vegetarian: A term with a variety of meanings: *vegans* avoid all foods of animal origin; *lacto-vegetarians* avoid flesh foods but eat dairy products; *ovo-vegetarians* avoid flesh foods but eat eggs; *lacto-ovo-vegetarians* avoid flesh foods but eat both dairy products and eggs; *pesco-vegetarians* avoid meat but eat fish, dairy products, and eggs; *semivegetarians* eat chicken, fish, dairy products, and eggs.

---

beyond the RNI. Vegan diets may be deficient in vitamins B2 (riboflavin), B12, and D. Riboflavin is found mainly in meat, eggs, and dairy products; but broccoli, asparagus, almonds, and fortified cereals are also good sources. Vitamins B12 and D are found only in dairy products and fortified products such as soy milk. Vegans are also at risk for calcium, iron, zinc, and other mineral deficiencies, but these nutrients can be obtained from supplements. Strict vegans have to pay much more attention to what they eat than the average person does, but by eating complementary combinations of plant products, they can receive adequate amounts of essential amino acids.

The Vegetarian Pyramid

Dr. Arlene Spark, a nutritionist at New York Medical College, devised a food guide pyramid in 1994 that conveys all the essentials of a vegetarian diet (see Figure 7.6). The vegetarian pyramid defines several categories. We include examples of single servings of foods in each category.

WHAT DO YOU THINK?

Have you ever considered becoming or are you currently a vegetarian? What was your reason for making this choice? Do you find it difficult to select vegetarian foods in restaurants/eating places on your campus? What actions can you take to help ensure more choices? From what you have learned here, what is one improvement you can make in your vegetarian eating behaviour?

IMPROVED EATING FOR THE UNIVERSITY STUDENT

University students often face a challenge when trying to eat healthy foods. Some students live in dorms and do not have their own cooking or refrigeration facilities. Others live in crowded apartments where everyone forages in the refrigerator for everyone else's food. Still others eat at university food services where food choices are limited. Most students have time constraints that make buying, preparing, and eating healthy food a difficult task. In addition, many lack the financial resources needed to buy many foods that their parents purchased while they lived at home. What's a student to do? While we can't come in and guard your refrigerator to make sure your roommates don't eat your food, we can offer some suggestions for choices that may make your eating experience more healthy.

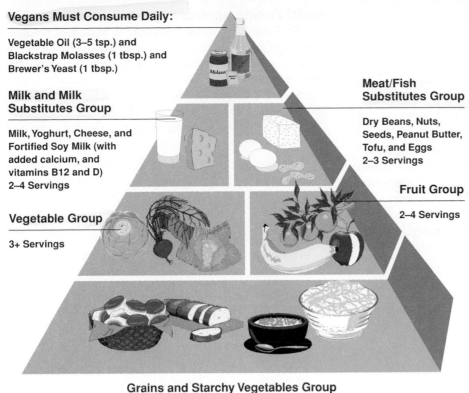

Vegans Must Consume Daily:

Vegetable Oil (3–5 tsp.) and
Blackstrap Molasses (1 tbsp.) and
Brewer's Yeast (1 tbsp.)

**Milk and Milk
Substitutes Group**

Milk, Yoghurt, Cheese, and
Fortified Soy Milk (with
added calcium, and
vitamins B12 and D)
2–4 Servings

Vegetable Group

3+ Servings

**Meat/Fish
Substitutes Group**

Dry Beans, Nuts,
Seeds, Peanut Butter,
Tofu, and Eggs
2–3 Servings

Fruit Group

2–4 Servings

Grains and Starchy Vegetables Group

Bread, Cereal, Rice, Pasta,
Potatoes, Corn, and Green Peas
6–11 Servings

FIGURE 7.6

New York Medical College Vegetarian Pyramid
Source: © 1994 New York Medical College. Adapted by permission.

Grains and Starchy Vegetables Group (6–11 servings/day)

- 1 slice bread
- 1/2 roll or bagel
- 1 tortilla (6"—10 cm)
- 30 g (1 ounce) cold cereal
- 125 mL (1/2 cup) cooked cereal, rice, or pasta
- 3–4 crackers
- 750 mL (3 cups) popcorn
- 125 mL (1/2 cup) corn
- 1 medium potato
- 125 mL (1/2 cup) green peas

Vegetable Group (3+ servings/day)

- 125 mL (1/2 cup) cooked or chopped raw vegetables
- 250 mL (1 cup) raw leafy vegetables
- 125 mL (1/2 cup) vegetable juice

Fruit Group (2–4 servings/day)

- 1 medium whole piece of fruit
- 125 mL (1/2 cup) canned, chopped, or cooked fruit
- 125 mL (1/2 cup) fruit juice

Milk and Milk Substitutes Group (3 servings/day for preteens and 4 for teens; 2–4 servings/day for adults)

- 250 mL (1 cup) milk or yoghurt
- 250 mL (1 cup) calcium- and vitamin-B12-fortified soy milk
- 45 g (1 1/2 ounces) hard cheese
- 45 g (1 1/2 ounces) calcium- and vitamin-B12-fortified soy cheese

Meat/Fish Substitutes Group (2–3 servings/day)

- 250 mL (1 cup) cooked dry beans, peas, or lentils
- 2 eggs
- 240 g (8 ounces) bean curd or tofu
- 125 mL (1/2 cup) shelled nuts
- 45–60 mL (3–4 tablespoons) peanut butter
- 45–60 mL (3–4 tablespoons) tahini
- 1/3 to 1/2 cup seeds

Vegans Must Consume Daily:

- 15–25 mL (3–5 teaspoons) vegetable oil + 15 mL (1 tablespoon) blackstrap molasses + 15 mL (1 tablespoon) brewer's yeast

Fast Foods: Eating on the Run

If your campus is like many others across the country, you've probably noticed a distinct move toward fast-food restaurants in your student unions so that they now resemble the food courts found in most major shopping malls. These new eating centres fit students' needs for a fast bite of food at a reasonable rate between classes and also bring in money to your school. Many fast foods are high in fat and sodium. But are all fast foods unhealthy?

You should recognize that not all fast foods are created equal and not all of them are bad for you. Even at the often-maligned burger chains, menus are healthier than ever before and offer excellent choices for the discriminating eater. The key word here is *discriminating*. It is possible to eat healthy food if you follow these suggestions:

- Ask for nutritional analyses of items. Most fast-food chains now have them.

- Order it "your way"—avoid mayonnaise or sauces and other add-ons. Some places even have fat-free mayonnaise if you ask.

- Hold the cheese. This extra contributes substantially to total fat while not adding a lot to taste.

- Order single, small burgers rather than large, high-calorie, bacon- or cheese-topped choices. Put on your own ketchup and keep portions small.

- Order salads and be careful how much dressing you put on. Many people think they are being health-smart by eating salad, only to load it with calorie- and fat-rich dressing. Try the vinegar and oil or low-fat alternative dressings. Stay away from eggs and other high-fat add-ons such as bacon bits.

- When ordering a chicken sandwich, order the skinless broiled version rather than the deep-fried version.

- Check to see what type of oil is used to cook fries if you must have them. Avoid lard-based or other saturated-fat products.

- Order whole-wheat buns/bread and ask them to hold the butter.

- Avoid fried foods in general, including hot apple pies and other crust-based fried foods.

- Opt for spots where foods tend to be broiled rather than fried.

Healthy Eating When Funds Are Short

Balancing the need for adequate nutrition with the many other activities that are part of college life can become a difficult task. Not surprisingly, it is often the nutritional part of the total picture that gets slighted. Maintaining a nutritious diet within the confines of student life is difficult. However, if you take the time to plan healthy diets, you may find that you are eating better, enjoying eating more, and actually saving money. Understanding the terminology used by the food industry may also help you eat a healthier diet; the Building Communication Skills box reviews some of these pertinent terms.

In addition, you can take these steps to help ensure a quality diet:

- Buy fruits and vegetables in season for their lower cost, higher nutrient quality, and greater variety.

- Use coupons and specials to get price reductions.

- Shop whenever possible at discount warehouse food chains; capitalize on volume discounts and no-frills products.

- Plan ahead to get the most for your dollar and avoid extra trips to the store. Make a list and stick to it.

- Purchase meats and other products in volume, freezing portions for future needs. Or purchase small amounts of meats and other expensive proteins and combine them with beans and plant proteins for lower total cost, lower calories, and lower fat.

- Cook large meals and freeze smaller portions for later use.

- If you find that you have no money for food, check with the local food bank or social service department. Assistance may be available.

Healthy Eating in the Dormitory

If you're like most university students, the meals provided in the student food service or in your dormitory may provide unique nutritional challenges and opportunities. Some food services have responded exceedingly well to new guidelines for low-fat, high-carbohydrate eating. Many offer vegetarian entrées; choices between broiled, baked, or fried foods; skim milks; nonfat yoghurts; and full-service salad and pasta bars. Unfortunately, there are many others that are still preparing foods as they have for years. Choices for students are limited and often provide only high- and higher-fat choices in foods.

If you find that you are in a health-conscious food service or dormitory, the guidelines and tips provided throughout this chapter should serve you well. If you are in a food service or dormitory that has a long way to go, here are some possible actions you might take to help them change their food choices and cooking practices.

- Ask your health instructor if anyone has ever done a food analysis of menu items at the food service or dorm. If they have, find out what happened to the information provided. If not, find out what you can do to get one done. Your student health service, health class, or local hospital may be a good resource.

- Once you've identified the nutrient content of these meals, take your findings to the student newspaper and the student government and try to find someone who is willing to help push for food service reform.

- If you are dissatisfied with cafeteria foods, make your complaints known in writing to the director of student services or the food service administrator. Be sure to include recommendations for improvements.

- Find out what is being done on other campuses throughout the country. Competition between universities often goes beyond the playing field. You may just spur someone to action.

- Use the suggestion box provided in the cafeteria. If there isn't one, try to get one.

- Be positive in your approach. More support is gained from providing suggestions for change rather than criticism of current practice.

*W*HAT DO YOU THINK?

What problems cause you the most difficulty when you try to eat more healthful foods? Are these problems that you noted in your family, too, or are they unique to your current situation as a student? What actions can you take that would help improve your current eating practices?

*I*S YOUR FOOD SAFE?

Irradiation

As we become increasingly worried that the food we put in our mouths may be contaminated with potentially harmful bacteria, insects, worms, or other not-so-nice substances, the food industry has come under fire. To convince us that our products are safe for consumption, some manufacturers have come up with "new and improved" ways of protecting our foods. One of these methods, food irradiation, has become the subject of much controversy. What is food irradiation? Should you buy irradiated foods?

Food irradiation involves treating foods with gamma radiation from radioactive cobalt 60, cesium-137, or some other source of X-rays at or below 5 MEV or electrons operated at or below 10 MEV. The killing effect on microorganisms rises with the power of the rays, which are measured in rads (radiant energy absorbed).[16] Irradiation lengthens food products' shelf life and prevents microor-

ganism and insect contamination. Because this results in less waste, the food industry can make higher profits while charging consumers lower prices. It is also claimed that irradiation will reduce the need to use many of the toxic chemicals now used to preserve foods and prevent contamination from external contaminants.

The following foods have already received approval for irradiation by Health Canada: onions, potatoes, wheat flour, whole wheat flour, whole or ground spices, and dehydrated seasoning preparations.

The long-term side-effects of irradiation are unknown. Although irradiation doesn't actually make your food radioactive, it does damage its molecular structure, creating new substances known as free radicals. Free radicals have been implicated in certain types of cancers, and diseases of the liver and kidney in animal studies, but, to date, no studies of the toxicity of irradiated foods on humans have been done. Because this radiation damages the molecular structure of foods, critics argue that it may lower the nutritional value of some foods by altering their protein structure, reducing their vitamin levels, or deactivating important enzymes. Some foods, such as apples, pears, and certain citrus fruits, have actually been shown to spoil faster after irradiation. While the health effects of irradiated food may not be known for many years, the long-term impact of the proliferation of radioactive material on our environment cannot be ignored.

Food-Borne Illness

Most of us have experienced the characteristic symptoms of diarrhea, nausea, cramping, and vomiting that prompt us to say, "It must be something I ate." The number of cases of food poisoning in Canada has been growing (there are 10 000 cases per year; for every reported case there are many unreported cases). In 1996, the Health Protection Branch issued a warning about certain Smith Snack Services products in Newfoundland. They produced foods in Mason jars that could be contaminated. The identified products were withdrawn.

Symptoms of food-borne illness vary tremendously according to the type of organism and the amount of contaminant eaten. These symptoms may appear as early as a half-hour after eating the food, or they may take several days or weeks to develop. In most people, they come on five to eight hours after eating and last only a day or two. In others, such as the very old and very young and those suffering from other illnesses, food-borne illness can be life-threatening.

Food irradiation: Treating foods with gamma radiation from radioactive cobalt, cesium, or some other source of X-rays to kill microorganisms.

Part of the responsibility for preventing food-borne illness lies with consumers, for over 30 percent of all such illnesses result from unsafe handling of food at home.

■ When shopping, pick up your packaged and canned foods first and save frozen foods and perishables such as meat, poultry, and fish till the last. Try to put these foods in separate plastic bags so that drippings don't run onto other foods in your cart, contaminating them.

■ Check for cleanliness at the salad bar and meat and fish counters. For instance, cooked shrimp lying on the same bed of ice as raw fish can easily be contaminated.

■ When shopping for fish, buy from markets that get their supplies from approved sources; stay clear of vendors who sell shellfish from roadside stands or the back of trucks. If you're planning to harvest your own shellfish, check the safety of the water in the area.

■ Remember that most cuts of meat, fish, and poultry should be kept in the refrigerator no more than one or two days. They shouldn't be in the grocery store meat counter beyond their dated shelf life, either. Check the shelf life of all products before buying. If expiration dates are close, freeze or eat immediately.

■ Leftovers should be eaten within three days.

■ Use a thermometer to ensure that meats are completely cooked. Remember that the rarer the steak, the greater the number of bacteria swarming on the plate. Beef and lamb should be cooked to at least 60°C, pork to 66°C, and poultry to 74°C. Don't eat poultry that is pink inside.

■ Fish is done when the thickest part becomes opaque and the fish flakes easily when poked with a fork.

■ Cooked food should never be left standing on the stove or table for more than two hours. Disease-causing bacteria grow in temperatures between 5°C and 60°C. Keep hot foods hot and cold foods cold.

■ Never thaw frozen foods at room temperature. Put in the refrigerator for a day to thaw, or thaw in cold water, changing the water every 30 minutes.

■ Wash your hands with soap and water between courses when preparing food, particularly after handling meat, fish, or poultry. Wash the countertop and all utensils before using them for other foods.[17]

Food Allergies

Up to 8 percent of children, and a smaller proportion of adults, are allergic to at least one food. People may also mistakenly believe they have allergies. If a person does not truly have allergies, treatments and diets designed to pre-

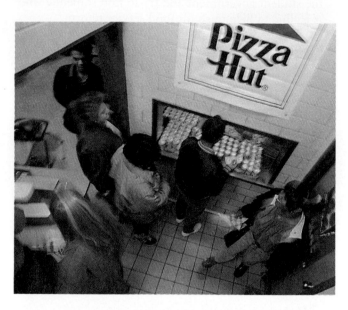

Maintaining a nutritious diet is often difficult for university students, but even fast-food chains now offer possibilities for healthy eating beyond the usual pizzas and burgers high in fat and calories.

vent allergies may be not only be worthless but shift efforts away from accurate diagnosis and appropriate actions.

True **food allergies** occur when the body overreacts to normally harmless proteins, perceiving them as allergens. The body then produces antibodies that activate immune cells known as *histamines*, thus triggering a variety of allergic symptoms. Such allergic reactions vary tremendously among individuals and may range from a case of the hives or a body rash to swelling of certain body parts (especially the lips), to pain, diarrhea, nausea, or vomiting. In more severe cases, irregularities in breathing and heartbeat are experienced, along with blood pressure fluctuations, shock, and, if untreated, even death. Symptoms may occur within minutes or over a two- to three-hour period.

The most common culprits are soybeans, legumes (including peanuts), nuts, shellfish, eggs, wheat, and milk. People are often allergic to a whole family of foods; this is called **cross-reactivity**. Unlike many other allergies, food allergies do not appear to be inherited. Breast-feeding babies seems to decrease their susceptibility to food allergies. If you think you may have a food allergy, have yourself tested by a trained allergist.

Some common reactions to food that may imitate allergies but do not involve the immune system are:

■ **Food intolerance**, which occurs in people who lack certain digestive chemicals and suffer adverse effects when they consume certain substances because their bodies have difficulty breaking them down. One of the most common examples is lactose intolerance, experi-

Checking Out Terms Used on Food Labels

Nutrition Claims

A nutrition claim highlights a nutritional feature of a product. It is known to influence consumers' buying habits. Nutrition claims are often positioned in a bold, banner format on the front panel of a package or, as in the cereal example, on the side panel along with the nutrition label. Since a nutrition claim must always be backed up by detailed facts relating to the claim, the consumer should look to the nutrition label to more information.

Popular Claims and What They Mean

The words used in claims are defined by government so that consumers can associate a claim with a particular standard. For instance:

- *Low* is always associated with a very small amount.

- *Less* is used to compare one product with another. For example, a box of crackers claiming to contain "50% less salt" will have half the salt of the food to which it's compared. It doesn't necessarily mean the produce is low in salt. Half the salt can still be a lot of salt.

- *Light* or *Lite* is a popular claim. If it is on a label, consumers should look further to find out which feature of the product is "light." This claim is often used to describe a food reduced in fat and energy but not always. Sometimes it describes the taste or texture of a food.

- *Low in Saturated Fat* or *Cholesterol-Free* may lead consumers to think the product is low in fat. It's not necessarily so. Vegetable oils may contain no cholesterol, may be low in saturated fat but are very high in total fat.

Percentage Fat Declaration

Most milk products list the fat content on the basis of weight as a percentage of butter fat (% B.F.) or milk fat (% M.F.) This information can be used to choose lower-fat milk products.

Source: Health and Welfare Canada, *Food Guide Facts* (Ottawa: Minister of Supply and Services, Cat. No. H39-253/01-1992E), 1992.

---

enced by people who do not have the digestive chemicals needed to break down the lactose in milk.

- *Reactions to food additives,* such as sulfites and MSG.

- *Reactions to substances occurring naturally in some foods,* such as tyramine in cheese, phenylethylamine in chocolate, caffeine in coffee, and some compounds in alcoholic beverages.

- *Food-borne illnesses.*

- *Unknown reactions* in people who have adverse symptoms that they attribute to foods and that may actually go away when treated as allergies but for which there is no evidence of a physiological basis.[18]

Organic Foods

Mounting concerns about food safety have caused many people to try to protect themselves by refusing to buy processed foods and mass-produced agricultural products. Instead, they purchase foods that are **organically grown**—foods reported to be pesticide- and chemical-free. Though they are sold at premium prices, many of these products are of only average quality. They are probably not worth the money, according to most experts, for several reasons. First, whether food has been exposed to pesticides at some time in the production cycle is not as important as the residual pesticides in the food at the time you consume it. Obviously, too much of anything is potentially harmful, but if a "nonorganic" food has been sprayed and the poison has since evaporated, changed into a nontoxic compound, or been diluted below the point at which it can do any harm, the food may be no more harmful than a product labelled as "organic."[19] Second, even though so-called organic foods generally claim to be pesticide-free, tests indicate that many contain pesticide residues in the same amounts as nonorganic foods.[20]

Food allergies: Overreaction by the body to normally harmless proteins, which are perceived as allergens. In response, the body produces antibodies, triggering allergic symptoms.

Cross-reactivity: Allergic reaction to a whole family of foods.

Food intolerance: Adverse effects resulting when people who lack the digestive chemicals needed to break down certain substances eat those substances.

Organically grown: Foods that are grown without use of pesticides or chemicals.

Managing Your Nutrition

Let's face it. Eating for health is not easy. It takes knowledge, careful thought and analysis, and the ability to put it all together and make the best decisions for your own lifestyle and personal goals within certain budgetary limits. There are no shortcuts, and what is true today may turn out to be false tomorrow. But by paying attention, reading, seeking help from reputable, trained professionals, and planning ahead, you can increase your own nutritional health. The following recommendations will help you improve your nutritional status:

Making Decisions for You

1. List the four biggest things about your current diet that you want to change.

2. Prioritize the items in the above list. Determine when you want to accomplish each item and outline a plan of action for accomplishing each goal.

3. List the little actions that you can take that may make a difference in your overall plan. List the big changes that you can make to accomplish your overall goals.

4. On the basis of your past history of trying to change these behaviours, what techniques do you think may be most likely to work for you? Indicate what you will use from these past tries and what you will do differently.

Checklist for Change: Making Personal Choices

✓ *Eat lower on the food chain.* Try to substitute fruits, vegetables, nuts, or grains for animal products at least once a day.

✓ *Eat seasonal foods whenever possible.* By eating foods at the peak of harvest, you are most apt to avoid nutrient losses incurred by storage, freezing, canning, and so on.

✓ *Eat lean.* The evidence against high-fat foods mounts daily. Pay attention to labels, assess your food intake, and balance high-fat meals with low-fat meals. Choose leaner cuts and bake, grill, boil, or broil whenever possible.

✓ *Increase your consumption of fruits and vegetables.* Use the real thing instead of juices and get more health for your money.

✓ *Combine foods for optimum nutrition.* Identify the best ways to combine grains, beans, fruits, vegetables, nuts, and other foods. You will then be able to optimize dietary returns. Ask your instructor or your local public health service for advice.

✓ *Practise responsible consumer safety.* Avoid unnecessary chemicals and buy, prepare, and store foods prudently to avoid food-borne illness.

✓ *Eat in moderation.* Learn to separate true hunger feelings from the food cravings that come from boredom. Recognize when your body is signalling that it is getting full, and stop eating. Don't undereat or overeat. Moderate your caloric consumption and reduce your consumption of sugars and other dietary "extras."

✓ *Keep your systems functioning well.* Even the best diets are doomed to failure if life problems are dragging your systems down, particularly your digestive system.

✓ *Keep dietary foods in balance.* Consume appropriate amounts of fats, carbohydrates, proteins, vitamins, minerals, amino acids, fatty acids, and water.

✓ *Pay attention to changing nutrient needs.* Various factors in your life, such as pregnancy or illness, may require you to adjust your nutritional intake. Prepare for these changes and remain informed about reputable sources of information concerning nutrient benefits and hazards.

Checklist for Change: Making Community Choices

✓ Evaluate the types of eating establishments available on your campus. If you don't have the options you think you should, take action. Involve your student newspaper and student organizations, talk with food service representatives, involve your student health service, and solicit the support of key campus representatives.

✓ Assess your elected officials' priorities regarding: nutrition as it pertains to the elderly, pregnant women, and the homeless. Are they supporting actions to help ensure adequate nutrition for high-risk groups? If not, why not? Write letters asking for clarification of their positions. Seek alternative candidates if these individuals do not represent your views.

✓ If you patronize certain food establishments, review the food choices. Tell them when they are doing a good job and request other options.

✓ Find out about government-subsidized foods. Who is eligible for these programs? What is their purpose? What are their limitations? Strengths? Be informed about these programs. Support or refute them on the basis of sound information rather than on emotional reactions.

✓ Be informed about key nutritional concepts. Speak up when you see information that is false and/or misleading. Demand accuracy in reported claims. Give advice only when you have taken the time to read and study the issues. Read reliable nutritional sources. When in doubt, seek help from professors or experts in the community.

Critical Thinking

Bill and Sarah have been married for almost six months. Sarah enjoys cooking large meals, many of them featuring fried foods. Bill, on the other hand, is more used to eating dishes built around rice, fruits, and vegetables. He is concerned about their eating habits, especially the higher fat and cholesterol content. But he doesn't want to say anything that would affect their otherwise perfect marriage.

Using the DECIDE model described in Chapter 1, decide how Bill can open up a discussion about better eating without hurting Sarah's feelings.

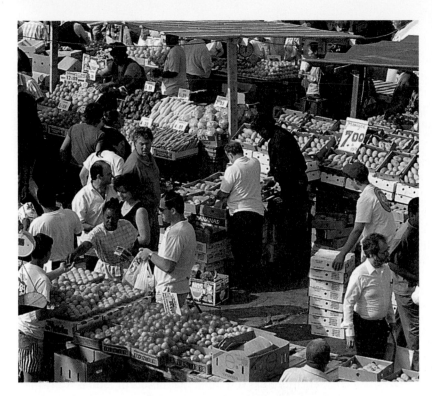

Learning to shop carefully for fresh, high-quality foods can help ensure that your food is safe and that you are maintaining good health.

These residues may be the result of pesticide drift from neighbouring farms and water supplies, sneak sprays by unscrupulous producers, or soils that have residue from previous growers.

The bottom line is what is really in the food, not whether it is labelled as "organic," "natural," or "healthy." In fact, these labels are often placed on foods that are far from healthy and may actually be of very low quality. Although the ideals upon which the organic movement was founded are sound, more testing and regulation are needed before people can be assured that what they are paying high prices for is the real unadulterated thing—a pesticide-free product.

Summary

◆ Recognizing that we eat for more reasons than just survival is the first step toward changing our health. *Canada's Food Guide* provides guidelines for healthy eating.

◆ The major nutrients that are essential for life and health include water, proteins, carbohydrates, fibre, fats, vitamins, and minerals. RNIs serve as guides to necessary amounts of nutrients.

◆ Vegetarianism can provide a healthy alternative for those wishing to cut fat from their diets or wanting to reduce animal consumption. The vegetarian pyramid provides dietary guidelines to help vegetarians obtain needed nutrients.

◆ University students face unique challenges in eating healthfully. Using the knowledge in this chapter, you can learn to make better choices at fast-food restaurants, eat healthily when funds are short, and eat nutritiously in the dorm.

◆ Food irradiation, food allergies, food-borne illnesses, and other food-safety and health concerns are becoming increasingly important to health-wise consumers. Recognition of potential risks and active steps taken to prevent problems are part of a sound nutritional plan.

Discussion Questions

1. What are several factors that may influence the dietary patterns and behaviours of the typical university student? What factors have been the greatest influences on your eating behaviours? Why is it important that you know about your dietary influences as you think about changing your eating behaviours?

2. What are the four major food groups in the new *Canada's Food Guide?* What groups might you find it difficult to get enough servings from? What can you do to increase/decrease your intake of selected food groups? What can you do to remember the four groups?

3. What are the major types of nutrients that you need to obtain from the foods you eat? What happens if you fail to get enough of some of these nutrients?

4. Distinguish between the different types of vegetarianism. Which types are most likely to lead to deficiencies? What can be done to ensure that even the most strict vegetarian receives enough of the major nutrients?

5. What are the major problems that many university students face when trying to eat the right foods? List five actions that you and your classmates could take immediately to improve your eating.

6. What are the potential benefits and risks of food irradiation? Why is it being used? What are the major risks for food-borne illnesses and what can you do to protect yourself? How are food illnesses and food allergies different?

Application Exercise

Reread the What Do You Think? scenario at the beginning of the chapter and answer the following questions:

1. Critique Jasper's eating habits. What suggestions could you make to help him? How could you make these suggestions in a way that won't offend him?

2. Is there anything Jasper can do to improve his eating situation? Do you think that his dorm food is really that unhealthy or that he just hasn't gotten used to it yet?

Health on the Net

Managing Your Weight
Finding a Healthy Balance

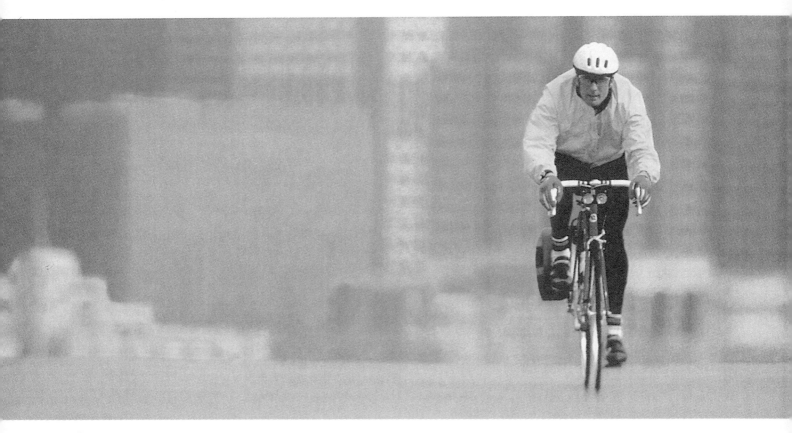

CHAPTER OBJECTIVES

◆ Describe how healthy weight is determined both by weight and in terms of body content; describe the major techniques for body content assessment.

◆ Describe those factors that place people at risk for problems with obesity.

◆ Discuss the roles of exercise, dieting, nutrition, "miracle diets," and other strategies in weight control.

◆ Describe the three major eating disorders and explain the health risks of these conditions.

Ray, aged 20, is desperately trying to lose the 25 pounds he put on in his first year at college. During that year, he spent much of his time studying, made little time for exercise, and often rewarded his hard work with lunch, dinner, and snack breaks with his friends. Because he wants to lose the extra weight fast and be buff in his trunks for spring break, Ray goes on a crash diet and begins an intense running and weightlifting program. After three weeks on the diet, all his friends tell him how cool he is starting to look, and, bolstered by their support, Ray decides to cut his already low food intake even more and to increase his exercise.

- ■ What risks are associated with Ray's plan for rapid weight loss? Is his thinking typical or atypical of people you know on similar "fast" weight loss plans? What are his motivations for losing weight, and how do the opinions of others appear to influence him? As a friend, what could you do to ensure that Ray doesn't harm himself during his quest to lose weight?

If you've never met a chocolate chip cookie you didn't like, you are probably one of the millions of Canadians who seem to be trapped in a constant battle of the bulge. By all accounts, in spite of being part of a generation of health and fitness buffs who exercise, forsake high-fat foods, and mesmerize ourselves with self-help diet and fitness books, we are not doing better in our quest for health and fitness. In fact, according to a 1995 study, 32 percent of Canadians are overweight enough to put their health at risk.[1]

What are all of these overweight Canadians doing to shed their excess poundage? Many of them opt for nutritionally balanced diets that include sufficient amounts of exercise to burn the calories they consume. Others elect to get help from weight-loss gurus, trained professionals, or weight-loss franchises. Still others purchase questionable products and services that claim to help people "shed unsightly pounds fast and effortlessly." Some are starving themselves in pursuit of the perfect body. Finally, there is a group that has made several attempts at weight loss before giving up.

In fact, in spite of good intentions, few people get beyond the first few days of a weight-loss effort. Those who do continue on their weight-loss programs and take off a significant number of pounds tend to gain most of them back. Follow-up studies of people on controlled diets indicate that at least half of the weight lost is regained within two to four years.[2]

This chapter focusses on the obsession with thinness and explores the reasons why so many of us seem to be trapped in overweight bodies that we can't escape from. It is designed to help you better understand what *overweight* and *obesity* really mean and why weight control is essential to your overall health. Finally, this chapter shows you how to develop strategies for controlling your own weight, losing weight, and yes, even for gaining weight if you are among that small group of underweight people who must struggle to put on needed pounds.

BODY IMAGE

Most of us think of the obsession with thinness as a phenomenon of recent years. Beginning with supermodel Twiggy in the 1960s and continuing with supermodel Kate Moss in the 1990s, the thin look seems to dominate fashion ads. And not only that: television, movies, and magazines constantly project images of lean, fit bodies. We have been led to believe that if we are thin, with shapely curves or well-defined muscles, we will be more desirable.

But the thin look has been around for a long time. Anorexia nervosa, an eating disorder, has been defined as a psychiatric disorder since 1873. During the Victorian era, corsets were used to achieve unrealistically tiny waists. By the 1920s, it was common knowledge that obesity was linked to poor health. The American Tobacco Company coined the phrase "Reach for a Lucky instead of a sweet" to promote the idea that cigarettes dulled appetite.

Today, beautiful female models in size 4 clothes and underweight Miss Americas exemplify desirability and success, delivering the subtle message that thin is in. In addition, we are bombarded with warnings that being overweight increases our risk of heart disease, certain types of cancer, arthritis, gallbladder disease, diabetes, poor emotional health, and a host of other problems that decrease our life expectancy. What's a body to do?

In response to our rational and emotional quests to be thin, a multibillion-dollar diet industry has developed, purveying liquid diets, freeze-dried foods, nonfat and low-fat foods, artificial sweeteners, diet books by the hundreds, and a host of weight-loss clinics. We are offered devices that are supposed to "melt away," "burn away," and "jiggle away" fat, and pills that claim to "burn fat" while you eat whatever you like and avoid exercise. While some advertised claims are valid, others are designed to make big profits at your expense.

How do you find a safe, effective means of losing those extra pounds? A good way to start is by gathering accurate information about weight-loss products and services, learning what triggers your "eat" buttons, and analyzing your lifestyle to determine your problem areas. Developing the skills to set rational weight-loss goals and taking advantage of social and community supports are also part of the process.

Determining the Right Weight for You

The answer to whether you are overweight is somewhat subjective and depends on your body structure and how your weight is distributed. Traditionally, people have compared their weight with data from some form of standard height-and-weight chart. These charts usually give the "ideal" weight for males and females of given height and frame size. In general, if you are 20 to 30 percent above your ideal weight, as indicated by the chart, you would be classified as obese.

One of the most reliable height-weight guides is the Metropolitan Life Height and Weight Table, which is reproduced in Table 8.1. Note that the tables do not indicate a relationship between weight and quality of life, total health, vitality, or appearance. Nor do they provide an indication of the ratio of body fat to lean muscle mass, which is the real indicator of how fat a person really is. Nevertheless, they are still the most commonly used measure of weight status.

TABLE 8.1 ■ Ideal Weights Based on Body Frame

Weights at ages 25 to 29 based on lowest mortality. Weights in pounds according to frame, in indoor clothing weighing 5 pounds for men and 3 pounds for women, shoes with 1-inch heels. Note that these heights and weights are given in imperial measures. To convert from a metric height, multiply centimetres by 0.4 for height in inches; to calculate a weight in kilograms, multiply weight in pounds by 0.454.

Men					Women				
Height		Small Frame	Medium Frame	Large Frame	Height		Small Frame	Medium Frame	Large Frame
Feet	Inches				Feet	Inches			
5	2	128–134	131–141	138–150	4	10	102–111	109–121	118–131
5	3	130–136	133–143	140–153	4	11	103–113	111–123	120–134
5	4	132–138	135–145	142–156	5	0	104–115	113–126	122–137
5	5	134–140	137–148	144–160	5	1	106–118	115–129	125–140
5	6	136–142	139–151	146–164	5	2	108–121	118–132	128–143
5	7	138–145	142–154	149–168	5	3	111–124	121–135	131–147
5	8	140–148	145–157	152–172	5	4	114–127	124–138	134–151
5	9	142–151	148–160	155–176	5	5	117–130	127–141	137–155
5	10	144–154	151–163	158–180	5	6	120–133	130–144	140–159
5	11	146–157	154–166	161–184	5	7	123–136	133–147	143–163
6	0	149–160	157–170	164–188	5	8	126–139	136–150	146–167
6	1	152–164	160–174	168–192	5	9	129–142	139–153	149–170
6	2	155–168	164–178	172–197	5	10	132–145	142–156	152–173
6	3	158–172	167–182	176–202	5	11	135–148	145–159	155–176
6	4	162–176	171–187	181–207	6	0	138–151	148–162	158–179

Source: Reproduced with permission of Metropolitan Life Insurance Company, *1983 Build Study*, Society of Actuaries and Association of Life Insurance Medical Directors of America, 1984.

Another formula for people between the ages of 18 and 25 establishes reasonable weights of 50 kilograms for a 152-centimetre-tall man and 45 kilograms for a 152-centimetre-tall woman. For each centimetre over 152, men and women should add 1 kilogram. In addition, a woman should subtract half a kilogram for each year under 25.

Redefining Obesity: Weight Versus Fat Content

In recent years, diagnosticians have revised their definition of obesity. Although body weight is certainly an important factor, they believe that the real indicator of **obesity** is how much fat your body contains (see Figure 8.1). A male weight lifter may be 30 to 40 percent overweight according to the charts and yet still not be obese because of the heaviness and relative density of his muscle tissue. Similarly, a 40-year-old woman who prides herself on weighing the same 60 kilograms that she did in high school may be shocked to learn that her body now contains over 40 percent fat compared to 15 percent fat in her high school days. Weight by itself, although a useful guide, is not a valid indicator of obesity.

A more accurate assessment of total body fat requires a different type of measurement. If traditional height-weight charts do not accurately define obesity, what general guidelines should be applied for determining acceptable levels of body fat? **Obesity** is generally defined as an accumulation of fat beyond what is considered normal for a person's age, sex, and body type. The difficulty lies in defining what is normal. To date, there are no universally accepted standards for the most "desirable" or "ideal" body weight or body composition (ratio of lean body mass to fat body mass). We will discuss body composition in more detail later in the chapter.

Although sources vary slightly, most agree that men's bodies should contain between 11 and 15 percent total body fat, and women should be within the range of 18 to 22 percent body fat. A man would be considered obese if his body fat exceeded 20 percent of his total body mass. A woman would be considered obese if her body fat exceeded 30 percent of her total body mass.[3] Table 8.2 provides general guidelines for determining how adults aged 18 to 30 compare in terms of overall percentages of body fat.

Why the difference between men and women? Much of it may be attributed to the normal structure of the female body and to sex hormones. As mentioned earlier, when considering how much or how little fat a person should have, it is important to think of body composition in terms of lean body mass and body fat. Lean body mass is made up of the structural and functional elements in cells, body water, muscle, bones, and other body organs such as the heart, liver, and kidneys. Body fat is composed of two types: essential fat and storage fat. Essential fat is necessary for normal physiological functioning, such as nerve conduction. Essential fat makes up approximately 3 to 7 percent of total body weight in men and approximately 15 percent of total body weight in women. Storage fat, the part that many of us are always trying to shed, makes up the remainder of our fat reserves. It accounts for only a small percentage of total body weight for very lean people and between 5 and 25 percent of body weight of most Canadian adults. Female bodybuilders, who are among the leanest of female athletes, may have body fat

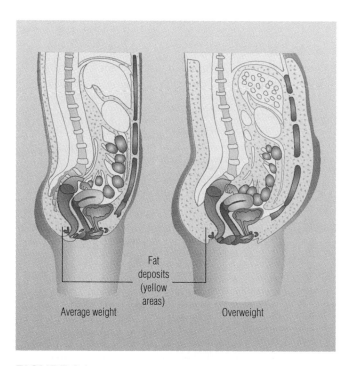

FIGURE 8.1

The figure compares an average-weight person and an overweight person. Note the fat deposits under the skin and around the internal organs.

TABLE 8.2 ■ General Ratings of Body Fat Percentages by Age and Sex

Rating	Males (ages 18–30) (%)	Females (ages 18–30) (%)
Athletic*	6–10	10–15
Good	11–14	16–19
Acceptable	15–17	20–24
Overfat	18–19	25–29
Obese	20 or over	30 or over

*The ratings in the athletic category are general guidelines for those athletes, such as gymnasts and long-distance runners, whose need for a "competitive edge" in selected sports may compel them to try to lose as much weight as possible. However, for the average person, such low body fat levels should be approached with caution.

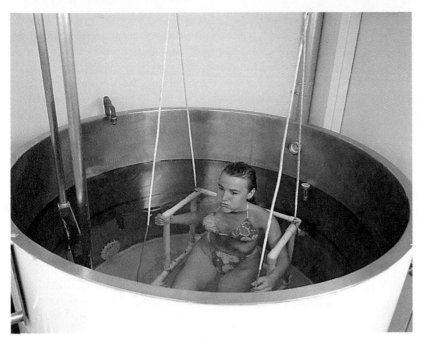

Hydrostatic weighing is the most sophisticated and accurate technique currently available to measure body fat.

percentages ranging from 8 to 13 percent, nearly all of which is essential fat.

Although most of us continually try to reduce our body fat, there are levels below which we dare not go. A minimal amount of body fat is necessary for insulation of the body, for cushioning between parts of the body and vital organs, and for maintaining body functions. In men, this lower limit is approximately 3 to 4 percent. Women should generally not go below 8 percent. Excessively low body fat in females may lead to amenorrhea, a disruption of the normal menstrual cycle. The critical level of body fat necessary to maintain normal menstrual flow is believed to be between 8 and 13 percent, but there are numerous exceptions to this rule and many additional factors that affect the menstrual cycle. Under extreme circumstances, such as starvation diets and certain diseases, the body often utilizes all available fat reserves and begins to break down muscle tissue as a last-ditch effort to obtain nourishment.

While some of us like to say that we are storing up fat to protect ourselves from the great food shortages of the future, there are limits to the plausibility of this argument! The fact is that too much fat and too little fat are both potentially harmful. The key is to find a level at which you are not at high risk for health problems and at which you are comfortable with your appearance.

Assessing Your Body Content

With all of the techniques available for calculating how fat you really are, how do you decide which is the best for you? Perhaps the best way is to ask yourself how much an exact measure of your body fat means to you. If you are interested in obtaining the most accurate measure before and after a program of diet and exercise, you may find the expense of some of the more sophisticated measures worth the investment. If you simply want a general idea of how much body fat you are carrying around, an inexpensive pinch test or skinfold measure may be all that you need. On the other hand, if you know, based on the bulges around your middle or the size and fit of your jeans, that you are obese, perhaps the exact amount of fat that you have does not matter as much as the fact that you need to take action.

Hydrostatic Weighing Techniques. From a clinical perspective, the most accurate method of measuring body fat is through **hydrostatic weighing techniques**. This method measures the amount of water a person displaces when completely submerged. Because fat tissue has a lower density than muscle or bone tissue, a relatively accurate indication of actual body fat can be computed by comparing a person's under-water and out-of-water weights. Although this method may be subject to error, it is one of the most sophisticated techniques currently available.

Obesity: A weight disorder generally defined as an accumulation of fat beyond that considered normal for a person's age, sex, and body type.

Hydrostatic weighing techniques: Methods of determining body fat by measuring the amount of water displaced when a person is completely submerged.

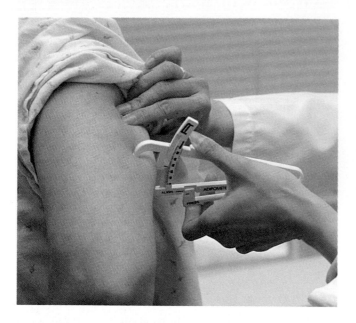

In the hands of a trained professional, the skinfold caliper can give an accurate measure of body fat for people who are not overly obese.

Pinch and Skinfold Measures. Perhaps the most commonly used method of body fat determination is the **pinch test**. Numerous studies have determined that the triceps area (located in the back of the upper arm) is one of the most reliable areas of the body for assessing the amount of fat in the subcutaneous (just under the surface) layer of the skin. In making this assessment, a person pinches a fold of skin just behind the triceps with the thumb and index finger. It is important to pinch only the fat layer and not the triceps muscle. After selecting a spot for measure, the person assesses the distance between the thumb and index finger. If the size of the pinch appears to be thicker than 2.5 centimetres, the person is generally considered overfat. Another technique, the **skinfold caliper test**, resembles the pinch test but is much more accurate. In this procedure, a person pinches folds of skin at various points on the body with the thumb and index finger. This technique uses a specially calibrated instrument called a *skinfold caliper* to take a precise measurement of the fat layer. Besides the triceps area, the points most often used in these measurements are the biceps area (front of the arm), the subscapular area (upper back), and the iliac crest (hip). Once these data points are assessed, special formulas are employed to arrive at a combined prediction of total body fat. In the hands of trained technicians, this procedure can be fairly accurate. If the person doing the test is inconsistent about the exact locations of the pinch or if there is difficulty in determining the difference between fat and muscle, the results may be inaccurate. In addition, the heavier a person is, the

more prone this technique is to error. For chronically obese people, difficulties in assessment are magnified because of problems with distinguishing between flaccid muscles and fat. Also, most currently available calipers do not expand far enough to obtain accurate measurements on the moderately obese (20 to 40 percent overweight) or the morbidly obese (more than 50 percent overweight). Additional errors in skinfold assessments may occur as a result of failure to account for certain age, sex, and ethnic differences in calibrations.

Girth and Circumference Measures. Another common method of body fat assessment is the use of **girth and circumference measures**. Diagnosticians use a measuring tape to take girth, or circumference, measurements at various body sites. These measurements are then converted into constants, and a formula is used to determine relative percentages of body fat. Although this technique is inexpensive, easy to use, and commonly performed, it is not as accurate as many of the other techniques listed here.

Body Mass Index. One of the more widely accepted approaches to weight assessment is a technique developed by the U.S. National Center for Health Statistics called the **body mass index (BMI)**. Because the BMI is an index of the relationship of weight to height, which is based on a norm of adults between the ages of 20 and 29, it is probably one of the best assessments for most university students.

The BMI is obtained by dividing your weight (in kilograms) by your height (in meters) squared. Weight should be taken without shoes or clothing, and height should be measured without shoes. In general, a BMI range of 20 to 24 is considered normal. The desirable range for females is 21 to 23; for males, it is 22 to 24. BMI values above 27.8 for men and 27.3 for women have been associated with increased health problems, including high blood pressure and diabetes. People with BMIs greater than 30 are considered obese and those having BMIs greater than 40 are considered morbidly obese and in need of prompt medical attention[4] (see Figure 8.2).

Soft-Tissue Roentgenogram. A relatively new technique for body fat determination, the **soft-tissue roentgenogram**, involves injecting a radioactive substance into the body and allowing this substance to penetrate muscle (lean) tissue so distinctions between fat and lean tissue can be made by means of imaging.

Bioelectrical Impedance Analysis. Another method of determining body fat levels, **bioelectrical impedance analysis (BIA)**, involves sending a small electric current through the subject's body. The amount of resistance to the current, along with the person's age, sex, and other physical characteristics, is then fed into a computer that uses special formulas to determine the total amount of lean and fat tissue.

Total Body Electrical Conductivity. One of the newest (and most expensive) assessment techniques is **total body electrical conductivity (TOBEC)**, which uses an electromagnetic force field to assess relative body fat. Although based on the same principle as impedance, this assessment requires much more elaborate, expensive equipment, and therefore is not practical for most people.

Although all of these methods can be useful, they can also be inaccurate and even harmful unless the testers are skillful and well trained. Before agreeing to any procedure, be sure you are aware of the expense, potential for accuracy, risks, and training of the tester.

*W*HAT DO YOU THINK?

Why is it important to consider your percentage of body fat rather than weight only when determining how fat you really are? Which of the above tests would you feel comfortable taking? Would any make you feel uncomfortable?

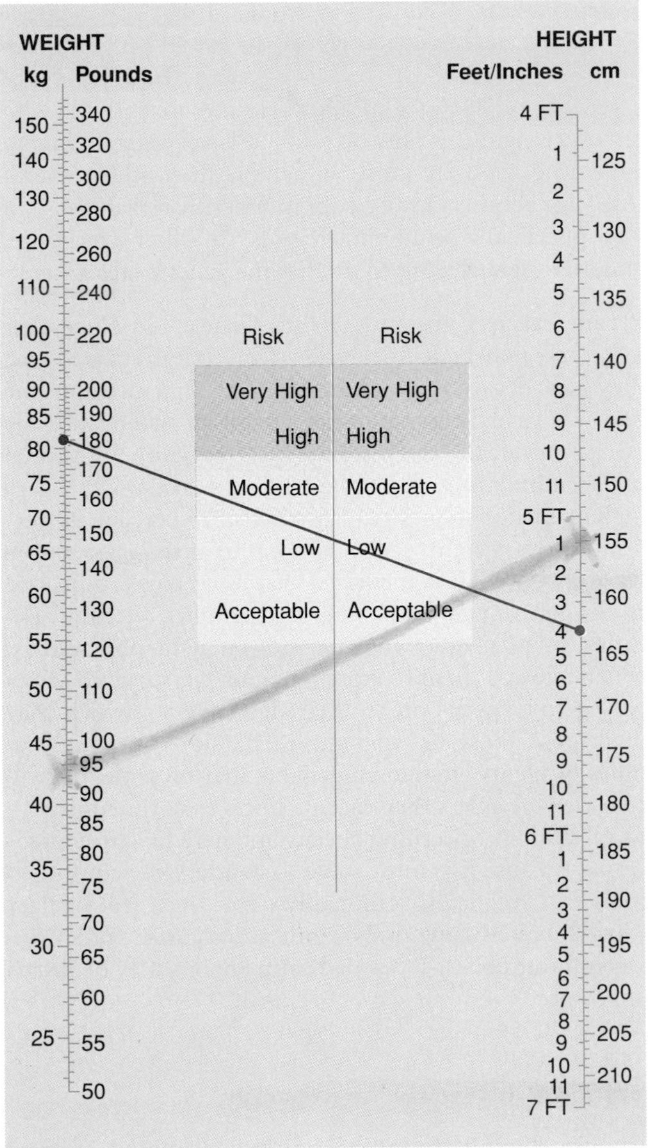

*R*ISK FACTORS FOR OBESITY

For many of us, the reason for obesity is quite simple: If you take in more calories than you burn up, you will gain weight. If you do this throughout your life, you will become increasingly obese. If we know what the cause is, we should be able to offer a simple prescription for preventing the problem. Right? Wrong.

Although the calorie explanation of obesity is certainly valid, it offers only one possible reason for a person's weight problem. It does not explain the many additional factors that contribute to the problem and that may make the possibility of permanent weight loss very unlikely.

FIGURE 8.2

Are you overweight? To find out if your current level of fatness increases your chances of dying early, angle a pencil or the edge of a piece of paper from your weight (on the left) to your height (on the right). Read your risk where the pencil crosses the centre line.

Pinch test: A method of determining body fat whereby a fold of skin just behind the triceps is pinched between the thumb and index finger to determine the relative amount of fat.

Skinfold caliper test: A method of determining body fat whereby folds of skin and fat at various points on the body are grasped between thumb and forefinger and measured with calipers.

Girth and circumference measures: A method of assessing body fat that employs a formula based on girth measurements of various body sites.

Body mass index (BMI): A technique of weight assessment based on the relationship of weight to height.

Soft-tissue roentgenogram: A technique of body fat assessment in which radioactive substances are used to determine relative fat.

Bioelectrical impedance analysis (BIA): A technique of body fat assessment in which electrical currents are passed through fat and lean tissue.

Total body electrical conductivity (TOBEC): Technique using an electromagnetic force field to assess relative body fat.

It also fails to answer many other critical questions. If we know that eating too much will cause us to gain weight, why do we continue to eat too much? Is there a metabolic explanation for obesity? Why do fewer than 5 percent of all people who go on a weight loss program achieve permanent success? Is pushing yourself away from the table the best exercise for maintaining your weight?

Heredity

Body Type and Genes. In some animal species, the shape and size of the individual's body is largely determined by the shape and size of its parents' bodies. Many scientists have explored the role of heredity in determining human body shapes. As early as 1940, Harvard psychologist William Sheldon analyzed weight problems in terms of genetically determined body types. His studies indicated that people having an ectomorphic body type, characterized by tall, slender frames, generally experienced few difficulties with weight control. People with an endomorphic body type, characterized by a rounded, soft appearance, often had a large abdomen and typically reported a history of weight problems beginning in childhood. Between these two extremes was the shorter, more muscular, and athletic-looking mesomorphic body type. Leaner and more active than endomorphs in early adulthood, mesomorphs demonstrated a strong tendency to gain weight later in life.[5]

Some researchers still support Sheldon's theories identifying body type as a major factor in the development of weight problems, but most contend that heredity plays a more subtle role in obesity. These researchers argue that obesity has a strong genetic determinant (it tends to run in families). They cite statistics showing that 80 percent of children having two obese parents are also obese.[6] But why is this the case? Can you really blame your parents for your problems with weight?

Twin Studies. Studies of identical twins who were separated at birth and raised in different environments have provided us with some of the most compelling evidence to date that obesity may be an inherited trait. Whether raised in family environments with fat or thin family members, twins with obese birth parents tend to be obese in later life.[7] According to another study, sets of identical twins who were separated and raised in different families and who ate widely different diets still grew up to weigh about the same.[8] So, if you are overweight, you cannot blame it all on your parents for overfeeding you as a child.

These studies contain the strongest evidence yet that the genes a person inherits are the major factor determining overweight, leanness, or average weight. Although the exact mechanics remain unknown, it is believed that genes set metabolic rates, influencing how the body handles calories.

Genetic Predisposition and Environmental Factors. Health professionals are concerned that these studies will convince many overweight people that they are doomed to be fat. However, Albert Stunkard, a psychiatrist at the University of Pennsylvania and author of one of these studies, believes that, on the contrary, their conclusions offer hope to those whose extra pounds have been blamed on their lack of willpower or hidden psychological needs. In Stunkard's study, early family environment had no apparent effect on adult weight. Based on this finding, Stunkard discounts previous theories that the amount children eat early in life helps determine whether they will be fat as adults. According to Stunkard, it is not the family environment in which you were raised but the environment in which you live as an adult that determines whether you will be a fat adult. He says that people who are overweight can now be told, "It is very largely due to your genes. You are more vulnerable than others; therefore your actions may be even more critical than those of your genetically prone thin friends." In other words, diet and exercise will work to modify the genetic effect.[9]

Errant Eating Cues and Thrifty Genes. In November 1994, researchers at Rockefeller University reported that they had discovered a defective gene that disrupts the body's "I've had enough to eat" signalling system and may be responsible for a least some types of obesity.[10] Research on Pima Indians in the United States, a group with a very high incidence of obesity (estimated at 75 percent; 90 percent are overweight) seems to point to an OB gene that is a *"thrifty gene."* It is theorized that as certain groups had to struggle during hard times and famines over the centuries, those people who had slower metabolic activity, which allowed them to store precious fat, survived. They passed their genes on to their descendents, which may predispose these descendents to be slow burners.[11] In times of plenty, it seems inevitable that these people will gain weight, unless they eat much less than the norm.

All studies concerning obesity and heredity are controversial because it is impossible to conduct the controlled trials that might prove heredity's role. It is still unclear whether any of these studies indicates a genetic predisposition toward obesity; learned eating habits may be just as important.

Hunger, Appetite, and Satiety

Theories abound concerning the mechanisms that regulate food intake. Some sources indicate that the hypothalamus (the part of the brain that regulates appetite) closely monitors levels of certain nutrients in the blood. When these levels begin to fall, the brain signals us to eat. In the obese person, it is possible that the monitoring system does not work properly and that the cues to eat are more frequent and intense than they are in people of normal weight.

Other sources indicate that thin people may send more effective messages to the hypothalamus. This concept, known as **adaptive thermogenesis**, states that thin people can often consume large amounts of food without gaining weight because the appetite centre of their brains speeds up metabolic activity to compensate for the increased consumption. More recent studies have indicated the possibility that specialized types of fat cells, called **brown fat cells**, may send signals to the brain, which controls the thermogenesis response.

The hypothesis that food tastes better to obese people, thus causing them to eat more, has largely been refuted. Scientists do distinguish, however, between **hunger**, an inborn physiological response to nutritional needs, and **appetite**, a learned response to food that is tied to an emotional or psychological craving for food often unrelated to nutritional need. Obese people may be more likely than thin people to satisfy their appetite and eat for reasons other than nutrition.

In some instances, the problem with overconsumption may be more related to **satiety** than to appetite or hunger. People generally feel satiated, or full, when they have satisfied their nutritional needs and their stomach signals "no more." For undetermined reasons, obese people may not feel full until much later than thin people.

Developmental Factors

Some obese people may have excessive numbers of fat cells. This type of obesity, **hyperplasia**, usually begins to develop in early childhood and perhaps, due to the mother's dietary habits, even prior to birth. The most critical periods for the development of hyperplasia seem to be the last two to three months of fetal development, the first year of life, and between the ages of 9 and 13. Parents who allow their children to eat without restrictions and to become overweight may be setting their children up for a lifelong excess of fat cells. Central to this theory is the belief that the number of fat cells in a person's body does not increase appreciably during adulthood. However, the ability of each of these cells to swell and shrink, known as **hypertrophy**, does carry over into adulthood. Weight gain may be tied to both the number of fat cells in the body and the capacity of each individual cell to enlarge.

An average-weight adult has approximately 25 billion to 30 billion fat cells, a moderately obese adult about 60 billion to 100 billion, and an extremely obese adult as many as 200 billion.[12] People who add large numbers of fat cells to their bodies in childhood may be able to lose weight by decreasing the size of each cell in adulthood, but the large numbers of cells remain, and with the next calorie binge, they fill up and sabotage weight loss efforts (see Figure 8.3). Additional research must be conducted to determine the accuracy of these theories.

Setpoint Theory

In 1982, nutritional researchers William Bennett and Joel Gurin presented a highly controversial theory concerning the difficulty some people have in losing weight. Their theory, known as the **setpoint theory**, states that a person's body has a setpoint of weight at which it is programmed to be comfortable. If your setpoint is around 70 kilograms, you will gain and lose weight fairly easily within a given range of that point. For example, if you gain 2 to 5 kilograms on vacation, it will be fairly easy to lose that weight and remain around the 70 kilogram mark for a long period of time. Some people have equated this point with the **plateau** that is sometimes reached after a person on a diet loses a certain amount of weight. The setpoint theory proposes that after losing a predetermined amount of weight, the body will actually sabotage additional weight loss by slowing down metabolism. In extreme cases, the metabolic rate will decrease to a point at which the body will maintain its weight on as little as 1000 calories per day. Can a person change this predetermined setpoint? Proponents of this theory argue that it is possible to raise one's setpoint over time by continually gaining weight and failing to exercise. Conversely, reducing caloric intake and exercising over a long period of time can slowly decrease one's setpoint. Exercise may be the most critical factor in readjusting your setpoint, although diet may also be important.

This theory, too, remains controversial. Perhaps its greatest impact was the sense of relief it provided for

Adaptive thermogenesis: Theoretical mechanism by which the brain regulates metabolic activity according to caloric intake.

Brown fat cells: Specialized type of fat cell that affects the ability to regulate fat metabolism.

Hunger: An inborn physiological response to nutritional needs.

Appetite: A learned response that is tied to an emotional or psychological craving for food that is often unrelated to nutritional need.

Satiety: The feeling of fullness or satisfaction at the end of a meal.

Hyperplasia: A condition characterized by an excessive number of fat cells.

Hypertrophy: The ability of fat cells to swell and shrink.

Setpoint theory: A theory of obesity causation that suggests that fat storage is determined by a thermostatic mechanism in the body that acts to maintain a specific amount of body fat.

Plateau: That point in a weight-loss program at which the dieter finds it difficult to lose more weight.

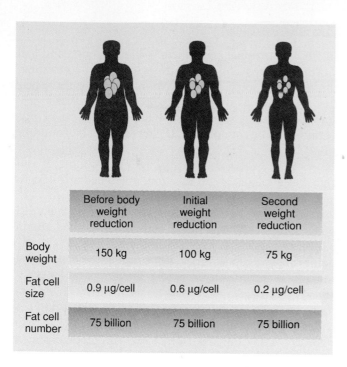

	Before body weight reduction	Initial weight reduction	Second weight reduction
Body weight	150 kg	100 kg	75 kg
Fat cell size	0.9 μg/cell	0.6 μg/cell	0.2 μg/cell
Fat cell number	75 billion	75 billion	75 billion

FIGURE 8.3

The figure depicts one person at various stages of weight loss. Note that, according to theories of hyperplasia, the number of fat cells remains constant but their size decreases.

people who have lost weight, plateaued, and regained weight time and time again. It told them that their failure was not due to a lack of willpower alone. The setpoint theory also prompted nutritional experts to look more carefully at popular methods of weight loss. If the setpoint theory is correct, a low-calorie or starvation diet, besides being dangerous, may cause the body to protect the dieter from "starvation" by slowing down metabolism and making weight loss more difficult.

Endocrine Influence

Over the years, many people have attributed obesity to problems with their **thyroid glands**. They claimed that an underactive thyroid impeded their ability to burn calories. This belief substituted an organic cause for individual responsibility for obesity. How many obesity problems may justifiably be blamed on a poorly functioning thyroid? Most authorities agree that only 3 to 5 percent of the obese population have a thyroid problem.

Psychosocial Factors

The relationship of weight problems to deeply rooted emotional insecurities, needs, and wants remains uncertain. Food is often used as a reward for good behaviour in childhood. As adults face unemployment, broken relationships, financial uncertainty, fears about health and

other problems, the bright spot in the day is often "what's on the table for dinner," or, "we're going to that restaurant tonight." Again, the research underlying this theory is controversial. What is certain is that in mainstream Canada, eating tends to be a focal point of people's lives. Eating is essentially a social ritual associated with companionship, celebration, and enjoyment.

Eating Cues: Targeted by the Food Industry

At least one major factor in our preoccupation with food is the pressure placed on us by the highly sophisticated, heavily advertised "eating" campaigns launched by the food industry. There may be salad bars at the local fast-food joints, but customers have to run the gauntlet of starchy, beefy delights and tasty high-fat super-size fries to find them. The food and restaurant industries spend billions every year on ads designed to entice hungry people to forgo fresh fruit and sliced vegetables for Whoppers and Happy Meals.[13] The average child, says psychologist Kelly Brownell, head of the Yale University Center for Eating and Weight Disorders, watches 10 000 food ads a year on TV. "And they're not seeing commercials for brussels sprouts," Brownell complains. "They're seeing soft drinks, candy bars, sugar-coated cereals and fast food."[14]

An increasing percentage (up over 13 percent in the 1980s) of the foods we eat are from fast-food restaurants. This is unfortunate because (1) fast food is high in calories, fat, sodium, and carbohydrates; (2) it tends to get eaten, even though portions are often much bigger than they should be; and (3) it tends to be eaten quickly, so there isn't enough time for the "I'm full" signal to get to your mouth before the last bite of food is there.[15] This is a particular problem for university students who now face the temptation of fast-food courts right on campus.

Dietary Myth and Misperception

You've all heard the story: "I eat like a bird, but I can't lose weight." Should you believe the person who says this? Probably not, according to a recent study analyzing the self-reported and actual caloric intakes and exercise expenditures of a group of overweight adults. The researchers carefully followed obese people who had been unsuccessful following as many as 20 diets, though they claimed that they consumed fewer than 1200 calories per day. They blamed their failure on "metabolism." It turned out that their metabolism levels were normal, but that they were actually eating nearly twice as much as they thought they were and exercising only three-quarters as much as they reported.[16] Does this mean that obesity is simply the result of gluttony and sloth? Are obese people the only ones who underestimate their caloric intake and overestimate the amount of exercise they do? No. In fact, many studies have shown that obese individuals do not eat much more than their normal-weight counterparts.

However, it should be noted that they do exercise less. The majority of overweight individuals are less active than people of normal weight. Of course, it could be argued that it is their obesity that leads to their sedentary lifestyle. Much more research is necessary before scientists really have a clear profile of both the obese and the nonobese.

Metabolic Changes

Even when completely at rest, the body needs a certain amount of energy. The amount of energy your body uses at complete rest is known as your **basal metabolic rate (BMR)**. About 60 to 70 percent of all the calories you consume on a given day go to support your basal metabolism: heartbeat, breathing, maintaining body temperature, and so on. So if you are consuming about 2000 calories per day, between 1200 and 1400 of those calories are burned without your doing any significant physical activity. But unless you exert yourself enough to burn the remaining 600 to 800 calories, you will gain weight. Your BMR can fluctuate considerably, with several factors influencing whether it slows down or speeds up. In general, the younger you are, the higher your BMR, partly because in young people cells undergo rapid subdivision, which consumes a good deal of energy. BMR is highest during infancy, puberty, and pregnancy, when bodily changes are most rapid. BMR is also influenced by body composition. Muscle tissue is highly active—even at rest—compared to fat tissue. In essence, the more lean tissue you have, the greater your BMR and the more fat tissue you have, the lower your BMR. Men have a higher BMR than women do, at least partly because of their greater tendency toward lean tissue.

Age is another factor that may greatly affect BMR. After the age of 30, your BMR slows down by about 1 to 2 percent a year. Therefore, people over 30 commonly find that they must work harder to burn off an extra helping of ice cream than they did when they were in their teens. "Middle-aged spread," a reference to the tendency to put on weight after the age of 30, is partly related to this change. A slower BMR, coupled with an inclination to be less active and priorities (family and career) that come before fitness and weight, puts many middle-aged people's weight in jeopardy.

In addition, the body has a number of self-protective mechanisms that signal BMR to speed up or slow down. For example, when you have a fever, the energy needs of your cells increase, and this increased activity generates heat and speeds up your BMR. In starvation situations, the body tries to protect itself by slowing down BMR to conserve precious energy. Thus, when people repeatedly resort to extreme diets, their bodies "reset" their BMRs at lower rates. **Yo-yo diets**, in which people repeatedly gain weight and then starve themselves to lose the weight, lowering their BMR in the process, are doomed to failure. When they begin to eat again after the weight loss, they have a BMR that is set lower, making it almost certain that they will regain the weight they just lost. After repeated cycles of such dieting/regaining, these people find it increasingly hard to lose weight and increasingly easy to regain it, so they become heavier and heavier.

According to a recent study by psychologist Kelly Brownell, middle-aged men who maintained a steady weight (even if they were overweight) had a lower risk of heart attack than men whose weight cycled up and down in a yo-yo pattern. Brownell found that smaller, well-maintained weight losses are more beneficial for reducing cardiovascular risk than larger, poorly maintained weight losses.[17]

Finally, certain hormones, particularly the stress hormones, may cause BMR to rise in response to increased nervous activity and energy requirements by the cells.

Lifestyle

Of all the factors affecting obesity, perhaps the most critical is the relationship between activity levels and calorie intake. Obesity rates are rising. But how can this be happening? Aren't more people exercising than ever before? While it may look like it, the facts are not so positive. According to Canada's Health Promotion Survey, just under half of Canadian adults (48 percent) scored high on an index of leisure-time physical activity in 1990—slightly fewer than five years earlier.[18] (See the Focus on Canada box.) Meanwhile, physical education has been made optional in many high schools.

You probably know someone who seems to be able to eat you under the table and does not appear to exercise more than you do, yet never seems to gain weight. You often do not understand how this person maintains a steady weight. With few exceptions, if you were to follow this person around for a typical day and monitor the level and intensity of activity, you would discover the answer to your question. Although the person's schedule may not include running or strenuous exercise, it probably includes a high level of activity. Walking up a flight of stairs rather than taking the elevator, speeding up the pace while mowing the lawn, getting up to change the TV channel rather than using the remote, and doing housework vigorously all

Thyroid gland: A two-lobed endocrine gland located in the throat region that produces a hormone that regulates metabolism.

Basal metabolic rate (BMR): The energy expenditure of the body under resting conditions at normal room temperature.

Yo-yo diet: Cycles in which people repeatedly gain weight, then starve themselves to lose weight. This lowers their BMR, which makes regaining weight even more likely.

While some people do burn calories and fat better than others, exercise and an active life style are the keys to balancing caloric intake and body weight.

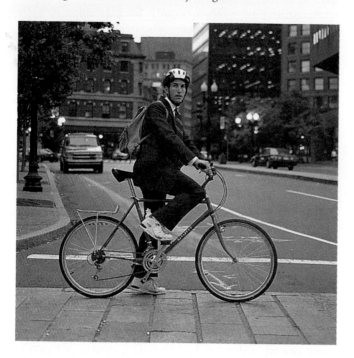

burn extra calories. Or, perhaps in some subtle ways, these people just manage to burn more calories through extra motions.

(Actually, there is a grain of truth to the notion of the person who burns up those calories without working at it. In studies of calorie burning by individuals placed in a controlled respiratory chamber environment where calories consumed, motion, and overall activity were measured, it was found that some people are better fat burners than others. It is possible that low fat burners may not produce as many of the enzymes needed to convert fat to energy. Or they may not have as many blood vessels supplying fatty tissue, making it tougher for them to deliver fat-burning oxygen. However, these differences do not appear to be as important a factor as activity levels.)

A major cause of low activity levels is the abundance of labour-saving devices in the modern household. Pushing vacuum cleaners rather than sweeping floors, typing on computer keyboards rather than manual typewriters, and using remote-control buttons on television and stereo equipment cause us to expend fewer calories than previous generations did. The automobile is a great convenience, but it has lowered our muscle tone and our cardiovascular efficiency.

Clearly, any form of activity that helps your body burn additional calories helps you maintain your weight. In fact, in a study conducted at Stanford University in 1987, a group of men who lost weight through exercise were far more successful at keeping the weight off than were a similar group who lost weight through dieting.

*W*HAT DO YOU THINK?

Based on the risk factors for obesity discussed thus far, which ones do you think pose the greatest risk for you? Which ones can you do something about? What actions can you take to reduce your risk?

Gender and Obesity

Throughout a woman's life, issues of appearance and beauty dominate her surroundings. Only recently have researchers begun to understand just how significant the quest for beauty and the perfect body really is.

In a recent U.S. study, researchers determined that being severely overweight in adolescence may predetermine one's social and economic future—particularly if you happen to be female. Researchers found that obese women complete about half a year less schooling, are 20 percent less likely to get married, and earn $6710 (U.S.) on average less per year than their slimmer counterparts. Obese women also have rates of household poverty 10 percent higher than those of women who are not overweight. In contrast, the study found that overweight men were 11 percent less likely to be married than thinner men but suffer few adverse economic consequences.

It is more likely that women will suffer such consequences of obesity simply because they are more likely than men to be overweight. Compared to men, women have a lower ratio of lean body mass to fatty mass, in part due to differences in bone size and mass, muscle size, and other variables. For all ages after sexual maturity, men have higher metabolic rates, making it easier for them to burn off excess calories than it is for women. Women also face greater potential for weight fluctuation due to hormonal changes, pregnancy, and other conditions that increase the likelihood of weight gain. Also, as a group, men are more socialized into physical activity from birth. Strenuous activity in both work and play are encouraged for men, while women's roles have typically been more sedentary and required a lower level of caloric expenditure to complete.

Not only are women more vulnerable to weight gain, but also pressures to maintain and/or lose weight make them more likely to take dramatic measures to lose weight. The predominance of eating disorders among women and the greater numbers of women than men taking diet pills is just one indicator of the female obsession with being thin and beautiful. However, males are also victims. As the male image becomes more associated with the bodybuilder shape and size and as men become more preoccupied with their own physical form, eating disorders,

How Active Are Canadians?

Canada's Health Promotion Survey in 1990 asked a sample of Canadians about their "leisure-time physical activity," or exercise, defined as "vigorous activities such as aerobics, jogging, racquet sports, team sports, dance classes, or brisk walking." They were asked about the frequency and duration of such activity. Those who reported activity of at least 15 minutes at least three times per week were considered "high" exercisers. The survey showed the following results:

- Just under half (48 percent) of Canadian adults are classified as high on the index of leisure-time physical activity. This is a slight decline from 1985.

- Women are as active as, or more active than, men between the ages of 25 and 64. However, men in the youngest and oldest age groups are more likely than women to be active.

- Daily physical activity decreases with age to middle adulthood and then increases after age 44 for both men and women. Canadians most likely to engage in daily exercise in their leisure time are men aged 65 and over.

- Active use of leisure time becomes more common as education, income, and occupational status increase. This is true for both men and women, across all age groups.

- For most working people, physical activity on the job does not make up for sedentary leisure time. Workers whose jobs are mostly sedentary are less likely than average to be high exercisers and more likely than average to be moderate or low exercisers, whereas those in more active jobs are more likely than average to be high exercisers.

- Canadians who reported increasing their exercise level in the year prior to the survey did so mainly because of increased knowledge of the risks of remaining sedentary. Commercial products and services played a very minor role in these changes. Most of these changes appear to have been from moderate to high levels of exercise rather than from sedentary to moderate levels.

- Two-thirds of the population express the belief that more exercise will benefit their future health. However, three-quarters of the sedentary population expressed no intention to exercise more in the year following the survey.

- For men and women of all ages, being more active is associated with better self-rated health status and lower stress levels. Being more sedentary is related to worse self-rated health status and higher stress levels.

Source: Thomas Stephens and Dawn Fowler, eds., *Canada's Health Promotion Survey, Technical Report*, Minister of Supply and Services Canada, 1993, Cat. No. H39-263/2-1990E.

---

exercise addictions, and other maladaptive responses among men are on the increase.

Managing Your Weight

At some point in our lives, almost all of us will decide to go on a diet. Whether dieting for vanity or for your health, it's important to begin by finding a program of exercise and healthy eating behaviours that will work for you now and in the long term. You are undoubtedly familiar with the saga of Oprah Winfrey's weight loss: Starting at 86 kilograms, she quickly lost 30 kilograms on a liquid diet. But failure to continue the maintenance program led to a weight gain of 38 kilograms. Are you ready to go on a weight-loss program? Take the Rate Yourself self-test and find out.

What Is a Calorie?

A *calorie* is a unit of measure that indicates the amount of energy we obtain from a particular food. A kilogram of body fat contains approximately 7500 calories. So each time you consume 7500 calories more than your body needs to maintain weight, you gain a kilogram (or, roughly, two pounds). Conversely, each time your body expends an extra 7500 calories, you lose a kilogram. So if you add a can of Coca-Cola (140 calories) to your diet and make no other changes in diet or activity, you would gain a kilogram in 54 days (7500 calories ÷ 140 calories/day = 53.6 days). Conversely, if you walked for half an hour each day at a pace of 9 minutes per kilometre (172 calories burned), you would lose a kilogram in 44 days (7500 calories ÷ 172 calories/day = 43.6 days).

The two ways to lose weight, then, are to lower caloric intake (through improved eating habits) and to increase exercise (expending more calories). First, determine your daily caloric intake. Then you can identify your daily intake and expenditure of calories until you reach a balance (to maintain weight), a decrease (for weight loss), or an increase (for weight gain). Table 8.3 lists the caloric output of varied activities.

Don't forget, it took time to gain weight; it will take time to lose it. As the opening of the chapter pointed out, don't plan on losing more than 500 grams a week if you want to be able to keep it off.

TABLE 8.3 ▪ Calories Expended in Various Activities

Activity	Calories per Hour*	Average Calories Used	Activity	Calories per Hour*	Average Calories Used
Sleeping	65	520 (for 8 h)	Running in place or		
Watching TV	80	80 (for 1 h)	skipping rope (50–60		
Driving a car	100	50 (for 1/2 h)	steps/min)	510	255 (for 1/2 h)
Dishwashing by hand	135	67 (for 1/2 h)	Downhill skiing	595	1190 (for 2 h
Bowling	190	190 (for 1 h)			on slope)
Washing and polishing			Swimming, 5.5 min/		
car	230	230 (for 1 h)	200 m	600	300 (for 1/2 h)
Dancing (waltz, rock,		105 (for 5	Hill climbing	600	300 (for 1/2 h)
fox-trot)	250	dances; 25 min)	Touch football	600	300 (for 1/2 h
Walking, 15 min/km	255	127 (for 1/2 h)			actual play)
Baseball (not pitching			Soccer	600	600 (for 1 h)
or catching)	280	560 (for 2 h)	Snow-shovelling, light	610	306 (for 1/2 h)
Weight training	300	150 (for 1/2 h)	Jogging, 7 min/km	655	327 (for 1/2 h)
Swimming,			Cross-country skiing,		
11 min/200 m	300	150 (for 1/2 h)	7.5 min/km	700	2800 (for 4 h)
Walking, 9 min/km	345	172 (for 1/2 h)	Basketball, full court	750	750 (for 1 h)
Volleyball, badminton	350	350 (for 1 h)	Squash, racquetball	775	775 (for 1 h)
Gardening	390	780 (for 2 h)	Martial arts (judo,		
Calisthenics	415	207 (for 1/2 h)	karate)	790	395 (for 1/2 h)
Bicycling, 3.5 min/km	415	207 (for 1/2 h)	Running, 4.5 min/km	800	400 (for 1/2 h)
Tennis	425	425 (for 1 h)	Ice hockey, lacrosse	900	900 (for 1 h)
Aerobic dancing (med.)	445	222 (for 1/2 h)			

*The bigger and more vigorous you are, the more calories your body uses for a given activity. The calories listed here are for the average, 72-kilogram adult. You will lose 1 kilogram for every 7500 calories of exercise, as long as you eat the same amount of food.

Source: Adapted by permission from C. Kuntzleman, *Diet Free!* (Spring Arbor, MI: Arbor Press, 1981).

Exercise

Approximately 90 percent of the daily calorie expenditures of most people occurs as a result of the **resting metabolic rate (RMR)**. The RMR is slightly higher than the BMR; it includes the BMR plus any additional energy expended through daily sedentary activities, such as food digestion, sitting, studying, or standing. The **exercise metabolic rate (EMR)** accounts for the remaining 10 percent of all daily calorie expenditures; it refers to the energy expenditure that occurs during physical exercise. For most of us, these calories come from light daily activities, such as walking, climbing stairs, and mowing the lawn. If we increase the level and intensity of our physical activity to moderate or heavy, however, our EMR may be 10 to 20 times greater than typical resting metabolic rates and can contribute substantially to weight loss.

Increasing BMR, RMR, or EMR levels will help burn calories. An increase in the intensity, frequency, and duration of your daily exercise levels may have significant impact on your total calorie expenditure.

Physical activity makes a greater contribution to BMR when large muscle groups are used. The energy spent on physical activity is the energy used to move the body's muscles—the muscles of the arms, back, abdomen, legs, and so on—and the extra energy used to speed up heartbeat and respiration rate. The number of calories spent depends on three factors:

1. the amount of muscle mass moved

2. the amount of weight being moved

3. the amount of time the activity takes

> **Resting metabolic rate (RMR):** The energy expenditure of the body under BMR conditions plus other daily sedentary activities.
>
> **Exercise metabolic rate (EMR):** The energy expenditure that occurs during exercise.

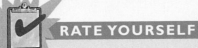

The Diet Readiness Test

To see how well your attitudes equip you for a weight-loss program, answer the questions that follow. For each question, circle the answer that best describes your attitude. As you complete each of the six sections, tally your score and analyze it according to the scoring guide.

I. Goals, Attitudes, and Readiness

1. Compared to previous attempts, how motivated are you to lose weight this time?

1	2	3	4	5
Not at all motivated	Slightly motivated	Somewhat motivated	Quite motivated	Extremely motivated

2. How certain are you that you will stay committed to a weight-loss program for the time it will take to reach your goal?

1	2	3	4	5
Not at all certain	Slightly certain	Somewhat certain	Quite certain	Extremely certain

3. Considering all outside factors at this time in your life—stress at work, family obligations, etc.—to what extent can you tolerate the effort required to stick to a diet?

1	2	3	4	5
Cannot tolerate	Can tolerate somewhat	Uncertain	Can tolerate well	Can tolerate easily

4. Think honestly about how much weight you hope to lose and how quickly you hope to lose it. Figuring a weight loss of 1 to 2 pounds per week, how realistic is your expectation?

1	2	3	4	5
Very unrealistic	Somewhat unrealistic	Moderately unrealistic	Somewhat realistic	Very realistic

5. While dieting, do you fantasize about eating a lot of your favourite foods?

1	2	3	4	5
Always	Frequently	Occasionally	Rarely	Never

6. While dieting, do you feel deprived, angry, and/or upset?

1	2	3	4	5
Always	Frequently	Occasionally	Rarely	Never

If you scored:

   6 to 16: This may not be a good time for you to start a diet. Inadequate motivation and commitment and unrealistic goals could block your progress. Think about what contributes to your unreadiness and consider changing these factors before undertaking a diet.

   17 to 23: You may be close to being ready to begin a program but should think about ways to boost your readiness.

   24 to 30: The path is clear: You can decide *how* to lose weight in a safe, effective way.

II. Hunger and Eating Cues

7. When food comes up in conversation or in something you read, do you want to eat, even if you are not hungry?

1	2	3	4	5
Never	Rarely	Occasionally	Frequently	Always

8. How often do you eat because of *physical hunger*?

1	2	3	4	5
Never	Rarely	Occasionally	Frequently	Always

(continued)

9. Do you have trouble controlling your eating when your favourite foods are around the house?

1	2	3	4	5
Never	Rarely	Occasionally	Frequently	Always

If you scored:

3 to 6: You might occasionally eat more than you should, but it does not appear to be due to high responsiveness to environmental cues. Controlling the attitudes that make you eat may be especially helpful.

7 to 9: You may have a moderate tendency to eat just because food is available. Dieting may be easier for you if you try to resist external cues and eat only when you are physically hungry.

10 to 15: Some or much of your eating may be in response to thinking about food or exposing yourself to temptations to eat. Think of ways to minimize your exposure to temptations so you eat only in response to physical hunger.

III. Control over Eating

If the following situations occurred while you were on a diet, would you be likely to eat *more* or *less* immediately afterward and for the rest of the day?

10. Although you planned on skipping lunch, a friend talks you into going out for a midday meal.

1	2	3	4	5
Would eat much less	Would eat somewhat less	Would make no difference	Would eat somewhat more	Would eat much more

11. You "break" your diet by eating a fattening, "forbidden" food.

1	2	3	4	5
Would eat much less	Would eat somewhat less	Would make no difference	Would eat somewhat more	Would eat much more

12. You have been following your diet faithfully and decide to test yourself by eating something you consider a treat.

1	2	3	4	5
Would eat much less	Would eat somewhat less	Would make no difference	Would eat somewhat more	Would eat much more

If you scored:

3 to 7: You recover rapidly from mistakes. However, if you frequently alternate between eating out of control and dieting very strictly, you may have a serious eating problem and should get professional help.

8 to 11: You do not seem to let unplanned eating disrupt your program. This is a flexible, balanced approach.

9 to 15: You may be prone to overeat after an event breaks your control or throws you off the track. Your *reaction* to these problem-causing events can be improved.

IV. Binge Eating and Purging

13. Aside from holiday feasts, have you ever eaten a large amount of food rapidly and felt afterward that this eating incident was excessive and out of control?

2	0
Yes	No

14. If yes to question 13, how often have you engaged in this behaviour during the last year?

1	2	3	4	5	6
Less than once a month	About once a month	A few times a month	About once a week	About three times a week	Daily

(continued)

15. Have you purged (used laxatives or diuretics, or induced vomiting) to control your weight?

5	0
Yes	No

16. If you answered yes to question 15, how often have you engaged in this behaviour during the last year?

1	2	3	4	5	6
Less than once a month	About once a month	A few times a month	About once a week	About three times a week	Daily

If you scored:

0: It appears that binge eating and purging are not problems for you.

2 to 11: Pay attention to these eating patterns. Should they arise more frequently, get professional help.

12 to 19: You show signs of having a potentially serious eating problem. See a counsellor experienced in evaluating eating disorders right away.

V. Emotional Eating

17. Do you eat more than you would like to when you have negative feelings such as anxiety, depression, anger, or loneliness?

1	2	3	4	5
Never	Rarely	Occasionally	Frequently	Always

18. Do you have trouble controlling your eating when you have positive feelings—do you celebrate feeling good by eating?

1	2	3	4	5
Never	Rarely	Occasionally	Frequently	Always

19. When you have unpleasant interactions with others in your life, or after a difficult day at work, do you eat more than you'd like?

1	2	3	4	5
Never	Rarely	Occasionally	Frequently	Always

If you scored:

3 to 8: You do not appear to let your emotions affect your eating.

9 to 11: You sometimes eat in response to emotional highs and lows. Monitor this behaviour to learn when and why it occurs and be prepared to find alternative activities.

12 to 15: Emotional ups and downs can stimulate your eating. Try to deal with the feelings that trigger the eating and find other ways to express them.

VI. Exercise Patterns and Attitudes

20. How often do you exercise?

1	2	3	4	5
Never	Rarely	Occasionally	Somewhat frequently	Frequently

21. How confident are you that you can exercise regularly?

1	2	3	4	5
Not at all confident	Slightly confident	Somewhat confident	Highly confident	Completely confident

22. When you think about exercise, do you develop a positive or negative picture in your mind?

1	2	3	4	5
Completely negative	Somewhat negative	Neutral	Somewhat positive	Completely positive

(continued)

23. How certain are you that you can work regular exercise into your daily schedule?

1	2	3	4	5
Not at all certain	Slightly certain	Somewhat certain	Quite certain	Extremely certain

If you scored:

4 to 10: You're probably not exercising as regularly as you should. Determine whether attitude about exercise or your lifestyle is blocking your way, then change what you must and put on those walking shoes!

11 to 16: You need to feel more positive about exercise so you can do it more often. Think of ways to be more active that are fun and fit your lifestyle.

17 to 20: It looks like the path is clear for you to be active. Now think of ways to get motivated.

After scoring yourself in each section of this questionnaire you should be able to better judge your dieting strengths and weaknesses. Remember that the first step in changing eating behaviour is to understand the conditions that influence your eating habits.

Source: Reprinted from "The Diet Readiness Test," in Kelly D. Brownell, "When and How to Diet," *Psychology Today,* June 1989, 41–46. Reprinted with permission from *Psychology Today* Magazine, ©1989 (Sussex Publishers, Inc.).

An activity involving both the arms and the legs burns more calories than one involving only the legs, an activity performed by a heavy person burns more calories than one performed by a lighter person, and an activity performed for 40 minutes requires twice as much energy as the same activity performed for only 20 minutes. Thus, obese persons walking for 1 kilometre burn more calories than slim people walking the same distance. It may also take overweight people longer to walk the mile, which means that they are burning energy for a longer time and therefore expending more overall calories than are thin walkers.[19]

*W*HAT DO YOU THINK?

Which of the methods for weight reduction discussed above do you think offers the lowest risk and the greatest chance for success?

Dieting: Is It Healthy?

Dieting can lead to improved health. It can also lead to serious physical problems and battered self-esteem. What seems to make the difference is whether a diet is part of an overall reappraisal of a person's attitudes about food and weight and part of an action plan that integrates improved nutrition and exercise or is just seen as a quick fix.

Most experts agree that the ultimate goal of weight-loss treatment should be improved quality of life and permanent weight control.[20] Weight goals should be set to reduce health risks and address medical problems and to help people improve their ability to perform daily tasks without undue stress and strain rather than merely to achieve an "ideal weight." In addition, experts agree that weight-loss programs that promote qualitative rather than quantitative changes in food intake improve health and long-term weight control and are more easily sustained than those that force people to severely restrict intake of calories or specific foods.[21] While the experts seem to agree on these points, many weight-loss programs fail to follow these basic premises. What happens to people who get caught up in "lose weight fast and furiously" campaigns? Researchers are increasingly concerned that

- dieting to lose weight may be more harmful than helpful in promoting health and psychological well-being[22]

- because dieting only rarely produces successful weight loss, the physical and psychological stress, damage to self-esteem, and other emotional disturbances associated with it are without purpose[23]

- dieting causes repeated cycles of weight loss and regain, changes in metabolic rates, increased risk for cardiovascular problems, and other conditions that are hazardous to health[24]

- dieting contributes to the development of eating disorders such as anorexia and bulimia[25]

Most health authorities recommend that, rather than going on a diet, a person should adopt nutritional dietary changes and a program of increased activity aimed at changing metabolic rates and increasing muscle strength.

Changing Your Eating Habits

Before you can change a given behaviour, you must first determine what causes that behaviour. Why do you suddenly find yourself at the refrigerator door eating everything in sight? Why do you take that second and third helping of potatoes or dessert when you know that you should be trying to lose weight?

Many people have discovered that one of the best ways of assessing their eating behaviour is to chart exactly when they feel like eating, where they are when they decide to eat, the amount of time they spend eating, other activities they engage in during the meal (watching television or reading), whether they eat alone or with others, what and how much they eat, and how they felt before they took their first bite. If you keep a detailed daily log of the triggers for at least a week, you will discover useful clues about what in your environment or in your emotional makeup causes you to want food. Typically, these dietary "triggers" centre on problems in everyday living rather than on real hunger pangs. As you record this information, your reasons for eating will often become apparent. Many people find that they eat compulsively when stressed or when they have problems in their relationships. For other people, the exact same circumstances diminish their appetite, causing them to lose weight.

Once you recognize the factors that cause you to eat, removing the triggers or substituting other activities for them will help you develop more sensible eating patterns. Here are some examples of substitute behaviours:

1. When eating dinner, turn off all distractions, including the television and radio.

2. Replace snack breaks or coffee breaks with exercise breaks.

3. Instead of gulping your food, force yourself to chew each bite slowly.

4. Vary the time of day when you eat. Instead of eating by the clock, do not eat until you are truly hungry.

5. If you find that you generally eat all that you can cram on a plate, use smaller plates.

6. If you find that you are continually seeking your favourite foods in the cupboard, stop buying them. Or place them in a spot that is very inconvenient to reach.

*W*HAT DO YOU THINK?

Based on what you have read so far, what can you do to maintain your current weight if you are satisfied with it, lose weight if you need to, or gain weight if you are too thin?

Selecting a Nutritional Plan That's Right for You

Once you have discovered what factors tend to sabotage your weight-loss efforts, you will be well on your way to successful weight control. To be successful, however, you must plan for success. By setting goals that are too far in the future or unrealistic for your current lifestyle, you will doom yourself to failure. Do not try to lose 20 kilograms in four months. Try, instead, to lose a healthy 500 grams to 1 kilogram during the first week, and stay with this slow and easy regimen. Reward yourself when you lose weight, and if you binge and go off your nutrition plan, get right back on it the next day. Remember that you did not gain 20 kilograms in eight weeks, so it is unrealistic to punish your body by trying to lose that amount of weight in such a short time.

Seek assistance from reputable sources in selecting a dietary plan that is easy to follow and includes adequate amounts of the basic nutrients. Registered nutritionists, some physicians (not all physicians have strong backgrounds in nutrition), health educators and exercise physiologists with nutritional backgrounds, and other health professionals can provide reliable information. Avoid quick weight-loss programs that promise miracle results. The majority are expensive, and most people regain the weight soon after completing the program. Ask questions about the credentials of the adviser in any weight-loss program, assess the nutrient value of the prescribed diet, verify that dietary guidelines are consistent with information from reliable dietary research, and analyze the suitability of the diet to your tastes, budget, and lifestyle to avoid putting yourself in a risky, expensive, or unhealthy dietary situation. Any diet that requires radical behaviour changes is doomed to failure. Nutritional plans that do not ask you to sacrifice everything you enjoy and that allow you to make choices are generally the most successful.

Ultimately, the decision to practise responsible weight management is yours. To be successful, you must choose a combination of exercise and eating that fits your needs and lifestyle. Find a workable plan, stick to it, and you will succeed.

General Tips for Managing Your Weight

When Eating at Home

- Eat only in the kitchen or dining room. Keep food out of your living room, bedroom, and study.

- Eat smaller meals four to five times a day rather than gorging yourself at dinner.

- Always leave some food on your plate.

- Use a smaller plate and fill it with low-calorie foods such as salad without dressing and pasta with a low-fat sauce.

- Take more time to eat; at least 20 minutes per meal is recommended. Chew each bit of food carefully, setting your fork down between bites and enjoying the taste of the food.

- Drink two to three glasses of water before a meal.

- Brush your teeth immediately after eating to avoid the temptation to take a second helping.

- Don't buy high-calorie and high-fat foods, even for guests. The temptation to eat them yourself will usually prove irresistible.

- If you must have desserts, make yourself go out for them.

- Get in tune with your true feelings of hunger. Eat only when you are really hungry, not by the clock.

- Don't skip meals or allow yourself to get too hungry before eating.

- Don't eat within three hours of going to bed.

- Put serving dishes on the counter or stove while you are eating. Leaving them on the table will only tempt you to take an extra bite.

When Eating Out

- Don't be afraid to ask for it "your way." Request that the cheese be left off, the sauce cut in half, etc.

- Ask for salad dressings, gravies, and sauces on the side. Then use only the smallest amount to flavour the food.

- Ask that entrées be broiled, steamed, baked, grilled, poached, or roasted, with only a small amount of fat used for the cooking process.

- When ordering omelets, ask for a one- or two-egg-yolk version containing only the whites of the other eggs. Avoid meat and cheese fillings in favour of low-fat vegetable fillings.

- Cut down on portion size. Order à la carte if possible, with a salad or fresh vegetable on the side. Even a baked potato is fine if you waive the butter and sour cream.

- Avoid the all-you-can-eat establishments. Even an all-you-can-eat salad bar is dangerous because of toppings loaded with fat and calories.

- Drink at least one glass of water before starting your meal. Try to relax while eating and make your mealtime last. Talk more, put your fork down more frequently, chew more, and generally slow down.

- Order fresh fruits in place of heavy desserts. If you have to have dessert, limit your portion size and only allow yourself to have it one or two times per week.

- Frequent restaurants that offer low-fat, high-complex-carbohydrate meals. All of us make better choices when there are more good options to choose from.

"Miracle" Diets

Fasting, starvation diets, and other forms of **very-low-calorie diets** (VLCDs) have been shown to cause significant health risks. Typically, when you deprive your body of food for prolonged periods, your body makes adjustments to save you from inevitable organ shutdown. It begins to deplete its energy reserves to obtain necessary fuels. One of the first reserves the body turns to to maintain its supply of glucose is lean, protein tissue. As this occurs, you lose weight rapidly, because protein contains only half as many calories per pound as fat. At the same time, significant water stores are lost. Over time, the body begins to run out of liver tissue, heart muscle, blood, and so on, as these readily available substances are burned to supply energy. Only after the readily available proteins from these sources are depleted will your body begin to burn fat reserves. In this process, known as **ketosis**, the body adapts to prolonged fasting or carbohydrate deprivation by converting body fat to ketones, which can be used as fuel for some brain cells. Within about ten days after the typical adult begins a complete fast, the body has used many of its energy stores and death may occur.

In very-low-calorie diets, powdered formulas are usually given to patients under medical supervision. These formulas have daily values of from 400 to 700 calories plus vitamin and mineral supplements. Although these diets may be beneficial for people who have failed at all conventional weight-loss methods and who face severe threats to their health that are complicated by their obesity, they should never be undertaken without strict medical supervision. Problems associated with fasting, VLCDs, and other forms of severe calorie deprivation include blood sugar imbalances, cold intolerance, constipation, decreased

BMR, dehydration, diarrhea, emotional problems, fatigue, headaches, heart irregularity, ketosis, kidney infections and failure, loss of lean body tissue, weakness, and weight gain due to the yo-yo effect and other variables.

Olestra, a fat substitute now being tested, has not yet been approved for sale in Canada. It has been linked to diarrhea and raised concerns about serious dehydration.[26]

Trying to Gain Weight

Although trying to lose weight poses a major challenge for many of us, there is a smaller group of people who, for a variety of metabolic, hereditary, psychological, and other reasons, can't seem to gain weight no matter how hard they try. If you are one of these individuals, determining the reasons for your difficulty in gaining weight is a must. Once you know what is causing you to have a daily caloric deficit, there are several things that you can do to help yourself gain extra weight:

- *Control your exercise.* Cut back if you are doing too much, slow down, and keep a careful record of calories burned.

- *Eat more.* Obviously, you are not taking in enough calories to support whatever is happening in your body. Eat more frequently, spend more time eating, eat the high-calorie foods first if you tend to fill up fast, and always start with the main course. Take time to shop, to cook, to eat slowly. Put extra spreads such as peanut butter, cream cheese, or cheese on your foods. Make your sandwiches with extra-thick slices of bread and add more filling. Take seconds whenever possible and eat high-calorie snacks during the day.

- *Try to relax.* Many people who are underweight also suffer from anxiety and the "hurry syndrome." Slow down and try to control stress.

*E*ATING DISORDERS

Obesity itself is neither a psychiatric disorder nor an eating disorder. An **eating disorder** consists of severe disturbances in eating behaviour, unhealthy efforts to control body weight, and abnormal attitudes about one's body and shape. The three main eating disorders are anorexia nervosa, bulimia nervosa, and binge eating disorder. The eating disorders are mostly associated with females.

Those with eating disorders generally suffer from low self-esteem. However, contrary to popular stereotypes, eating disorders are not restricted to middle-class white females with overprotective or over-perfectionist parents. Eating disorders span social classes and many ethnic groups.

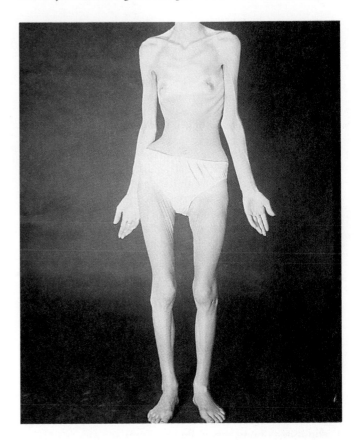

The self-starvation associated with eating disorders like anorexia nervosa can damage bones, muscles, and organs and create a host of other serious and, in some cases, life-threatening medical problems.

Eating disorders have been reported to occur with roughly similar frequencies in most industrialized countries, including Canada, the United States, Europe, Australia, Japan, New Zealand, and South Africa. Emigrants from cultures in which the disorders are rare to cultures in which the disorders are more prevalent may develop anorexia nervosa as they assimilate thin-body ideals.

Very-low-calorie diets (VLCDs): Diets with caloric value of 400 to 700 calories.

Ketosis: A condition in which the body adapts to prolonged fasting or carbohydrate deprivation by converting body fat to ketones, which can be used as fuel for some brain activity.

Eating disorder: Disorder consisting of severe disturbances in eating behaviour, unhealthy efforts to control body weight, and abnormal attitudes about one's body and shape.

Gender and Eating Disorders

Eating disorders occur predominantly in women. Anorexia nervosa and bulimia nervosa are rare among men. What explains this striking gender difference?

At the sociocultural level, it is clear that physical attractiveness is more important for women than for men. Numerous studies have demonstrated this societal double standard. The cultural pressure to be thin influences the developmental psychology of women.

One researcher argues that two aspects of our contemporary female sex-role stereotype have particular relevance to women's risk for eating disorders. First, beauty is a central aspect of "femininity"; girls learn early on that being "pretty" is what draws attention and praise from others, and girls in books and on television focus on their appearance while boys play and "do." As early as in fourth grade, body build and self-esteem are correlated for girls but not for boys.

A second aspect is women's interpersonal orientation. Theorists about the psychology of women argue that self-worth is closely tied to the establishment and maintenance of close relationships. Thus, women's self-concept is interpersonally constructed: girls' self-descriptions at age seven have been found to be more based on the perceptions of others than are boys'. Consequently, women are said to derive self-worth from other's opinions and approval of them, and in our culture, social approval is related to physical attractiveness. Research has consistently shown a significant correlation between self-esteem and feelings about one's body, especially in women, for whom it is significantly related to how they are evaluated by others. Even lesbians, who generally take a more critical stance than other women towards sociocultural norms regarding women and female sex-role stereotypes, do not seem to differ much from heterosexual women in their attitudes about weight. In one study, self-esteem was strongly related to feelings about one's body, and the prevalence of bulimia nervosa among lesbians was similar to that among heterosexual women.

The ideal standard of physical attractiveness has become thinner over the past few decades. This has made it harder for women to meet the standard, so they resort to such extreme methods as rigid dieting rules and purging. Some men also rely on these extreme measures to achieve a leaner body; examples include jockeys and wrestlers. Both jockeys and wrestlers report some of the features of eating disorders during their competitive season. But these features disappear when they are not competing. Why do dieting and purging affect these men only temporarily but trap so many women in a life-threatening downward spiral?

There is a crucial difference between these male athletes and women. The men wish to lose weight to improve their athletic performance. Their concern with body weight is secondary to their goal of performing well. For women, dieting to achieve an ideal weight has more profound psychological meaning. It is related to their self-identity and self-evaluation. Biological factors may also help to explain the gender gap. Women not only diet more than men do, but may also suffer more serious effects of dieting than do men. Studies of dieting by normal, healthy male and female university students show a differential effect on brain serotonin function. The men were unaffected. But the women showed reduced serotonin activity.

Source: Adapted from G. Terrence Wilson, Peter Nathan, K. Daniel O'Leary, and Lee Anna Clark, *Abnormal Psychology.* © 1996 by Allyn & Bacon. Reprinted by permission.

The disorders usually begin during early adolescence, although rare cases occur even after the age of 40. Over 90 percent of cases occur in women. To learn more about why females have higher rates of eating disorders, see the Global Perspectives box.

Anorexia Nervosa

Anorexia nervosa is characterized by self-starvation motivated by an intense fear of gaining weight and a severe disturbance in the perception of one's body. When anorexia develops in childhood or early adolescence, the symptom may be the failure to gain weight associated with normal growth rather than the loss of weight. About 0.5 to 1 percent of females in late adolescence or early adulthood meet the criteria for full diagnosis of anorexia nervosa.

Those diagnosed with anorexia weigh less than 85 percent of normal weight. Their unusual weight is accomplished primarily through reduction in total food intake. Usually, they begin by restricting high-calorie foods, and eventually exclude almost all foods from their diet. In addition, they lose weight through *purging*—self-induced vomiting or the misuse of laxatives or diuretics—and through exercise.

Individuals with this disorder have an intense fear of gaining weight or becoming fat. This intense fear is usually not alleviated by weight loss. In fact, concern about weight gain often increases as actual weight continues to decrease.

Helping Someone with an Eating Disorder

When a family member or a friend has an eating disorder, that person needs serious medical help. You can take a proactive role in getting help. Here are some suggestions:

- **Speak up.** Don't encourage denial of the problem by ignoring it.

- **Base what you say on your own observations and keep the tone affectionate, not accusing:** "I've noticed you're skipping a lot of meals, and I'm worried about you." Or, "I can smell that you have been vomiting, and I'm concerned about your health." Make yourself available to the individual to discuss emotional concerns and anxieties.

- **Inform yourself about the disorder, and share your information with the other person.** For many women, recovery has started with a book or a pamphlet provided by a friend or relative. Consult an eating disorders clinic in your area. Clinics in teaching hospitals are the most likely to offer counselling and programs free or at a low cost.

- **Attend a support group for help with your own pain resulting from the situation and for advice on how to interact with your family member or friend.**

- **If the person with the disorder agrees to seek help, be supportive in constructive ways.** Offer to accompany him or her to appointments; express interest and concern without trying to take over.

- **If a relative has an eating disorder, consider family therapy to explore some of the emotional roots of the disorder.** Jean Rubel, Ph.D., founder of Anorexia Nervosa and Related Eating Disorders, says, "Ignore tears, tantrums, and promises." If the relative is younger than 18, get him or her to a doctor and tell him or her what you suspect; this is no time for guessing games. Get educational counselling and therapy. Rubel also believes that the whole family should be involved in the therapy to deal with the root issues: "You can't send her off to be fixed like a car to a garage."

- **Do not nag or bully.** You can't recover for someone else, and you may create more problems by monitoring someone else's eating habits.

- **Do not tell a recovering bulimic or anorexic that he or she is looking better.** No matter how carefully you phrase it, he or she will hear, "You got fat."

Source: Adapted with permission from Suanne Kelman, "The Way Back," *Shape*, March 1995, 113.

People with this illness have a distorted view of the experience and significance of body weight and shape. Some feel globally overweight; others feel that parts (particularly the abdomen, buttocks, and thighs) are "too fat." They may constantly weigh themselves, measure themselves, and look at themselves in the mirror to check for fat. This is because their self-esteem is highly dependent on their body shape and weight. Weight loss is viewed as an impressive achievement and a sign of extraordinary self-discipline; weight gain is perceived as unacceptable failure of self-control.[27]

The medical problems associated with anorexia are appalling. Starvation can damage the bones, the muscles, and the organs as well as the immune, nervous, and digestive systems. The acid in vomit may cause tooth enamel to dissolve. People with anorexia often either lose hair or develop excessive, fine facial and body hair. Worse, between 5 and 18 percent of victims die as a result of suicide or of the medical complications of this disorder.[28]

Bulimia Nervosa

The essential features of **bulimia nervosa** are binge eating followed by inappropriate compensating measures taken to prevent weight gain, such as induced vomiting. Binge eating normally occurs in secrecy and is accompanied by a lack of control. It is difficult for a person with bulimia to stop the binge once it has started. About 1 to 3 percent of adolescent and young adult females are bulimic; the rate among men is about 10 percent that among females.

As with anorexic individuals, those with bulimia place an excessive emphasis on body shape and weight in their self-evaluation, and these factors are critical in determining their self-esteem. Unlike the anorexic individual's body weight, the bulimic's body weight is typically within the normal weight range (some may be underweight or overweight). In addition, treatment of bulimia nervosa is effective in the majority of cases, with good prospects for a full and lasting recovery.[29]

Anorexia nervosa: Eating disorder characterized by excessive preoccupation with food, self-starvation, and/or extreme exercising to achieve weight losses.

Bulimia nervosa: Eating disorder characterized by binge eating followed by inappropriate compensating measures taken to prevent weight gain.

Managing Your Weight

Managing your weight is not an easy task. To ensure success, you must make a real change in the way you eat and consider it a lifelong commitment rather than a diet. Analyzing where you are right now and then taking the steps outlined below will help you lose excess weight.

Making Decisions for You

The first step in managing your weight is an honest self-assessment of where you are. You don't need sophisticated fat-measurement techniques. What you need is a scale. Your university probably has a gym that has body-content assessment equipment available. Next you need to set a realistic goal. Ask yourself, why do I want to meet this goal? What will I do when I reach this goal? Then set out a plan to reach your goal. Keep in mind what you enjoy doing. If you like taking walks, you might make walking part of your weight-loss program. If you absolutely love chocolate chip cookies, you might consider limiting yourself to two cookies per day.

Checklist for Change: Making Personal Choices

✓ *Design your plan for your needs.* Your plan must fit your personality, your priorities, and your work and recreation schedules. It should allow for sufficient rest and relaxation.

✓ *Plan for nutrient-dense foods.* Attempt to get the most from the foods you eat by selecting foods with high nutritional value.

✓ *Balance food intake throughout the day.* Although the evidence is controversial, research indicates that the body may burn calories more efficiently in small amounts than in excessive quantities.

✓ *Plan for plateaus.* If you prepare yourself psychologically for plateaus you will be less likely to become discouraged. Exercise is probably the critical factor in getting past a plateau.

✓ *Chart your progress.* For many people, the daily "weigh-in" is a critical factor in maintaining their program. However, particularly for those who have reached a weight plateau, it may be necessary to think in terms of weekly weigh-ins to avoid frustration.

✓ *Chart your setbacks.* Rather than thinking in terms of failure and punishment, think in terms of temporary setbacks and how to accommodate them. By carefully recording your emotional states when eating, eating habits, environmental cues, and feelings, you may determine why you needed that ice cream cone or why you chose a pizza instead of a salad. Successful weight-loss plans may have to accommodate hormonal fluctuations as an influence on dietary habits.

✓ *Become aware of your feelings of hunger and fullness.* For many of us, eating is time-dependent, and we stop eating only when the food is gone (the "clean your plate" syndrome). Long years of "eating when it is time" instead of eating when it is necessary cost us the ability to tell when we really are hungry and when we really are full. By training yourself to become more aware of the eating process, by learning to recognize true hunger pangs and the first signals that you have eaten enough, you will be able to change your eating patterns.

✓ *Accept yourself.* For many people, this is the most important aspect of successful weight management. Although our culture can certainly oppress fat people, many overweight people are their own worst enemies. It is important to keep your weight in perspective. Unless you feel good about who you are inside, exterior changes will not help you very much.

✓ *Exercise, exercise, exercise.* Different people benefit from different types of activities. Just because your friends are into jogging or jazzercise does not mean that that type of exercise program is best for you. Select an exercise program that you consider fun, not a daily form of punishment for overeating. Variety may be the key here. Planning a program that includes friends and family may also improve your chances of success. It is important to remember that every little effort contributes toward long-term results.

Checklist for Change: Making Community Choices

✓ Identify volunteer organizations that provide physical fitness opportunities for teens.

✓ What opportunities for volunteering at nutrition- or weight-related programs does your campus provide?

Critical Thinking

Until university, your girlfriend Tami had taken ballet very seriously, practising several hours a day. Now that the time pressures of university, a part-time job, and your relationship are starting to get to her, Tami rarely has time to work out on the dance floor. You notice that she has consequently been more and more concerned about her weight. She rarely eats on your dates, but she says that that's because she wants the two of you to save money for a nice trip during spring break. When you find a laxative hidden under her pillow, she says, "Doesn't everyone get constipated now and then?" Then a mutual female friend tells you that she's heard Tami in the bathroom throwing up on several occasions after meals; Tami denies it.

Using the DECIDE model in Chapter 1, decide how you can approach Tami with your concern that she has an eating disorder. What help is available in your local area? Should you involve Tami's family? If Tami denies she has an eating disorder, what can you do?

Binge Eating Disorder

People afflicted with **binge eating disorder (BED)** engage in recurrent binge eating but, unlike bulimics, do not take excessive measures to lose the weight gained during binges. Neither do BED patients report abnormal attitudes about dieting or body weight and shape. Binge eating disorder occurs predominantly in obese patients. This disorder is often referred to in the popular literature as "compulsive overeating." Studies show that obese patients with BED consume significantly more food than do obese people who don't binge. Take note that, as of the date of this writing, binge eating disorder is only under consideration as a psychiatric diagnosis.[30]

Treating Eating Disorders

The most effective treatments for eating disorders combine different approaches into a package that involves the patient and his or her family and friends. Eating disorder patients usually come to the attention of medical personnel because someone else shows concern. To learn about how you could help someone you suspect has a disorder see the Building Communication Skills box.

Treatment options for eating disorders vary. Due to the medical complications brought on by dangerous weight loss, anorexia often requires hospitalization, and the first goal of treatment is to restore patients to near-normal body weight. For all eating disorders, individual psychotherapy provides an opportunity for the patient to develop self-confidence, self-esteem, and feelings of power and control. In therapy, the person learns new, more effective ways to handle stress so that it is no longer necessary to turn to or away from food to deal with problems. In addition, eating disorder patients often exhibit depression and other clinical illnesses, and these problems can also be treated.

Support groups are useful for providing a social network, emotional support, and self-help techniques. Family therapy can also be useful.

Binge eating disorder (BED): Eating disorder characterized by recurrent binge eating. However, BED sufferers do not take excessive measures to lose the weight gained during binges.

---

*W*HAT DO YOU THINK?

Why do college students in particular seem to have so many problems with eating disorders? What factors place young women at risk? Why do you think there are fewer eating disorders among men? What programs or services on your campus would you recommend for a friend with an eating disorder?

Summary

- Overweight, obesity, and weight-related problems appear to be on the rise in Canada. Obesity is now defined in terms of fat content rather than in terms of weight alone. There are many different methods of assessing body fat. Body fat percentages give you a more accurate indication of how fat versus lean you really are.

- Many factors contribute to your risk for obesity. Included among these factors are genetics, developmental factors, your setpoint, endocrine influences, psychosocial factors, eating cues, lack of awareness, metabolic changes, lifestyle, and gender.

- Exercise, dieting, diet pills, and other strategies are used to maintain or lose weight. However, sensible eating behaviour and adequate exercise probably offer the best options.

- Eating disorders consist of severe disturbances in eating behaviours, unhealthy efforts to control body weight, and abnormal attitudes about body and shape. Anorexia nervosa, bulimia nervosa, and binge eating disorder are the three main eating disorders. Eating disorders occur mainly in adolescent and young adult women in industrialized countries.

Discussion Questions

1. Discuss the pressures, if any, you feel to improve your personal body image. Do these pressures come from TV shows, movies, ads, and other external sources or from concern for your personal health?

2. List the risk factors for obesity. Evaluate which seem to be most important in determining whether you will be obese in middle age.

3. Create a plan to help someone lose over the summer vacation the weight he has put on over the year. Assume that the person is male, weighs 82 kilograms, and wants to lose 7 kilograms over the next 15 weeks.

4. Differentiate among the three eating disorders. Then give reasons why females might be more prone than males to anorexia and bulimia.

Application Exercise

Reread the What Do You Think? scenario at the beginning of the chapter and answer the following questions:

1. What motivates someone like Ray to try to spiff up and look good at certain times of the year? How could someone like Ray change his behaviours so as to be more healthy nutritionally and to avoid the diet syndrome so many of us find ourselves in?

2. Why is dieting to lose weight probably not such a good idea in the long run?

Health on the Net

Health Canada: Food Program
www.hwc.ca/datahpb/datafood/english/main_e.html

Mental Health Net: Eating Disorders
www.cmhc.com/guide/eating.htm

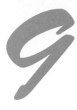

Personal Fitness

Improving Your Health Through Exercise

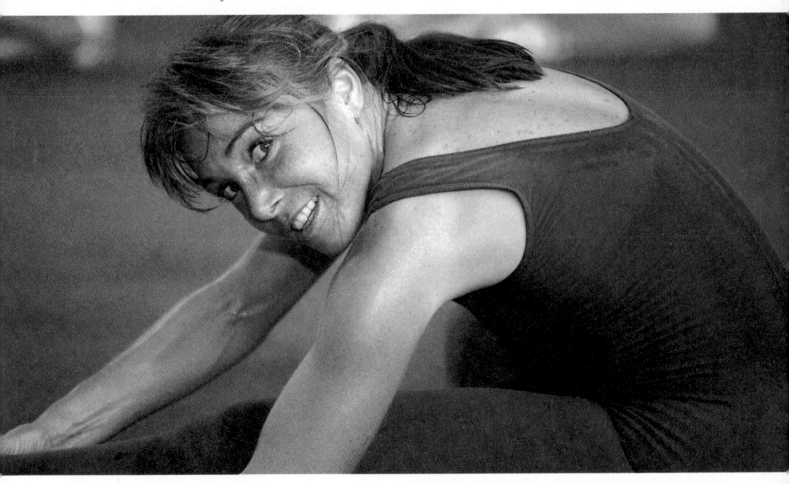

CHAPTER OBJECTIVES

◆ Describe the benefits of physical activity, including improved cardiorespiratory efficiency, skeletal mass, weight control, health and life span, mental health and stress management, and physical fitness.

◆ Describe the components of an aerobic exercise program and how to determine proper exercise frequency, intensity, and duration.

◆ Describe the different stretching exercises designed to improve flexibility.

◆ Compare the various types of resistance training programs, including the methods of providing external resistance and intended physiological benefits.

◆ Describe common fitness injuries, suggest ways to prevent injuries, and list the treatment process.

◆ Summarize the key components of a personal fitness program.

While in high school, Georgia participated in many school activities, including gymnastics, soccer, and track. Among the many lifestyle changes she encountered during her first year in college was the need for much more time spent reading and writing. Georgia had seen some of her older friends struggle to control their weight during their college years; she liked the way she looked and didn't want that to change. Despite the academic and social demands of her first semester at college, Georgia was determined to make time for fitness activities and worked out at least five times a week. Instead of gaining weight, she lost eight pounds by the end of the first semester. She studied hard and got good grades, but averaged less than six hours of sleep a night. By the end of the day, Georgia usually felt tired and stressed out.

■ Was Georgia overdoing it? What potential problems can you foresee if she continues her first-semester schedule? What changes should Georgia make in her lifestyle to reverse the effects of her first semester at college?

More than 30 years ago, Sport Canada was created because of concerns about the poor fitness levels of Canadian children. Participation in regular fitness activity gradually increased during the 1960s, 1970s, and early 1980s, but has levelled off in recent years. Research indicates that your physical activity level as a child is a good predictor of your physical activity level as an adult.[1] But if you spent your childhood or adolescence as a couch potato, don't despair. University is an excellent place to make a break with the past and develop exercise habits that can increase both the quality and the duration of your life. Especially when combined with a healthy diet, regular physical activity combats obesity and thus reduces your likelihood of coronary artery disease, high blood pressure, diabetes, and other chronic diseases.[2]

Regular physical activity improves more than 50 different physiological, metabolic, and psychological aspects of human life[3]—which is why more and more Canadians are getting serious about exercising. Unfortunately, millions more have not abandoned their sedentary lifestyles.

BENEFITS OF PHYSICAL FITNESS

Physical activity is any force exerted by skeletal muscles that results in energy usage above the level used when the body's systems are at rest.[4] Among adults, higher levels of physical activity have been associated with a lower incidence of coronary artery disease, the leading cause of death in Canada for both men and women.[5] Regular physical activity has also been linked to lower incidence of high blood pressure (hypertension), cancers of the colon and reproductive organs, bone fractures produced by os-

teoporosis, and depression.[6] A recent study reported that regular exercise (four hours a week or more) beginning in adolescence and continuing into adulthood can significantly reduce the risk of breast cancer in women 40 and younger.[7]

Many of the risk factors for coronary artery disease, hypertension, and osteoporosis first appear during childhood and adolescence.[8] In one study of middle-class children, average fat intake was 35 percent of daily consumption.[9] Fortunately, if identified during childhood, adolescence, or young adulthood, many of these risks can be reduced through exercise and modifications in diet. Many physiological and psychological benefits of regular exercise have been demonstrated.

Improved Cardiorespiratory Efficiency

A regular program of aerobic exercise improves the efficiency of your cardiovascular and respiratory systems. As a benefit of regular exercise, the heart is able to pump more blood with each stroke, thus lowering resting heart rate. Additionally, the body's capacity to distribute oxygen to working muscles is improved, while the muscles responsible for respiration are strengthened.

Reduced Risk of Heart Disease. Your heart is a muscle made up of highly specialized tissue. Because muscles become stronger and more efficient with use, regular exercise strengthens the heart, enabling it to pump more blood with each beat. This increased efficiency means that your heart requires fewer beats per minute to circulate blood throughout your body. A stronger, more efficient heart is better able to meet the ordinary and extraordinary demands of life.

Reduced risk of disease and new dimensions for living are among the benefits of physical fitness that are available to people of all ages and all capabilities.

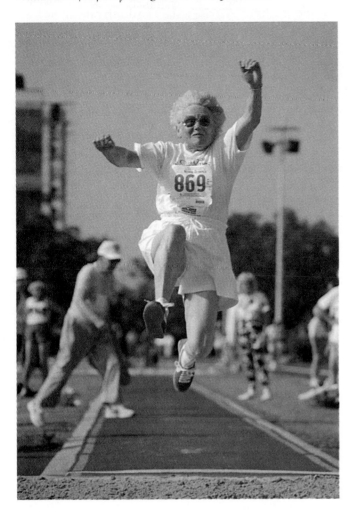

Prevention of Hypertension.   Hypertension is the medical term for abnormally high blood pressure. It is a significant risk factor for cardiovascular disease and stroke. If your resting **systolic blood pressure** is consistently 160 millimeters of mercury (mm Hg) or higher, your risk of coronary heart disease is four times greater than normal. If your resting **diastolic blood pressure** regularly exceeds 95 mm Hg, your risk of heart disease is six times greater than normal.[10] Low to moderate exercise training lowers both systolic and diastolic blood pressure by about 10 mm Hg in people with mild to moderate hypertension.[11] Regular physical activity can also reduce both systolic and diastolic blood pressure in people with normal and high blood pressures.[12]

Improved Blood Lipid and Lipoprotein Profile.   Lipids are fats that circulate in the bloodstream and are stored in various places in your body. Regular exercise is known to reduce the levels of low-density lipoproteins (LDLs—

"bad cholesterol") while increasing the number of high-density lipoproteins (HDLs—"good cholesterol") in the blood. Higher HDL levels are associated with lower risk for artery disease because they remove some of the "bad cholesterol" from artery walls and hence prevent clogging. The net effect of these two physiological responses to exercise is a diminished risk of cardiovascular disease.

Improved Skeletal Mass

Osteoarthritis is a nonfatal but incurable disease characterized by degeneration of joint cartilage and irritation of surrounding bone and soft tissues. Affecting one in ten, or 2.9 million Canadians, osteoarthritis is the most prevalent chronic joint condition in Canada. Women are afflicted more frequently than men.[13] Several recent studies have demonstrated that supervised fitness walking and weight-loss programs can improve physical capacity while reducing knee joint osteoarthritis symptoms.[14]

A common affliction of older women is **osteoporosis**, a disease characterized by low bone mass and deterioration of bone tissue, which increase fracture risk. One of the physical activities recommended most frequently to women wanting to improve their bone health is walking. While walking is an excellent activity for overall fitness, there is currently no evidence that it can significantly increase bone mass in healthy women.[15] Bone, like other human tissues, responds to the demands placed upon it, and unless the mechanical stresses placed on bone by a particular physical activity exceed the level of stress the bone has adapted to, there is no stimulus to increase bone mass.[16] Women (and men) have much to gain by remaining physically active as they age—bone mass levels have been found to be significantly higher among active than among sedentary women.[17] However, it appears that exercise's full benefit can only be achieved when proper hormone levels (estrogen in women, testosterone in men) are present. Regular exercise, when combined with a balanced diet containing adequate calcium, will help maintain skeletal mass, although this benefit is harder to achieve as we age.

Systolic blood pressure: The pressure in the arteries during a heartbeat; abnormal if consistently 160 mm Hg or above.

Diastolic blood pressure: The pressure in the arteries during the period between heartbeats; abnormal if consistently 95 mm Hg or above.

Osteoarthritis: A disease characterized by degeneration of joint cartilage and irritation of surrounding bone and soft tissue.

Osteoporosis: A disease characterized by low bone mass and deterioration of bone tissue, which increase fracture risk.

Improved Weight Control

For many people, the desire to lose weight is the main purpose for starting an exercise program. Exercise does have a direct effect upon metabolic rate, even raising it for a few hours following a vigorous workout. If you are planning to lose weight through exercise alone, without decreasing the amount of food you eat, you'll have to exercise frequently (at least three days a week) for extended time periods (at least 20 to 30 minutes at 60 percent of maximum heart rate per workout). A more effective method for losing weight combines regular endurance-type exercises with a moderate decrease (about 500 to 1000 calories per day) in food intake. Decreasing daily caloric intake beyond this range ("severe dieting") appears to decrease metabolic rate by up to 20 percent, making weight loss more difficult.

Improved Health and Life Span

Prevention of Diabetes. Diabetes is a complex disorder that affects 1.5 million Canadians; with perhaps another 750 000 undiagnosed. Of these, 90 percent have type 2 diabetes (also called non-insulin-dependent diabetes, although people with this disorder may indeed need insulin). The strongest predisposing factors for this type of diabetes are obesity, increasing age, and a family history of diabetes. Lesser risk factors include high blood pressure and high cholesterol.[18] Physicians suggest exercise combined with weight reduction and proper diet for the management of this form of diabetes. A recent large epidemiological study found that for every 2000 calories of energy expended during leisure-time activities, the incidence of diabetes was reduced by 24 percent. Perhaps the most encouraging finding was that the protective effect of excrcise was greatest among those individuals who were at the highest risk for non-insulin-dependent diabetes.[19]

Increased Longevity. Experts have long debated the relationship between exercise and longevity. For decades, most research failed to show that we could increase our life expectancy through exercise alone. Then, a landmark study conducted at the Institute for Aerobics Research in Texas found that exercise does increase longevity. More

than 13 000 white middle- to upper-middle-class men and women aged 20 to 80 were followed for eight years to discover how physical fitness relates to death rates. Participants were assigned fitness levels based upon their age, sex, and results of exercise tests. The death rate in the least physically fit group was more than three times higher than the death rate in the most fit group. How much exercise was required to produce a difference? Participants who changed from a sedentary lifestyle to one that included a brisk 30- to 60-minute walk each day experienced significant increases in their life expectancies.[20]

Improved Immunity to Disease. Will regular exercise make you more immune to disease, and if so, how does this occur? Recent research suggests that regular moderate exercise makes people less susceptible to disease, but that this potential benefit may depend upon whether they perceive exercise as pleasurable or stressful.[21] While current evidence suggests that moderate exercise improves immunity, more extreme forms of exercise may be detrimental. For example, athletes engaging in marathon-type events or very intense physical training programs have been shown to be at increased risk of upper respiratory tract infections (e.g., colds and flu).[22] In a recent study of 2300 marathon runners, those who ran more than 100 kilometres per week suffered twice as many upper respiratory tract infections as those who ran fewer than 35 kilometres per week.[23]

Just how exercise alters immunity is not well understood. We do know that brisk exercise temporarily increases the number of white blood cells (WBCs), the blood cells responsible for fighting infection. Generally speaking, the less fit the person and the more intense the exercise, the greater the increase in WBCs.[24] After brief periods of exercise (without injury), the number of WBCs typically returns to normal levels within one to two hours. After exercise bouts lasting longer than 30 minutes, WBCs may be elevated for 24 hours or more before returning to normal levels.[25] An increased number of WBCs suggests increased immunity to disease and infection.

Improved Mental Health and Stress Management

People who engage in regular physical activity may be unaware of all the beneficial changes in their physiological functions, but most notice the psychological benefits. While these psychological benefits are difficult to quantify, they are frequently mentioned as reasons for continuing to exercise. Regular vigorous exercise has been shown to "burn off" the chemical by-products released by our nervous system during normal response to stress. Elimination of these biochemical substances reduces our stress levels by accelerating the neurological system's return to a balanced state. For this reason, exercise should be an integral component of your stress management plan.

Physical fitness: A set of attributes related to the ability to perform normal physical activity.

Exercise: Physical activity at higher-than-normal levels of exertion.

Exercise training: The systematic performance of exercise at a specified frequency, intensity, and duration to achieve a desired level of physical fitness.

Exercise and Socioeconomic Status

Physical activity level increases with education and income. People with a university degree tend to be more active than others. Those who have not completed their secondary education are the least active.

When employment status is considered, students are the most likely to be active, followed by full-time and part-time workers, homemakers, and unemployed individuals. Retired people are the least active; they are half as likely to be active as students.

The largest increases in physical activity levels since 1988 occurred in people with high school and university education. Unfortunately, the gap in physical activity levels between the least and the most educated has widened since 1981 and 1988.

Higher education levels tend to accompany higher income levels. It is no surprise, then, that households with annual incomes over $60 000 also have the highest reported physical activity levels. In this income bracket, four in ten are active, as against three in ten of those earning between $20 000 and $60 000.

The results for education and employment status are influenced by age-related patterns of physical activity. For example, adults completing only primary education tend to be in the older age groups. Some of the education-related differences may therefore reflect age-related differences. Similarly, the pattern of employment status between students, workers, homemakers, and retired Canadians likely reflects age-related patterns of physical activity.

Source: Canadian Fitness and Lifestyle Research Institute, "How Active Are Canadians?" *Bulletin* No. 1, 1995, 3.

Regular exercise improves physical appearance by toning and developing muscles and, in combination with dieting, reducing body fat. Feeling good about personal appearance can provide a tremendous boost to self-esteem. At the same time, as people come to appreciate the improved strength, conditioning, and flexibility that accompany fitness, they often become less obsessed with physical appearance.[26] Through regular physical activity, they learn new skills and develop increased abilities in favourite recreational activities, which also help improve self-esteem.

WHAT DO YOU THINK?

Do you know your resting heart rate? Blood pressure? Cholesterol level? Who could provide you with this information? Based upon what you've read, what are the health benefits you'd like to achieve as the result of regular physical activity?

Improved Physical Fitness

Physical fitness can be defined as a set of attributes related to the ability to perform normal physical activity.[27] The individual fitness components are listed and described in Table 9.1. In contrast, **exercise** is defined as physical activity at higher-than-normal levels of exertion. **Exercise training** is the systematic performance of exercise at a specified frequency, intensity, and duration to achieve a desired level of physical fitness.[28]

Almost any regular exercise program will help you lose weight, but achieving some idealized form is nearly impossible for many people. Participation in a comprehensive physical fitness program, in contrast, is healthy, realistic, and respectful of your own unique physical traits. It will help you to achieve a better body—*your* optimal body, not some celebrity's.

Although physical fitness has many facets, it is most commonly measured by four interdependent components: (1) cardiorespiratory endurance, (2) flexibility, (3) muscular strength, and (4) muscular endurance.

To be considered physically fit, you generally need to attain (and then maintain) certain minimum standards for each component that have been established by exercise physiologists and other fitness experts. Some people have physical limitations that make achieving one or more of these standards impossible. That doesn't mean they can't attain physical fitness. For example, a woman who needs to use a wheelchair will be unable to run or walk a mile, as is required in some fitness tests, but may achieve physical fitness by playing wheelchair basketball. Our definition of physical fitness should be adapted to address individual differences in capabilities.

WHAT DO YOU THINK?

Which of the key aspects of physical fitness do you currently possess? Which ones would you like to improve or develop? What types of activities will you do to improve your fitness level?

Physical Activity Levels of Canadians

1995 Physical Activity Monitor

	Active (≥3 KKD[1])	Moderately Active (1.5–2.9 KKD)	Somewhat Active (0.5–1.4 KKD)	Sedentary (<0.5 KKD)
Total, Adults (18+)	37%	28%	23%	12%
Women	34	28	24	14
Men	40	28	23	9
18–24	54	23	16	—
Women	54	20	17	—
Men	54	—	—	—
25–44	37	28	25	10
Women	33	29	26	11
Men	40	27	24	8
45–54	32	30	24	13
Women	32	30	25	13
Men	33	30	24	—
65+	24	30	22	24
Women	18	29	22	31
Men	33	—	—	—
Education Level				
Less than secondary	28	28	24	20
Secondary	36	31	20	12
College	37	27	26	11
University	45	26	23	6
Household Income				
< $ 20 000	36	28	21	15
$ 20 000–29 999	31	25	32	11
$ 30 000–39 999	33	29	27	—
$ 40 000–59 999	34	26	26	13
$ 60 000–79 999	47	30	16	—
$ 80 000–99 999	44	—	—	—
≥ $100 000	44	32	—	—
Employment Status				
Full-time worker	38	29	24	9
Part-time worker	34	32	26	—
Unemployed	37	33	—	—
Homemaker	39	21	19	—
Student	53	—	—	—
Retired	29	28	21	22

[1]Kilocalories/kilogram of body weight/day; an energy expenditure of three KKD is equivalent to walking one hour every day.

—: Data unavailable because of insufficient sample size.

Source: Canadian Fitness and Lifestyle Research Institute, "How Active Are Canadians?" *Bulletin* No. 1, 1995.

Self-Assessment of Cardiovascular Fitness

Once you've been exercising regularly for several weeks, you might want to assess your cardiovascular fitness level. Find a local track, typically one-quarter mile per lap, to perform your test. You may either run/walk for 2.4 kilometres and measure how long it takes to reach that distance, or run/walk for 12 minutes and determine the distance you covered in that time. Use the chart below to estimate your cardiovascular fitness level based upon your age and sex. Note that females have lower standards for each fitness category because of their higher levels of essential fat.

Age*	2.4 Kilometre Run (min:sec)		12-Minute Run (kilometres)	
	Female	Male	Female	Male
Good				
15–30	<12:00	<10:00	>2.4	>2.7
35–50	<13:30	<11:30	>2.25	>2.4
55–70	<16:00	<14:00	>1.9	>2.1
Adequate for Most Activities				
15–30	<13:30	<11:50	>2.25	>2.4
35–50	<15:00	<13:00	>2.1	>2.25
55–70	<17:30	<15:30	>1.8	>2.1
Borderline				
15–30	<15:00	<13:00	>2.1	>2.25
35–50	<16:30	<14:30	>1.9	>2.1
55–70	<19:00	<17:00	>1.6	>1.9
Need Extra Work on Cardiovascular Fitness				
15–30	>17:00	>15:00	<1.9	<2.1
35–50	>18:30	>16:30	<1.8	<1.9
55–70	>21:00	>19:00	<1.4	<1.6

*Cardiovascular fitness declines with age.

If you are now at the Good level, your emphasis should be on maintaining this level for the rest of your life. If you are now at lower levels, you should set realistic goals for improvement.

Source: Adapted from Edward T. Howley and B. Don Franks, *Health/Fitness Instructor's Handbook* (Champaign, IL: Human Kinetics Publishers, 1986), 85. Copyright 1986 by Edward T. Howley and B. Don Franks. Reprinted by permission.

TABLE 9.1 ■ Physical Fitness Components

Agility	Speed in changing direction or in changing body positions.
Anaerobic power	Maximum rate of work performance.
Balance	Maintenance of a stable body position.
Body composition	Fatness: ratio of fat weight to total body weight.
Cardiorespiratory endurance	Ability to sustain moderate-intensity whole-body activity for extended time periods.
Flexibility	Range of motion in a joint or series of joints.
Muscular endurance	Ability to perform repeated high-intensity muscle contractions.
Muscular strength	Maximum force applied with a single muscle contraction.

Source: Reprinted by permission of Williams and Wilkins from T. Baranowski et al., "Assessment, Prevalence, and Cardiovascular Benefits of Physical Activity and Fitness in Youth," *Medicine and Science in Sports and Exercise* 24 (June 1992): supplement, S238.

IMPROVING CARDIOVASCULAR FITNESS

The number of walkers, joggers, bicyclists, step aerobics participants, and swimmers is tangible evidence of Canadians' increased awareness of the most important aspect of physical fitness: **cardiovascular fitness**, which refers to the ability of your heart, lungs, and blood vessels to function efficiently. Our very lives depend on our cardiovascular system's ability to deliver oxygenated blood and nutrients to our body tissues and to remove carbon dioxide and other metabolic waste products.

The primary category of physical activity known to improve cardiovascular fitness is **aerobic exercise**. The term *aerobic* means "with oxygen" and describes any type of exercise, typically performed at moderate levels of intensity for extended periods of time, that increases your heart rate. Aerobic activities such as walking, jogging, bicycling, and swimming are among the best exercises for improving overall health status as well as cardiovascular fitness. A person said to be in "good cardiovascular shape" has an above-average *aerobic capacity*—a term used to describe the current functional status of the cardiovascular system (i.e., heart, lungs, blood vessels). **Aerobic capacity** (commonly written $VO_{2\ max}$) is defined as the volume of oxygen consumed by the muscles during exercise.

To measure your maximal aerobic capacity, an exercise physiologist or physician will typically have you exercise on a treadmill. He or she will initially ask you to walk or run at an easy pace, and then, at set time intervals during this **graded exercise test**, will gradually increase the workload (i.e., a combination of running speed and the angle of incline of the treadmill) to the point of maximal exertion. Generally, the higher your cardiovascular fitness level, the more oxygen you can transport to exercising muscles and the longer you can maintain a high intensity of exercise prior to exhaustion. In healthy individuals, the higher the $VO_{2\ max}$ value, the higher the level of aerobic fitness. According to the Canadian Society for Exercise Physiology, physician approval for fitness testing is required for many people; check with the person conducting the test. Other, less reliable but safer methods of measuring aerobic capacity are frequently employed to estimate $VO_{2\ max}$. These submaximal tests may use stationary bicycles, walk/run tests, or walk tests to quantify the aerobic fitness levels in people of all ages. You may have performed one of these aerobic capacity tests as part of a high school or college physical education course.

You can conduct your own submaximal test of your aerobic capacity by using either the 2.4 kilometre run or the 12-minute run endurance test described in the Rate Yourself box. However, you should not use these endurance-run tests when you are just beginning an exercise program.[29] Progress slowly through a walking/jogging program at low intensities before you attempt to measure your aerobic capacity with one of these tests. It is also important for you to consult a doctor before beginning an exercise program if you have certain medical conditions, such as asthma, diabetes, heart disease, or obesity.

Aerobic Fitness Programs

Researchers tell us that a physically active lifestyle is the key to improved cardiovascular health, but what level of activity is required to improve aerobic fitness? There are numerous variables in any particular aerobic activity, but comfortable aerobic exercise that works your heart at a moderate intensity (approximately 60 to 70 percent of your maximum heart rate, or about 115 to 145 beats per minute) for prolonged periods of time (20 to 30 minutes of continuous activity) will improve your fitness level.

The most beneficial aerobic exercises are total body activities involving all the large muscle groups of your body. If you have been sedentary for quite a while, simply initiating a physical activity program may be the hardest task you'll face. The key is to begin your exercise program at a very low intensity, progress slowly . . . and stay with it! For example, if you choose an aerobic fitness program that involves jogging, you'll need several weeks of workouts combining jogging and walking before you will reach a fitness level that enables you to jog continuously for 15 to 20 minutes.

You will need to adjust the frequency, intensity, and duration of your aerobic activity program to accommodate your level of cardiovascular fitness. As you progress,

---

Cardiovascular fitness: The ability of the heart, lungs, and blood vessels to function efficiently.

Aerobic exercise: Any type of exercise, typically performed at moderate levels of intensity for extended periods of time (20 to 30 minutes or longer), that increases heart rate.

Aerobic capacity: The current functional status of a person's cardiovascular system; measured as $VO_{2\ max}$.

Graded exercise test: A test of aerobic capacity administered by a physician, exercise physiologist, or other trained person; two common forms are the treadmill running test and the stationary bike test.

Target heart rate: Calculated as a percentage of maximum heart rate (220 minus age); heart rate (pulse) is taken during aerobic exercise to check if exercise intensity is at the desired level (e.g., 70 percent of maximum heart rate).

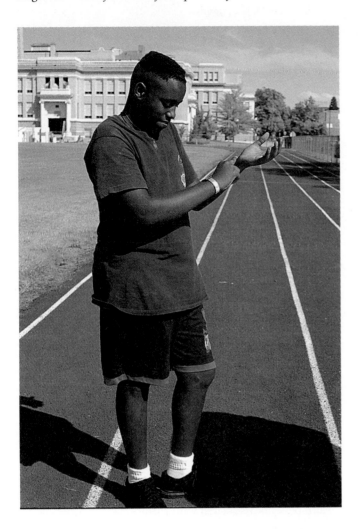

An aerobic fitness program starts with setting a target heart rate and then adjusting the frequency, intensity, and duration of exercise in order to maintain that target heart rate for a beneficial period of time.

add to your exercise load by increasing exercise duration or intensity, but do not increase both at the same time.

Determining Exercise Frequency. If you are a newcomer to regular physical activity, the frequency of your aerobic exercise bouts should be at least three times per week. If you exercise less frequently, you will achieve fewer health benefits. The proper frequency of exercise is affected by the intensity and duration of the individual exercise periods. Three to five days per week is a good schedule for most aerobic exercise programs. As your fitness level improves, your goal should be to exercise five days a week. To avoid overuse injuries and monotony, vary your activities and take a day off when you need a rest.

Determining Exercise Intensity. An aerobic exercise program must employ prolonged, moderate-intensity workouts to improve cardiorespiratory fitness. The measure of such a workout is your **target heart rate**, which is a percentage of your maximum heart rate. To calculate target heart rate, subtract your age from 220 for females or from 226 for males. The result is your maximum heart rate. You determine your target heart rate by calculating a desired percentage of maximum heart rate, often 60 to 70 percent. If you are a 20-year-old female, your maximum heart rate is 200 (220 − 20). Your target heart rate would be somewhere between 120 (200 × 0.60) and 140 (200 × 0.70). People in poor physical condition should set a target heart rate between 40 and 50 percent of maximum. As your condition improves, you can gradually increase your target heart rate. Increases should be made in small increments: increase from 40 to 45 percent; then from 45 to 50 percent. It is not recommended that most people exceed 80 to 85 percent of maximum heart rate.

Once you know your target heart rate, you can determine how close you are to this value during your workout. You'll need to stop exercising briefly in order to measure your heart rate. To take your pulse, lightly place your index and middle fingers (don't use your thumb) over one of the major (carotid) arteries in your neck, along either side of your Adam's apple, or on the artery in the inside wrist. Be sure to start counting your pulse immediately after you stop exercising, as your heart rate will decrease quickly. Using a watch or clock, take your pulse for six seconds and multiply this number by 10 (just add a zero to your count) to get the number of beats per minute. Your pulse should be within a range of about 5 bpm above or below your target heart rate. If necessary, increase or decrease the pace or intensity of your workout to achieve your target heart rate.

A target heart rate of 70 percent of maximum is sometimes called the "conversational level of exercise" because you are able to talk with a partner while exercising.[30] If you are a novice and you are breathing so hard that talking is difficult, your intensity of exercise is too high. If you can sustain a conversational level of aerobic exercise for 20 to 30 minutes, you will improve your cardiovascular fitness.

Determining Exercise Duration. Duration refers to the number of minutes of exercise performed during any one session. Every adult should accumulate 30 minutes or more of moderate-intensity physical activity over the course of most days of the week.[31] Activities that can contribute to this 30-minute total include dancing, walking up stairs (instead of taking the elevator), gardening, and raking leaves as well as planned physical activities such as jogging, swimming, and cycling. One way to meet this recommendation is to walk 3 kilometres briskly.

Here are general-purpose stretching techniques to be used as part of your warmup and cool-down. Hold each stretch for 10 seconds, and repeat three times on each limb.

After only a few weeks of regular stretching, you'll begin to see improvements.

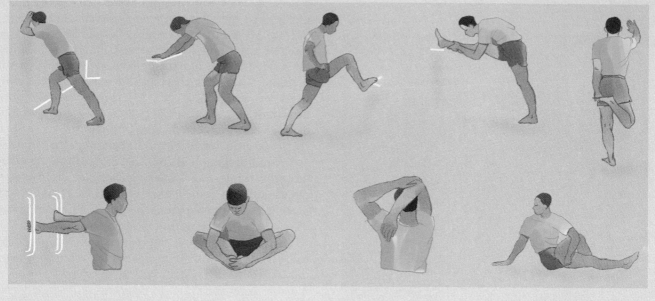

Source: R. A. Anderson, *Stretching* (Bolinas, CA: Sheller Publishing, 1990), 132.

FIGURE 9.1

Stretching Exercises That Will Help You Improve Your Flexibility

Source: Excerpted from *Stretching,* © 1980 by Bob and Jean Anderson. $12.00 Shelter Publications, Inc., P.O. Box 279, Bolinas, CA 94924. Distributed in bookstores by Random House. Reprinted by permission.

The lower the intensity of the activity, the longer the duration you'll need to get the same caloric expenditure. For example, an 82-kilogram man will expend 288 calories per hour of playing golf if he carries his clubs, but will burn 805 calories per hour if he is cross-country skiing.[32] Your goal should be to expend 300 to 500 calories per exercise session, with an eventual weekly goal of 1500 to 2000 calories. As you age and your basal metabolic rate decreases, the weight-control (caloric expenditure) benefits of longer-duration, low-intensity exercise can become increasingly important.

A program of repeated bouts of exercise over several months or years—exercise training—causes changes in the way your cardiovascular system meets your body's oxygen requirements at rest and during exercise. Since many of the health benefits associated with cardiovascular fitness activities take about one year of regular exercise to achieve, you shouldn't expect an immediate reduction in your risk of cardiovascular disease when you start an exercise program.[33] However, any low-to-moderate-intensity physical activity, even if it does not meet all the cardiovascular exercise characteristics mentioned in this chapter, will benefit your overall health almost from the start.

Flexibility: The measure of the range of motion, or the amount of movement possible, at a particular joint.

Static stretching: Techniques that gradually lengthen a muscle to an elongated position (to the point of discomfort) and hold that position for 10 to 30 seconds.

*W*HAT DO YOU THINK?

Calculate your maximum heart rate. Pick an intensity of exercise that suits your fitness level, for example, 50 percent, 60 percent, or 70 percent of your maximum heart rate. Using a familiar physical activity and monitoring your pulse, experiment by exercising at three different intensities. Do you notice any difference in the way you felt while exercising? Afterward?

IMPROVING YOUR FLEXIBILITY

Flexibility is a measure of the range of motion, or the amount of movement possible, at a particular joint. This component of fitness is commonly overshadowed by the muscular strength and aerobic capacity components, but muscles that lack elasticity and resiliency are more susceptible to injury. Improving your range of motion through stretching exercises will enhance your efficiency of movement and your posture. A regular program of stretching exercises also can enhance psychological as well as physical well-being.

Stretching for Flexibility

Flexibility is enhanced by the controlled stretching of muscles that act on a particular joint. The primary strategy is to decrease the resistance to stretch (tension) within a tight muscle that you have targeted for increased range of motion.[34] To do this, you repeatedly stretch the muscle and its two tendons of attachment to elongate them. Flexibility can also be increased temporarily by having a whole-body massage that results in widespread muscle relaxation.

The safest techniques for improving flexibility employ **static stretching.** Static stretching techniques involve the slow, gradual lengthening of a muscle or group of muscles. Various positions and postures are used to lengthen the tight muscle or muscle group to a point where a mild

burning sensation is felt within the muscle. This end position is held for 10 to 30 seconds, and is repeated two or three times in close succession for each muscle or muscle group. With each repetition of a static stretch, range of motion improves temporarily. When static stretching is done properly, it stimulates the tension receptors within the muscle being stretched to allow the muscle to be stretched to greater length.[35]

A major goal of static stretching is to cause permanent elongation of the targeted muscle or muscle group, thus permitting greater range of motion at a given joint. To achieve this goal, a regular program of stretching exercises must be performed at least three (preferably five) days a week. If you are just beginning a program to improve your flexibility, proceed cautiously. Follow the diagrams in Figure 9.1 to stretch all the major muscle groups of your body. Hold each static stretch at the point of discomfort for 10 to 30 seconds initially.

IMPROVING MUSCULAR STRENGTH AND ENDURANCE

Muscular strength refers to the amount of force a muscle is capable of exerting. The most common way to assess strength in a resistance exercise program is to measure the maximum amount of weight you can lift one time. This value is known as the **one repetition maximum**, and is written as **1RM. Muscular endurance** is defined as a muscle's ability to exert force repeatedly without fatiguing. The more repetitions of a certain resistance exercise you can perform successfully (e.g., a bench press of 0.50 kilograms), the greater your muscular endurance.

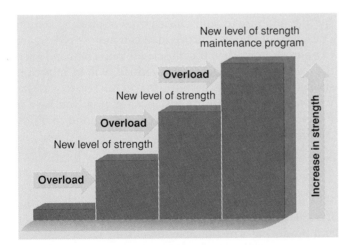

FIGURE 9.2

The overload principle contributes to an increase in strength. Notice that once the muscle has adapted to the original overload, a new overload must be placed on the muscle for subsequent gains in strength to occur.

Source: From Philip A. Sienna, *One Rep Max: A Guide to Beginning Weight Training*, Fig. 2.1, 8. © 1989. Wm. C. Brown Communications, Inc., Dubuque, Iowa. Reprinted by permission of Times Mirror Higher Education Group, Inc., Dubuque, Iowa. All rights reserved.

Muscular strength: The amount of force that a muscle is capable of exerting.

One repetition maximum (1RM): The amount of weight/resistance that can be lifted/moved one time, but not twice; a common measure of strength.

Muscular endurance: A muscle's ability to exert force repeatedly without fatiguing.

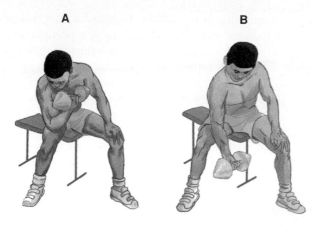

A   **B**

FIGURE 9.3

The figure depicts concentric and eccentric muscle actions. In A, the bicep shortens while producing tension in the upward phase of a curl. This is called a concentric muscle action. In B, the bicep lengthens while producing tension and permitting the controlled lowering of the weight. This is known as an eccentric muscle action.

Principles of Strength Development

There are three key principles to understand if you intend to maximize muscular strength and endurance benefits from your **resistance exercise program**.[36] Unless you follow these principles, you are likely to be disappointed in the results of your program.

The Tension Principle. The key to developing strength is to create tension within a muscle. The more tension you can create in a muscle, the greater your strength gain will be. The most common recreational way to create tension in a muscle is by lifting weights. While weight lifting is one method of producing tension in a muscle, any activity that creates muscle tension—for example, using weight machines with pulleys and cables or riding a bike up a steep hill—will result in greater strength. It really does not matter what type of equipment you choose to develop

tension in your muscles; what matters is that you use the equipment in such a way as to produce the desired strength and endurance.

The Overload Principle. The overload principle is the most important of the three key principles for improving muscular strength. Everyone begins a resistance training program with an initial level of strength. To increase that level of strength, you must regularly create a degree of tension in your muscles that is greater than they are accustomed to. This overloading of your muscles, most commonly accomplished with weights of some type, will cause your muscles to adapt to the level of overload. As your muscles respond to a regular program of overloading by getting larger (**hypertrophy**), they become capable of generating more tension. Figure 9.2 illustrates how a continual process of overload and adaptation to the overload improves strength. If you fail to provide an overload—if you "underload" your muscles—you will not increase your strength. But if you provide too great an overload, you may experience muscle injury, muscle fatigue, and even a loss of strength.[37]

Once you have reached your strength goal, no further overloading is necessary. Your next challenge is to maintain that level of strength by continuing to participate in a regular (at least three times per week) resistance exercise program.

The Specificity of Training Principle. This principle refers to the manner in which a specific body system responds to the physiological demands placed upon it. According to the specificity principle, you'll get a very specific response to your chosen type of physical activity or exercise. If the specific overload you impose is designed to improve strength in the muscles of your chest and back, the response to that demand (overload) will be improved strength in those muscles only. As you can see, to get what you want and need from resistance training, you have to understand how your body is going to respond to different types of resistance exercises.

Types of Muscle Activity

When your skeletal muscles receive a stimulus from your nervous system to act, they respond by developing tension and producing a measurable force. Your skeletal muscles act in three different modes—isometric, concentric, and eccentric—to produce this force.[38] An **isometric muscle action** is one in which force is produced by the muscle without any resulting muscle movement. Isometric muscle actions do not create any joint motion. Muscles act isometrically to stabilize a particular body part while another body part is moving, or when a maximal resistance is met and the force produced by your muscles cannot overcome the resistance. Isometric exercise routines were popular in the 1960s and can develop strength, but they are not commonly used today.

Resistance exercise program: A regular program of exercises designed to improve muscular strength and endurance in the major muscle groups.

Hypertrophy: Increased size (girth) of a muscle.

Isometric muscle action: Force produced without any resulting muscle movement.

Concentric muscle action: Force produced while shortening the muscle.

Eccentric muscle action: Force produced while lengthening the muscle.

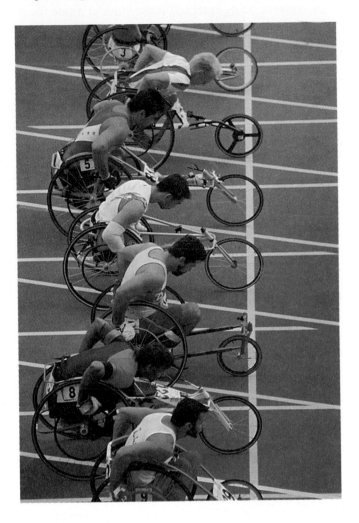

People with physical disabilities can attain the levels of cardiovascular fitness and muscular strength necessary to participate in physical activities they enjoy—including competitive sports.

One example of an isometric muscle action is the unsuccessful attempt to push a car out of snow or mud. Although you push with all your might, the car (as well as your joints) does not move. The muscles involved are all producing forces, but in an isometric way. Another example, and one more related to resistance training, is attempting to lift a barbell too heavy for you. The more you try, the more tired your muscles become, but the barbell never leaves the floor.

A **concentric muscle action** is one in which force is produced while the muscle shortens. Joint movement is always produced during concentric muscle actions. Raising a 20-pound dumbbell in an elbow flexion movement (curl) is an example of a concentric action of the elbow flexor muscles (biceps). In general, concentric muscle actions produce movement in a direction opposite of the downward pull of gravity (Figure 9.3A).

Eccentric muscle action describes a muscle's ability to produce force while lengthening. Typically, eccentric muscle actions occur when movement is in the same direction as the pull of gravity. If you want to be sure that a given resistance exercise has an eccentric phase, you must use the type of resistance training equipment that requires you to perform an eccentric action in order to achieve the starting position prior to your next repetition. For example, with a 20-pound dumbbell biceps curl, you lower the weight slowly to the starting point of the exercise in an eccentric action of the elbow flexors. Even though the motion produced during this phase of the curl is elbow extension, it is the force exerted by the controlled lengthening of the elbow flexors (biceps) that is responsible for the motion, *not* the elbow extensor muscles (triceps) (Figure 9.3B).

All factors being equal, the greatest amount of force is produced during eccentric muscle actions, followed by isometric and then concentric muscle actions. Changes in muscle size and strength are affected both by the type of resistance exercise you employ and by the type of muscle action(s) you use during your workout. When using free weights (barbells, dumbbells), the typical sequential pattern of concentric-eccentric muscle actions during resistance training contributes to improved muscle strength and muscle fibre size. According to current research, if your resistance exercise program uses only concentric muscle actions, you'll need to perform at least twice as many concentric-only repetitions to achieve the same results as you would attain by using concentric-eccentric combinations.[39]

Methods of Providing Resistance

There are four commonly used methods of applying resistance to develop strength and endurance.

Body Weight Resistance. Many different techniques can be used to develop skeletal muscle fitness without relying on resistance equipment. Most of these methods use part or all of your body weight to offer the resistance during exercise. While these techniques are not as effective as external resistance in developing muscular strength, they are quite adequate for improving general muscular fitness. Many common exercises require your muscles to lift your body weight off the floor. Activities such as sit-ups, push-ups, and pull-ups use both concentric and eccentric muscle actions.

Fixed Resistance. Fixed resistance exercises provide a constant amount of resistance throughout the full range of movement. Barbells and dumbbells provide fixed resistance because their weight (amount of resistance) does not change as you exercise. Unfortunately, due to the biomechanics of human motion, the muscle forces that must be exerted to move the weight are lower at some joint angles and higher at others. Any given muscle generates its least amount of force at the beginning and ending positions of a weightlifting exercise and can create the

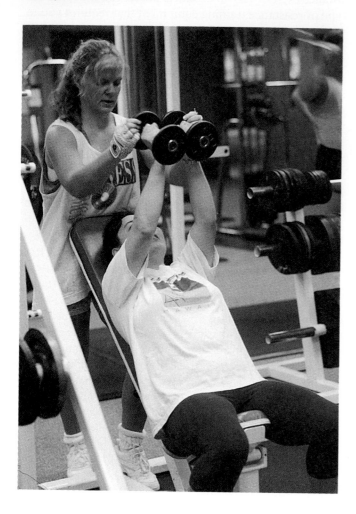

Lifting free weights to build muscular strength and endurance has many advantages, but reaching strength and endurance goals without injury requires skills that are best learned from a certified trainer.

most force when the joint involved in the exercise approximates a right angle (90 degrees). As a result, the disadvantage of fixed resistance exercises is that the extent to which a muscle is overloaded varies throughout the exercise, and the exercise may not fully develop the muscle.

Variable Resistance.   Whether found at a health club or in your home workout area, variable resistance equipment alters the resistance encountered by a muscle at various joint angles so that the effort by the muscle is more consistent throughout the full range of motion. Variable resistance machines are typically single-station devices (e.g., Nautilus), but some have multiple stations at which muscles of the upper and lower extremities can be exercised (e.g., Soloflex).

Accommodating Resistance.   With accommodating resistance devices, the resistance changes according to the amount of force generated by the individual. There is no external weight to move or overcome. Resistance is provided by having the exerciser perform at maximal level of effort, while the exercise machine controls the speed of the exercise and does not allow any faster motion. The body segment being exercised must move at a rate faster than or equal to the set speed to encounter resistance. One way to distinguish between accommodating and variable resistance is to recall that with variable resistance, the resistance increases from the beginning to the end of the repetition. In contrast, accommodating resistance can become more or less difficult depending on the input (muscular force exerted by the exerciser) into the machine.[40]

Getting Started

You will find some general principles useful whatever your resistance exercise goals. If sufficient tension is generated within a muscle, it will respond by becoming stronger regardless of the type of muscle action or resistance employed. You need to determine your 1RM for each muscle or muscle group you plan to exercise in order to design your program, but the strategies you use in resistance training sessions will vary according to your specific goals.

Strength Training.   There are almost as many ways to develop muscular strength as there are participants in strength training exercises. It is important to select at least one resistance exercise for each major muscle group in the body to ensure development of comprehensive muscular strength. To develop strength, you should perform a relatively low number of repetitions of each exercise using a relatively high resistance. Strength training exercises are done in a *set*, or a single series of multiple repetitions using the same resistance. Strength training with 85 percent of the 1RM increases the risk of injury, while training with 65 percent of the 1RM decreases the overload on the muscle(s) exercised.[41] Therefore, to improve strength, the amount of resistance employed is typically 70 to 80 percent of the 1RM for a given exercise, with 8 to 12 repetitions of the exercise performed per set.

Resistance training exercises cause microscopic damage (tears) to muscle fibres, and the rebuilding process that increases the size and capacity of the muscle takes about 24 to 48 hours. Thus, resistance training exercise programs require at least one day of rest (and recovery) between workouts to make overloading the same muscle group safe again.

Muscular Endurance Training.   To develop muscular endurance, you should perform a relatively high number of repetitions (10 to 30 per set) using a relatively low resistance (50 to 60 percent of the 1RM for a particular exercise). Instead of using traditional resistance exercise equipment to develop muscular endurance, consider adding variety to your training program with devices

Suggested Exercises for Strength Development

When you perform a series of strength exercises, we suggest that you begin each workout by exercising the larger muscle groups in the legs first and then perform exercises using the smaller muscle groups of the trunk and arms. This strategy permits performance of the most demanding exercises when muscle fatigue levels are lowest.

Days of the Week: Monday, Thursday, and Saturday (3 Times/Week)

Major Muscles/Muscle Group	*Free Weight/Machine Strength Training Exercise(s)*
1. Quadriceps (front of thigh)	Leg extension
2. Hamstrings (back of thigh)	Leg curl
3. Calf muscles	Heel raises
4. Quadriceps, gluteal muscles	Squat
5. Pectoralis major	Bench press
6. Deltoids	Shoulder/military press
7. Biceps	Arm curl
8. Latissimus dorsi	Lat pulldowns, bent-over row
9. Triceps	Arm extension

Days of the Week: Sunday, Tuesday, Wednesday, and Friday (4 Times/Week)

One to three sets of 25 repetitions each:

Major Muscles/Muscle Group	*Body-Weight Resistance Exercises*
1. Pectoralis major	Push-ups
2. Triceps	Chair or parallel bar dips
3. Abdominal muscles	Abdominal curl-ups (partial sit-ups)
4. Biceps	Chin-ups

Source: Reprinted by permission from W. L. Westcott, "Muscular Strength and Endurance," *Personal Trainer Manual—The Resource for Fitness Instructors* (San Diego: American Council on Exercise, 1991), 250–274.

equipped with an ergometer, such as a stationary bicycle, rowing machine, or stair-climbing machine. With these and other devices, you can control the cadence of the activity and/or adjust the amount of resistance you encounter. Performing thousands of repetitions during a 20-minute (or longer) workout using a relatively low resistance will quickly develop muscular endurance in the muscles exercised. This type of workout will also have cardiorespiratory benefits if you select an intensity that allows you to reach your target heart rate.

There is no one resistance exercise program perfect for everyone. Experiment with different resistance exercise devices and programs to find what works best for you. Once you gain strength and endurance, they are fairly easy to maintain. Maintenance resistance training consists of two to three workouts per week. You can consult with a fitness professional or hire a credentialed personal trainer to set up a program to meet your personal needs. The Skills for Behaviour Change box gives you more tips on strength training.

WHAT DO YOU THINK?

What types of resistance equipment can you currently access? Based on what you've read, what specific actions can you take to increase your muscular strength? Muscular endurance? How would you measure your improvement?

TABLE 9.2 ■ Proper Shoe Selection for Running

- Shop in the afternoon to get the right fit.

- Try on both shoes with the same type of sock you will wear when running.

- Try on several different models to make a good comparison. Walk or jog around the store in the shoes.

- Check the quality of the shoes. Look at the stitching, eyelets, gluing. Feel for bumps inside the shoe.

- The sole should flex where your foot flexes. Look for shoes with removable insoles to accommodate orthotic devices.

- Allow a centimetre between the end of the shoe and your longest toe when you stand up.

- The heel counter should fit snugly so that there is no slipping at the heel.

- Shoes should be comfortable on the day you buy them. Don't rely on a break-in period.

- Consult the staff at running specialty stores for help in selecting the correct shoe.

Source: Adapted by permission from Injury Prevention Information Series, "Proper Shoe Selection," American Running and Fitness Association, 1993.

FITNESS INJURIES

Overtraining is the most frequent cause of injuries associated with fitness activities. Enthusiastic but out-of-shape beginners often injure themselves by doing too much activity too soon. While participating in your personal fitness program, listen to your body's injury warning signs. Muscle stiffness and soreness, bone and joint pains, and whole-body fatigue are a few of the common warning signs of an impending overuse injury. One strategy to prevent overuse injury to a particular muscle group or body part is to vary your fitness activities throughout the week to give muscles and joints a rest. Setting appropriate short-term and long-term training goals is another good strategy for preventing overtraining injuries. Establishing realistic but challenging fitness goals can help you maintain a high level of motivation while ensuring that you do not attempt to do too much exercise too soon.

Overtraining injuries occur most often in repetitive activities like swimming, running, bicycling, and aerobic dance exercise. Progress slowly, set realistic exercise goals, vary your fitness activities to keep your workouts fun and fresh, and schedule rest days. Simply put, use common sense, and you're likely to remain injury-free.

Causes of Fitness-Related Injuries

There are two basic types of injuries stemming from participation in fitness-related activities: overuse and traumatic. **Overuse injuries** occur because of cumulative, day-after-day stresses placed on body parts (e.g., tendons, bones, and ligaments) during exercise. The forces that occur normally during physical activity are not enough to

cause a ligament sprain or muscle strain, but when these forces are applied on a daily basis for weeks or months they can result in an injury. That is why people who sustain this type of injury typically cannot pinpoint a particular time or day when they were injured. Common sites of overuse injuries are the leg, knee, shoulder, and elbow joints.

Traumatic injuries, which occur suddenly and violently, typically by accident, are the second major type of fitness-related injuries. Typical traumatic injuries are broken bones, torn ligaments and muscles, contusions, and lacerations. Most traumatic injuries are unavoidable—for example, spraining your ankle by landing on another person's foot after jumping up for a rebound in basketball. If your traumatic injury causes a noticeable loss of function and immediate pain or pain that does not go away after 30 minutes, you should have a physician examine it.

Prevention

For personal fitness activities, the function of your exercise clothing is far more important than the fashion statement it makes. For some types of physical activity, you will need clothing that allows maximal body heat dissipation—for example, light-coloured nylon shorts and mesh tank top while running in hot weather. For other types, you will need clothing that permits significant heat reten-

Overuse injuries: Injuries that result from the cumulative effects of day-after-day stresses placed on tendons, muscles, and joints.

Traumatic injuries: Injuries that are accidental in nature; they occur suddenly and violently (e.g., fractured bones, ruptured tendons, and sprained ligaments).

tion without getting you sweat-soaked—for example, layers of polypropylene and/or wool clothing while cross-country skiing.

Appropriate Footwear.   When you are purchasing running shoes, look for several key components. Biomechanics research has revealed that running is a "collision" sport—that is, the runner's foot collides with the ground with a force three to five times the runner's body weight with each stride.[42] The 68-kilogram runner who takes 620 strides per kilometre might apply a cumulative force to his or her body of 127 000 kilograms per kilometre. The force not absorbed by the running shoe is transmitted upward into the foot, leg, thigh, and back. Our bodies are able to absorb forces such as these, but may be injured by the cumulative effects of repetitive impacts (e.g., running 65 kilometres per week). Therefore, the ability of running shoes to absorb shock is a critical factor to consider when you are sampling shoes at the store.

The midsole of a running shoe must absorb impact forces, but must also be flexible. One method used to evaluate the flexibility of the midsole is to hold the shoe between the index fingers of your right and left hand. When you push on both ends of the shoe with your fingers, the shoe should bend easily at the midsole. If the force exerted by your index fingers cannot bend the shoe, its midsole is probably too rigid and may cause irritation of your Achilles tendon, among other problems.[43] Other basic characteristics of running shoes include: a rigid plastic insert within the heel of the shoe (known as a heel counter) to control the movement of your heel; a cushioned foam pad surrounding the heel of the shoe to prevent Achilles tendon irritation; and a removable thermoplastic innersole that customizes the fit of the shoe by using your body heat to mould it to the shape of your foot. Shoes are the runner's most essential piece of equipment, so carefully select appropriate footwear before you start a running program. See Table 9.2 for more information on how to choose a running shoe.

Appropriate Exercise Equipment.   It is essential to use correctly fitted, appropriate athletic equipment for your personal fitness activities. For some activities, there is specialized protective equipment that will reduce your chances of injury. In tennis, for example, the use of proper equipment helps prevent the general inflammatory condition known as tennis elbow. Excessive racquet string tension, repetitive use of the forearm muscles during hours of daily practice, and poor flexibility cause this problem in experienced tennis players. To avoid tennis elbow, consult an instructor or skilled salesperson to assist you in selecting the correct tennis racquet and string tension for you.

Eye injuries can occur in virtually all fitness-related activities, though the risk of injury is much greater in some activities than in others. As many as 90 percent of the eye injuries resulting from racquetball and squash are preventable with the use of appropriate eye protection—for example, goggles with polycarbonate lenses.[44] One-eyed participants should wear polycarbonate prescription or non-prescription eyeglasses for all recreational activities.[45]

According to the Canadian Cycling Association, in 1992, cycling was the third-most-popular year-round sport for those 18 and over. The selection of the right-size bicycle frame and seat height, coupled with the use of a bicycle helmet, padded grips/handlebars, and padded biking gloves, can significantly reduce the number of injuries that occur in this extremely popular activity. Head injuries used to account for 85 percent of all deaths attributable to bicycle accidents; however, the wearing of bike helmets has significantly reduced the number of skull fractures and facial injuries among recreational cyclists.[46] Bicycle helmets that meet the standards established by the Canadian Standards Association (CSA) should be worn by all cyclists.

𝓦HAT DO YOU THINK?

Given your activity level, what are some injury risks that you are exposed to on a regular basis? What changes can you make in your equipment or clothing to reduce these risks?

Common Overuse Injuries

Body movements in physical activities such as running, swimming, and bicycling are highly repetitive, so participants are susceptible to overuse injuries. In fitness activities, the joints of the lower extremities (foot, ankle, knee, and hip) tend to be injured more frequently than the upper-extremity joints (shoulder, elbow, wrist, and hand). Three of the most common injuries from repetitive overuse during exercise are plantar fasciitis, "shin splints," and "runner's knee."

Plantar Fasciitis.   Plantar fasciitis is an inflammation of the plantar fascia, a broad band of dense, inelastic tissue (fascia) that runs from the heel to the toe on the bottom of your foot. The main function of the plantar fascia is to protect the nerves, blood vessels, and muscles of the foot from injury. In repetitive, weight-bearing fitness activities such as walking and running, the plantar fascia may become inflamed. Common symptoms of this condition are pain and tenderness under the ball of the foot, at the heel, or at both locations. The pain of plantar fasciitis is particularly noticeable during your first steps out of bed in the morning. If not treated properly, this injury may progress in severity to the point that weight-bearing exercise is too painful to endure. Uphill running is not advised for anyone suffering from this condition, since each uphill stride severely stretches (and thus irritates) the already inflamed plantar fascia. This injury can often be prevented by regularly stretching the plantar fascia prior to exercise and by wearing athletic shoes with good arch support and shock absorbency. The plantar fascia are stretched by slowly pulling all five toes upward toward your head, holding for 10 to 15 seconds, and repeating this three to five times on each foot prior to exercise.

Shin Splints. A general term for any pain that occurs below the knee and above the ankle is shin splints. More than 20 different medical conditions have been identified within the broad description of shin splints. Problems range from stress fractures of the tibia (shinbone) to severe inflammation in the muscular compartments of the lower leg, which can interrupt the flow of blood and nerve supply to the foot. The most common type of shin splints occurs along the inner side of the tibia and is usually a combination of a muscle irritation and irritation of the tissues that attach the muscles to the bone in this region. Typically, there is pain and swelling along the middle one-third of the posteromedial tibia in the soft tissues, not the bone.

Sedentary people who start a new weight-bearing exercise program are at the greatest risk for shin splints, though well-conditioned aerobic exercisers who rapidly increase their distance or pace may also develop shin splints.[47] Running is the most frequent cause of shin splints, but those who do a great deal of walking (e.g., waitresses) may also develop this injury.

To help prevent shin splints, wear athletic shoes that have good arch support and shock absorbency. If the severity of this lower-leg condition increases to the point that you cannot comfortably complete your desired fitness activity, see your physician. Specific pain on the tibia or on the adjacent, smaller fibula should be examined by a doctor for possible stress fracture. Reduction of the frequency, intensity, and duration of weight-bearing exercise may be required. You may be advised to substitute a non-weight-bearing activity, such as swimming, for weight-bearing exercise during your recovery period.

Runner's Knee. An overuse condition known as runner's knee describes a series of problems involving the muscles, tendons, and ligaments about the knee. The most common problem identified as runner's knee is abnormal movement of the patella (kneecap).[48] Women are more commonly affected by this condition than are men because their wider pelvis makes abnormal lateral pull on the patella by the muscles that act at the knee more likely. In women (and some men), this causes irritation to the cartilage on the back side of the patella as well as to the nearby tendons and ligaments.

RICE: Acronym for the standard first-aid treatment for virtually all traumatic and overuse injuries: rest, ice, compression, and elevation.

The main symptom of this kind of runner's knee is the pain experienced when downward pressure is applied to the patella after the knee is straightened fully. Additional symptoms may include swelling, redness, and tenderness around the patella, and a dull, aching pain felt in the centre of the knee.[49] If you have these symptoms in your knee, your physician will probably recommend that you stop running for a few weeks and reduce daily activities that put compressive forces on the patella (e.g., exercise on a stair-climbing machine or doing squats with heavy resistance) until you no longer have any pain around your kneecap.

Treatment

First-aid treatment for virtually all personal fitness injuries involves **RICE: r**est, **i**ce, **c**ompression, and **e**levation. *Rest,* the first component of this treatment, is required to eliminate the risk of further irritation of the injured body part. *Ice* is applied to relieve the pain of the injury and to constrict the blood vessels in order to slow and stop any internal or external bleeding associated with the injury. Never apply ice cubes, reusable gel ice packs, chemical cold packs, or other forms of cold directly to your skin. Instead, place a layer of wet towelling between the ice and your skin. Ice should be applied to a new injury for approximately 20 minutes every hour for the first 24 to 72 hours. *Compression* of the injured body part can be accomplished with a 10- or 15-centimetre-wide elastic bandage; this applies

While appropriate clothing and equipment help prevent injuries in any fitness activity, a workout partner is also an important safeguard when exercising outdoors in cold weather.

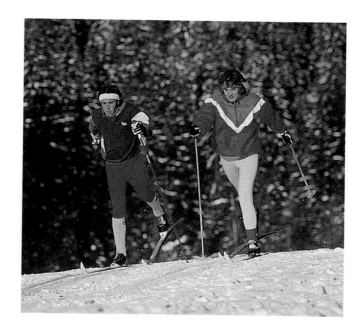

TABLE 9.3 ■ The Humidex (What It Feels Like)

RELATIVE HUMIDITY (%)

Temp. (°C)	100	95	90	85	80	75	70	65	60	55	50	45	40	35	30	25	20
D 43														56	54	51	49	47
R 42												56	54	52	50	48	46
Y 41											57	54	52	51	49	47	44
40										57	54	53	51	49	47	45	43
B 39									56	54	53	51	49	47	45	43	41
U 38							57	56	54	52	51	49	47	46	43	42	40
L 37					58	57	55	53	51	50	49	47	45	43	42	40	
B 36			58	57	56	54	53	51	50	48	47	45	43	42	40	38	
35		58	57	56	54	52	51	49	48	47	45	43	42	41	38	37	
T 34	58	57	55	53	52	51	49	48	47	45	43	42	41	39	37	36	
E 33	55	54	52	51	50	48	47	46	44	43	42	40	38	37	36	34	
M 32	52	51	50	49	47	46	45	43	42	41	39	38	37	36	34	33	
P 31	50	49	48	46	45	44	43	41	40	39	38	36	35	34	33	31	31
E 30	48	47	46	44	43	42	41	40	38	37	36	35	34	33	31	31	
R 29	46	45	44	43	42	41	39	38	37	36	34	33	32	31	30		
A 28	43	42	41	41	39	38	37	36	35	34	33	32	31	29	28	28	
T 27	41	40	39	38	37	36	35	34	33	32	31	30	29	28	28		
U 26	39	38	37	36	35	34	33	32	31	31	29	28	28	27			
R 25	37	36	35	34	33	33	32	31	30	29	28	27	27	26			
E 24	35	34	33	33	32	31	30	29	28	28	27	26	26	25			
23	33	32	32	31	30	29	28	27	27	26	25	24	23				
°C 22	31	29	29	28	28	27	26	26	24	24	23	23					
21	29	29	28	27	27	26	26	24	24	23	23	22					

Humidex (°C)	Degree of Comfort
20–29	Comfortable
30–39	Varying degrees of discomfort
40–45	Almost everyone uncomfortable
46 and over	Many types of labour must be restricted

The chart measures the apparent temperature at various temperatures and humidity levels. A humidex of 20–29° is comfortable; at 30–35° levels of discomfort vary; almost everyone is uncomfortable when the humidex rises over 40°; and many types of labour (and exercise) must be restricted at levels over 46°. Heat cramps and heat exhaustion are also possible with exertion at humidex levels as low as 32–40°; pay close attention to your body's signals.

Source: J. M. Masterton and F. A. Richardson, *Humidex: A Method of Quantifying Human Discomfort* (Downsview, ON: Environment Canada, 1979).

indirect pressure to damaged blood vessels to help stop bleeding. Be careful, though, that the compression wrap does not interfere with normal blood flow. A throbbing, painful hand or foot is an indication that the compression wrap was applied too tightly and should be loosened. *Elevation* of the injured extremity above the level of your heart also helps to control internal or external bleeding by making the blood flow uphill to reach the injured area.

Exercising in the Heat

Exercising in extreme temperatures may increase your risk for a heat-related injury. Fortunately, if you are in good physical condition and wear appropriate clothing for outdoor physical activities, you can safely withstand a wide range of temperatures and humidity levels. Heat stress, which includes several potentially fatal illnesses resulting from excessive core body temperatures, should be a constant concern when you are exercising in warm, humid weather. In these conditions, your body's rate of heat production often exceeds its ability to cool itself.

You can help prevent heat stress by following certain precautions. First, proper acclimatization to hot and/or humid climates is essential. The process of heat acclimatization, which increases your body's cooling efficiency, requires about 10 to 14 days of gradually increased exercise in a hot environment. Second, heat stress can be prevented by avoiding dehydration, accomplished through proper fluid replacement during and following exercise. Third, wear clothing appropriate for the fitness activity and the environment. Finally, use common sense when exercising in hot and humid conditions—for example,

Playing to Win

Each of us has a different personal health style. Whether you are beginning or maintaining your exercise plan, it's important that it be something you believe in. Here is what two tennis professionals say about their workouts, self-motivation, and fitness and winning advice. Note how they communicate with themselves to keep going. Self-talk, introduced in Chapter 1, is an important component of your exercise program.

Gabriela Sabatini

On Working Out

I do lots of sit-ups. A couple of years ago, I started lifting weights. Since my upper body is very strong, I'm now concentrating on strength training my legs. That gives me lots of power on the court. It's made a difference. If I'm not playing tennis so much I play soccer, I run . . . . I have to do something. I have lots of energy.

Self-Motivation

Of course you should talk to yourself if you're doing badly, to encourage and give yourself energy and power—but you should also talk to yourself when you're doing well—just to keep in touch so you keep going strong.

Fitness and Winning Advice

Choose tennis, choose whatever, because you love it. Run, do aerobics, play sports—it's important to do something.

It takes work, but it makes you feel great. I myself have to keep active. It's the best. I highly recommend it.

Arantxa Sanchez Vicario

On Working Out

I have a personal trainer and we run and lift weights. Mostly though, I like to practise my tennis. There has never been a day yet when I haven't wanted to get out on the court. Maybe that sounds weird, but it's true. I just love the game so much.

Self-Motivation

If something goes wrong, I try to learn from it. I stop for a while, think, figure out what's happening, and then try to change. Staying positive is very important.

Fitness and Winning Advice

You have to work really hard. It takes a lot of work and a lot of sacrifice. Choose something you love, something you enjoy. That's the most important thing.

Source: All but the opening paragraph excerpted with permission from Lisa Klein, "Playing To Win," *Shape*, June 1993, 20.

---

when the temperature is 30°C and the humidity 90 percent, postpone your usual lunchtime run until the cool of evening.

The three different heat stress illnesses are progressive in their level of severity: heat cramps, heat exhaustion, and heat stroke. The least serious problem, heat-related muscle cramps (**heat cramps**), is easily prevented by adequate fluid replacement and a diet that includes the elec-

trolytes lost during sweating (sodium and potassium). **Heat exhaustion** is caused by excessive water loss resulting from intense or prolonged exercise or work in a warm and/or humid environment. Symptoms of heat exhaustion include nausea, headache, fatigue, dizziness and faintness, and, paradoxically, "goosebumps" and chills. If you are suffering from heat exhaustion, your skin will be cool and moist. Heat exhaustion is actually a mild form of shock, in which the blood pools in the arms and legs away from the brain and major organs of the body, causing nausea and fainting. **Heat stroke**, often called sunstroke, is a life-threatening emergency condition having a 20 to 70 percent death rate.[50] Heat stroke occurs during vigorous exercise when the body's heat production significantly exceeds your body's cooling capacities. Body core temperature can rise from normal (37°C) to 40.5°C to 43°C within minutes after the body's cooling mechanism shuts down. With no cooling taking place, rapidly increasing core temperatures can cause brain damage, permanent disability, and death. Common signs of heat stroke are dry, hot, and usually red skin; very high body temperature; and a very rapid heart rate.

Heat cramps: Muscle cramps that occur during or following exercise in warm/hot conditions.

Heat exhaustion: A heat stress illness caused by significant dehydration resulting from exercise in warm/hot conditions; frequent precursor to heat stroke.

Heat stroke: A deadly heat stress illness resulting from dehydration and overexertion in warm/hot conditions; can cause body core temperature to rise from normal to 40.5°C to 43°C in just a few minutes.

Heat stress illnesses may occur in situations in which the danger is not obvious. Serious or fatal heat strokes may result from prolonged sauna or steam baths, prolonged total immersion in a hot tub or spa, or by exercising in a plastic or rubber head-to-toe "sauna suit." If, while exercising, you experience any of the symptoms mentioned here, you should stop exercising immediately, move to the shade or a cool spot to rest, and drink large amounts of cool fluids. See Table 9.3 for a quick way to compute the risks of exercising under various heat and humidity conditions.

Exercising in the Cold

When you exercise in cool to cold weather, especially in windy conditions, your body's rate of heat loss is frequently greater than its rate of heat production. Under these conditions, **hypothermia**—a potentially fatal condition resulting from abnormally low body core temperature, which occurs when body heat is lost faster than it is produced—may result. Hypothermia can occur as a result of prolonged, vigorous exercise (e.g., snowboarding or rugby) in 4°C to 10°C temperatures, particularly if there is rain, snow, or a strong wind.

In mild cases of hypothermia, as your body core temperature drops from the normal 37°C to 34°C, you will begin to shiver. Shivering—the involuntary contraction of nearly every muscle in your body—is designed to increase your body temperature by using the heat given off by muscle activity. During this first stage of hypothermia, you may also experience cold hands and feet, poor judgement, apathy, and amnesia.[51] Shivering ceases in most hypothermia victims as their body core temperatures drop to between 30C° and 32°C, a sign that the body has lost its ability to generate heat. Death from hypothermia usually occurs at body core temperatures between 24°C and 26.5°C.

Hypothermia: Potentially fatal condition caused by abnormally low body core temperature.

TAKING CHARGE

Managing Your Fitness Behaviours

The decision to be physically fit is easy to make but not always easy to put into action. Physical fitness should be enjoyable. In addition to the health benefits, you should choose activities that make you happy.

Making Decisions for You

Begin by making a list of a variety of your favourite physical activities that may increase strength, flexibility, and cardiorespiratory efficiency. Your list may include walking, gardening, or mowing the lawn, as well as athletic endeavours such as weight lifting and swimming. Which would you like to make part of your health program? Next, you need to find time to exercise. Do you have extra time you could set aside? If not, how could exercise become part of your daily activities? Could you, for example, leave for class a few minutes earlier and walk a few blocks instead of taking the bus all the way?

Checklist for Change: Making Personal Choices

✓ *Start slowly as a beginning exerciser.* For the sedentary, first-time exerciser, any type and amount of physical activity will be a step in the right direction. If you are extremely overweight or out of condition, you may only be able to walk for five minutes at a time. Don't be discouraged: you're on your way!

✓ *Make only one life change at a time.* Attempting too many major changes in your lifestyle at once invites failure. Success at one major behaviour change will encourage you to make other positive changes.

✓ *Have reasonable expectations for yourself and your fitness program.* Many people become exercise dropouts because their expectations are too high to begin with. Have patience with yourself and your body. Allow sufficient time to reach your fitness goals.

✓ *Choose a specific time to exercise and stick with it.* Learning to establish priorities and keeping to a schedule are vital steps toward improved fitness. Experiment by exercising at different times of the day to learn what schedule works best for you.

✓ *Exercise with a friend.* Reneging on an exercise commitment is more difficult if you do not exercise alone. Enjoy the relaxed, social aspects of exercising with a friend. Partners can motivate and encourage one another, provided they remember that progress will not be the same for them both.

✓ *Make exercise a positive habit.* Usually, if you are able to practise a desired activity for three weeks, you will be able to incorporate it into your lifestyle. But also be aware that for some highly fit individuals exercise can become a negative habit (addiction).

(continued)

✓ *Keep a record of your progress.* A personal fitness journal can be a good motivator. Your journal could include various facts about your physical activities (duration, intensity) and chronicle your emotions and personal achievements as you progress in your fitness program.

✓ *Take lapses in stride.* Physical deconditioning—a decline in fitness level—occurs at about the same rate as does physical conditioning. If you have not exercised for three or more weeks after having developed a regular exercise habit, you will notice some lower levels of cardiovascular and muscular fitness. First, renew your commitment to fitness, and then restart your exercise program.

Checklist for Change: Making Community Choices

✓ Does your university have facilities for exercise? Is the use of facilities included in your student fees? What hours are those facilities available?

✓ What community facilities does your home town have available for exercise? Have you ever considered using these facilities?

✓ What opportunities are available for you to volunteer at a local exercise facility? Have you considered volunteering to help out low-income individuals? Why or why not?

Critical Thinking

Your friend Joan catches everyone's eye: five years of intense bodybuilding have created a sleek, "ripped-up," hard body. She even plans to start entering bodybuilding contests within the next year. Joan started working out in high school after her father had a heart attack at age 38. Her family doctor pointed out that her family had a history of cardiovascular disease and that she should take steps to lower her own risk. Cardiovascular exercise was his suggestion. Now Joan works out two to three hours a day in the weight room, usually powerlifting to build bigger muscles for competition. When she had a higher-than-normal blood pressure reading last week, she became convinced that she must work out harder. From what you have learned in your health class, you want to suggest that she add some elements of aerobic exercise to her workout. However, because you do little more than jog 20 minutes a day, you are afraid she won't take your suggestion seriously.

Using the DECIDE model described in Chapter 1, decide how you could approach Joan to urge her to take a more balanced approach to her workout.

To prevent hypothermia, follow these common sense guidelines: analyze weather conditions and your risk of hypothermia before you undertake your planned outdoor physical activity, remembering that wind and humidity are as significant as temperature; use the "buddy system"—that is, have a friend join you for your cold-weather outdoor activities; wear layers of appropriate clothing to prevent excessive heat loss (e.g., polypropylene or woolen undergarments, Gore-Tex windbreaker, and wool hat and gloves); and finally, don't allow yourself to become dehydrated.

*W*HAT DO YOU THINK?

Given what you've read about the symptoms of common fitness injuries, are you currently developing any overuse injuries? If so, what specific actions can you take to prevent these problems from getting more serious?

*P*LANNING YOUR FITNESS PROGRAM

You now know that regular physical activity and exercise can help you avoid preventable diseases and add to both the quality and the length of your life. You should also be aware of the importance of creating a program you love and of motivating yourself through self-talk, as the Building Communication Skills box discusses.

Identifying Your Fitness Goals

Before you embark on a fitness program, analyze your personal needs, limitations, physical activity likes and dislikes, and daily schedule. Your primary reason for exercising may be to lower your risks for health problems. This goal is prudent, particularly if you have a family history of cardiovascular diseases (heart attack, stroke, high blood pressure), diabetes, obesity, and/or substance abuse. If you have inherited no major risks for fatal or debilitating diseases, then your primary reason for exercising may be to improve the quality of your life. Your specific goal may be to achieve (or maintain) healthy levels of body fat, cardiovascular fitness, muscular strength and endurance, or flexibility/mobility. But your most vital goal should be to become committed to fitness for the long haul—to establish a realistic schedule of diverse exercise activities that you can maintain and enjoy throughout your life.

Designing Your Fitness Program

Once you commit yourself to exercise, you must decide what type of fitness program is best suited to your needs. The amounts and types of exercises required to yield beneficial results vary with the age and physical condition of the exerciser. Men over 40 and women over 50 should consult their physicians before beginning a fitness program.

Good fitness programs are designed to improve or maintain cardiorespiratory endurance, flexibility, muscular strength, and muscular endurance. A comprehensive program could include a warmup period of easy walking followed by stretching activities to improve flexibility, then selected strength development exercises, followed by performance of an aerobic activity for 20 minutes or more,

Cross-training: Regular participation in two or more types of exercises (e.g., swimming and weight lifting).

and concluding with a cool-down period of gentle flexibility exercises.

The greatest proportion of your exercise time should be spent developing cardiovascular fitness, but you should not exclude the other components. Choose an aerobic activity you think you will like. Many people find **cross-training**—alternate-day participation in two or more aerobic activities (i.e., jogging and swimming)—less monotonous and more enjoyable than long-term participation in only one aerobic activity. Cross-training is also beneficial because it strengthens a variety of muscles, thus helping you avoid overuse injuries to muscles and joints.

Jogging, walking, cycling, rowing, step aerobics, and cross-country skiing are all excellent activities for developing cardiovascular fitness. Responding to the exercise boom, fitness equipment manufacturers have made it easy for you to participate in these activities. Most colleges and universities now have recreation centres where students can use weights, stationary bicycles, and other exercise equipment.

*W*HAT DO YOU THINK?

You now have the ability to design your own fitness program. What two activities would you select for a cross-training program? Do the activities you selected exercise different major muscle groups? What may happen to you if they don't?

Summary

- The physiological benefits of regular physical activity include reduced risk of heart attack, prevention of hypertension, improved blood profile, improved skeletal mass, improved weight control, prevention of diabetes, increased life span, improved immunity to disease, improved mental health and stress management, and improved physical fitness.

- An aerobic exercise program improves cardiovascular fitness. Exercise frequency begins with three days per week and eventually moves up to five. Exercise intensity involves working out at your target heart rate. Exercise duration should increase to 30 to 45 minutes; the longer the exercise period, the more calories burned and the bigger improvement in cardiovascular fitness.

- Flexibility exercises should involve static stretching exercises performed in sets of three repetitions held for

10 to 30 seconds at least three days a week in order for progress to be made.

- The key principles for developing muscular strength and endurance are the tension principle, the overload principle, and the specificity of training principle. The different types of muscle actions include isometric, concentric, and eccentric. Resistance training programs include fixed, variable, and accommodating resistance.

- Fitness injuries are generally caused by overuse or trauma; the most common are plantar fasciitis, shin splints, and runner's knee. Limited prevention can be achieved with proper footwear and equipment. Exercise in the heat or cold requires special precautions.

- Planning your fitness program involves setting goals and designing a program to achieve these goals.

Application Exercise

Reread the What Do You Think? scenario at the beginning of the chapter and answer the following questions:

1. Assuming that Georgia's workouts were about 30 to 45 minutes long, five times a week, was there really anything wrong with what she was doing? What amount of workout is too much? Too little? Just right?

2. Given that Georgia is still tired and stressed out even though she regularly works out, what advice would you give her? Is stress simply a part of university life, or can it be controlled?

Health on the Net

Canadian Sport, The Centre (also has web links to many national sports organizations)
www.cdnsport.ca/

Canadian Heritage Sport Canada
www.pch.gc.ca/sportcanada

Sports Medicine and Science Council of Canada
www.smscc.ca/

Licit and Illicit Drug Use
Understanding Addictions

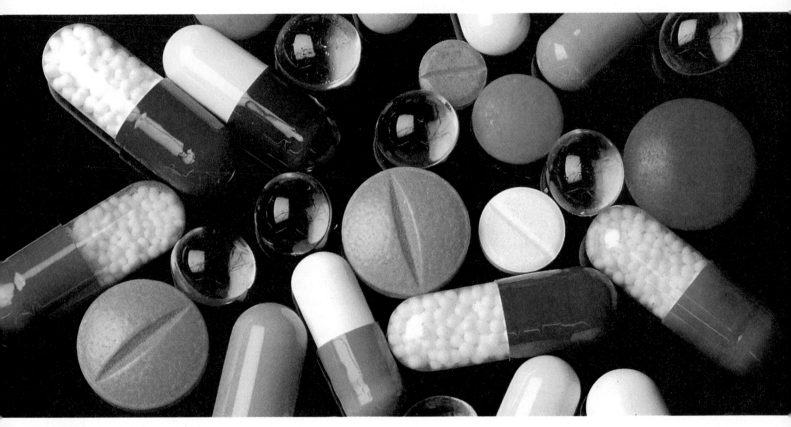

CHAPTER OBJECTIVES

◆ Distinguish addictions from habits and identify the signs of addiction.

◆ List the six categories of drugs and explain the routes of administration that drugs take into the body.

◆ Discuss proper drug use and explain how hazardous drug interactions occur.

◆ Discuss the types of over-the-counter drugs and general precautions to be taken with them.

◆ Discuss the key questions you should ask in order to make intelligent decisions about drug use.

◆ Discuss patterns of illicit drug use, including who uses illicit drugs and why they use them.

◆ Describe the use and abuse of controlled substances, including cocaine, amphetamines, marijuana, opiates, psychedelics, deliriants, designer drugs, and inhalants.

◆ Profile overall illegal drug use in the Canada, including frequency, financial impact, arrests for drug offences, and impact on the workplace.

The company for which Richard works as a machine operator recently introduced random drug testing for all employees. At a party last weekend, Richard smoked a little marijuana, unaware that the drug would remain in his body for a few days. On Monday, he tested positive for drug use and was suspended from work without pay for a week. He was informed that he would receive a dismissal warning if he tested positive again. Richard argues that his personal life is his own business as long as he can perform his job.

■ Is Richard justified in maintaining that his use of drugs off the job is his own business? Is his attitude toward drug use a potential danger to co-workers? Is random drug testing in the workplace a viable deterrent?

If you pick up the newspaper, watch TV, or listen to the radio, you're certain to hear about the devastating personal and social consequences of substance abuse. Few people would challenge the idea that chemical dependency is a major health threat in Canada. But while the war on drugs rages on, it is increasingly clear that chemical dependency represents only one part of Canada's problem with addiction. Indeed, it seems that millions of Canadians are struggling with compulsive and harmful behaviours that are not only conventional but also actually enhance the lives of people who can engage in them moderately.

DEFINING ADDICTION

The Addiction Foundation of Manitoba[1] defines a "dependency syndrome," commonly called **addiction**, as

> Patterned use that carries with it a dependence on mind or mood altering substances which has attained such a degree as to disrupt academic or work performance, interfere with family and interpersonal relationships, disrupt social and economic functioning and impair the state of physical and/or mental health.

A person with a dependency syndrome will generally exhibit at least three of the following behaviour patterns:

■ overuse a substance: that is, use a larger quantity or over a longer period than intended

Addiction: Patterned use involving dependence on mind- or mood-altering substances that interferes with academic/work performance, family and interpersonal relationships, social and economic functioning, and/or physical and mental health.

■ express a persistent desire or make unsuccessful efforts to cut down or control use

■ spend a great deal of time to get or use the substance, or to recover from its aftereffects

■ frequently be intoxicated or incapacitated by withdrawal when expected to fulfill major obligations

■ give up activities for substance use

■ continue to use the substance despite problems

■ develop a physical tolerance for the substance

■ display signs of withdrawal when not using the substance

■ use the substance to relieve or avoid withdrawal symptoms

Physiological dependence is only one indicator of addiction. Psychological dynamics play an important role, which explains why behaviours not related to the use of chemicals—gambling, for example—may also be addictive. In fact, psychological and physiological dependence are so intertwined that it is not really possible to separate the two. For every psychological state, there is a corresponding physiological state. In other words, everything you feel is tied to a chemical process occurring in your body.[2] Thus, addictions once thought to be entirely psychological in nature are now understood to have physiological components.

To be addictive, a behaviour must have the potential to produce a positive mood change. Chemicals are responsible for the most profound addictions, not only because they produce dramatic mood changes, but also because they cause cellular changes to which the body adapts so well that it eventually requires the chemical in order to function normally. Yet other behaviours, such as gambling, spending, working, and sex, also create changes at the cellular level along with positive mood changes. Although the mechanism is not well understood, all forms of addiction probably reflect dysfunction of certain biochemical systems in the brain.[3]

The Physiology of Addiction

Virtually all mental, emotional, and behavioural functions occur as a result of biochemical interactions between nerve cells in the body. Biochemical messengers, called **neurotransmitters**, exert their influence at specific receptor cites on nerve cells. Drug use and chronic stress can alter these receptor sites and cause the production and breakdown of neurotransmitters.

Mood-altering chemicals, for example, fill up the receptor sites for the body's natural "feel-good" neurotransmitters (endorphins) so that nerve cells are fooled into believing they have enough neurotransmitters and shut down production of these substances temporarily. When the drug use is stopped, those receptor sites become emptied, resulting in uncomfortable feelings that remain until the body resumes neurotransmitter production or the person consumes more of the drug. Some people's bodies always produce insufficient quantities of these neurotransmitters, so they naturally seek out chemicals like alcohol as substitutes, or they pursue behaviours like exercise that increase natural production. Thus we may be "wired" to seek out substances or experiences that increase pleasure or reduce discomfort.

Mood-altering substances and experiences produce **tolerance**, a phenomenon in which progressively larger doses of a drug or more intense involvement in an experience are needed to obtain the desired effects. All of us develop some degree of tolerance to any mood-altering experience. But because addicts tend to seek intense mood-altering experiences, they eventually require amounts of mood-altering substances or experiences large enough to cause negative side-effects.

Withdrawal is another phenomenon associated with mood-altering experiences. The drug or activity replaces or causes an effect that the body should normally provide on its own. If the experience is repeated often enough, the body makes an adjustment: it comes to require the drug or experience to obtain the effect it used to be able to produce itself, but no longer can. Stopping the behaviour will therefore cause a withdrawal syndrome. Withdrawal symptoms of chemical dependencies are generally the opposite of the effects of the drug being withdrawn. For example, a cocaine addict experiences a characteristic "crash" (depression and lethargy), while a barbiturate addict experiences trembling, irritability, and convulsions upon withdrawal. Withdrawal symptoms for addictive behaviours are usually less dramatic. They usually involve psychic discomforts such as anxiety, depression, irritability, guilt, anger, and frustration, with an underlying preoccupation with or craving for another exposure to the behaviour. Withdrawal syndromes range from mild to severe. The severest form of withdrawal syndrome is delirium tremens (DTs), which occurs in approximately 5 percent of alcoholics withdrawing from alcohol.

The Addictive Process

Addiction is a process that evolves over time. It begins when a person repeatedly seeks the illusion of relief to avoid unpleasant feelings or situations. This pattern is known as **nurturing through avoidance** and is a maladaptive way of taking care of emotional needs.[4] As a person becomes increasingly dependent on the addictive behaviour, there is a corresponding deterioration in relationships with family, friends, and co-workers; in performance at work or school; and in personal life. Eventually, addicts do not find the addictive behaviour pleasurable but consider it preferable to the unhappy realities they are seeking to escape.

Signs of Addiction

Although there are different opinions as to the cause of addiction, most experts agree that there are some universal signs of addiction. All addictions are characterized by four common symptoms: (1) **compulsion**, which is characterized by **obsession**, or excessive preoccupation with

Neurotransmitters: Biochemical messengers that exert influence at specific receptor sites on nerve cells.

Tolerance: Phenomenon in which progressively larger dose of a drug or more intense involvement in a behaviour is needed to produce the desired effects.

Nurturing through avoidance: Repeatedly seeking the illusion of relief to avoid unpleasant feelings or situations, a maladaptive way of taking care of emotional needs.

Compulsion: Obsessive preoccupation with a behaviour and an overwhelming need to perform it.

Obsession: Excessive preoccupation with an addictive object or behaviour.

Loss of control: Inability to predict reliably whether any isolated involvement with the addictive object or behaviour will be healthy or damaging.

Native American Rite of Purification

The important role of spiritual health in the treatment of addictions has been clear for most of this century. Alcoholics Anonymous and other 12-step programs rely heavily on spiritual belief to help the addict maintain control. Culturally specific religious beliefs and rituals can also play a role both in the healing process and in gaining acceptance by the addict for the medical portions of therapy.

At the St. Cloud Veterans Hospital, therapists take a novel approach in the treatment of alcoholism among Native Americans. The Native American *onikane,* or sweat lodge, is used in conjunction with the 12 steps of the Alcoholics Anonymous program. The sweat lodge is the setting for a rite of purification that Native Americans believe can purge their past and reunite them with the earth and its goodness.

The sweat lodge itself is a small tent covered with blankets and tarpaulins. A group of five or six Native Americans enter the sweltering tent, followed by a "spiritual advisor"—called a "medicine man" by hospital officials. The spiritual advisor uses a pair of reindeer antlers (only natural objects are allowed in the tent) to rake red-hot rocks into a small pit in the centre of the tent. Pouring water on the rocks, the medicine man transforms the darkened tent into a steamy oven, with temperatures soaring to over 100 degrees.

Participants are first urged to block out impure thoughts and to imagine that they are returning to their mothers' wombs to recall their very first thoughts. If that fails, "impure thoughts" are considered to be blocking their minds. The men remain in the tent for more than two hours, chanting songs in their native tongues, confessing to misdeeds in English, and imploring "the Great Spirit" to help them return to their traditional roots. It is a demanding ordeal.

The ceremony is an attempt to help addicted Native Americans to deal with themselves. It harkens back to tribal traditions and helps them touch base with their heritage. Most importantly, it makes them more receptive to the medical therapy offered in conjunction with the traditional part of the hospital's therapy.

_____

Source: Adapted from Bill McAllister, "At VA Hospital, 'Medicine Man' Helps Indians Try to Beat an Old Nemesis," *Washington Post,* June 9, 1991, A3. © 1991 The Washington Post. Reprinted with permission.

---

the behaviour and an overwhelming need to perform it; (2) **loss of control**, or the inability to predict reliably whether any isolated occurrence of the behaviour will be healthy or damaging; (3) **negative consequences**, such as physical damage, legal trouble, financial problems, academic failure, and family dissolution, which do not occur with healthy involvement in any behaviour; and (4) **denial**, or the inability to perceive that the behaviour is self-destructive. These four components are present in all addictions, whether chemical or behavioural.

Negative consequences: Physical damage, legal trouble, financial ruin, academic failure, family dissolution, and other severe problems associated with addiction.

Denial: Inability to perceive or accurately interpret the effects of the addictive behaviour.

Withdrawal: A series of temporary physical and biopsychosocial symptoms that occurs when the addict abruptly abstains from an addictive chemical or behaviour.

Relapse: The tendency to return to the addictive behaviour after a period of abstinence.

Traditionally, diagnosis of an addiction was limited to drug addiction and was based on three criteria: (1) the presence of an abstinence syndrome, or **withdrawal**; (2) an associated pattern of pathological behaviour (deterioration in work performance, relationships, and social interaction); and (3) **relapse**, the tendency to return to the addictive behaviour after a period of abstinence. Furthermore, until recently, health professionals were unwilling to diagnose an addiction until medical symptoms appeared in the patient. Now we know that although withdrawal, pathological behaviour, relapse, and medical symptoms are valid indicators of addiction, they do not characterize all addictive behaviour.

DRUG DYNAMICS

Have you ever walked into a drugstore looking for some cough syrup or an antacid and become overwhelmed by the number of choices available? Although there are literally tens of thousands of drugs at our disposal, these choices cannot be made lightly. All drugs are chemical substances that have the potential to alter the structure and function of our bodies. Quite simply, any drug use in-

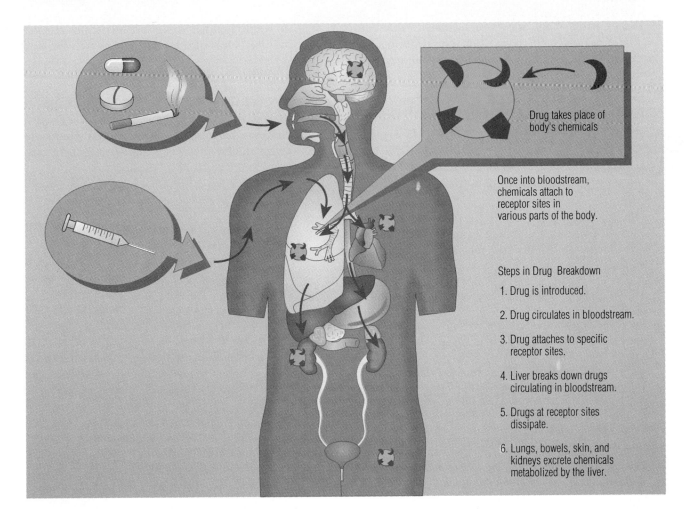

FIGURE 10.1

How the Body Metabolizes Drugs

volves risks. You can best minimize the risks by asking appropriate questions of health care providers and by being an educated consumer of over-the-counter (OTC) drugs.

Drugs work because they physically resemble the chemicals produced naturally within the body (see Figure 10.1). For example, many painkillers resemble the endorphins ("morphine within") that are manufactured in the body. Most bodily processes result from chemical reactions or from changes in electrical charge. Because drugs possess an electrical charge and a chemical structure similar to chemicals that occur naturally in the body, they can affect physical functions in many different ways.

A current explanation of drug actions is the *receptor site* theory, which states that drugs attach themselves to specific **receptor sites** in the body. These sites are specialized cells to which a drug is able to attach because of its size, shape, electrical charge, and chemical properties. Most drugs can attach at multiple receptor sites located throughout the body in such places as the heart and blood system, the lungs, liver, kidneys, brain, and gonads (testi-

cles or ovaries). The physiology of drug activity and its effect on human behaviour is very complex.

Types of Drugs

Drugs may be divided into six categories: prescription drugs, OTC preparations, recreational substances, herbal preparations, illicit drugs, and commercial drugs. Each category includes some drugs that stimulate the body, some that depress body functions, and others that produce hallucinations. Each category also includes **psychoactive drugs**, which have the potential to alter a person's mood or behaviour.

Receptor sites: Specialized cells to which drugs can attach themselves.

Psychoactive drugs: Drugs that have the potential to alter mood or behaviour.

- **Prescription drugs** are those substances that can be obtained only with the written prescription of a licensed physician. Approximately 228 million prescriptions were written in Canada in 1995.

- **Over-the-counter (OTC) drugs** can be purchased in pharmacies, supermarkets, and discount stores without a physician's prescription. Each year, Canadians spend over $85 million on OTC products.[5]

- **Recreational drugs** belong to a somewhat vague category whose boundaries depend upon how people define *recreation*. Generally, drugs in this category contain chemicals used to help people relax or socialize. Most of them are legally sanctioned even though they are psychoactive. Alcohol, tobacco, coffee, tea, and chocolate products are usually included in this category.

- **Herbal preparations** form another vague category. Included among these approximately 750 substances are herbal teas and other products of botanical origin that are believed to have medicinal properties.

- **Illicit (illegal) drugs** are the most notorious substances. Although laws governing their use, possession, cultivation, manufacture, and sale differ from country to country, illicit drugs are generally recognized as harmful. Most of these substances are psychoactive.

- **Commercial preparations** are the most universally used yet least commonly recognized chemical substances having drug action. More than 1000 of these substances exist, including such seemingly benign items as perfumes, cosmetics, household cleansers, paints, glues, inks, dyes, gardening chemicals, pesticides, and industrial by-products.

Routes of Administration of Drugs

Route of administration refers to the way in which a given drug is taken into the body. Common routes are oral ingestion, injection, inhalation, inunction, and suppository.

Oral ingestion is the most common route of administration. Drugs that you swallow include tablets, capsules, and liquids. Oral ingestion of a drug generally results in relatively slow absorption compared to other methods of administration, because the drug must pass through the stomach, where it is acted on by digestive juices, and then move on to the small intestine before it enters the bloodstream.

Many oral preparations are coated to keep them from being dissolved by corrosive stomach acids before they reach the intestine as well as to protect the stomach lining from irritating chemicals in the drugs. If your stomach contains food, absorption will be slower than if your stomach is empty. Some drugs must not be taken with certain foods because the food will inhibit the drug's action. Others must be taken with food to prevent stomach irritation.

Injection, another common form of drug administration, involves the use of a hypodermic syringe to introduce a drug into the body. This method can result in rapid absorption, depending on the type of injection. **Intravenous injection**, or injection directly into a vein, puts the chemical in its most concentrated form directly into the bloodstream. Effects will be felt within three minutes, making this route extremely effective, particularly in medical emergencies. But injection of many substances into the bloodstream may cause serious or even fatal reactions. In addition, some serious diseases, such as hepatitis and HIV infection, can be transferred in this way. For this reason, intravenous injection can be one of the most dangerous routes of administration.

Intramuscular injection results in much slower absorption than intravenous injection. This type of injection places the hypodermic needle into muscular tissue, usually in the buttocks or the back of the upper arm. Normally used to administer antibiotics and vaccinations, this route of administration ensures a slow and consistent dispersion of the drug into the body tissues.

Subcutaneous injection puts the drug into the layer of fat directly beneath the skin. Its common medical uses are

Prescription drugs: Medications that can be obtained only with the written prescription of a licensed physician.

Over-the-counter (OTC) drugs: Medications that can be purchased in pharmacies or supermarkets without a physician's prescription.

Recreational drugs: Legal drugs that contain chemicals that help people to relax or socialize.

Herbal preparations: Substances of plant origin that are believed to have medicinal properties.

Illicit (illegal) drugs: Drugs whose use, possession, cultivation, manufacture, and/or sale are against the law because they are generally recognized as harmful.

Commercial preparations: Commonly used chemical substances including cosmetics, household cleaning products, and industrial by-products.

Route of administration: The manner in which a drug is taken into the body.

Oral ingestion: Intake of drugs through the mouth.

Injection: The introduction of drugs into the body via a hypodermic needle.

Intravenous injection: The introduction of drugs directly into a vein.

Intramuscular injection: The introduction of drugs into muscles.

Subcutaneous injection: The introduction of drugs into the layer of fat directly beneath the skin.

for administration of local anesthetics and for insulin replacement therapy. A drug injected subcutaneously will circulate even more slowly than an intramuscularly injected drug because it takes longer to be absorbed into the bloodstream.

Inhalation refers to administration of drugs through the nostrils. This method transfers the drug rapidly into the bloodstream through the alveoli (air sacs) in the lungs. Some examples of illicit inhalation are cocaine sniffing and the inhalation of aerosol sprays, gases, or fumes from solvents. Effects are frequently noticed immediately after inhalation, but they do not last as long as with the slower routes of administration because only small amounts of a drug can be absorbed and metabolized in the lungs.

Inunction introduces chemicals into the body through the skin. A common example of this method of drug administration is the small adhesive patches that are used to alleviate motion sickness. These patches, which contain a prescription medicine, are applied to the skin behind one ear, where they slowly release their chemicals to provide relief for nauseated travelers. Another example is the nicotine patch.

Suppositories are drugs that are mixed with a waxy medium designed to melt at body temperature. The most common type of suppository is inserted into the anus until it is past the rectal sphincter muscles, which hold it in place. As the wax melts, the drug is released and absorbed through the rectal walls into the bloodstream. Since this area of the anatomy contains many blood vessels, the effects of the drug are usually felt within 15 minutes. Other types of suppositories are for use in the vagina. Vaginal suppositories usually release drugs, such as antifungal agents, that treat problems in the vagina itself as opposed to drugs meant to travel in the bloodstream.

*W*HAT DO YOU THINK?

What types of drugs have you used or experimented with? Why are some drugs administered differently than others?

*D*RUG USE, ABUSE, AND INTERACTIONS

Many people fail to take the time needed to make intelligent decisions when considering the use of a drug. Although drug abuse is usually referred to in connection with illicit and recreational psychoactive drugs, many people abuse and misuse prescription and over-the-counter medications. **Drug misuse** is generally considered to be the use of a drug for a purpose for which it was not intended. For example, using a friend's high-powered prescription painkiller for your headache is a misuse of that drug. This is not too far removed from **drug abuse**, or the excessive use of any drug. The misuse and abuse of drugs may lead to *addiction,* the habitual reliance on a substance or behaviour to produce a desired mood.

There are risks and benefits to the use of any type of chemical substance. Intelligent decision making requires a clear-headed evaluation of these risks and benefits. If, after considering all the facts, you feel that the benefits outweigh the potential problems associated with a particular drug, you may decide to use it. But sometimes unforeseeable reactions or problems arise even after the most careful deliberation.

In order to compare drug risks to benefits, you may want to create a profile for each drug you use or are considering using. A *drug profile* consists of a set of answers to specific questions about a drug. You should identify the chemicals in the drug, receptor sites that will be affected, main effects, side-effects, and any potential adverse reactions.

Individual Response to Psychoactive Drugs: Set and Setting

Individuals differ in how they respond to psychoactive drugs. Two environmental factors that bear on both the main effects and the side-effects of psychoactive drugs are set and setting. **Set** is the total internal environment, or mindset, of a person at the time a drug is taken. Physical, emotional, and social factors work together or against one another to influence the drug's effect on that particular person. Expectations of what the drug will or will not do are also part of the set. For example, a young woman who reads two pages of reported side-effects for a particular drug may experience more side-effects after taking that drug than someone who was not exposed to this information. In other cases, set may be related to the user's

---

Inhalation: The introduction of drugs through the nostrils.

Inunction: The introduction of drugs through the skin.

Suppositories: Mixtures of drugs and a waxy medium designed to melt at body temperature that are inserted into the anus or vagina.

Drug misuse: The use of a drug for a purpose for which it was not intended.

Drug abuse: The excessive use of a drug.

Set: The total internal environment, or mindset, of a person at the time a drug is taken.

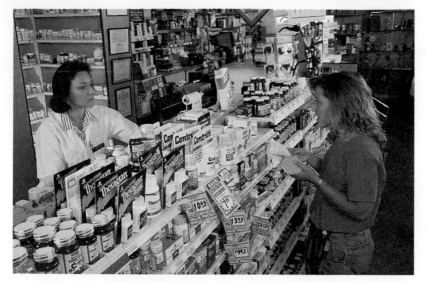

Whenever you take more than one medication at a time, you should consider how the medications will interact. For example, women who rely on oral contraceptives need to understand that dosage instructions must be strictly followed and that medicines such as penicillin can alter the contraceptive's effectiveness. Asking a pharmacist is a good way to learn about drug interactions.

mood. A depressed person using marijuana for a lift may find that the drug actually deepens the depression. Similarly, someone who is already giddy may become even sillier after using the drug. In addition, drugs do not necessarily have the same effect on the elderly.

If set refers to the internal environment, **setting** is the drug user's total external environment. It encompasses both the physical and the social aspects of that environment at the time the person takes the psychoactive drug. If the user is surrounded by wild colours, heavy-metal rock music, and a noisy crowd of people, the drug will generally produce a very different effect than when it is taken in a quiet place with soft music and relaxed company.

Drug Interactions

Sharing medications, using outdated prescriptions, taking higher doses than recommended, or using medications as

---

Setting: The total external environment of a person at the time a drug is taken.

Polydrug use: The use of multiple medications or illicit drugs simultaneously.

Synergism: An interaction of two or more drugs that produces more profound effects than would be expected if the drugs were taken separately.

Antagonism: A type of interaction in which two or more drugs work at the same receptor site.

Inhibition: A type of interaction in which the effects of one drug are eliminated or reduced by the presence of another drug at the receptor site.

Intolerance: A type of interaction in which two or more drugs produce extremely uncomfortable symptoms.

Cross-tolerance: The development of a tolerance to one drug that reduces the effects of another similar drug.

---

a substitute for dealing with personal problems may result in serious health consequences. But so may engaging in **polydrug use:** taking several medications or illegal drugs simultaneously may result in very dangerous problems associated with drug interactions. The most hazardous interactions are synergism, antagonism, inhibition, and intolerance. Hazardous interactions may also occur between drugs and nutrients.

Synergism, also known as potentiation, is an interaction of two or more drugs in which the effects of the individual drugs are multiplied beyond what would normally be expected if they were taken alone. Synergism can be expressed mathematically as: $2 + 2 = 10$.

A synergistic interaction is most likely to occur when *central nervous system depressants* are combined. Included in this category are alcohol, opiates (morphine, heroin), antihistamines (cold remedies), sedative hypnotics (Quaaludes), minor tranquillizers (Valium, Librium, and Xanax), and barbiturates. The worst possible combination is alcohol and barbiturates (sleeping preparations such as Seconal and phenobarbital) because the combination of these depressants leads to a slowdown of the brain centres that normally control vital functions. Respiration, heart rate, and blood pressure can drop to the point of inducing coma and even death.

Prescription drugs carry special labels warning the user not to combine the drug with certain other drugs or with alcohol. Many OTC preparations carry similar warning labels. Because the dangers associated with synergism are so great, you should always verify any possible drug interactions before using a prescribed or OTC drug. Pharmacists, physicians, drug information centres, or community drug education centres can answer your questions. Even if one of the drugs in question is an illegal substance, you should still attempt to determine the dangers involved in combining it with other drugs. Health-care professionals are legally bound to maintain

Asking the Right Questions

At one time or another you will probably use prescriptions or OTC drugs to help restore or maintain your health. How can you be certain that you need a medication in the first place, that you are taking the right medication for you, and that your medication is not robbing you of vital nutrients or being rendered ineffective by other products or foods you are ingesting? Only by asking the right questions of the right people can you be sure. Listed below are 13 questions to pose to your physician, your pharmacist, or yourself before you begin to take any drug.

1. Do you know the diagnosis of your condition?

2. Is your doctor or pharmacist aware of all other drugs that you are taking, both prescription and/or OTC? (Don't forget that birth control pills are drugs.)

3. Do you know the name of the medication you are taking? Is it the chemical name, a generic name, or a brand name?

4. Are you certain of how often you should take the medication, how long you should take it, and in what dosage?

5. Do you know when your medication should be taken in relation to meals?

6. Do you know if you can drink alcohol while on your medication?

7. What are the known side-effects of the medication? What should you do if you experience any of the side-effects?

8. Can you stop taking your medication when you start feeling better, or is it important that you continue taking the drug until the prescription is finished?

9. Do you know what you should do if you forget to take your medication at the scheduled time?

10. Do you know what signs and symptoms signal that you are allergic to the medication?

11. Do you know how and where to store your medication properly?

12. Are there any drug-nutrient interactions that you should be aware of with your medication?

13. Are there any adverse consequences of long-term use of the medication?

---

confidentiality even when they know that a client is using illegal substances. The Building Communication Skills box suggests questions you should ask before taking any drug.

Antagonism, although not usually as serious as synergism, can produce unwanted and unpleasant effects. In an antagonistic reaction, drugs work at the same receptor site so that one drug blocks the action of the other. The "blocking" drug occupies the receptor site, preventing the other drug from attaching, and this creates alterations in absorption and action.

Inhibition is a type of interaction in which the effects of one drug are eliminated or reduced by the presence of another drug at the receptor site. One common inhibitory reaction occurs between antacid tablets and aspirin. The antacid inhibits the absorption of aspirin, making it less effective as a pain reliever. Other inhibitory reactions occur between alcohol and contraceptive pills and between antibiotics and contraceptive pills. Alcohol and antibiotics may diminish the effectiveness of birth control pills in some women.

Intolerance occurs when drugs combine in the body to produce extremely uncomfortable reactions. The drug Antabuse, used to help alcoholics give up alcohol, works by producing this type of interaction. It binds liver enzymes (the chemicals the liver produces to break down alcohol), making it impossible for the body to metabolize alcohol.

As a result, the user of Antabuse who drinks alcohol experiences nausea, vomiting, and, occasionally, fever.

Cross-tolerance occurs when a person develops a physiological tolerance to one drug and shows a similar tolerance to selected other drugs as a result. Taking one drug may actually increase the body's tolerance to another drug. For example, cross-tolerance can develop between alcohol and barbiturates, two depressant drugs.

WHAT DO YOU THINK?

What are common expectations university students have when using drugs? What is the difference between drug abuse and drug misuse? Are people who abuse or misuse drugs addicts?

PRESCRIPTION DRUGS

Even though prescription drugs are administered under medical supervision, the wise consumer still takes precautions. Hazards and complications arising from the use of prescription drugs are common. Responsible decision making about prescription drug use requires the consumer to acquire basic drug knowledge.

Types of Prescription Drugs

Prescription drugs can be divided into dozens of categories. Those of most interest to university students are discussed later; others are explored in the chapters on birth control, infectious diseases and sexually transmitted infections, cancer, and cardiovascular disease. Some of the most common are discussed here.

Antibiotics are drugs used to fight bacterial infection. They may be dispensed by intramuscular injection or in tablet or capsule form. Some, called broad-spectrum antibiotics, are designed to control disease caused by a number of bacterial species. These medications may also kill off helpful bacteria in the body, thus triggering secondary infections. For example, some types of vaginal infections are related to long-term use of antibiotics.

Analgesics are pain relievers. The earliest pain relievers were made of derivatives manufactured from the opium poppy. Today narcotic pain relievers, such as codeine, Demerol (meperidine), and morphine, are the most frequently used type of prescription drugs in Canada. In 1993, 8.2 percent of Canadians aged 15 and older reported using these drugs, with use highest in British Columbia (12.4 percent) and lowest in Quebec (3.2 percent).[6] Most pain relievers work at receptor sites by interrupting pain signals. Some analgesics are available as OTC drugs.

Some analgesics are called **prostaglandin inhibitors**. Prostaglandins are chemicals that resemble hormones and are released by the body in response to pain. When a painful stimulus such as a cut or scrape occurs, nerve cells near the site of the pain release prostaglandins. (Scientists believe that the additional pain caused by the release of prostaglandins signals the body to begin the healing process.) Prostaglandin inhibitors restrain the release of prostaglandins, thereby reducing the pain. The most commonly used prostaglandin inhibitors are ibuprofen (Motrin) and sodium naprosyn (Anaprox). Both are used in prescription strength to relieve arthritis pain and menstrual cramps.

Most analgesics have side-effects, the most common of which is drowsiness due to the depression of the central nervous system. Label warnings are, as usual, important. Some labels caution specifically against driving or operating heavy machinery when using the drug, and most state that analgesics should not be taken with alcohol.

Sedatives are central nervous system depressants that induce sleep and relieve anxiety. Used heavily in the 1950s and 1960s in the form of phenobarbital or Seconal, they gradually fell out of favour because of the risks associated with their use. The potential for addiction is high. Detoxification can be life-threatening and must be medically supervised. Because doctors do not prescribe sedatives as frequently as they did in past decades, users often purchase them illegally.

Tranquillizers are another form of central nervous system depressant. They are classified as major tranquillizers and minor tranquillizers. The most powerful tranquillizers are used in the treatment of major psychiatric illnesses. When used appropriately, these strong sedatives are capable of reducing violent aggressiveness and self-destructive impulses. About 4 percent of Canadians aged 15 and older reported using sleeping pills, and 3.8 percent reported using tranquillizers. Of all of the provinces, Quebec has the highest reported levels of use of sleeping pills (6.1 percent) and tranquillizers (7.4 percent).[7]

Antidepressants are powerful substances used to treat clinically diagnosed cases of depression. These drugs inhibit the release of certain neurotransmitters in the brain, thereby elevating the user's mood.

Amphetamines are stimulants that are prescribed less commonly now than in the past. Like many psychoactive drugs, they are purchased both legally and illegally. Amphetamines suppress appetite and elevate respiration, blood pressure, and pulse rate.

Tolerance to these powerful stimulants develops rapidly, and the user trying to cut down or quit may experience unpleasant **rebound effects.** These severe withdrawal symptoms, peculiar to stimulants, include depression, irritability, violent behaviour, headaches, nausea, and deep fatigue.

Antibiotics: Prescription drugs designed to fight bacterial infection.

Analgesics: Pain relievers.

Prostaglandin inhibitors: Drugs that inhibit the production and release of prostaglandins associated with arthritis or menstrual pain.

Sedatives: Central nervous system depressants that induce sleep and relieve anxiety.

Tranquillizers: Central nervous system depressants that relax the body and calm anxiety.

Antidepressants: Prescription drugs used to treat clinically diagnosed depression.

Amphetamines: Prescription stimulants not commonly used today because of the dangers associated with them.

Rebound effects: Severe withdrawal effects experienced by users of stimulants, including depression, nausea, and violent behaviour.

Generic drugs: Drugs marketed by their chemical name rather than by a brand name.

Use of Generic Drugs

Generic drugs, medications sold under a chemical name rather than under a brand name, have gained popularity in recent years. These alternatives to more expensive brand-name drugs contain the same active ingredients as their brand-name counterparts.

There is some controversy about the effectiveness of some generic drugs because substitutions are often made in minor ingredients and these can affect the way the drug is absorbed, causing discomfort or even an allergic reaction in some users. Therefore, you must note any allergic reactions you have to medications and tell your doctor, who can prescribe an alternative drug. A list of medicines that can be interchanged has been approved in Canada.

If your doctor or pharmacist fails to offer you the option of using a generic drug, you should ask if such a substitute exists and if it would be safe for you to use it.

OVER-THE-COUNTER (OTC) DRUGS

Over-the-counter (OTC) drugs are nonprescription drugs we use in the course of self-diagnosis and self-medication. In an effort to cure themselves, Canadians spend many millions yearly on OTC preparations for relief of everything from runny noses to ingrown toenails. Most OTC drugs are manufactured from a basic group of 1000 chemicals. The many different OTC drugs available to us are produced by combining as few as two and as many as ten substances.

Despite a common belief that OTC products are both safe and effective, indiscriminate use and abuse can occur with these drugs just as with all others. In fact, many OTC drugs have the potential to produce dependency, tolerance, and addiction as well as adverse toxic reactions.

Types of OTC Drugs

Analgesics. Although these pain relievers come in several forms, aspirin and acetaminophen are the two most commonly used ingredients in OTC analgesics.

In 1993, more than two of every three Canadians aged 15 and older (69.8 percent) reported using ASA (acetylsalicylic acid, or aspirin) in the month before the survey. Quebeckers were least likely to use ASA (59.1 percent), and people in Saskatchewan, Prince Edward Island, and Nova Scotia were most likely (about 75 percent each).[8]

ASA relieves pain by inhibiting the body's production of prostaglandins. It brings down fever by increasing the flow of blood to the skin surface, which causes sweating and therefore cooling of the body. ASA has also long been used to reduce the inflammation and swelling of arthritis. Recently it has been discovered that ASA's anticoagulant (interference with blood clotting) effects make it a useful medication for reducing the chances of repeat heart attacks in people who have already had one heart attack.

Despite the fact that ASA has been commonly used as a medication for nearly a century, it is not as harmless as many people think. Possible side-effects include allergic reactions, ringing in the ears, stomach bleeding, and ulcers. Combining ASA with alcohol can compound the drug's gastric irritant properties.

In addition, research has linked ASA to a potentially fatal condition called Reye's syndrome. Children, teenagers, and young adults (up to age 25) who are treated with ASA while recovering from the flu or chicken pox are at risk for developing the syndrome. ASA substitutes are recommended for people in these age groups.

Acetaminophen is an ASA substitute found in Tylenol and related medications. Like ASA, acetaminophen is an effective analgesic and antipyretic (fever-reducing drug). It does not, however, provide relief from inflamed or swollen joints. The side-effects associated with acetaminophen are generally minimal, though overdose can cause liver damage.

Cold, Cough, Allergy, and Asthma Relievers. These substances are popular OTC remedies for the symptoms that affect millions of sufferers. The operative word in their titles is *reliever*. Most of these medications are designed to alleviate some or all of the discomforting symptoms associated with these upper-respiratory-tract maladies. Unfortunately, no drugs exist to cure the actual diseases. The drugs available provide only temporary relief until the sufferer's immune system prevails over the disease. Aspirin or acetaminophen is used in some cold preparations, as are several other ingredients. The basic types of OTC cold, cough, and allergy relievers are:

- *Expectorants.* These drugs are formulated to loosen phlegm, allowing the user to cough it up and clear congested respiratory passages. Reviewers have found no expectorants to be both safe and effective.

- *Antitussives.* These OTC drugs are used to calm or curtail the cough reflex. They are most effective when the cough is "dry," or does not produce phlegm.

- *Antihistamines.* These are central nervous system depressants that dry runny noses, clear postnasal drip, clear sinus congestion, and reduce tears.

- *Decongestants.* These remedies are designed to reduce nasal stuffiness due to colds.

- *Anticholinergics.* These substances are often added to cold preparations to reduce nasal secretions and tears. Some cold compounds contain alcohol in concentrations that may exceed 40 percent.

Stimulants. Nonprescription stimulants are sometimes used by university students who have neglected assignments and other obligations until the last minute. The active ingredient in OTC stimulants is caffeine (see Chapter 11). It acts to heighten wakefulness, increase alertness, and relieve fatigue.

Sleeping Aids and Relaxants. These drugs are often used to induce the drowsy feelings that precede sleep. The principal ingredient in OTC sleeping aids is an antihistamine called pyrilamine maleate. Chronic reliance on sleeping aids may lead to addiction; people accustomed to using these products may find it impossible to sleep without them.

Dieting Aids. Many drugs designed to help people lose weight are available over the counter. Some of these drugs are advertised as "appetite suppressants." Their active chemical is phenylpropanolamine. Its stimulant effects can cause dangerous reactions in people suffering from diabetes or heart or thyroid ailments.

Phenylpropanolamine is a **sympathomimetic**, a drug that affects the sympathetic nervous system, causing reactions similar to those we experience when we are angry or excited. These reactions include a dry mouth and a lack of appetite.

Most manufacturers of appetite suppressants include a written diet to complement their drug. The majority of these diets contain 1200 calories. On this number of calo-ries, most people will lose weight without appetite suppressants.

Some people rely on **laxatives** and **diuretics** ("water pills") to aid weight reduction. Frequent use of laxatives to aid weight loss disrupts the body's natural elimination patterns and may cause constipation or even obstipation (inability to have a bowel movement). The use of laxatives to produce weight loss has generally unspectacular results and can rob the body of needed fluids, salts, and minerals.

Use of diuretics as part of a weight-loss plan is also dangerous. Not only will the user gain the weight back upon drinking fluids, but diuretic use may contribute to dangerous chemical imbalances. The potassium and sodium eliminated by diuretics play important roles in maintaining electrolyte balance. Depletion of these vital minerals may cause weakness, dizziness, fatigue, and sometimes death. (See Table 10.1 for a description of possible side-effects of OTC drugs.)

TABLE 10.1 ■ Some Side-Effects of OTC Drugs

Drug	Possible Hazards
Acetaminophen	• Bloody urine, painful urination, skin rash, bleeding and bruising, yellowing of the eyes or skin (even for normal doses) • Difficulty in diagnosing overdose because reaction may be delayed up to a week • Severe liver damage and death (for dose of about 50 tablets) • Liver damage from chronic low-level use
Antacids	• Reduced mineral absorption from food • Possible concealment of ulcer • Reduction of effectiveness for anticlotting medications • Prevention of certain antibiotics' functioning (for antacids that contain aluminum) • Worsening of high blood pressure (for antacids that contain sodium) • Aggravation of kidney problems
ASA	• Stomach upset and vomiting, stomach bleeding, worsening of ulcers • Enhancement of the action of anticlotting medications • Potentiation of hearing damage from loud noise • Severe allergic reaction • Association with Reye's syndrome in children and teenagers • Prolonged bleeding time (when combined with alcohol)
Cold medications	• Loss of consciousness (if taken with prescription tranquillizers)
Diet pills, caffeine, decongestants	• Organ damage or death from cerebral hemorrhage
Ibuprofen	• Allergic reaction in some people with aspirin allergy • Fluid retention or edema • Liver damage similar to that from acetaminophen • Enhancement of action of anticlotting medications • Digestive disturbances (half as often as with ASA)
Laxatives	• Reduced absorption of minerals from food • Creation of dependency
Toothache medications	• Destruction of the still-healthy part of a damaged tooth (for medications that contain clove oil)

ILLICIT DRUGS

Illicit drug abuse is a problem in our society. We need to understand how these drugs work and why people use them. The drug problem touches us all. While some people become addicted to prescription drugs and painkillers, we focus our attention here on **illicit drugs**—those drugs that are illegal to possess, produce, or sell.

On June 19, 1996, the Senate passed Bill C-8, the Controlled Drugs and Substances Act. The Act came into force on May 14, 1997. It replaces Canada's main laws on illicit drugs—the Narcotic Control Act and parts of the Food and Drugs Act.

The Controlled Drugs and Substances Act significantly expands the reach of Canada's drug laws and continues Canada's heavy reliance on a failed policy of criminal prohibition.[9]

Illicit drug users come from all walks of life. Not all illicit drug use occurs in dilapidated crack houses and not all users fit the stereotype of the crazed junkie.

The reasons for using drugs vary from one situation to another and from one person to another. A person's age, gender, genetic background, physiology, personality, experiences, and expectations are all factors.

The 1997 Canadian profile found that 23.1 percent of respondents had used cannabis at some point and 7.4 percent are current users; 3.8 percent had used cocaine, and 5.9 percent had used LSD, speed (amphetamines), or heroin at some point. Altogether, an estimated 23.9 percent of the population have used illicit drugs at some point; 7.7 percent are current users.[10] In particular, the proportion of students using LSD has more than doubled since 1988, from 3.2 per cent to 7 percent. Heroin use increased from 0.3 per cent in 1988 to 1.1 per cent in 1993. Use of anabolic steroids, which were almost unknown at the time of the first survey, increased from 0.6 per cent in 1988 to 1.5 per cent in 1993. Over the same period, however, use of powdered cocaine, cannabis, non-prescription stimulants, and prescription tranquillizers declined significantly.[11] Cocaine use increased from 0.3 percent in 1993 to 0.7 percent in 1994, and the proportion of people who report using LSD, heroin, or speed in the prior year increased from 0.3 percent in 1993 to 1.1 percent in 1994.[12]

Why is illicit drug use increasing after such a long period of decline? There is no clear answer. Rebellion against a decade of postwar materialism and conservative thinking fuelled the drug revolution of the 1960s. Today's economic despair, collapse of the family and community, and a general sense of hopelessness may be even more powerful engines of abuse, particularly when combined with greater availability and variety of drugs than we could have imagined 30 years ago, and, some have argued, more liberal parental attitudes.

Social policy also affects drug use, although its effects are extremely hard to measure and evaluate. We can observe that drug use declined significantly during the first five years of Canada's Drug Strategy, when the focus was on the general public. It started rising again during Phase II, when the focus shifted to street youth and high-risk groups. The resurgence of drug use we are now witnessing is led largely by mainstream youth, indicating that we may be paying a heavy price for changing our focus and neglecting this group in Phase II. Ultimately we must aim our prevention messages at all youth. According to the Canadian Centre on Substance Abuse, all young people, dropouts and A students alike, are vulnerable to drug use and should be viewed as an at-risk population.[13]

Antidrug programs have been developed to deal with the problems of illegal drug use. The major drawback of most of these programs is their failure to take a multidimensional approach. The tendency has been to focus on only one aspect of drug abuse rather than to examine all factors that contribute to the problem. For example, many programs consider the drugs themselves the culprits. Others oversimplify the problem by exhorting potential users to "just say no," ignoring the fact that drugs are an integral part of many people's social or cultural lives. The pressures to take drugs are often tremendous, and the reasons for using them are complex.

People who develop drug problems generally begin with the belief that they can control their drug use. Initially, they often view drug taking as a fun and controllable pastime. Peer influence is a strong motivator, especially among adolescents, who greatly fear not being accepted as part of the group. Other people use drugs to cope with feelings of worthlessness and despair or to battle depression and anxiety. Drugs are seen as the quick answer to life's difficulties in our society. Since the majority of illegal drugs produce physical and psychological dependence, the idea that a person can use these substances regularly without becoming addicted is foolish. To find out if you are controlled by drugs, see the Rate Yourself box.

Canada's Drug Strategy, launched in 1987 and renewed in 1992, closed on March 31, 1997. Health programming developed under the Strategy merged with many other

Sympathomimetics: Drugs found in appetite suppressants that affect the sympathetic nervous system.

Laxatives: Medications used to soften stool and relieve constipation.

Diuretics: Drugs that increase the excretion of urine from the body.

Illicit drugs: Drugs that are illegal to possess, produce, or sell.

Older Canadians and Medications

Drug use, and possible attendant problems, present a somewhat different picture among seniors than among the Canadian population as a whole.

Medication Use

- Use of medications, including psychoactive drugs such as tranquillizers and sleeping pills, is higher among older Canadians than younger Canadians.

- Use of medications is higher among older women than older men. Among young seniors (55–64), 5 percent report using sleeping pills in the month prior to the survey, in comparison with 11 percent of older seniors (65 years and over).

- Tranquillizers are used by 6 percent of younger seniors and 5 percent of older seniors.

- A prescription or non-prescription pain reliever was the most frequently reported medication used by older Canadians. In the month prior to the survey, 53 percent of women and 49 percent of men reported using at least one pain reliever.

- Multiple drug use (three or more drugs) was most common among seniors who reported that their lives were stressful, that their health was poor, or that they lacked the support of family and friends.

- Among older adults, 12–14 percent report experiencing the effects of medications. Seniors may be more vulnerable to adverse drug reactions because of many factors, including an increased sensitivity to drugs and an increase in the number of drugs used.

Other Drugs

- Less than 1 percent of seniors report using illegal drugs such as marijuana, cocaine, and heroin.

- Currently, 31 percent of young seniors and 19 percent of older seniors smoke.

- Older women are less likely to smoke than men. Seventy-five percent of men versus 33 percent of women over 65 smoked in the past or are current smokers.

Source: Health Canada, *Seniors and Medication, Alcohol, and Other Drugs.*

health and social issues under the label of population health. It is not clear what priority drug and alcohol programs will be given within this new framework, or what level of funding they will receive. Current indications are that they will be severely cut back.[14]

WHAT DO YOU THINK?

Would you change any of the current laws governing drugs? If so, what would you consider legitimate and illegitimate use of a drug? What types of changes do you think are needed to help reduce the level of substance abuse in Canada?

Cocaine: A powerful stimulant drug made from the leaves of the South American coca shrub.

CONTROLLED SUBSTANCES

Hundreds of illegal drugs exist. For general purposes, they can be divided into five representative categories: stimulants, like cocaine; marijuana and its derivatives; depressants, like the opiates; psychedelics and deliriants; and so-called designer drugs.

Cocaine

Cocaine is a crystalline white alkaloid powder derived from the leaves of the South American coca shrub (not related to cocoa plants). The leaves had been chewed exclusively for their stimulant effects for thousands of years by the Incas and their descendants until 1860, when a German pharmacology graduate student "invented" cocaine. Despite a few chemical similarities to less potent stimulants, such as those found in coffee and tea, cocaine is very dangerous and cannot be compared with these substances.

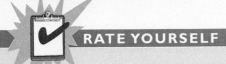

Recognizing a Drug Problem

Are You Controlled by Drugs?

How do you know whether you are chemically dependent? A dependent person can't stop using drugs. This abuse hurts the user and everyone around him or her. Take the following assessment. The more "yes" checks you make, the more likely you have a problem.

Yes	No	
☐	☐	Do you use drugs to handle stress or escape from life's problems?
☐	☐	Have you unsuccessfully tried to cut down or quit using your drug?
☐	☐	Have you ever been in trouble with the law or been arrested because of your drug use?
☐	☐	Do you think a party or social gathering isn't fun unless drugs are available?
☐	☐	Do you avoid people or places that do not support your usage?
☐	☐	Do you neglect your responsibilities because you'd rather use your drug?
☐	☐	Have your friends, family, or employer expressed concern about your drug use?
☐	☐	Do you do things under the influence of drugs that you would not normally do?
☐	☐	Have you seriously thought that you might have a chemical dependency problem?

Are You Controlled by a Drug User?

Is your life controlled by a chemical abuser? Your love and care (codependency) may actually be enabling the chemical abuser to continue the abuse, hurting you and others. Try this assessment; the more "yes" checks you make, the more likely there's a problem.

Yes	No	
☐	☐	Do you often have to lie or cover up for the chemical abuser?
☐	☐	Do you spend time counseling the person about the problem?
☐	☐	Have you taken on additional financial or family responsibilities?
☐	☐	Do you feel that you have to control the chemical abuser's behavior?
☐	☐	At the office, have you done work or attended meetings for the abuser?
☐	☐	Do you often put your own needs and desires after the user's?
☐	☐	Do you spend time each day worrying about your situation?
☐	☐	Do you analyze your behavior to find clues to how it might affect the chemical abuser?
☐	☐	Do you feel powerless and at your wit's end about the abuser's problem?

Source: Reprinted by permission of Krames Communications, 1100 Grundy Lane, San Bruno, CA 94066–3030.

Cocaine is generally sold on the street as a hydrochloride salt—a fine, white crystalline powder known as coke, C, snow, flake, or blow. Street dealers dilute it with inert (non-psychoactive) but similar-looking substances such as cornstarch, talcum powder, and sugar, or with active drugs such as procaine and benzocaine (used as local anesthetics), or other central nervous system (CNS) stimulants such as amphetamines. Nevertheless, illicit cocaine has actually become purer over the years; according to RCMP figures, in 1988 its purity averaged about 75 percent.[15]

According to the 1997 Canadian Profile, 3.8 percent of the population used cocaine at some point and 1.4 percent are regular users.[16]

Cocaine can affect mood, judgement, and motor skills. The most dramatic effects of cocaine with respect to driving are on vision. Cocaine may cause a higher sensitivity to light, halos around bright objects, and difficulty focussing. Users have also reported blurred vision, glare problems, and hallucinations, particularly "snow lights"— weak flashes or movements of light in the peripheral field of vision, which tend to make drivers swerve toward or away from the lights. Some users have also reported auditory hallucinations (e.g., ringing bells) and olfactory hallucinations (e.g., smell of smoke or gasoline).

Many users say that cocaine actually improves their driving ability, which is not surprising because the drug induces euphoria and feelings of increased mental and physical abilities. Such self-reports must be accepted with caution, however, since these effects of cocaine are short-lived and are often followed by fatigue and lassitude.

Cocaine can also heighten irritability, excitability, and startle response. Users have reported that sudden sounds, such as horns or sirens, have caused them severe anxiety coupled with rapid steering or braking reactions, even when the source of the sound was not in the immediate vicinity of their vehicles. Suspiciousness, distrust, and paranoia—other reactions to cocaine—have prompted users to flee in their cars or drive evasively. Everyone surveyed reported attention lapses while driving and ignoring relevant stimuli such as changes in traffic signals.[17]

Methods of Cocaine Use.   Cocaine can be taken in several ways. The powdered form of the drug is "snorted" through the nose. Smoking (freebasing) and intravenous injections are more dangerous means of ingesting cocaine.

When cocaine is snorted, it can cause both damage to the mucous membranes in the nose and sinusitis. It can destroy the user's sense of smell, and occasionally it even creates a hole in the septum. Smoking cocaine can cause lung and liver damage. Freebasing has become more popular than injecting in recent years because people fear contracting diseases such as AIDS and hepatitis by sharing contaminated needles. But freebasing involves other dangers. Because the volatile mixes it requires are very explosive, some people have been killed or seriously burned.

Many cocaine users still occasionally "shoot up." Injecting allows the user to introduce large amounts of cocaine into the body rapidly. Within seconds, there is an incredible sense of euphoria. This intense high lasts only 15 to 20 minutes, and then the user heads into a "crash." To prevent the unpleasant effects of the crash, users must shoot up frequently, which can severely damage their veins. Besides AIDS and hepatitis, injecting users place themselves at risk for skin infections, inflammation of the arteries, and infection of the lining of the heart.

Physical Effects of Cocaine.   The effects of cocaine are felt rapidly. Snorted cocaine enters the bloodstream through the lungs in less than one minute and reaches the brain in less than three minutes. When cocaine binds at its receptor sites in the central nervous system, it produces intense pleasure. The euphoria quickly abates, however, and the desire to regain the pleasurable feelings makes the user want more cocaine.

Cocaine is both an anesthetic and a central nervous system stimulant. In tiny doses, it can slow heart rate. In larger doses, the physical effects are dramatic: increased heart rate and blood pressure, loss of appetite that can lead to dramatic weight loss, convulsions, muscle twitching, irregular heartbeat, even eventual death due to overdose. Other effects of cocaine include temporary relief of depression, decreased fatigue, talkativeness, increased alertness, and heightened self-confidence. Again, however, as the dose increases, users become irritable and apprehensive and their behaviour may turn paranoid or violent.

Cocaine-Affected Babies.   Because cocaine rapidly crosses the placenta (as virtually all drugs do), the foetus is vulnerable when a pregnant women snorts or shoots up. The most threatening problem during pregnancy is the increased risk of a miscarriage.

Many cocaine-exposed babies are born with brain damage, heart defects, kidney problems, and malformed heads, arms, and fingers. They tend to show signs of withdrawal at birth, including irritability, jitteriness, and the inability to eat or sleep properly. They seem to be unable to respond or to relate to people the way normal babies do, and they are difficult to console and comfort. Because it is so difficult for adults to interact with them, their social and emotional development is negatively affected.

Freebase Cocaine.   Freebase is a form of cocaine that is more powerful and costly than the powder or chip (crack) form. Street cocaine (cocaine hydrochloride) is converted to pure base by removing the hydrochloride salt and many of the "cutting agents." The end product, freebase, is smoked through a water pipe.

Because freebase cocaine reaches the brain within seconds, it is more dangerous than cocaine that is snorted. It produces a quick, intense high that disappears quickly, leaving an intense craving for more. Freebasers typically increase the amount and frequency of the dose. They often become severely addicted and experience serious health problems and financial ruin.[18]

Side-effects of freebasing cocaine include weight loss, increased heart rate and blood pressure, depression, paranoia, and hallucinations. Freebase is an extremely dangerous drug and is responsible for a large number of cocaine-related hospital emergency-room visits and deaths.

Crack.   Crack is the street name given to freebase cocaine that has been processed from cocaine hydrochloride using ammonia or sodium bicarbonate (baking soda) and water and heating the substance to remove the hydrochloride. Crack can also be processed with ether, but this is much riskier because ether is a flammable solvent.

The mixture (90-percent-pure cocaine) is then dried. The soapy-looking substance that results can be broken up into "rocks" and smoked. These rocks are approximately five times as strong as cocaine. Crack gets its name from the popping noises it makes when burned.

Freebase: The most powerful distillate of cocaine.

Crack: A distillate of powdered cocaine that comes in small, hard "chips" or "rocks."

A crack user may quickly become addicted to the drug. Addiction is accelerated by the speed at which crack is absorbed through the lungs (it hits the brain within seconds after use) and by the intensity of the high. It is not uncommon for crack addicts to spend over $1000 a day on their habits.

Cocaine Addiction and Society. Cocaine addicts often suffer both physiological damage and serious disruptions of their lifestyle, including loss of employment and self-esteem.

Amphetamines

The amphetamines include a large and varied group of synthetic agents that stimulate the central nervous system. Small doses of amphetamines improve alertness, lessen fatigue, and generally elevate mood. With repeated use, however, physical and psychological dependence develops. Sleep patterns are affected (insomnia); heart rate, breathing rate, and blood pressure increase; restlessness, anxiety, appetite suppression, and vision problems are common. High doses over long time periods can produce hallucinations, delusions, and disorganized behaviour. Abusers become paranoid, fearing everything and everyone. Some become very aggressive or antisocial.

Amphetamines for recreational use are sold under a variety of names. "Bennies" (amphetamine/Benzedrine), "dex" (dextroamphetamine/Dexedrine), and "meth" or "speed" (methamphetamine/Methedrine) are some of the most common. Other street terms for amphetamines are "cross tops," "crank," "uppers," "wake-ups," "lid poppers," "cartwheels," and "blackies." Amphetamines do have therapeutic uses (see Chapter 2) in the treatment of attention deficit-hyperactivity disorder in children (Ritalin, Cylert) and of obesity (Pondimin).

Newer-Generation Stimulants

Illicit stimulants such as **crank** and **ice** have created further concerns because their effects last considerably longer than those produced by crack and cocaine. The elevated mood and excitability caused by crank, an amphetamine-like stimulant, last from two to four hours. For this reason, crank is becoming more and more popular among people whose occupations require long periods of wakefulness, such as truck drivers.

Ice is an even more potent stimulant that has begun to gain popularity.[19] Called *shabu* by the Japanese and *hiroppon* by the Koreans, ice can be manufactured in the laboratory using easily obtained chemicals. Purer and more crystalline than crank, most ice comes from Asia, particularly South Korea and Taiwan. Because it is odourless, public use of ice often goes unnoticed.

Typically, ice quickly becomes addictive. Some users have reported severe cravings after using the drug only once. Addicts call the sensation from smoking ice *amping*, for the amplified euphoria it gives them. However, as is true of other *methamphetamines* (sympathetic nervous system stimulants), the "down" side of this drug can be devastating. Prolonged use can cause fatal lung and kidney damage as well as long-lasting psychological damage. In some instances, major psychological dysfunction has lasted as long as two and a half years after last use. Aggressive behaviour is also associated with the drug's use, as evidenced by the dramatic increase in the number of ice-related violent crimes.[20] The number of babies born severely addicted to the drug is also increasing at an alarming rate.

Marijuana

Although archaeological evidence documents **marijuana** ("grass," "weed," "pot") use as far back as 6000 years ago, the drug did not become popular in North America until the 1960s. Marijuana receives less media attention today than it did then, but it is still the most extensively used illicit drug by far.

Physical Effects of Marijuana. Marijuana is derived from either the cannabis sativa or cannabis indica (hemp) plants. Today's top-grade cannabis packs a punch very similar to hashish. **Tetrahydrocannabinol (THC)** is the psychoactive substance in marijuana, and the key to determining how powerful a high the marijuana will produce.

Crank: An amphetamine-like stimulant having effects that last longer than those of crack or cocaine.

Ice: A potent, inexpensive stimulant that has long-lasting effects.

Marijuana: Chopped leaves and flowers of the cannabis indica or cannabis sativa plant (hemp); a psychoactive stimulant that intensifies reactions to environmental stimuli.

Tetrahydrocannabinol (THC): The chemical name for the active ingredient in marijuana.

Whereas marijuana from two decades ago ranged in potency from 1 to 5 percent THC, today's crop averages 8 percent, although concentrations as high as 15 percent may be found.

Hashish, a potent cannabis preparation derived mainly from the thick, sticky resin of the plant, contains high concentrations of THC. Hash oil, a substance produced by percolating a solvent such as ether through dried marijuana to extract the THC, is a tarry liquid that may contain up to 70 percent THC.

Marijuana has been brewed and drunk in tea and baked into quick breads or brownies. THC concentrations in such products are impossible to estimate. Most of the time, however, marijuana is rolled into cigarettes (joints) or packed firmly into a pipe. Some people smoke marijuana through water pipes called bongs. Effects are generally felt within 10 to 30 minutes and usually wear off within three hours.

The most noticeable effect of THC is the dilation of the eyes' blood vessels, which produces the characteristic bloodshot eyes. Smokers of the drug also exhibit coughing, dry mouth and throat ("cotton mouth"), increased thirst and appetite, lowered blood pressure, and mild muscular weakness, primarily exhibited in drooping eyelids. Those users who take a high dose in an unfamiliar or uncomfortable setting are more likely to experience anxiety and the paranoid belief that their companions are ridiculing or threatening them.

Effects of Chronic Marijuana Use. Because the use of marijuana is illegal, and because the drug has only been widely used since the 1960s, long-term studies of its effects are difficult to conduct. Also, studies conducted in the 1960s involved marijuana with THC levels that were only a fraction of the levels found in plants today. Thus the results of these studies may not be relevant to the more toxic forms of the drug presently in use. Most of the current information gathered about chronic marijuana use has been obtained from countries such as Jamaica and Costa Rica, where the drug is not illegal. These studies of chronic users (people who have used the drug for 10 or more years) indicate that long-term use of marijuana causes lung damage comparable to that caused by tobacco smoking. Smoking a single joint may be as damaging to

the lungs as smoking five tobacco cigarettes. The chemicals do not damage the heart, but the effects of inhaling burning material do. Inhalation of marijuana transfers carbon monoxide to the bloodstream. Because the blood has a greater affinity for carbon monoxide than it does for oxygen, the oxygen-carrying capacity of the blood is diminished. The heart must then work harder to pump the vital element to oxygen-starved tissues.

Other suspected risks associated with marijuana include suppression of the immune system, blood pressure changes, and impaired memory function. Recent studies suggest that pregnant women who smoke marijuana are at a higher risk for stillbirth or miscarriage and for delivering low-birthweight babies and babies with abnormalities of the nervous system. Babies born to women who use marijuana during pregnancy are five times more likely to have features similar to those exhibited by children with foetal alcohol syndrome.

Debates concerning the effects of marijuana on the reproductive system have yet to be resolved. Studies conducted in the mid-1970s suggested that marijuana inhibited testosterone (and thus sperm) production in males and caused chromosomal breakage in both ova and sperm. Subsequent research in these areas is inconclusive. The question of whether the high-level THC plants currently available will increase the risks associated with this drug is, as yet, unanswered.

Marijuana and Medicine. Marijuana has at least two medical purposes. It has been used to help control the side-effects, such as severe nausea, produced by chemotherapy (chemical treatment for cancer). Some reports claim that marijuana also reduces the pressure in the eyeball caused by glaucoma (a progressive disease characterized by increased fluid pressure in the eyeball).

Marijuana and Driving. Marijuana use presents clear hazards for drivers of motor vehicles as well as for others on the road. The drug substantially reduces a driver's ability to react and to make quick decisions.

Opiates

The opiates are among the oldest analgesics known to humans. These drugs cause drowsiness, relieve pain, and induce euphoria. Also called **narcotics,** they are derived from the parent drug **opium,** a dark, resinous substance made from the milky juice of the opium poppy. Other opiates include *morphine, codeine, heroin,* and *black tar heroin.*

The word *narcotic* comes from the Greek word for "stupor" and is generally used to describe sleep-inducing substances. For many years, opiates were widely used by the medical community to relieve pain, induce sleep, curb nausea and vomiting, stop diarrhea, and sedate psychiatric patients. During the late nineteenth and early twentieth centuries, many patent medicines contained opiates.

Hashish: The sticky resin of the cannabis plant, which is high in THC.

Narcotics: Drugs that induce sleep and relieve pain; primarily the opiates.

Opium: The parent drug of the opiates; made from the milky juice of the opium poppy.

Battling Addictions

For individuals shackled by an addiction, the road to recovery is a process that begins with recognition of a problem. Recognition is one of the most difficult steps in the process due to individual levels of denial. Denial, or the inability to see the truth, is the hallmark of addiction. It can be so powerful that intervention sometimes may be necessary to break down the addict's denial system. Intervention is a planned process of confrontation by significant others. Its purpose is to break down the denial compassionately so that the addict can see the destructive nature of the addiction. The addict must come to perceive that the addiction is destructive and requires treatment. Once this has been accomplished, treatment and recovery can begin.

Treatment and recovery for any addiction begin with abstinence—refraining from the addictive behaviour. But abstinence does little to change the personality and psychological dynamics or the biological and environmental influences behind the addictive behaviour. Without a recovery, an addict is apt to relapse time and again or simply to change addictions. Recovery involves learning new ways of looking at oneself, others, and the world. It may require exploration of a traumatic past so that psychological wounds can be healed. It requires new ways of taking care of oneself, physically and emotionally. It involves developing communication skills and new ways of having fun. Recovery programs are the fuel that gives addicts the energy to resist relapsing. For a large number of addicts, recovery begins with a period of formal treatment. A good treatment program should have the following characteristics:

- professional staff familiar with the specific addictive disorder for which help is being sought
- a flexible schedule of both inpatient and outpatient services
- access to medical personnel who can assess the addict's medical status and provide treatment for all medical concerns as needed
- medical supervision of addicts who are at high risk for a complicated detoxification
- involvement of family members in the treatment process
- a team approach to treatment of the addictive disorders (e.g., medical personnel, counsellors, psychotherapists, social workers, clergy, educators, dietitians, and fitness counsellors)
- both group and individual therapy options
- integration of peer-led support groups into its programs and encouragement of the addict to continue involvement after treatment ends
- structured after-care and relapse-prevention programs
- a clean and attractive environment
- a cordial and helping staff

Highly structured treatment programs help their clients get started on a lifetime program of personal recovery. They include wellness programs to teach critical self-care skills, educational programs to formulate a deep understanding of the addiction, self-help groups to provide a foundation of support after treatment, and several forms of therapy, including those listed below.

Individual Therapy. Therapy in the company of a trained addictions specialist provides a safe environment in which recovering addicts can identify and experience feelings they have been chronically medicating with their addictive behaviour. During sessions, addicts begin to deal with issues related to their addiction.

Group Therapy. Group therapy is a safe environment in which to relearn relationship skills that were lost during addiction or that were never developed. A critical skill developed in group therapy is learning how to give and receive feedback. The group provides an opportunity for developing communication skills and offers an environment where addicts learn how to be honest with themselves and others. The standard care in a treatment program is to combine group therapy with individual therapy.

Family Therapy. Addiction inevitably affects the addict's entire family. If the family receives no attention during the addict's recovery process, family members will continue to function as codependents because that's all they know. Family therapy helps all members of the family to recover.

12-Step Programs. One of the most common types of peer support groups is a 12-step program, patterned after Alcoholics Anonymous. Such programs use a series of 12 steps to guide individuals through a process of personal growth. They are designed to keep addicts free of their addictions through honest acknowledgement of their shortcomings and through the mutual support of others who have had similar experiences. There are 12-step programs for every addiction, as well as for families and others who have a relationship with an addict.

Alternatives to 12-Step Programs. Because many 12-step programs adhere to a spiritual basis in the recovery process, some recovering addicts have sought out or started alternative groups.

Recovery is an ongoing process that must continue after an individual leaves any formal treatment program. Ideally, all recovering addicts develop personal recovery programs that they follow indefinitely. Such programs may involve self-help and reeducation programs. Many continue on with therapy and attend meetings of peer groups dealing with similar addictions. Good treatment facilities integrate many of these maintenance programs into their treatment plans to reinforce long-term recovery.

Suppliers advertised these concoctions as cures for everything from menstrual cramps to teething pains.

Among the opiates once widely used by medical practitioners was **morphine.** First manufactured in the early nineteenth century, morphine was named after Morpheus, the Greek god of sleep, and is more powerful than opium. Codeine, a less powerful analgesic derived from morphine, also became popular.

As opiate use became more common, physicians noted that patients tended to become dependent on these substances. Contrary to earlier belief, all of the opiates are highly addictive. Growing concern about addiction led to government controls of narcotic use. Subsequent legislation required physicians prescribing opiates to keep careful records. Physicians are still subject to audits of their prescriptions of these agents.

Some of the opiates are still used today for medical purposes. Morphine is sometimes prescribed by doctors in hospital settings for relief of severe pain. **Codeine** is found in prescription cough syrups and in other painkillers. Several prescription drugs, including Percodan, Demerol, and Dilaudid, contain synthetic opiates. All opiate use is strictly regulated.

Physical Effects of Opiates. Opiates are powerful central nervous system depressants. In addition to relieving pain, these drugs lower heart rate, respiration, and blood pressure. Side-effects include weakness, dizziness, nausea, vomiting, euphoria, decreased sex drive, visual disturbances, and lack of coordination. Of all the opiates, heroin is the most notorious. Because all opiate addiction follows a similar progression, we will use heroin as a model for narcotic abuse.

Heroin Addiction. **Heroin** and **black tar heroin** are powerful opiates. Heroin is a white powder derived from morphine. Black tar heroin is a sticky, dark brown, foul-smelling substance, also made from morphine.

Once considered a cure for morphine dependency, heroin was later discovered to be even more addictive and potent than morphine.

Morphine: A derivative of opium; sometimes used by medical practitioners to relieve pain.

Codeine: A drug derived from morphine; used in cough syrups and certain painkillers.

Heroin: An illegally manufactured derivative of morphine, usually injected into the bloodstream.

Black tar heroin: A dark brown, sticky substance made from morphine.

Methadone maintenance: A treatment for people addicted to opiates that substitutes methadone, a synthetic narcotic, for the opiate of addiction.

Heroin is a depressant. It produces a dreamy, mentally slow feeling and drowsiness in the user. In addition to its depressant effects, it can cause drastic mood swings in some users, with euphoric highs followed by depressive lows. Heroin also slows respiration and urinary output and constricts the pupils of the eyes. In fact, pupil constriction is a classic sign of narcotic intoxication; hence the image of the stereotypical drug user hiding his eyes behind a pair of dark sunglasses. Symptoms of tolerance and withdrawal can appear within three weeks of the first use of the drug.

The most common route of administration for heroin addicts is "mainlining"—intravenous injection of powdered heroin mixed in a solution—though fear of HIV infection has induced some people to avoid needles. Many users describe the "rush" they feel when injecting themselves as intensely pleasurable, whereas others report unpredictable and unpleasant side-effects. The temporary nature of the rush contributes to the drug's high potential for addiction—many addicts shoot up four or five times a day. Mainlining can cause veins to become scarred, and if this practice is frequent enough, the veins collapse. Once a vein has collapsed, it can no longer be used to introduce heroin into the bloodstream. Addicts become expert at locating new veins to use: in the feet, the legs, even the temples. When they do not want their needle tracks (scars) to show, they inject themselves under the tongue or in the groin.

Treatment for Heroin Addiction. Programs to help heroin addicts kick their habits have not been very successful. The rate of recidivism (tendency to return to previous behaviours) is high. Some addicts resume their drug use even after years of drug-free living because the craving for the injection rush is very strong. It takes a great deal of discipline to seek alternative, non-drug highs.

Heroin addicts experience a distinct pattern of withdrawal. They begin to crave another dose four to six hours after their last dose. Symptoms of withdrawal include intense desire for the drug, yawning, a runny nose, sweating, and crying. About 12 hours after the last dose, addicts experience sleep disturbance, dilated pupils, loss of appetite, irritability, goose bumps, and muscle tremors. The most difficult time in the withdrawal process occurs 24 to 72 hours following last use. All of the preceding symptoms continue, along with nausea, abdominal cramps, restlessness, insomnia, vomiting, diarrhea, extreme anxiety, hot and cold flashes, elevated blood pressure, and rapid heartbeat and respiration. Once the peak of withdrawal has been passed, all these symptoms begin to subside. Still, the recovering addict has many hurdles to jump.

Methadone maintenance is one type of treatment available for people addicted to heroin or other opiates. Methadone is a synthetic narcotic that blocks the effects of opiate withdrawal. It is chemically similar enough to the opiates to control the tremors, chills, vomiting, diarrhea, and severe abdominal pains of withdrawal. Methadone dosage is decreased over a period of time until the addict is weaned off the drug.

Methadone maintenance is controversial because of the drug's own potential for addiction. Critics contend that the program merely substitutes one addiction for another. Proponents argue that people on methadone maintenance are less likely than heroin addicts to engage in criminal activities to support their habits. For this reason, many methadone maintenance programs are state- or federally financed and are available to clients free of charge or at reduced costs.

Psychedelics

The term **psychedelic** was adapted from a Greek phrase meaning "mind manifesting." Psychedelics are a group of drugs whose primary pharmacological effect is to alter feelings, perceptions, and thoughts in the user. The major receptor sites for most of these drugs are in the part of the brain that is responsible for interpreting outside stimuli before allowing these signals to travel to other parts of the brain. This area is called the **reticular formation** and is located in the brain stem at the upper end of the spinal cord (see Figure 10.2). When a psychedelic drug is present at a reticular formation receptor site, messages become scrambled, and the user may see wavy walls instead of straight ones or may smell colours or hear tastes. This mixing of sensory messages is known as **synesthesia.**

In addition to synesthetic effects, users may recall events long buried in the subconscious mind or become less inhibited than they are in a non-drug state. Some psychedelic drugs are erroneously labelled "hallucinogens." Hallucinogens are substances that are capable of creating auditory or visual **hallucinations**, or images that are perceived but are not real. Not all of the psychedelic drugs are capable of producing hallucinations. The most widely recognized psychedelics are LSD, mescaline, psilocybin, and psilocin. All are illegal and carry severe penalties for manufacture, possession, transportation, or sale.

LSD. Of all the psychedelics, **lysergic acid diethylamide (LSD)** has achieved the most notoriety. This chemical was first synthesized in the late 1930s by the Swiss chemist Albert Hoffman. It resulted from experiments aimed at deriving medically useful drugs from the ergot fungus found on rye and other cereal grains. Because LSD seemed capable of unlocking the secrets of the mind, psychiatrists initially felt it could be beneficial to patients unable to remember and recognize suppressed traumas. From 1950 through 1968, the drug was used for such purposes.

Media attention was drawn to LSD in the late 1960s. Young people were using the drug to "turn on" and "tune out" the world that gave them the war in Vietnam, race

Cultivation of the opium poppy—from which opium, morphine, codeine, and heroin are produced—has been a staple of the economy of many underdeveloped countries.

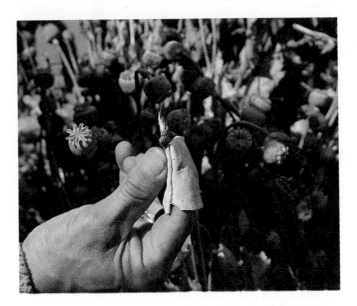

riots, and political assassinations. Although the drug was made illegal, its popularity remained high until the early 1970s, then tapered off, primarily because of users' inability to control dosages accurately.

Because of the recent wave of nostalgia for the 1960s, this dangerous psychedelic drug has been making a comeback. Known on the street as "acid," LSD is now widely available, and its availability is increasing.

An odourless, tasteless, white crystalline powder, LSD is most frequently dissolved in water to make a solution that can then be used to manufacture the street forms of the

Psychedelics: Drugs that distort the processing of sensory information in the brain.

Reticular formation: An area in the brain stem that is responsible for relaying messages to other areas in the brain.

Synesthesia: A (usually) drug-created effect in which sensory messages are incorrectly assigned—for example, hearing a taste or smelling a sound.

Hallucination: An image (auditory or visual) that is perceived but is not real.

Lysergic acid diethylamide (LSD): Psychedelic drug causing sensory disruptions; also called acid.

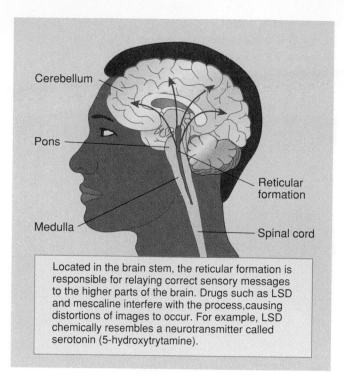

Cerebellum

Pons

Medulla

Reticular formation

Spinal cord

Located in the brain stem, the reticular formation is responsible for relaying correct sensory messages to the higher parts of the brain. Drugs such as LSD and mescaline interfere with the process,causing distortions of images to occur. For example, LSD chemically resembles a neurotransmitter called serotonin (5-hydroxytrytamine).

FIGURE 10.2

The Reticular Formation

The psychological effects of LSD vary from person to person. The set and setting in which the drug is used are very influential factors. Euphoria is the common psychological state produced by the drug, but *dysphoria* (a sense of evil and foreboding) may also be experienced. The drug also shortens attention span, causing the mind to wander. Thoughts may be interposed and juxtaposed as well. The user may thus be able to experience several different thoughts simultaneously. Synesthesia occurs occasionally. Users become introspective, and suppressed memories may surface, often taking on bizarre symbolism. Many more effects are possible, including decreased aggressiveness and enhanced sensory experiences.

While there is no evidence that LSD creates a physical dependence, it may well create a psychological dependence. Many LSD users become depressed for one or two days following a trip and turn to the drug to relieve this depression. The result is a cycle of LSD use to relieve post-LSD depression, which often leads to psychological addiction.

*W*HAT DO YOU THINK?

Discuss the reasons for use of LSD during the 1960s. Discuss the prevalence of LSD's use in the 1990s. What are the similarities and differences between the two periods and the use of this drug during them?

drug: tablets, blotter acid, and windowpane. What the LSD consumer usually buys is blotter acid—small squares of blotter-like paper that have been impregnated with the liquid. The blotter is swallowed or chewed briefly. LSD also comes in tiny thin squares of gelatin called windowpane and in tablets called microdots, which are less than an eighth of an inch across (it would take 10 or more of these to add up to the size of an ASA tablet).

LSD is one of the most powerful drugs known to science and can produce strong effects in doses as low as 20 micrograms. (To give you an idea of how small a dose this is, the average-sized postage stamp weighs approximately 60 000 micrograms.) The potency of the typical dose of LSD currently ranges from 20 to 80 micrograms, compared to 150 to 300 micrograms commonly used in the 1960s.

Despite its reputation for being primarily a psychedelic, LSD produces a large number of physical effects, including slightly increased heart rate, elevated blood pressure and temperature, goose flesh (roughened skin), increased reflex speeds, muscle tremors and twitches, perspiration, increased salivation, chills, headaches, and mild nausea. Since the drug also stimulates uterine muscle contractions, it can lead to premature labour and miscarriage in pregnant women.

Research into the effects of long-term LSD use has been inconclusive. As with any illegally purchased drug, users run the risk of purchasing an impure product.

Mescaline. **Mescaline** is one of the hundreds of chemicals derived from the **peyote** cactus. The small, buttonlike cactus grows in the southwestern United States and parts of Latin America. Natives of these regions have long used the dried peyote buttons during religious ceremonies. In fact, members of the Native American Church (a religion practised by thousands of North American Indians) have been granted special permission to use the drug during religious ceremonies in some U.S. states.

Users normally swallow 10 to 12 dried peyote buttons. These buttons taste bitter and generally induce immediate nausea or vomiting. Long-time users claim that the nausea becomes less noticeable with frequent use.

Those who are able to keep the drug down begin to feel the effects within 30 to 90 minutes, when mescaline reaches maximum concentration in the brain. (It may persist for up to 9 or 10 hours.) Unlike LSD, mescaline is a powerful hallucinogen. It is also a central nervous system stimulant.

Products sold on the street as mescaline are likely to be synthetic chemical relatives of the true drug. Street names of these products include DOM, STP, TMA, and MMDA. Any of these can be toxic in small quantities.

Psilocybin. **Psilocybin** and *psilocin* are the active chemicals in a group of mushrooms sometimes called "magic mushrooms." Psilocybe mushrooms, which grow throughout the world, can be cultivated from spores or can be harvested wild. Because many mushrooms resemble the psilocybe variety, people who use wild mushrooms for any purpose should be certain of what they are doing. Mushroom varieties can easily be misidentified, and mistakes can be fatal. Psilocybin is similar to LSD in physical effects. These effects generally wear off within 4 to 6 hours.

The Deliriants

Delirium is an agitated mental state characterized by confusion and disorientation. Almost all of the psychoactive drugs will produce delirium at high doses, but the **deliriants** produce this condition at relatively low (subtoxic) levels.

PCP. **Phencyclidine**, or **PCP**, is one of the best-known deliriants. It is a synthetic substance that became a black-market drug in the early 1970s. PCP was originally developed as a "disassociative anesthetic," which means that patients administered this drug could keep their eyes open, apparently remain conscious, and feel no pain during a medical procedure. Patients would afterward experience amnesia for the time the drug was in their system. Such a drug had obvious advantages as an anesthetic during surgery, but its unpredictability and drastic effects (postoperative delirium, confusion, and agitation) made doctors abandon it and it was withdrawn from the legal market.

On the illegal market, PCP is a white, crystalline powder that users often sprinkle onto marijuana cigarettes. It is dangerous and unpredictable regardless of the method of administration. Common street names for PCP are "angel dust" for the crystalline powdered form and "peace pill" and "horse tranquillizer" for the tablet form.

The effects of PCP depend on the dosage. A dose as small as 5 milligrams will produce effects similar to those of strong central nervous system depressants. These effects include slurred speech, impaired coordination, reduced sensitivity to pain, and reduced heart and respiratory rate. Doses between 5 and 10 milligrams cause fever, salivation, nausea, vomiting, and total loss of sensitivity to pain. Doses greater than 10 milligrams result in a drastic drop in blood pressure, coma, muscular rigidity, violent outbursts, and possible convulsions and death.

Psychologically, PCP may produce either euphoria or dysphoria. It is also known to produce hallucinations as well as delusions and overall delirium. Some users experience a prolonged state of "nothingness." The long-term effects of PCP use are unknown.

Designer Drugs

Designer drugs are structural analogues (drugs that produce similar effects) of more familiar illicit drugs. These illegal drugs are manufactured by underground chemists to mimic the psychoactive effects of controlled drugs.

At present, at least three types of synthetic drugs are available on the illegal drug market: analogues of phencyclidine (PCP), analogues of *fentanyl* and *meperidine* (both synthetic narcotic analgesics), and analogues of amphetamine and methamphetamine, which have hallucinogenic and stimulant properties.[21]

Although PCP analogues have been identified in street samples of drugs, they are less frequently used today than are other forms of designer drugs. Analogues of fentanyl are much more common. The pharmacological properties of most fentanyl analogues are similar to those of heroin or morphine. These analogues are known as "synthetic heroin," "china white," or "new heroin." These designer drugs may be addictive and carry the risk of overdose.

Amphetamine and methamphetamine analogues are the most common forms of designer drugs on university campuses today. These analogues often cause hallucinations and euphoria. *Ecstasy*, which was dubbed the "LSD of the 80s," is one such analogue that became popular on many campuses in the 1980s. It is actually a chemical called methylene dioxymethylamphetamine, or MDMA, and it is similar to the hallucinogen MMDA.

Users claim that Ecstasy provides the rush of cocaine combined with the mind-expanding characteristics of the hallucinogens. Psychological effects of MDMA include confusion, depression, anxiety, and paranoia. Physical symptoms may include muscle tension, nausea, blurred vision, faintness, chills, and sweating. MDMA also increases heart rate and blood pressure and may destroy neurons that regulate aggression, mood, sexual activity, and sensitivity to pain.[22]

Mescaline: A hallucinogenic drug derived from the peyote cactus.

Peyote: A cactus with small "buttons" that, when ingested, produce hallucinogenic effects.

Psilocybin: The active chemical found in psilocybe mushrooms; it produces hallucinations.

Delirium: An agitated mental state characterized by confusion and disorientation that can be produced by psychoactive drugs.

Deliriant: Any substance that produces delirium at relatively low doses, including PCP and some herbal substances.

Phencyclidine (PCP): A deliriant commonly called "angel dust."

Designer drug: A synthetic analogue of an existing illicit drug—i.e., a drug that has effects similar to those of an illicit drug.

Inhalants

Inhalants are chemicals that produce vapours that, when inhaled, can cause hallucinations as well as create intoxicating and euphoric effects. They are not commonly recognized as drugs. They are legal to purchase and universally available but are potentially dangerous when used incorrectly. These drugs are generally used by young people who can't afford illicit substances.

Some of these agents are organic solvents representing the chemical by-products of the distillation of petroleum products. Rubber cement, model glue, paint thinner, lighter fluid, varnish, wax, spot removers, and gasoline belong to this group. Most of these substances are sniffed by users in search of a quick, cheap high.

Because they are inhaled, the volatile chemicals in these products reach the bloodstream within seconds. An inhaled substance is not diluted or buffered by stomach acids or other body fluids and thus is more potent and dangerous than the same substance would be if swallowed. This characteristic, along with the fact that dosages are extremely difficult to control because everyone has unique lung and breathing capacities, makes inhalants particularly dangerous.

An overdose of fumes from inhalants can cause unconsciousness. If the user's oxygen intake is reduced during the inhaling process, death can result within five minutes.

Amyl Nitrite.   Sometimes called "poppers" or "rush," **amyl nitrite** is often prescribed to alleviate chest pain in heart patients. It is packaged in small, cloth-covered glass capsules that can be crushed to release the active chemical. The drug relieves chest pains because it causes rapid dilation of the small blood vessels and reduces blood pressure. That same dilation of blood vessels in the genital area is thought to enhance sensations or perceptions of orgasm. It also produces fainting, dizziness, warmth, and skin flushing.

Nitrous Oxide.   "Laughing gas" is the popular term for **nitrous oxide.** It is sometimes used as an adjunct to den-

tal anesthesia or minor surgical anesthesia. It is also used as a propellant chemical in aerosol products such as whipped toppings. Users experience a state of euphoria, floating sensations, and illusions. Effects also include pain relief and a "silly" feeling, demonstrated by laughing and giggling (hence the term *laughing gas*). Regulating dosages of this drug can be difficult. Sustained inhalation can lead to unconsciousness, coma, and death.

Steroids

Public awareness of **anabolic steroids** has recently been heightened by media stories about their use by amateur and professional athletes, including Ben Johnson, who lost the gold he had won for Canada at the Seoul Olympics when he failed a urine test. Anabolic steroids are artificial forms of the male hormone testosterone that promote muscle growth and strength. These **ergogenic drugs** are used primarily by young men to increase their strength, power, bulk (weight), and speed. These attributes are sought either to enhance athletic performance or to develop the physique that users perceive will make them more attractive and increase their sex appeal.

Most steroids are obtained through black market sources. Steroids are available in two forms: injectable solution and pills.[23] Anabolic steroids produce a state of euphoria, diminished fatigue, and increased bulk and power in both sexes. These qualities give steroids an addictive quality. When users stop, they appear to undergo psychological withdrawal, mainly caused by the disappearance of the physique they have become accustomed to.

Several adverse effects occur in both men and women who use steroids. These drugs cause mood swings (aggression and violence), sometimes known as "roid rage"; acne; liver tumours; elevated cholesterol levels; hypertension; kidney disease; and immune system disturbances. There is also a danger of HIV transmission through shared needles. In women, large doses of anabolic steroids trigger masculine changes, including lowered voice, increased facial and body hair, male pattern baldness, enlarged clitoris, decreased breast size, and changes in or absence of menstruation. When taken by healthy males, anabolic steroids shut down the body's production of testosterone, causing men's breasts to grow and testicles to atrophy.

A new and alarming trend is the use of other drugs to achieve the "performance-enhancing" effects of steroids. These steroid alternatives are sought in order to avoid the penalties (such as being banned from sports) for illicit use of anabolic steroids.

The two most common steroid alternatives are gamma hydroxybutyrate (GHB) and clenbuterol. GHB is a deadly,

---

Inhalants: Products that are sniffed or inhaled in order to produce highs.

Amyl nitrite: A drug that dilates blood vessels and is properly used to relieve chest pain.

Nitrous oxide: The chemical name for "laughing gas," a substance properly used for surgical or dental anesthesia.

Anabolic steroids: Artificial forms of the hormone testosterone that promote muscle growth and strength.

Ergogenic drug: Substance that enhances athletic performance.

The use of steroids to increase bulk and power carries many health risks, including disturbance of the immune system from the drug itself, plus the risk of AIDS transmission through the use of shared needles.

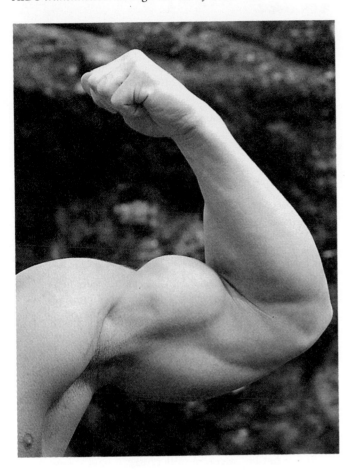

Drugs in the Workplace

The cost of drug and alcohol use in the workplace has been estimated at $18.45 billion in 1992 or about 2.7 percent of the total gross domestic product. Illicit drugs cost the Canadian economy $1.4 billion. The balance were due to smoking ($9.6 billion) and alcohol ($7.5 billion).

The largest economic costs of substance abuse are for lost productivity due to morbidity and premature mortality, direct health care costs, and law enforcement. There is considerable variation in the costs of substance abuse between the provinces.[24]

It is becoming more and more common for companies to have employee assistance programs (EAP), which offer drug and personal counselling. Large companies can contract with an EAP provider. Smaller companies will find this benefit offered under most insurance benefit packages.[25]

WHAT DO YOU THINK?

What is the cost society pays for drug use? Have you ever personally known someone who has suffered because of addiction to drugs? How did you respond?

Solutions to the Problem

In 1993, there were 56 811 drug-related offences, a slight decrease of 0.6 percent from the previous year. Cannabis-related offences accounted for 63 percent of the total while cocaine-related offences accounted for an additional 22 percent.

In general, researchers in the field of drug education agree that a multimodal approach to drug education is best. Students should be taught the difference between drug use and abuse. Factual information that is free from scare tactics must be presented; moralizing about drug use and abuse does not work. Programs that teach people to control drugs, as opposed to allowing drugs to control them, are needed, as are programs that teach about the influences of set and setting. Reinforcement of self-esteem is mandatory. It is not adequate to urge people to "just say no." Alternatives to drugs should be taught.

All drug abuse prevention approaches probably help up to a point, but neither alone nor in combination do they offer a total solution to the problem. Drug abuse has been a part of human behaviour for thousands of years, and it is not likely to disappear in the near future. For this reason, it is necessary to educate ourselves and to develop the self-discipline necessary to avoid dangerous drug dependencies.

illegal drug that is a primary ingredient in many of these "performance-enhancing" formulas. GHB does not produce a high. It does, however, cause headaches, nausea, vomiting, diarrhea, seizures and other central nervous system disorders, and possibly death. Clenbuterol, another steroid alternative, has become an extremely popular item on the black market.

WHAT DO YOU THINK?

How do you think reports in the media about the use of stimulants and/or steroids by athletes affect the popularity of these drugs? Would you consider using such a drug to improve your appearance?

Managing Drug Use Behaviour

After reading this chapter, you know that addictions can be devastating to both the user's life and the lives of his or her family and friends. Addictions usually progress gradually, and it is difficult to know for certain when a person crosses the line from habit to addiction. Keep in mind that a behaviour is problematic when it causes a person to incur negative consequences. If a person continues to abuse a drug despite negative consequences, chances are that he or she is addicted.

Making Decisions for You

When you have a medical problem (even a minor one such as a headache), you need to decide how best to treat it. What are the medical symptoms from which you are seeking relief? What questions would you like to ask your pharmacist or physician? What drugs (legal or illegal) are you currently using that could cause interactions? What are the pros and cons of each alternative? Which alternative is the best solution for you?

Checklist for Change: Making Personal Choices

✓ Do you know what key questions to ask to create a drug profile for any drugs you may decide to use?

✓ Do you read the warning labels on the medications that you use?

✓ Do you take medication only for the problem for which it is being prescribed?

✓ Do you ask your doctor or pharmacist if you should avoid alcohol—or any foods, beverages such as coffee or caffeinated soft drinks, or other medications—while taking a drug?

✓ Do you purchase generic medications instead of brand-name products?

✓ Do you know what resources exist in the community to help people answer questions about medications?

Checklist for Change: Making Personal Choices

✓ What illicit drugs are you familiar with? How did you become familiar with them? What drugs are most popular among your peers? What is it about these drugs that makes them popular?

✓ How do you and your peers feel about illicit drug use? Is it condoned or condemned? Has that changed in the last few years? What has led to these feelings?

✓ Have you thought of recreational activities that you can do in place of using drugs?

✓ Are you prepared for the challenge of refusing to use illicit drugs that you may be offered and for dealing with the consequences associated with that decision?

✓ Do you practise assertiveness? Do you practise speaking up and voicing your opinion regardless of the subject?

✓ Are you someone who takes pride in your accomplishments? Do you view setbacks as times for growth?

✓ Do you have strategies for coping with stress? Do you use exercise, meditation, or some other healthy activity as a method of stress reduction?

Checklist for Change: Making Community Choices

✓ Do you take the time to find out what the current drug problems on your campus and in your community are?

✓ Would you be willing to assist a friend in combatting his or her substance abuse problem? Would you accompany him or her to support groups?

✓ Would you be willing to be a role model in community programs such as Big Brothers or Big Sisters?

✓ Do you volunteer your time for any campus or community organizations that provide opportunities for high-risk youth?

✓ Would you be willing to volunteer to help out at an addiction hotline or community centre?

Critical Thinking

You have a major term paper due in three days, and you've just completed the reading for it. You're worried about how you'll get it done, and realize you may have to pull an all-nighter. If you don't get at least a B, you'll lose your academic scholarship and will be forced to leave university. A friend tells you that, last semester, she took a few lines of coke; it not only helped her stay awake, but also stimulated her thinking. She got an A– on the paper and experienced no side-effects. She suggests you try it, too.

Using the DECIDE model described in Chapter 1, decide how you will keep yourself awake to finish your paper. What stimulant, if any, are you willing to take to stay awake?

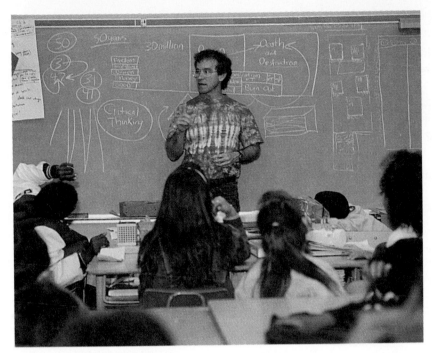

Many people believe that the most effective strategy for fighting illicit drug use is educating young people, particularly if they can learn about its dangers and consequences from someone who has "been there."

Summary

◆ Habits are repetitious behaviours whereas addiction is behaviour resulting from compulsion; without the behaviour, the addict experiences withdrawal. Addicts have four common symptoms: compulsion, loss of control, negative consequences, and denial.

◆ Addiction is a process, evolving over time through a pattern known as nurturing through avoidance. Mood-altering substances and experiences produce biochemical reactions that make the body feel good; when absent, the person feels a withdrawal effect. The biopsychosocial model of addiction takes into account biological (genetic) factors as well as social and psychological influences in understanding the addiction process.

◆ The six categories of drugs are prescription drugs, OTC drugs, recreational drugs, herbal preparations, illicit drugs, and commercial preparations. Routes of administration include oral ingestion, injection (intravenous, intramuscular, and subcutaneous), inhalation, inunction, and suppositories.

◆ Hazardous drug interactions may occur when a person takes several medications or illegal drugs simultaneously. The most hazardous interactions are synergism, antagonism, inhibition, and intolerance.

◆ Prescription drugs are administered under medical supervision. Categories include antibiotics, analgesics, prostaglandin inhibitors, sedatives, tranquillizers, antidepressants, and amphetamines. Generic drugs can often be substituted for more expensive brand-name drugs.

◆ Over-the-counter drug categories include analgesics; cold, cough, allergy, and asthma relievers; stimulants; sleeping aids and relaxants; and dieting aids. Consumers should exercise personal responsibility by reading directions for OTC drugs and asking their pharmacist or doctor if any special precautions are advised when taking these substances.

◆ People from all walks of life use illicit drugs, although university students report higher usage rates than does the general population.

◆ Controlled substances include cocaine and its derivatives, amphetamines, newer-generation stimulants, marijuana, the opiates, the psychedelics, the deliriants, designer drugs, inhalants, and steroids. Users tend to become addicted quickly to such drugs.

◆ The drug problem reaches everyone through crime and elevated health care costs. Drugs are a major problem in the workplace; workplace drug testing is one proposed solution to this problem.

Discussion Questions

1. What factors distinguish a habit from an addiction? Is it possible for you to tell if someone else is really addicted?

2. Compare and contrast the varied methods of treatment. Which do you think would be most effective for you? For your best friend? For your parents? What accounts for the differences?

3. What environmental factors influence the main effects and side-effects of psychoactive drugs?

4. What are *prostaglandin inhibitors*? What are some examples of these analgesics?

5. What are rebound effects? What are the severe symptoms of withdrawal from stimulants?

6. What general precautions should OTC users consider?

7. Create an antidrug program aimed at grade-school children. Think about what antidrug message would have reached you.

8. List the varied types of drugs. Then discuss their physiological and psychological effects. Why is it that newer, purer forms of drugs (like crack cocaine) are developed?

9. List non-drug alternative behaviours to drug use. Are these realistic? What could make them more enticing?

Application Exercise

Reread the What Do You Think? scenario at the beginning of the chapter and answer the following questions.

1. Do you think employers have the right to require drug screenings? How about potential employers? Would you want airline pilots or train engineers to be tested regularly? How about cafeteria workers?

2. Do you think that university athletes should be tested for drugs? Why or why not? Which drugs would you test for?

Health on the Net

Canadian Centre for Substance Abuse (also has links to various addictions agencies across Canada)
www.ccsa.ca

Canadian Substance Abuse Network
www.ccsa.ca/special.htm

Model Programs for Drug and Alcohol Abuse (WHO)
www.who.ch/programmes/psa/idada97/mob1.htm

Alcohol, Tobacco, and Caffeine

Unacknowledged Addictions

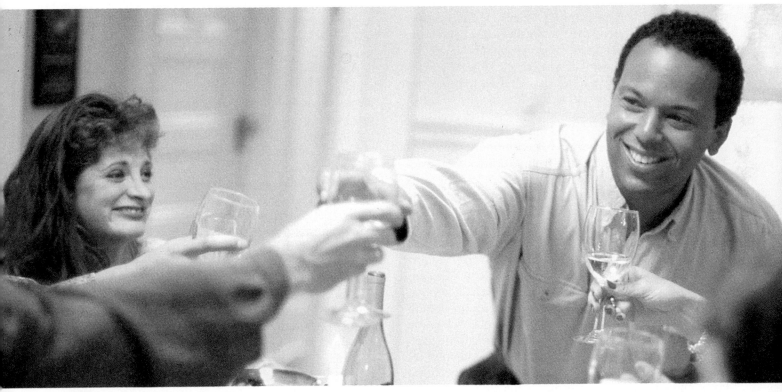

CHAPTER OBJECTIVES

◆ Summarize the alcohol use patterns of university students and discuss overall trends in consumption.

◆ Explain the physiological and behavioural effects of alcohol, including blood alcohol concentration, absorption, metabolism, and immediate and long-term effects of alcohol consumption.

◆ Explain the symptoms and causes of alcoholism, its cost to society, and its effects on the family.

◆ Explain the treatment of alcoholism, including the family's role, varied treatment methods, and whether or not alcoholics can be cured.

◆ Discuss the social issues involved in tobacco use, including advertising and the medical costs associated with tobacco use.

◆ Review how smoking affects a smoker's risk for cancer, cardiovascular disease, and respiratory diseases, and how it adversely affects the health of a foetus.

◆ Discuss the risks associated with using smokeless tobacco.

◆ Evaluate the risks to nonsmokers associated with environmental tobacco smoke.

◆ Describe strategies people adopt to quit using tobacco products, including strategies aimed at breaking the nicotine addiction as well as habit.

◆ Compare the benefits and risks associated with caffeine, and summarize the health consequences of long-term caffeine use.

Teresa is a waitress at a restaurant. In the entryway of the building, there is a large warning sign about the dangers of drinking alcohol while pregnant. While taking a drink order from a woman, Teresa notices that she is in maternity clothes and in the advanced stages of pregnancy. Teresa takes the order and tells the restaurant manager that she feels uneasy serving alcohol to a pregnant woman. The manager says, "Mind your own business," and orders her to bring the woman the drink. Teresa delivers the drink. During the course of the evening, she brings several more drinks to the same woman.

■ Should Teresa refuse to serve the pregnant woman? Why? If the baby is born with alcohol-related problems, should the mother be sued for endangering her child?

When you hear references to the dangers of drugs, what comes to mind? Usually the term *drugs* conjures up images of people abusing cocaine, heroin, marijuana, LSD, PCP, and other illegal substances. We conveniently use the word *drugs* to refer to one set of dangerous substances, but we steadfastly refuse to categorize alcohol as a drug, primarily because it is socially accepted.

Canadians consumed an average of 7.1 litres of alcohol per capita in 1991. How does this compare with other countries? The average person in Luxembourg consumed 12.3 litres; Algerians consumed only 0.02 litres. Countries with comparable levels include Argentina (7.5), Australia (7.7), and the United States (7.4). Europeans generally consume more: between 8 and 11 litres per capita.[1]

Most of us think of alcohol the way it is portrayed in ads or in the movies: a way of having fun in company, an important adjunct to a romantic dinner or a cozy evening in front of the fireplace. Moderate use of alcohol can enhance celebrations or special times. Research shows that very low levels of use may actually lower some health risks. But you should remember that alcohol is a chemical substance that affects your physical and mental behaviour. The tragedies associated with alcohol addiction receive far less attention than cocaine-related deaths, drug busts, and efforts to eradicate marijuana crops. Nevertheless, they are more common and may have devastating effects on people of all ages.

ALCOHOL: AN OVERVIEW

An estimated 58 percent of Canadians consume alcoholic beverages regularly, though consumption patterns are unevenly distributed throughout the drinking population. Occasional drinkers (less than once per month) made an additional 21 percent of users; 12 percent were former drinkers; and 10 percent had never used alcohol.[2] Alcohol use peaks at ages 25–29 for men (79 percent). There were several peaks for women, at ages 20–24, 35–39, and 40–44 (54 percent)

Alcohol use does appear to be declining. A 1989 survey of adults in Ontario found that 83 percent reported ever having used alcohol, with 55 percent saying they have five drinks or more at a single sitting and 10 percent reporting daily drinking.[3] In a 1990 nation-wide Gallup poll, 79 percent of adults reported that they had at some point drunk alcohol.

Total alcohol consumption in Canada during 1988/89 reached 202.9 million litres. This corresponds to an average annual consumption of 9.9 litres of alcohol for each Canadian over the age of 15 (11 drinks per week, or a little under two drinks a day). Beer was the most popular drink, making up 52 percent of the total volume, with spirits in second place at 31 percent, and wine a distant third at 17 percent.[4] The average adult drank the equivalent of 7.58 litres of absolute alcohol in 1992/93, a decline of 5 percent from the previous year. Young adults, males, and those with higher incomes drink more than other Canadians.[5]

Alcohol and University Students

Alcohol is the most widely used (and abused) recreational drug in our society. It is also the most popular drug on university campuses, where approximately 94.5 percent of students consume alcoholic beverages. The Addiction Research Foundation estimates that one-third of Ontario university students take more than 15 drinks per week: a level that puts them at risk for health and other problems. A greater number of alcohol users live in residence (41 percent) are between 17 and 22 years of age (65 percent) and have lower grades (49.5 percent D, 22.6 percent A) (see Table 11.1).[6]

While alcohol has long been seen as a "social lubricant" by college students, alcohol abuse and reckless driving have become serious problems on many campuses.

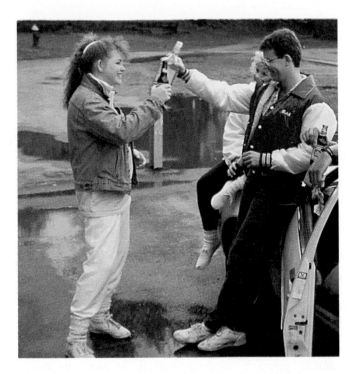

University is a critical time to become conscious of and responsible about your drinking. A number of social factors are involved in campus drinking. There is little doubt that alcohol is a part of campus culture and tradition. It is used to help relieve tensions and to celebrate. Its ability to lower inhibitions makes it the "social lubricant" of choice for many students, giving them an easy way to initiate conversations and create friendships.

How do students view the drinking patterns of their peers? Students consistently report that their friends drink much more than they do and that average drinking within their own social living group is higher than actual self-reports. Such misinformation may promote or be used to excuse excessive drinking practices among college students.

Binge drinking on university campuses has become a big problem. **Binge drinking** is defined as the consumption of five drinks in a row by men or four in a row by women on a single occasion. The express purpose of binge drinking is to become intoxicated.

Although everyone is at some risk for alcoholism and alcohol-related problems, university students seem to be particularly vulnerable:

- Alcohol exacerbates their already high risk for suicide, automobile crashes, and falls.

TABLE 11.1 ■ Alcohol Use Among University Students by Selected Characteristics, Ontario, 1993

	Current Drinkers	Daily Drinkers	15+/Week
TOTAL:	94.5 percent	1.8 percent	31.1 percent
Gender			
Male	94.5	3.1	8.2
Female	94.4	0.6	20.7
Age			
17–19	94.6	2.7	32.4
20–22	95.3	1.2	32.4
23–25	92.5	2.5	22.8
26 and over	93.1	2.3	17.3
Grade			
A	93.6	1.8	22.6
B	94.5	1.6	29.5
C	95.0	12.7	37.1
D	98.9	1.8	49.5
Place of Residence			
Residence	96.1	2.0	41.1
Parents	93.3	1.8	21.8
Off-campus	95.3	1.7	30.9
Other	87.1	3.0	25.5
Program			
Arts	95.0	1.7	33.7
Science	93.1	1.0	24.6
Social Science	96.4	1.7	31.3
Business	94.2	3.5	25.3
Other	93.3	1.8	28.4

Source: L. Gliksman, B. Newton-Taylor, E. Adlaf, D. Dewit, and N. Giesbrecht, *University Student Drug Use & Lifestyle Behaviours: Current Patterns and Changes from 1988 to 1993* (Toronto: Addiction Research Foundation, 1995).

- Many university customs, norms, traditions, and mores encourage certain dangerous practices and patterns of alcohol use.

- University campuses are heavily targeted by advertising and promotions from the alcohol industry.

- It is more common for university students than for their peers to drink recklessly and to engage in drinking games and other dangerous drinking practices.

- University students are particularly vulnerable to peer influences and have a strong need to be accepted by their peers.

In an effort to prevent alcohol abuse, many universities are instituting strong policies against drinking. At the same time, they are making more help available to students with drinking problems. Today, both individual and group counselling are offered on most campuses, and more attention is being directed toward the prevention of alcohol abuse.[7] Student organizations also promote responsible drinking and responsible party hosting.

Rights Versus Responsibilities

Most of us recognize the dangers associated with alcohol consumption in general, yet we tend to deny that such things could happen to us. We are aware of the relationship between alcohol and traffic accidents, spouse battering and child abuse, violent crimes, and family disruption, but we like to believe that these tragedies happen only to other people.

People who drink often argue that drinking is their inalienable right. Many refuse to acknowledge that alcohol is a drug simply because they do not wish to see themselves as drug users. Our society condones, approves, and often encourages the consumption of alcoholic beverages but neglects to teach us how to use alcohol responsibly.

In 1993, there were 194 916 liquor act offences in Canada, representing 63 percent of offences reported under provincial statutes (excluding traffic offences). There were 117 567 drinking and driving offences in Canada during 1993. The number has generally been declining since 1983. The rate per 100 000 age 16 or older has declined an average 4.6 percent per year over the period 1984 to 1993.[8]

If you make the choice to drink, you should do so judiciously, with complete information about the risks. The

Binge drinking: Drinking for the express purpose of becoming intoxicated; five drinks in a single sitting for men and four drinks in a sitting for women.

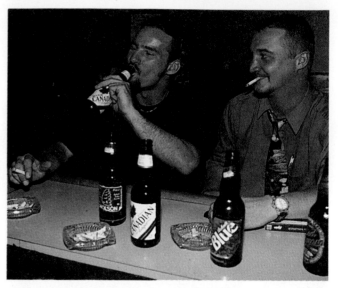

When drinking alcohol, it is important to remember that choosing wine or beer and keeping food in the stomach are ways to minimize alcohol's negative effects on the mind and body.

physiological and psychological reactions of the human organism to alcohol are strong. For this reason, you should approach the drug carefully. To avoid the devastating effects of alcohol abuse, you must adhere to the same principles of prevention that apply to any potentially harmful substance.

*W*HAT DO YOU THINK?

Have you ever thought about how much you drink in comparison to your friends? If you are not drinking more than your friends, does that mean that your drinking is not a problem?

*P*HYSIOLOGICAL AND BEHAVIOURAL EFFECTS OF ALCOHOL

The intoxicating substance found in beer, wine, liquor, and liqueurs is **ethyl alcohol**, or **ethanol**. It is produced during a process called **fermentation**, whereby plant sugars are broken down by yeast organisms, yielding ethanol and carbon dioxide. Fermentation continues until the solution of plant sugars (called mash) reaches a concentration of 14 percent alcohol. At this point, the alcohol kills the yeast and halts the chemical reactions that produce it.

Manufacturers then add other ingredients that dilute the alcohol content of the beverage. Other alcoholic beverages are produced through further processing called **distillation**, during which alcohol vapours are released from the mash at high temperatures. The vapours are then condensed and mixed with water to make the final product.

The **proof** of an alcoholic drink is a measure of the percentage of alcohol in the beverage. "Proof" comes from "gunpowder proof," a reference to the gunpowder test, whereby potential buyers would test the distiller's product by pouring it on gunpowder and attempting to light it. If the alcohol content was at least 50 percent, the gunpowder would burn; otherwise the water in the product would put out the flame. Thus, alcohol percentage is 50 percent of the given proof. For example, 80 proof whiskey or scotch is 40 percent alcohol by volume. The proof of a beverage provides an indication of its strength. Lower-proof drinks will produce fewer alcohol effects than the same amounts of higher-proof drinks.

Most wines are between 12 and 15 percent alcohol, and ales are between 6 and 8 percent. The alcoholic content of beers is between 2 and 6 percent, varying according to type of beer.

Behavioural Effects

Behavioural changes caused by alcohol vary with the setting and with the individual. Alcohol may make shy people less inhibited and more willing to talk to others. It may make a depressed person even more depressed. In people reluctant to share emotions, it may bring out violence and aggression. In many cases, alcohol will do for the drinker what the drinker expects and wants it to do, making it possible for the user to blame his or her inappropriate behaviour on the alcohol.

Blood alcohol concentration (BAC) is the ratio of alcohol to total blood volume. It is the factor used to measure the physiological and behavioural effects of alcohol. Despite individual differences, alcohol produces some general behaviour effects depending on BAC (see Table 11.2). At a BAC of 0.02, a person feels slightly relaxed and in a good mood. At 0.05, relaxation increases, there is some motor impairment, and a willingness to talk becomes apparent. At 0.08, the person feels euphoric and there is further motor impairment. At 0.10, the depressant effects of alcohol become apparent, drowsiness sets in, and motor skills are further impaired, followed by a loss of judgement. Thus a driver may not be able to estimate distances or speed, and some drinkers lose their ability to make value-related decisions and may do things they would not do when sober. As BAC increases, the drinker suffers increased physiological and psychological effects. All these changes are negative. No skills or functions are enhanced because of alcohol ingestion. Rather, physical and mental functions are all impaired.

People can acquire physical and psychological tolerance to the effects of alcohol through regular use. The nervous system adapts over time, so greater amounts of alcohol are required to produce the same physiological and psychological effects. Some people can learn to modify their behaviour so that they appear to be sober even when their BAC is quite high. This ability is called **learned behavioural tolerance.**

Absorption and Metabolism

Alcohol is rapidly absorbed into the bloodstream from the small intestine, and less rapidly from the stomach and colon. In proportion to its concentration in the bloodstream, alcohol decreases activity in parts of the brain and spinal cord. The drinker's blood alcohol concentration depends on:

- the amount consumed in a given time
- the drinker's size, sex, body build, and metabolism
- the type and amount of food in the stomach

Once the alcohol has passed into the blood, however, no food or beverage can retard or interfere with its effects. Fruit sugar, however, in some cases can shorten the duration of alcohol's effect by speeding up its elimination from the blood.

In the average adult, the rate of metabolism is about 8.5 grams of alcohol per hour (i.e., about two-thirds of a regular beer or about 30 millilitres of spirits an hour). This

Ethyl alcohol (ethanol): An addictive drug produced by fermentation and found in many beverages.

Fermentation: The process whereby yeast organisms break down plant sugars to yield ethanol.

Distillation: The process whereby mash is subjected to high temperatures to release alcohol vapours, which are then condensed and mixed with water to make the final product.

Proof: A measure of the percentage of alcohol in a beverage.

Blood alcohol concentration (BAC): The ratio of alcohol to total blood volume; the factor used to measure the physiological and behavioural effects of alcohol.

Learned behavioural tolerance: The ability of heavy drinkers to modify their behaviour so that they appear to be sober even when they have high BAC levels.

TABLE 11.2 ■ Psychological and Physical Effects of Various Blood Alcohol Concentration Levels*

Number of Drinks†	Blood Alcohol Concentration	Psychological and Physical Effects
1	0.02%–0.03%	No overt effects, slight mood elevation.
2	0.05%–0.06%	Feeling of relaxation, warmth; slight decrease in reaction time and in fine-muscle coordination.
3	0.08%–0.09%	Balance, speech, vision, and hearing slightly impaired; feelings of euphoria, increased confidence; loss of motor coordination; legal intoxication.
4	0.11%–0.12%	Coordination and balance becoming difficult; distinct impairment of mental faculties, judgement.
5	0.14%–0.15%	Major impairment of mental and physical control; slurred speech, blurred vision, lack of motor skills.
7	0.20%	Loss of motor control—must have assistance in moving about; mental confusion.
10	0.30%	Severe intoxication; minimum conscious control of mind and body.
14	0.40%	Unconsciousness, threshold of coma.
17	0.50%	Deep coma.
20	0.60%	Death from respiratory failure.

*For each hour elapsed since the last drink, subtract 0.015 percent blood alcohol concentration, or approximately one drink.

† One drink = one beer (4 percent alcohol, 12 ounces), one highball (1 ounce whiskey), or one glass table wine (5 ounces).

Source: Modified from data given in Ohio State Police Driver Information Seminars and the National Clearinghouse for Alcohol and Alcoholism Information, Rockville, MD.

rate can vary dramatically among individuals, however, depending on usual amount of drinking, physique, sex, liver size, and genetic factors.[9]

Mood is another influence on the rate of absorption, since emotions affect how long it takes for the contents of the stomach to empty into the intestine. Powerful moods, such as stress and tension, are likely to cause the stomach to "dump" its contents into the small intestine. That is why alcohol is absorbed much more rapidly when people are tense than when they are relaxed.

Alcohol is metabolized in the liver, where it is converted by the enzyme alcohol dehydrogenase to acetaldehyde. It is then rapidly oxidized to acetate, converted to carbon dioxide and water, and eventually excreted from the body. Acetaldehyde is a toxic chemical that can cause immediate symptoms such as nausea and vomiting as well as long-term effects such as liver damage.

Like food, alcohol contains calories. Proteins and carbohydrates (starches and sugars) each contain 4 kilocalories per gram. Fat contains 9 kilocalories per gram. Alcohol, although similar in structure to carbohydrates, contains 7 kilocalories per gram. The body uses the calories in alcohol in the same manner it uses those found in carbohydrates: for immediate energy or for storage as fat if not immediately needed.

A drinker's BAC depends on weight and body fat, the water content in body tissues, the concentration of alcohol in the beverage consumed, the rate of consumption, and the volume of alcohol consumed. Heavier people have larger body surfaces through which to diffuse alcohol; therefore, they have lower concentrations of alcohol in their blood than do thin people after drinking the same amount. Because alcohol does not diffuse as rapidly into body fat as into water, alcohol concentration is higher in a person with more body fat. Because a woman is likely to have more body fat and less water in her body tissues than a man of the same weight, she will be more intoxicated than a man after drinking the same amount of alcohol.

TABLE 11.3 ▪ Calculation of Estimated Blood Alcohol Concentration (BAC) for Men and Women

Males					Number of Drinks					
Body Weight (lb.)	1	2	3	4	5	6	7	8	9	10
100	0.043	0.870	0.130	0.174	0.217	0.261	0.304	0.348	0.391	0.435
125	0.034	0.069	0.103	0.139	0.173	0.209	0.242	0.278	0.312	0.346
150	0.029	0.058	0.087	0.116	0.145	0.174	0.203	0.232	0.261	0.290
175	0.025	0.050	0.075	0.100	0.125	0.150	0.175	0.200	0.225	0.250
200	0.022	0.043	0.065	0.087	0.108	0.130	0.152	0.174	0.195	0.217
225	0.019	0.039	0.058	0.078	0.097	0.117	0.136	0.156	0.175	0.195
250	0.017	0.035	0.052	0.070	0.087	0.105	0.122	0.139	0.156	0.173

Females					Number of Drinks					
Body Weight (lb.)	1	2	3	4	5	6	7	8	9	10
100	0.050	0.101	0.152	0.203	0.253	0.304	0.355	0.406	0.456	0.507
125	0.040	0.080	0.120	0.162	0.202	0.244	0.282	0.324	0.364	0.404
150	0.034	0.068	0.101	0.135	0.169	0.203	0.237	0.271	0.304	0.338
175	0.029	0.058	0.087	0.117	0.146	0.175	0.204	0.233	0.262	0.292
200	0.026	0.050	0.076	0.101	0.126	0.152	0.177	0.203	0.227	0.253
225	0.022	0.045	0.068	0.091	0.113	0.136	0.159	0.182	0.204	0.227
250	0.020	0.041	0.061	0.082	0.101	0.122	0.142	0.162	0.182	0.202

Body weight: Calculations are for people who have a normal body weight for their height, who are free of drugs or other affecting medications, and who are neither unusually thin nor obese.

Drink equivalents: 1 drink equals:
1 1/2 oz. of rum, rye, scotch, brandy, gin, vodka, etc.
1 12-oz. bottle of normal-strength beer
3 oz. of fortified wine
5 oz. of table wine

Using the chart: Find the appropriate figure using the proper chart (male or female), body weight, and number of drinks consumed. Then subtract the time factor (see Time Factor Table) from the figure on the chart to obtain the approximate BAC. For example, for a 150-lb. man who has had 4 drinks in 2 hours, take the figure 0.116 (from the chart for males) and subtract 0.030 (from the Time Factor Table) to obtain a BAC of 0.086%.

Time Factor Table

Hours since first drink	1	2	3	4	5	6
Subtract from BAC	0.015	0.030	0.045	0.060	0.075	0.090

Source: From *The Encyclopedia of Alcoholism* by Glen Evans and Robert O'Brien. © 1991 Facts on File and Greenspring Inc. Reprinted with permission of Facts on File, Inc., New York.

WHAT DO YOU THINK?

Have you thought that BAC is only based upon the amount of alcohol you drink? What other factors contribute to BAC? Are these factors different for men and women?

Women and Alcohol. Body fat is not the only contributor to the differences in alcohol's effects on men and women. Compared to men, women appear to have half as much alcohol hydrogenase, the enzyme that breaks down alcohol in the stomach before it has a chance to get to the bloodstream and the brain. Therefore, if a man and a woman both drink the same amount of alcohol, the woman's BAC will be approximately 30 percent higher than the man's, leaving her more vulnerable to slurred speech, careless driving, and other drinking-related impairments. Table 11.3 compares blood-alcohol levels by sex, weight, and consumption. Although this table can provide an estimate of probable BAC levels, many additional factors may cause considerable variation in these rates. For this reason, you should always err on the side of caution when gauging your blood alcohol level.

Breathalyzer and Other Tests. The breathalyzer tests used by law enforcement officers are designed to determine BAC based on the amount of alcohol exhaled in the breath. Urinalysis can also yield a BAC based on the concentration of unmetabolized alcohol in the urine. Both breath analysis and urinalysis are used to determine whether a driver is legally intoxicated, but blood tests are more accurate measures.

Immediate Effects

The most dramatic effects produced by ethanol occur within the central nervous system (CNS). The primary action of the drug is to reduce the frequency of nerve transmissions and impulses at synaptic junctions. This reduction of nerve transmissions results in a significant depression of CNS functions, with resulting decreases in respiratory rate, pulse rate, and blood pressure. As CNS depression deepens, vital functions become noticeably depressed. In extreme cases, coma and death can result.

Alcohol is a diuretic, causing increased urinary output. Although this effect might be expected to lead to automatic **dehydration** (loss of water), the body actually retains water, most of it in the muscles or in the cerebral tissues. This is because water is usually pulled out of the **cerebrospinal fluid** (fluid within the brain and spinal cord), leading to what is known as mitochondrial dehydration at the cell level within the nervous system. Mitochondria are miniature organs within cells that are responsible for specific functions. They rely heavily upon fluid balance. When mitochondrial dehydration occurs from drinking, the mitochondria cannot carry out their normal functions, resulting in symptoms that include the "morning-after" headaches suffered by some drinkers.

Alcohol is also an irritant to the gastrointestinal system and may cause indigestion and heartburn if taken on an empty stomach. Long-term use of alcohol causes repeated irritation that has been linked to cancers of the esophagus and stomach. In addition, people who engage in brief drinking sprees during which they consume unusually high amounts of alcohol put themselves at risk for irregular heartbeat or even total loss of heart rhythm, which can cause disruption in blood flow and possible damage to the heart muscle.

A **hangover** is often experienced the morning after a drinking spree. The symptoms of a hangover are familiar to most of you who drink: headache, upset stomach, anxiety, depression, thirst, and, in severe cases, an almost overwhelming desire to crawl into a hole and die. People who get hangovers often also smoke too much, stay up too late, or engage in other behaviours likely to leave them feeling unwell the next day. The causes of hangovers are not well known, but the effects of **congeners** are suspected. Congeners are forms of alcohol that are metabolized more slowly than ethanol and are more toxic. Your body metabolizes the congeners after the ethanol is gone from your system, and their toxic by-products are thought to contribute to the hangover. It usually takes 12 hours to recover from a hangover. Bed rest, solid food, and ASA may help relieve the discomforts of a hangover, but unfortunately, nothing cures it but time.

Drug Interactions. When you use any drug (and alcohol is a drug), you need to be aware of the possible interactions with any prescription drugs, over-the-counter

---

TABLE 11.4 ■ Drugs and Alcohol: Actions and Interactions

Drug Class/Trade Name(s)	Effects with Alcohol
Anti-alcohol: Antabuse	Severe reactions to even small amounts: headache, nausea, blurred vision, convulsions, coma, possible death.
Antibiotics: penicillin, Cyantin	Reduces therapeutic effectiveness of antibiotics.
Antidepressants: Elavil, Sinequan, Tofranil, Nardil	Increased central nervous system (CNS) depression, blood pressure changes. Combined use of alcohol and MAO inhibitors, a specific type of antidepressant, can trigger massive increases in blood pressure, even brain hemorrhage and death.
Antihistamines: Allerest, Dristan	Drowsiness and CNS depression. Impairs driving ability.
ASA: aspirin, Anacin, Excedrin, Bayer	Irritates stomach lining. May cause gastrointestinal pain, bleeding.
Depressants: Valium, Ativan, Placidyl	Dangerous CNS depression, loss of coordination, coma. High risk of overdose and death.
Narcotics: heroin, codeine, Darvon	Serious CNS depression. Possible respiratory arrest and death.
Stimulants: caffeine, cocaine	Masks depressant action of alcohol. May increase blood pressure, physical tension.

Source: Adapted by permission from *Drugs and Alcohol: Simple Facts About Alcohol and Drug Combinations* (Phoenix: DIN Publications, 1988), No. 121.

drugs, or other drugs you are taking or considering taking. Table 11.4 summarizes some possible interactions. Note that alcohol may cause a negative interaction even with ASA.

Long-Term Effects

Effects on the Nervous System. The nervous system is especially sensitive to alcohol. Even people who drink moderately experience shrinkage in brain size and weight and a loss of some degree of intellectual ability. The damage that results from alcohol use is localized primarily in the left side of the brain, which is responsible for written and spoken language, logic, and mathematical skills. The degree of shrinkage appears to be directly related to the amount of alcohol consumed. In terms of memory loss, the evidence suggests that having one drink every day is better than saving up for a binge and consuming seven or eight drinks in a night. The amount of alcohol consumed at one time is critical. Alcohol-related brain damage can be partially reversed with good nutrition and staying sober.

Cardiovascular Effects. The cardiovascular system is affected by alcohol in a number of ways. Evidence suggests that the effect of alcohol on the heart is not all bad. Studies in the United States by the National Heart, Lung, and Blood Institute suggest that moderate drinkers suffer fewer heart attacks, have less cholesterol buildup in their arteries, and are less likely to die of heart disease than either nondrinkers or heavy drinkers.[10] However, drinking is not recommended as a preventive measure against heart disease because there are many more cardiovascular health hazards than benefits from alcohol consumption. Alcohol contributes to high blood pressure and slightly increased heart rate and cardiac output. Those who report drinking three to five drinks a day, regardless of race or sex, have higher blood pressure than those who drink less.

People who engage in brief drinking sprees, during which they consume unusually large amounts of alcohol, also suffer some risks, including irregular heartbeat or total loss of heart rhythm. This condition has been called *holiday heart syndrome* because it typically occurs after such holidays as Thanksgiving, Christmas, and New Year's Eve, occasions when drinkers are likely to overindulge. It can cause disruption in blood flow and possible damage to the heart muscle. Prolonged drinking can also lead to deterioration of the heart muscle, a condition called *cardiomyopathy.*

Liver Disease. One of the most common diseases related to alcohol abuse is **cirrhosis** of the liver. It is among the top ten causes of death in Canada. One result of heavy drinking is that the liver begins to store fat—a condition known as *fatty liver.* If there is insufficient time between drinking episodes, this fat cannot be transported to storage sites and the fat-filled liver cells stop functioning. Continued drinking can cause a further stage of liver deterioration called *fibrosis,* in which the damaged area of the liver develops fibrous scar tissue. Cell function can be partially restored at this stage with proper nutrition and abstinence from alcohol. If the person continues to drink, however, cirrhosis results. At this point, the liver cells die and the damage is permanent. **Alcoholic hepatitis** is a serious condition resulting from prolonged use of alcohol. A chronic inflammation of the liver develops, which may be fatal in itself or progress to cirrhosis.

Cancer. Heavy drinkers are at higher risk for certain types of cancer, particularly cancers of the gastrointestinal tract. The repeated irritation caused by long-term use of alcohol has been linked to cancers of the esophagus, stomach, mouth, tongue, and liver. Research has also shown a link between breast cancer and moderate levels of alcohol consumption in women. A study conducted in 1987 found that women between the ages of 34 and 59 who consumed between three and nine drinks a week were 30 percent more likely than nondrinkers to develop breast cancer.[11] The 1994 study by the Harvard Medical School of male drinkers showed a 12 percent increased risk for cancer for those who had only one drink a day and 123 percent for those who had two drinks a day. It is unclear how alcohol exerts its carcinogenic effects, though it is thought that it inhibits the absorption of carcinogenic substances, permitting them to be taken to sensitive organs.

Other Effects. An irritant to the gastrointestinal system, alcohol may cause indigestion and heartburn if ingested on an empty stomach. It also damages the mucous membranes and can cause inflammation of the esophagus, chronic stomach irritation, problems with intestinal absorption, and chronic diarrhea.

Dehydration: Loss of fluids from body tissues.

Cerebrospinal fluid: Fluid within and surrounding the brain and spinal cord tissues.

Hangover: The physiological reaction to excessive drinking, including such symptoms as headache, upset stomach, anxiety, depression, diarrhea, and thirst.

Congeners: Forms of alcohol that are metabolized more slowly than ethanol and produce toxic by-products.

Cirrhosis: The last stage of liver disease associated with chronic heavy use of alcohol during which liver cells die and damage is permanent.

Alcoholic hepatitis: Condition resulting from prolonged use of alcohol in which the liver is inflamed. It can result in death.

Alcohol and the Older Canadian

Alcohol is the most commonly used drug by older Canadians. Overall, older Canadians are more likely to be frequent but low-volume drinkers. Sixteen percent of young seniors and 22 percent of older seniors drink four or more times a week, in comparison with 11 percent of all adults. In contrast, 29 percent of young seniors and 19 percent of older seniors report drinking five or more drinks on one occasion during the previous year, in comparison with 50 percent of all adults.

- Older seniors are more likely to be lifetime abstainers (15 percent) than younger seniors (6 percent) or all adults (7 percent). They are also more likely to be former drinkers.

- Older men are more likely to be current drinkers (70 percent) than older women (46 percent). Older men also drink more frequently and consume greater quantities than older women.

- Older adults most often do their drinking at home or with friends, but in comparison with younger Canadians, they are more likely to drink alone.

The reasons older Canadians drink are similar to those of other age groups. The most common reasons are to be sociable and to enjoy meals. The least common reasons are to facilitate mood-change, such as to forget worries, to feel less shy, or to feel good. The mood-change reasons for drinking are more likely to be reported by older men than older women.

Older adults are less likely than other age groups to report alcohol-related problems, and they are also less likely to drink and drive in comparison to younger Canadians. Current drinkers are more likely to be current smokers than nondrinkers.

Sources: Addiction Research Foundation, Statistical Information Service. This information was taken from the following documents: Health and Welfare Canada (1992), *Alcohol and Other Drugs Use by Canadians: A National Alcohol and Other Drugs Survey* (1989), technical report; M. Bergob, Statistics Canada, "Drug Use Among Senior Canadians," *Canadian Social Trends,* Summer 1994; Health Canada, *Older Canadians, Alcohol and Other Drug Use: Increasing Our Understanding,* unpublished.

Alcohol abuse is a major cause of chronic inflammation of the pancreas, the organ that produces digestive enzymes and insulin. Chronic abuse of alcohol inhibits enzyme production, which further inhibits the absorption of nutrients. Drinking alcohol can block the absorption of calcium, a nutrient that strengthens bones. This should be of particular concern to women, for as women age their risk for osteoporosis (bone thinning and calcium loss) increases. Heavy consumption of alcohol worsens this condition.

Evidence also suggests that alcohol impairs the body's ability to recognize and fight foreign bodies such as bacteria and viruses. The relationship between alcohol and AIDS is unclear, especially since some of the populations at risk for HIV infection are also at risk for alcohol abuse. But any effect on the immune system would probably contribute to the development of the disease.

Foetal Alcohol Syndrome

Alcohol can have harmful effects on foetal development. A disorder called **foetal alcohol syndrome (FAS)** is associated with alcohol consumption throughout pregnancy. Alcohol consumed during the first trimester poses the greatest threat to organ development; exposure during the last trimester, when the brain is developing rapidly, is most likely to affect CNS development.

FAS occurs when alcohol ingested by the mother passes through the placenta into the infant's bloodstream. Because the foetus is so small, its BAC will be much higher than that of the mother. Thus, consumption of alcohol during pregnancy can affect the infant far more seriously than it does the mother.

FAS is the leading cause of developmental delay in Canada and North America. In addition, FAS children may suffer from a wide variety of physical and behavioural effects. One-fifth of FAS children have difficulty sleeping and are hyperactive. Many have severe learning disabilities and are dyslexic. Congenital heart problems are more common than in normal babies, as are genitourinary problems. There is an increased incidence of spina bifida, hip dislocation, and delayed skeletal maturation.

The term **foetal alcohol effects (FAE)** is used to describe children with prenatal exposure to alcohol, but only some FAS characteristics.

It is estimated that one to three children in every 1000 in industrialized countries will be born with FAS. The rate of FAE may be several times higher. There are no statistics regarding the extent of FAS/FAE in Canada.

As there is no definitive information regarding a safe quantity of alcohol use during pregnancy, women who are or may become pregnant should abstain from alcohol. However, health professionals should reassure women who have consumed small amounts of alcohol occasionally during pregnancy that the risk is likely minimal. Pregnant women should also know that stopping any time will have benefits for both foetus and mother.

In June, 1992, the Standing Committee on Health and Welfare, Social Affairs, Seniors, and the Status of Women released its report, "Foetal Alcohol Syndrome, A Preventable Tragedy." Since then, Health Canada has worked with health care professionals to identify and implement prevention strategies; has produced pamphlets and videos on FAS; and, with the Association of Canadian Distillers and the Brewers' Association of Canada, sponsors a national information service resource centre providing links to support groups, prevention projects, and experts on FAS/FAE (1-800-559-4514).

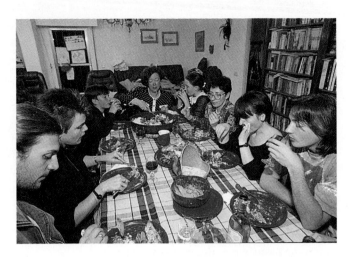

𝒲HAT DO YOU THINK?

Why do we hear so little about FAS when it is the leading cause of developmental delay in North America? Is this a reflection of our society's denial of alcohol as a dangerous drug?

Drinking and Driving

The leading cause of death for all age groups from 5 to 34 years old (including university students) is traffic accidents. Young people between 15 and 29 account for 38 percent of motor vehicle fatalities. The rate is highest for 20- to 24-year-olds, at 14.7 percent.[12] A high proportion of traffic fatalities are alcohol-related. Impaired driving is a major cause of death; among fatally injured drivers, 45 percent had some alcohol in their blood, and 38 percent were over the legal limit of 0.08 percent BAC.[13]

𝒜LCOHOLISM

Alcohol use becomes **alcohol abuse** or **alcoholism** when it interferes with work, school, or social and family relationships or when it entails any violation of the law, including driving with a blood alcohol level over the legal limit.

Alcoholism is one of many addictions or dependencies on substances or behaviours that have mood-altering consequences. The Canadian Centre for Studies in Addiction estimates that in 1989 there were 1900 alcoholics per 100 000 population in Canada, ranging from a high of 2100 in Ontario to a low of 1100 in New Brunswick.[14]

According to the 1993 General Social Survey, nearly one in ten adult Canadians (9.2 percent) said they have problems with their drinking. The most common problems affect physical health (5.1 percent) and financial position (4.7 percent). Almost half of Canadians (43.9 percent) say they have had problems from other people's drinking, such as being disturbed by loud parties (23.8 percent), being insulted or humiliated (20.9 percent) and having a serious argument (15.6 percent). There were 6701 deaths and 86 076 hospitalizations attributed to alcohol in 1992. Motor vehicle accidents accounted for the largest number of alcohol-related deaths, while accidental falls and alcohol dependence syndrome accounted for the largest number of alcohol-related hospitalizations.

Foetal alcohol syndrome (FAS): A disorder that may affect the foetus when the mother consumes alcohol during pregnancy. Among its effects are mental retardation, small head, tremors, and abnormalities of the face, limbs, heart, and brain.

Foetal alcohol effects (FAE): A syndrome describing children with a history of prenatal alcohol exposure but without all the physical or behavioural symptoms of FAS. Among its symptoms are low birthweight, irritability, and possible permanent mental impairment.

Alcohol abuse (alcoholism): Use of alcohol that interferes with work, school, or personal relationships or that entails violations of the law.

Am I Severely Dependent on Alcohol?

Most people who are severely dependent on alcohol experience the symptoms described below. Review each point carefully and check any statements that apply to you.

Wlthdrawal symptoms

In the past six months, after I had been drinking I sometimes experienced:

☐ shakes (a coarse tremor in my hands, tongue, or eyelids)

☐ a lot of sweating and fever

☐ panic (strong anxiety)

☐ hallucinations (I saw, heard, or felt things that were not really there)

Drinking to Relieve Withdrawal Symptoms

In the past six months, more than once:

☐ I needed alcohol to relieve withdrawal symptoms (for instance, I drank in the morning, or when I woke up, to calm the shakes or other unpleasant feelings).

☐ I needed alcohol to avoid experiencing withdrawal symptoms.

If you checked any of the symptoms in the two sections above, you should seek professional assistance.

Do I Have Other Signs of Dependence?

If an expert were assessing how dependent you are on alcohol, he or she would also judge to what degree the following statements were true or not true about you.

In the past six months:

☐ I often drank larger amounts of alcohol than I intended, or I drank for longer periods than I intended.

☐ I often felt that I should cut down or control my alcohol use, or I made one or more unsuccessful efforts to control it.

☐ I spent a great deal of time trying to get alcohol, drinking alcohol, or recovering from the effects of drinking.

☐ I was often intoxicated, or suffering the effects of drinking during my work, while taking care of my child, or during school. Or I put myself and others at risk (for example, by driving under the influence of alcohol).

☐ I have given up, or reduced my involvement in important social, work-related, or recreational activities because of my drinking.

☐ I continued to use alcohol in spite of one or more persistent or recurring problems that were being made worse because of my drinking.

☐ My tolerance for alcohol has increased. I need to drink at least 50 percent more to get the effect I want, or I get much less effect if I drink at my previous level.

If you experienced three, four, or even five of these symptoms, but not to an extreme degree, your alcohol dependence is mild or moderate. If you are not sure about your answers, you may consider:

☐ consulting a specialist to help you with this assessment

☐ starting this program, but keeping in mind that if you do not make progress, it would be wise to consider more intensive help

Am I Enduring a Personal Crisis?

Personal crises make it difficult to change drinking habits without extra help.

I am:

☐ in the middle of a separation or divorce

☐ in the middle of a child custody dispute

☐ charged with a serious offence

☐ unemployed after losing a good job

☐ filing for bankruptcy or having serious financial problems

☐ severely depressed

☐ mourning the recent loss of someone I loved

If you checked any of the above, you should get appropriate professional advice to help you cope with your crisis and your drinking. When you get over the crisis, if you are still concerned about your drinking, a program such as Saying When can help you.

Am I Having Problems with Other Drugs?

These are some of the drugs that can make a drinking problem even worse:

☐ tranquillizers (such as Valium, Librium, and Ativan)

☐ sleeping pills (such as Seconal and Halcyon)

☐ painkillers (such as codeine, Percodan, and Demerol)

☐ marijuana or hashish

☐ amphetamines or "uppers" (such as speed)

☐ cocaine

You have a problem with drugs other than alcohol if one of these statements is true of you:

☐ I am taking a prescription drug, but not according to the recommendation of my doctor—usually I take more.

☐ I occasionally use an illicit drug, sometimes with problems and sometimes without problems.

☐ I frequently use an illicit drug.

If you have problems with any of the drugs mentioned above, you should seek professional help.

Source: Adapted from *Saying When: How to Quit Drinking or Cut Down,* by Martha Sanchez-Craig, Addiction Research Foundation, 1993.

How, Why, Who?

As with other drug addicts, tolerance, psychological dependence, and withdrawal symptoms must be present to qualify a drinker as an addict. Addiction results from chronic use over a period of time that may vary from person to person. Problem drinkers or irresponsible users are not necessarily alcoholics. The stereotype of the alcoholic on skid row applies to only 5 percent of the alcoholic population. The remaining 95 percent of alcoholics live in some type of extended family unit. They can be found at all socioeconomic levels and in all professions, ethnic groups, geographical locations, religions, and races. You have a 1 in 10 risk of becoming an alcoholic.

Alcoholics tend to have a number of behaviours in common. Some of the indicators of this disease are listed in the Rate Yourself box. People who recognize one or more of these behaviours in themselves may wish to seek professional help to determine whether alcohol has become a controlling factor in their lives.

Women are the fastest-growing component of the population of alcohol abusers. They tend to become alcoholic at a later age and after fewer years of heavy drinking than do male alcoholics. Women at highest risk for alcohol-related problems are those who are unmarried but living with a partner, are in their 20s or early 30s, or have a husband or partner who drinks heavily.

The Causes of Alcoholism

We know that alcoholism is a disease with biological, psychological, and social/environmental components, but we do not know what role each of these components plays in the disease.

Biological and Family Factors.   Research into the hereditary and environmental causes of alcoholism has found higher rates of alcoholism among family members of alcoholics. In fact, according to researchers, alcoholism is four to five times more common among the children of alcoholics than in the general population.

Male alcoholics, especially, are more likely than nonalcoholics to have alcoholic parents and siblings. Two distinct subtypes of alcoholism have provided important information about the inheritance of alcoholism. *Type 1 alcoholics* are drinkers who had at least one parent of either sex who was a problem drinker and who grew up in an environment that encouraged heavy drinking. Their drinking is reinforced by environmental events during which there is heavy drinking. Type 1 alcohol abusers share certain personality characteristics. They avoid novelty and harmful situations and are concerned about the thoughts and feelings of others. *Type 2 alcoholism* is seen in males only. These alcoholics are typically the biological sons of alcoholic fathers who have a history of both violence and drug use. Type 2 alcoholics display the opposite characteristics of Type 1 alcoholics. They do not seek so-

cial approval, they lack inhibition, and they are prone to novelty-seeking behaviour.[15]

A 1984 study found a strong relationship between alcoholism and alcoholic patterns within the family.[16] Children with one alcoholic parent had a 52 percent chance of becoming alcoholics themselves. With two alcoholic parents, the chances of becoming alcoholic jumped to 71 percent. These findings are controversial today.

Scientists are on the trail of an "alcohol gene," but so far they have not managed to find one. In 1990, it appeared that a specific gene linked to alcoholism had been discovered. The gene was reportedly a receptor for dopamine, a chemical that plays a crucial role in cell communication and pleasure-seeking behaviour. It turned out, however, that not only was the gene not found consistently in every alcoholic studied but it also existed in some individuals who were not alcoholics.[17]

Because the effects of heredity and environment are so difficult to separate, some scientists have chosen to examine the problem through twin and adoption studies. So far, these studies have produced inconclusive results, although a slightly higher rate of similar drinking behaviours has been demonstrated among identical twins. Moreover, sons living away from their alcoholic parents tend to more nearly resemble them in drinking behaviour than they do their adoptive or foster parents.

Social and Cultural Factors.   Although a family history of alcoholism may predispose a person to problems with alcohol, there are numerous other factors that may mitigate or exacerbate that tendency. Furthermore, researchers now believe that social and cultural factors may trigger the affliction for many people who are not genetically predisposed to alcoholism. Some people begin drinking as a way to dull the pain of an acute loss or an emotional or social problem. For example, students may drink to escape the stress of university life, disappointment over unfulfilled expectations, difficulties in forming relationships, or loss of the security of home, loved ones, and close friends. Unfortunately, the emotional discomfort that causes many people to turn to alcohol also ultimately causes them to become even more uncomfortable as the depressant effect of the drug begins to take its toll. Thus, the person who is already depressed may become even more depressed, antagonizing friends and other social supports until they begin to turn away.

Family attitudes toward alcohol also seem to influence whether or not a person will develop a drinking problem. It has been clearly demonstrated that people who are raised in cultures in which drinking is a part of religious or ceremonial activities or in which alcohol is a traditional part of the family meal are less prone to alcohol dependency. In contrast, in societies in which alcohol purchase is carefully controlled and drinking is regarded as a rite of passage to adulthood, the tendency for abuse appears to be greater.[18]

Certain social factors have been linked with alcoholism as well. These include urbanization, the weakening of links to the extended family and a general loosening of kinship ties, increased mobility, and changing religious and philosophical values. Apparently, then, some combination of heredity and environment plays a decisive role in the development of alcoholism.

WHAT DO YOU THINK?

What were the attitudes in your family toward drinking? Are those attitudes reflected in your current drinking behaviour?

Effects of Alcoholism on the Family

Only recently have people begun to recognize that it is not only the alcoholic but the alcoholic's entire family that suffers from the disease of alcoholism. Although most research focusses on family effects during the late stages of alcoholism, the family unit actually begins to react early on as the person starts to show symptoms of the disease.

Dealing with the far-reaching effects of alcoholism strains the alcoholic's entire family. Many families affected by alcoholism have no idea what normal family life is like. Family members unconsciously adapt to the alcoholic's behaviour by adjusting their own behaviour. To minimize their feelings about the alcoholic or out of love for him or her, family members take on various abnormal roles. Unfortunately, these roles actually help keep the alcoholic drinking. Children in such dysfunctional families generally assume at least one of the following roles:

- *Family hero:* tries to divert attention from the problem by being too good to be true

- *Scapegoat:* draws attention away from the family's primary problem through delinquency or misbehaviour

- *Lost child:* becomes passive and quietly withdraws from upsetting situations

- *Mascot:* disrupts tense situations by providing comic relief

For children in alcoholic homes, life is a struggle. They have to deal with constant stress, anxiety, and embarrassment. Because the alcoholic is the centre of attention, the children's wants and needs are often ignored. It is not uncommon for these children to be victims of violence, abuse, neglect, or incest. As we have seen, when such children grow up, they are much more prone to alcoholic behaviours themselves than are children from nonalcoholic families.

In the last decade, we have come to recognize the unique problems of adult children of alcoholics whose difficulties in life stem from a lack of parental nurturing during childhood. Among these problems are an inability to develop social attachments, a need to be in control of all emotions and situations, low self-esteem, and depression.

Fortunately, not all individuals who have grown up in alcoholic families are doomed to have lifelong problems. Many of these people as they mature develop a resiliency in response to their families' problems. They thus enter adulthood armed with positive strengths and valuable career-oriented skills, such as the ability to assume responsibility, strong organizational skills, and realistic expectations of their jobs and others.

Costs to Society

The entire society suffers the consequences of individuals' alcohol abuse. The figure of $18.45 billion, or 2.7 percent of GDP, represents the most optimistic estimate of the cost of addiction to society. The actual number could be significantly higher. Of this amount, alcohol accounts for $7.5 billion in costs.[19]

Women and Alcoholism

In the past, women have consumed less alcohol and have had fewer alcohol-related problems than have men. But now, greater percentages of women, especially university-aged women, are choosing to drink and are drinking more heavily.

Studies indicate that there are now almost as many female as male alcoholics. However, there appear to be differences between men and women when it comes to alcohol abuse.[20]

1. Women attribute the onset of problem drinking to a specific life stress or traumatic event more frequently than do men.

2. Women's alcoholism starts later and progresses more quickly than men's alcoholism, a phenomenon called telescoping.

3. Women tend to be prescribed mood-altering drugs more often than are men; women thus face the risks of drug interaction or cross-tolerance more often.

4. Nonalcoholic males tend to divorce their alcoholic spouses nine times more often than they do their nonalcoholic spouses; alcoholic women are thus not as likely to have a family support system to aid them in their recovery attempts.

5. Female alcoholics do not tend to receive as much social support as do males in their treatment and recovery.

6. Unmarried, divorced, or single-parent women tend to have significant economic problems that may make entry into a treatment program especially difficult.[21]

Talking to the Drinker

Friendship is not all fun and games. There are tough times in any relationship. Sometimes that means directly confronting a problem and giving support when your friend is having trouble coping. If you think a friend has a drinking problem, it may mean getting involved in some embarrassing discussions or situations. But you can help. Don't step back and pretend it's none of your business. Many problem drinkers say that talking with friends helped them seek professional guidance or gain better control of their drinking.

How to Talk to the Drinker

If you care, show your concern. Don't be too polite to bring up the topic, but be tactful. Ask whether the person feels he or she has a drinking problem and continue asking questions that encourage frankness. Avoid sermons, lectures, and verbal attacks. Keep an open mind about how the person evaluates his or her situation.

Dealing with Defensiveness. Make it clear to the problem drinker that you dislike the behaviour, not the person. Understand that the person's defensiveness is based on fear of facing the problem and isn't directed at you.

Dealing with Denial. If your discussions have no effect on your friend's drinking behaviour, you should still tell him or her how the drinking problem affects you. For example, you can say how hard it is for you to enjoy going out together to a party because you are afraid he or she will get sick, pass out, or otherwise embarrass you both.

Dealing with Agreement. If at some point your friend agrees that drinking is creating personal problems, you may want to ask:

1. Why do you think you have a problem with alcohol?
2. What do you think you can do about it?
3. What are you going to do about it?
4. What kinds of support do you need from me to stop or limit your drinking?

You may also want to have some referrals ready for your friend. Most campuses and communities have discussion groups and/or counselling services.

Progress, Not Perfection

In some cases, even though the drinker agrees there is a problem, he or she may be unable or unwilling to act as quickly or directly as you'd like. Keep in mind that alcohol-related habits are hard to end or control. If your friend is struggling, try to

- remain supportive by recognizing the effort the person puts into even small attempts to limit drinking
- be prepared for some steps backward as well as forward
- help your friend make contact with recovering alcoholics
- encourage nondrinking behaviour by planning activities not related to alcohol and by curbing your own drinking when you are with your friend

Source: From "How to Help a Friend with a Drinking Problem," by permission of American College Health Association, P.O. Box 28937, Baltimore MD 21240 - 8937 (phone 410 - 859 - 1500).

*W*HAT DO YOU THINK?

Why have women started to drink more heavily? Do we look at men's and women's drinking problems in the same way? Can you think of ways to increase support for women in their recovery process?

*R*ECOVERY

Most alcoholics and problem drinkers who seek help have experienced a turning point or dramatic occurrence, such as a failed relationship or confrontation at work. Regardless of the reasons for seeking help, the alcoholic has finally recognized that alcohol controls his or her life. The first step on the road to recovery is to regain that control and to begin to assume responsibility for personal actions.

The Family's Role

Family members of an alcoholic sometimes take action before the alcoholic does. They may go to an organization or a treatment facility to seek help for themselves and their relative. An effective method of helping an alcoholic to confront the disease is a process called **intervention.**

Intervention: A planned confrontation with an alcoholic in which family members or friends express their concern about the alcoholic's drinking.

Essentially, an intervention is a planned confrontation with the alcoholic that involves several family members plus professional counsellors. For more on how to plan an intervention, see the Building Communication Skills box. The family members express their love and concern, telling the alcoholic that they will no longer refrain from acknowledging the problem and affirming their support for appropriate treatment. A family intervention is the turning point for a growing number of alcoholics.

Treatment Programs

There are 262 residential care facilities in Canada for the treatment of alcohol and drug addiction, funded by a mix of municipal, provincial, and federal sources. There are also outpatient, detox, walk-in, and crisis centres. Treatment programs are based on various models and are offered in many languages besides French and English, from Cree to Norwegian to Urdu. A pamphlet is available describing all the facilities.[22]

Upon admission to a treatment facility, the patient is given a complete physical exam to determine whether there are underlying medical problems that will interfere with treatment. Alcoholics who decide to quit drinking will experience withdrawal symptoms, including:

- hyperexcitability
- confusion
- sleep disorders
- convulsions
- agitation
- tremors of the hands
- brief hallucinations
- depression

- headache
- seizures

In a small percentage, alcohol withdrawal results in a severe syndrome known as **delirium tremens (DTs)**. Delirium tremens is characterized by confusion, delusions, agitated behaviour, and hallucinations.

For any long-term addict, medical supervision is usually necessary. *Detoxification*, the process by which addicts end their dependence on a drug, is commonly carried out in a medical facility, where patients can be monitored to prevent fatal withdrawal reactions. Withdrawal takes from 7 to 21 days. Shortly after detoxification, alcoholics begin their treatment for psychological addiction. Most treatment facilities keep their patients from three to six weeks. Treatment at private treatment centres costs several thousand dollars, but some insurance programs or employers will assume most of this expense.

Family Therapy, Individual Therapy, and Group Therapy. Various individual and group therapies are also available. In family therapy, the person and family members gradually examine the psychological reasons underlying the addiction. In individual and group therapy with fellow addicts, alcoholics learn positive coping skills for use in situations that have regularly caused them to turn to alcohol. On some university campuses, the problems associated with alcohol abuse are so great that student health centres are opening their own treatment programs.

Other Types of Treatment. Two other treatments are drug and aversion therapy. Disulfiram (trade name: Antabuse) is the drug of choice for treating alcoholics. If alcohol is consumed, the drug causes such unpleasant effects as headache, nausea, vomiting, drowsiness, and hangover. These symptoms discourage the alcoholic from drinking. Aversion therapy is based on conditioning therapy. It works on the premise that the sight, smell, and taste of alcohol will acquire aversive properties if repeatedly paired with a noxious stimulus. For a period of ten days, the alcoholic takes drugs that induce vomiting when combined with several drinks. These treatments work best in conjunction with some type of counselling.

Alcoholics Anonymous (AA) is a private, nonprofit, self-help organization founded in 1935. The organization, which relies upon group support to help people stop drinking, currently has over one million members and has branches all over the world. People attending their first AA meeting will find that no last names are ever used. Neither is anyone forced to speak. Members are taught to believe that their alcoholism is a lifetime problem. They share their stories with the group and are asked to place their faith and control of the habit into the hands of a "higher power." The road to recovery is taken one step at a time. AA offers specialized meetings for gay, atheist, HIV-positive, and professional individuals with alcohol problems.

Delirium tremens (DTs): A state of confusion brought on by withdrawal from alcohol. Symptoms include hallucinations, anxiety, and trembling.

Alcoholics Anonymous: An organization whose goal is to help alcoholics stop drinking; includes auxiliary branches such as Al-Anon and Alateen.

Snuff: A powdered form of tobacco that is sniffed and absorbed through the mucous membranes in the nose or placed inside the cheek and sucked.

Chewing tobacco: A stringy type of tobacco that is placed in the mouth and then sucked or chewed.

Nicotine: The stimulant chemical in tobacco products.

Tar: A thick, brownish substance condensed from particulate matter in smoked tobacco.

Alcoholics Anonymous also has auxiliary groups to help spouses or partners, friends, and children of alcoholics. *Al-Anon* is the group dedicated to helping adult relatives and friends of alcoholics understand the disease and learn how they can contribute to the recovery process.

The support gained from talking with others who have similar problems is one of the greatest benefits derived from participation in Al-Anon. Many members learn how to exert greater control over their own lives. Some are able to rid themselves of the guilt they feel about their participation in their loved one's alcoholism.

Alateen, another AA-related organization, is designed to help adolescents live with an alcoholic parent or parents. They are taught that they are not at fault for their parents' problems. They learn skills to develop their self-esteem so they can function better socially. Alateen also helps them to overcome their guilt feelings.

Relapse

Success in recovery from alcoholism varies with the individual. A return to alcoholic habits often follows what appears to be a successful recovery. Some alcoholics never recover. Some partially recover and improve other parts of their lives, but remain dependent on alcohol. Many alcoholics refer to themselves as "recovering" throughout their lifetime; they never use the word *cured.*

Roughly 60 percent of alcoholics relapse (resume drinking) within the first three months of treatment. Why is the relapse rate so high? Treating an addiction requires more than getting the addict to stop using; it also requires getting the person to break a pattern of behaviour that has dominated his or her life.

People who are seeking to regain a healthy lifestyle must not only confront their addiction, but also guard against the tendency to relapse. Drinkers with compulsive personalities need to learn to understand themselves and take control. Others need to view treatment as a long-term process that takes a lot of effort beyond attending a weekly self-help group meeting. In order to work, a recovery program must offer the alcoholic ways to increase self-esteem and resume personal growth.

$\mathcal{S}$MOKING

Canadians are smoking less since 1966, when 54 percent of men and 28 percent of women were smokers. The rate in 1991 was 26 percent for both sexes. (See the Global Perspectives box for a comparison with rates in other countries.)

Smoking remains, however, the number one preventable cause of death and disease in Canada. In 1991, smoking-related deaths accounted for about 62 percent of the overall increase in deaths from 1989. Female smoking-related deaths are rising faster than those of their male counterparts. The number of smoking deaths among women increased from 9009 in 1985 to 13 541 in 1991. The number of deaths among men remained relatively constant throughout this period.[23]

$\mathcal{W}$HAT DO YOU THINK?

What would it be like if Canada were smoke-free? What types of repercussions would there be? Who would be affected? What do you think needs to be done to further reduce the number of smokers in Canada?

$\mathcal{T}$OBACCO AND ITS EFFECTS

Tobacco is available in several forms: cigarettes, cigars, and pipes are used for burning and inhaling tobacco. **Snuff** is a finely ground form of tobacco that can be inhaled, chewed, or placed against the gums. **Chewing tobacco,** also known as "smokeless tobacco," is placed between the gums and teeth for sucking or chewing.

The chemical stimulant **nicotine** is the major psychoactive substance in all these tobacco products. In its natural form, nicotine is a colourless liquid that turns brown upon oxidation (exposure to oxygen). When tobacco leaves are burned in a cigarette, pipe, or cigar, nicotine is released and inhaled into the lungs. Sucking or chewing a quid of tobacco releases nicotine into the saliva, and the nicotine is then absorbed through the mucous membranes in the mouth.

Smoking is the most common form of tobacco use. Smoking delivers a strong dose of nicotine to the user, along with an additional 4000 chemical substances. Among these chemicals are various gases and vapours that carry particulate matter in concentrations that are 500 000 times as great as the most air-polluted cities in the world.[24]

Particulate matter condenses in the lungs to form a thick, brownish sludge called **tar.** Tar contains various carcinogenic (cancer-causing) agents such as benzopyrene and chemical irritants such as phenol. Phenol has the potential to combine with other chemicals to contribute to the development of lung cancer.

In healthy lungs, millions of tiny hairlike tissues called cilia sweep away foreign matter. Once the foreign material is swept up and collected by the cilia, it can be expelled from the lungs by coughing. Nicotine impairs the cleansing function of the cilia by paralyzing them for up to one hour following the smoking of a single cigarette. Tars and other solids in tobacco smoke are thus allowed to accumulate and irritate sensitive lung tissue.

Tar and nicotine are not the only harmful chemicals in cigarettes. In fact, tars account for only 8 percent of the components of tobacco smoke. The remaining 92 percent is made up of various gases, the most dangerous of which is **carbon monoxide.** In tobacco smoke, the concentration of carbon monoxide is 800 times higher than the level considered safe. In the human body, carbon monoxide reduces the oxygen-carrying capacity of the red blood cells by binding with the receptor sites for oxygen. Smoking thus diminishes the capacity of the circulatory system to carry oxygen, causing oxygen deprivation in many body tissues.

The heat from tobacco smoke, which can reach 880°C, is also harmful to the smoker. Inhaling hot gases and vapours exposes sensitive mucous membranes to irritating chemicals that weaken the tissues and contribute to the development of cancers of the mouth, larynx, and throat.

Filtred cigarettes designed to reduce levels of gases such as hydrogen cyanide and hydrocarbons may actually deliver more hazardous carbon monoxide to the user than do non-filtred brands. Some smokers use low-tar and nicotine products as an excuse to smoke more cigarettes. This practice is self-defeating, because such smokers wind up exposing themselves to more harmful substances than they would if they smoked regular-strength cigarettes.

Clove cigarettes contain about 40 percent ground cloves (a spice) and about 60 percent tobacco. Many users mistakenly believe that these products are made entirely of ground cloves and that smoking them eliminates the risks associated with tobacco. In fact, clove cigarettes contain higher levels of tar, nicotine, and carbon monoxide than do regular cigarettes. In addition, the numbing effect of eugenol, the active ingredient in cloves, allows smokers to inhale the smoke more deeply.

Nicotine is a powerful central nervous system stimulant that produces an aroused, alert mental state. Nicotine also stimulates the adrenal glands, increasing the production of adrenaline. The physical effects of nicotine stimulation include increased heart and respiratory rate, constriction of blood vessels, and subsequent increased blood pressure because the heart must work harder to pump blood through the narrowed vessels.

Nicotine decreases the stomach contractions that signal hunger. It also decreases blood sugar levels. These factors, along with decreased sensation in the taste buds, reduce appetite. For this reason, many smokers eat less than nonsmokers do and weigh, on average, three kilograms less than nonsmokers. Beginning smokers usually feel the effects of nicotine with their first puff. These symptoms, called **nicotine poisoning**, include dizziness, lightheadedness, rapid, erratic pulse, clammy skin, nausea, vomiting, and diarrhea. The effects of nicotine poisoning cease as soon as tolerance to the chemical develops. Medical research indicates that tolerance develops almost immediately in new users, perhaps after the second or third cigarette. In contrast, tolerance to most other drugs, such as alcohol, develops over a period of months or years.

SMOKING—A LEARNED BEHAVIOUR

Taking up smoking is a gradual process. It begins with forming a predisposition to smoking: that is, a perception that smoking is a normal behaviour that is acceptable and pervasive in society or one's peer group. Trying smoking can lead to an experimental stage when smoking happens repeatedly but irregularly; regular use and addiction follow. The transition from trying smoking to daily use takes an average of two to three years.

About 85 percent of smokers start before age 16. New smokers do not expect to become addicted, believing instead that they will be able to quit whenever they want to, and tend to discount the prospect of addiction and the potential adverse health effects of that future addiction.

Tobacco product promotions are intended to convey a positive brand image and convey as many "impressions" (exposures to the consumer) as possible in order to create and maintain the perception that tobacco use is desirable, socially acceptable, healthy, and more pervasive in society than it really is.

This positive image of tobacco use is precisely the perception that people need in order to feel reassured about smoking. Promotion affects tobacco consumption in three interrelated ways:

- by influencing the smoking decision process among starters through helping to shape and reinforce their belief that it's okay to smoke

- by influencing the amount consumed by smokers

- by hindering the quitting decision process among those who are addicted by acting as a reassuring cue to smoke[25]

Carbon monoxide: A gas found in cigarette smoke that binds at oxygen receptor sites in the blood.

Nicotine poisoning: Symptoms often experienced by beginning smokers; they include dizziness; diarrhea; lightheadedness; rapid, erratic pulse; clammy skin; nausea; and vomiting.

WHAT DO YOU THINK?

Given the unpleasant effects of smoking when people begin to smoke, why do they continue? Do you think people would buy cigarettes if they were nicotine-free? Why or why not?

Global Smoking Patterns

Globally, it is estimated that 47 percent of men and 12 percent of women smoke. In developing countries, there is a marked difference between male and female patterns: available data suggest that about 48 percent of men and 7 percent of women smoke. For developed countries, the corresponding figures are 42 percent for men and 24 percent for women. The rate for men varies substantially among regions, from less than 30 percent in the African Region to 60 percent in the Western Pacific Region, primarily due to a 61 percent rate in China. In countries with established market economies, male smoking rates average 37 percent, compared to 60 percent in the formerly socialist countries of Central and Eastern Europe.

In many countries, smoking begins at younger and younger ages, with the median age of initiation under 15 in many countries. For example, in South Africa, over half of young men under the age of 35 are smokers. Over 40 percent of young people age 18–24 in both France and Spain are smokers. In Canada, for the 15–19 age group, 20 percent of women and 12 percent of men are smokers.

Starting to smoke at younger ages increases the risk of death from a smoking-related cause. Data from the mid-1990s show that smoking causes many more deaths than was previously estimated: smokers have a threefold higher death rate than nonsmokers in middle age (35–69), and at least a twofold excess mortality from all causes in old age. In fact, the data suggest that at least one in two regular smokers who begin smoking during adolescence will eventually be killed by tobacco, half in middle age, half in old age.

Per capita cigarette consumption in the developed countries rose steadily from around 600 cigarettes per adult per year (mainly among males) in the early 1920s, to reach a peak of over 3000 cigarettes per adult in the 1970s. As consumption levels rose, smoking-related mortality increased, with an approximate 30-to-40-year lag between onset of persistent smoking and deaths from smoking. By 1955, smoking was claiming around 500 000 deaths per year in the developed countries, mostly among men. Since that time, smoking-attributable deaths have risen dramatically and by 1995, almost 2 million people (1.5 million men, 500 000 women) in developed countries were dying each year from tobacco. In populations where tobacco use has been common for several decades (e.g., men in the United States and the United Kingdom), tobacco is likely to be the most important risk of death in middle age. For example, in the United Kingdom, on average, among 1000 20-year-olds who smoke cigarettes regularly:

- About one will die from homicide (murder) before age 70.

- About six will die from motor vehicle accidents prior to age 70.

- About 250 will die from smoking before age 70 (plus about another 250 deaths from smoking after age 70).

Sources: World Health Organization, *Health Effects;* World Health Organization, *Health Hazards of Tobacco.*

FINANCING THE HEALTH COSTS OF SMOKING

Of the estimated $18.45 billion addictions cost society, smoking accounted for $9.6 billion—more than alcohol and drugs combined.[26] How can this cost be met?

Since 1987, the state of Victoria, in Australia, has taken a leading role in creatively undermining tobacco promotions and sponsorship. The state has legislation which not only bans tobacco sponsorship, but has also created a Health Promotion Foundation (VicHealth) funded by revenue from a special levy on cigarettes. In addition to funding numerous other health promotion activities and an ongoing QUIT smoking campaign, a portion of this revenue also provides funding to sports and cultural associations that might otherwise have depended upon tobacco companies for support.[27]

In Canada, the Tobacco Demand Reduction Strategy, announced in February 1994, is being implemented cooperatively with the provinces and territories and with Canada's health community. The three-year initiative combines targeted activities including legislation, communication action initiatives, research, public education, and awareness for groups at risk. Financed by a surtax on tobacco manufacturing profits, the Strategy provides funding for activities designed to reduce tobacco use.[28]

HEALTH HAZARDS OF SMOKING

An estimated 27 867 male and 13 541 female deaths in Canada in 1994 were attributable to smoking, for a total of 41 408 deaths. This number includes 171 infants under the age of one who died of smoking-related causes.

Cardiovascular diseases accounted for the greatest number of deaths. with 16 393, while cancers accounted for 16 268 deaths and respiratory diseases for 8157 deaths.

Of the deaths caused by smoking-related disease, lung cancer accounted for 31 percent of male deaths and 26 percent of female deaths; ischemic heart disease (heart attacks) accounted for 25 percent of male deaths and 20 percent of female deaths.

Eighty-five deaths altogether occurred as a result of fires caused by careless smoking.

Twenty-one percent of all deaths were attributable to smoking. The deaths reported in the study were generally the result of smoking habits which began in the 1950s and 1960s.[29]

---

*W*HAT DO YOU THINK?

Given all the dramatic health hazards related to cigarette smoking, why is it difficult for people to stop smoking? Do you think tobacco companies should be held liable for damages resulting from tobacco use?

---

*S*MOKELESS TOBACCO

In the wake of strong antismoking campaigns, tobacco companies have increased their production of chewing tobacco products.

"Smokeless tobacco" is used by a number of teenage and young adult males, who are often emulating a professional sports figure or a family member. Chewing tobacco comes in the form of loose leaf, plug, or twist, and contains tobacco leaves treated with molasses and other flavourings. The user places a "quid" of tobacco in the mouth between the teeth and gums and then sucks or

---

Leukoplakia: A condition characterized by leathery white patches inside the mouth produced by contact with irritants in tobacco juice.

Environmental tobacco smoke (ETS): Smoke from tobacco products, including sidestream and mainstream smoke.

Mainstream smoke: Smoke that is drawn through tobacco while inhaling.

Sidestream smoke: The cigarette, pipe, or cigar smoke breathed by nonsmokers; also called secondhand smoke.

Nicotine withdrawal: Symptoms, including nausea, headaches, and irritability, suffered by smokers who cease using tobacco.

---

chews it to release the nicotine. Once the quid becomes ineffective, the user spits it out and inserts another. Dipping is another method of using chewing tobacco. The dipper takes a small amount of tobacco and places it between the lower lip and teeth to stimulate the flow of saliva and release the nicotine. Dipping rapidly releases the nicotine into the bloodstream.

Risks of Smokeless Tobacco

Smokeless tobacco is just as addictive as cigarettes due to its nicotine content. There is nicotine in all tobacco products, but smokeless tobacco contains more nicotine than do cigarettes. Holding an average-sized dip or chew in your mouth for 30 minutes gives you as much nicotine as smoking four cigarettes. A two-can-a-week snuff dipper gets as much nicotine as a one-and-a-half-pack-a-day smoker.

One of the major risks of chewing tobacco is **leukoplakia**, a condition characterized by leathery white patches inside the mouth produced by contact with irritants in tobacco juice.

Smokeless tobacco also impairs the senses of taste and smell, causing the user to add salt and sugar to food, which may contribute to high blood pressure and obesity. Some smokeless tobacco products contain high levels of sodium (salt), which also contributes to high blood pressure. In addition, dental problems are common among users of smokeless tobacco. Contact with tobacco juice causes receding gums, tooth decay, bad breath, and discoloured teeth. Damage to both the teeth and jawbone can contribute to early loss of teeth. Users of all tobacco products may not be able to use the vitamins and other nutrients in food effectively. In some cases, vitamin supplements may be recommended by a physician.

---

*W*HAT DO YOU THINK?

Why do you think chewing tobacco has attracted athletes? Do you think the use of smokeless tobacco should be banned in high school and university athletics? Should its use be forbidden in residence halls and classrooms just as cigarettes are banned?

---

*E*NVIRONMENTAL TOBACCO SMOKE

As the population of nonsmokers rises, so does the demand for the right to breathe clean air. Although fewer than 30 percent of Canadians are smokers, air pollution from smoking in public places continues to be a problem.

Environmental tobacco smoke (ETS) is divided into two categories: mainstream smoke and sidestream smoke

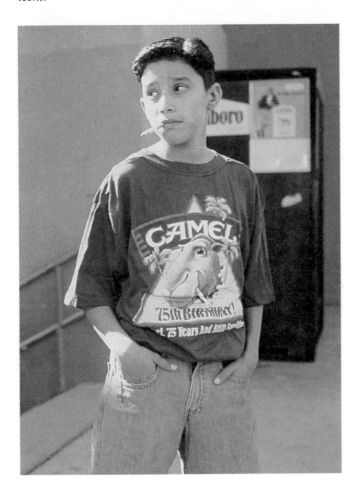

The likelihood of developing cancer and other smoking-related illnesses increases for smokers who start in their teens.

(also called secondhand smoke). **Mainstream smoke** refers to smoke drawn through tobacco while inhaling; **sidestream smoke** refers to smoke from the burning end of a cigarette or to smoke exhaled by a smoker. People who breathe smoke from someone else's smoking product are said to be *involuntary* or *passive* smokers.

Although involuntary smokers breathe less tobacco than active smokers do, they still face risks from exposure to tobacco smoke. Sidestream smoke actually contains more carcinogenic substances than the smoke that a smoker inhales—about twice as much tar and nicotine, five times as much carbon monoxide, and 50 times as much ammonia. A report from the U.S. Environmental Protection Agency (EPA) released in January 1993, following a four-year study of sidestream cigarette smoke, stated that lung cancer caused by cigarette smoke kills about 3000 nonsmokers a year in the United States.[30] There is also recent evidence that sidestream smoke poses an even greater risk for death due to heart disease than for death due to lung cancer.[31] Sidestream smoke is estimated to cause more deaths per year than any other environmental pollutant.[32]

Lung cancer and heart disease are not the only risks involuntary smokers face. Sidestream smoke increases the risk of pneumonia and bronchitis in children.[33] Children exposed to sidestream smoke also have a greater chance of developing other respiratory problems, such as cough, wheezing, asthma, and chest colds, along with a decrease in pulmonary performance. The greatest effects of sidestream smoke are seen in children under the age of five.

Cigarette, cigar, and pipe smoke in enclosed areas present other hazards to nonsmokers. An estimated 10 to 15 percent of nonsmokers are extremely sensitive (hypersensitive) to cigarette smoke.[34] These people experience itchy eyes, difficulty in breathing, painful headaches, nausea, and dizziness in response to minute amounts of smoke. The level of carbon monoxide in cigarette smoke contained in enclosed places is 4000 times higher than the standard recommended by the U.S. EPA for a definition of clean air.

Efforts to reduce the hazards associated with passive smoking have been gaining momentum in recent years. Smoking is now illegal in most public places, including government buildings. Hotels and motels now set aside rooms for nonsmokers, and car rental agencies designate certain vehicles for nonsmokers. Smoking has been banned on all domestic airline flights. In 1996 the City of Toronto brought in a law banning smoking altogether from restaurants, rather than requiring a nonsmoking section as it had until then. Although the bylaw was hailed by environmentalists and health groups, opposition from smokers and restaurant owners led the city to back down—for the moment. The city plans to reintroduce smoke-free restaurants in stages.

QUITTING

Quitting smoking isn't easy. To stop smoking requires breaking an addiction and a habit. Smokers must break the physical addiction to nicotine.

From what we know about successful quitters, quitting is often a lengthy process involving several unsuccessful attempts before success is finally achieved. Even successful quitters suffer occasional slips, emphasizing the fact that quitting smoking is a dynamic process that occurs over time.

Breaking the Nicotine Addiction

Nicotine addiction may be one of the toughest addictions to overcome. Smokers' attempts to quit often lead to **nicotine withdrawal**, which includes irritability, restlessness, nausea, vomiting, and intense cravings for tobacco. The person who wishes to quit has several options.

Nicotine Replacement Products.   Non-tobacco products that replace depleted levels of nicotine in the bloodstream have helped some people stop using tobacco. The two most common nicotine-replacement products are nicotine chewing gum and the nicotine patch, both available by prescription.

Some patients use a prescription chewing gum containing nicotine, called Nicorette, to help them reduce their nicotine consumption over time. Under the guidance of a physician, the user chews between 12 and 24 pieces of gum per day for up to six months. Nicorette delivers about as much nicotine as a cigarette does, but because it is absorbed through the mucous membrane of the mouth, it doesn't produce the same rush as inhaling a cigarette does. Users experience no withdrawal symptoms and fewer cravings for nicotine as the dosage is reduced until they are completely weaned.

There is some controversy surrounding the use of nicotine replacement gum. Opponents believe that it substitutes one addiction for another. Successful users counter that it is a valid way to help break a deadly habit without suffering the unpleasant withdrawal symptoms and cravings that often lead ex-smokers to resume smoking.

The nicotine patch, first marketed in 1991, is the hottest new method for those attempting to quit smoking. It is generally used in conjunction with a comprehensive smoking-behaviour cessation program. A small, thin 24-hour patch placed on the smoker's upper body delivers a continuous flow of nicotine through the skin, helping to relieve the body's cravings. The patch is worn for 8 to 12 weeks under the guidance of a physician. During this time, the dose of nicotine is gradually reduced until the smoker is fully weaned from nicotine. Occasional side-effects include mild skin irritation, insomnia, dry mouth, and nervousness. The patch costs the equivalent of two packs of cigarettes a day—about four dollars—and some insurance plans will pay for it.

Breaking the Habit

For many smokers, the road to quitting includes some type of antismoking therapy. Among the more common therapy techniques are aversion therapy, operant conditioning, and self-control therapy. Prospective quitters must decide which method or combination of methods will work best for them. Programs that combine several approaches have shown the most promise. The Skills for Behaviour Change box takes a light-hearted look at some of the attitudinal aspects of quitting.

Benefits of Quitting

Many tissues damaged by smoking can repair themselves. As soon as smokers stop, their bodies begin the repair

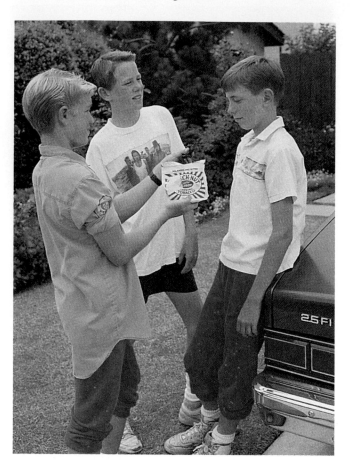

In the wake of anti-smoking campaigns, consumption of smokeless chewing tobacco, particularly by young males, has increased dramatically despite the fact that it can be more hazardous than cigarettes.

process. Within eight hours, carbon monoxide and oxygen levels return to normal, and "smoker's breath" disappears. Within a few days of quitting, the mucus clogging airways is broken up and eliminated. Circulation and the senses of taste and smell improve within weeks. Many ex-smokers who have kicked the cigarette habit say they have more energy, sleep better, and feel more alert. By the end of one year, the risk for lung cancer and stroke decreases. Within two years, the risk for heart attack drops to near-normal. At the end of ten smoke-free years, the ex-smoker can expect to live out his or her normal life span. Figure 11.1 shows the health benefits of quitting smoking.

*W*HAT DO YOU THINK?

What could you personally do to help someone quit smoking? What are the most common barriers to quitting tobacco use? When trying to stop smoking, why do people often interpret a relapse as a total failure?

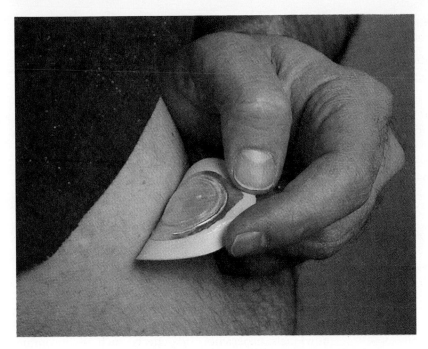

Many smokers find that the unpleasant symptoms of nicotine withdrawal can be mitigated by a nicotine patch that delivers nicotine through the skin, but the success rates for quitting are highest when the patch is combined with counselling or a behaviour modification program.

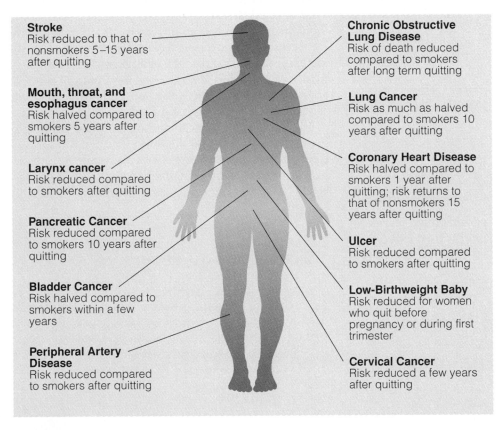

Stroke
Risk reduced to that of nonsmokers 5–15 years after quitting

Mouth, throat, and esophagus cancer
Risk halved compared to smokers 5 years after quitting

Larynx cancer
Risk reduced compared to smokers after quitting

Pancreatic Cancer
Risk reduced compared to smokers 10 years after quitting

Bladder Cancer
Risk halved compared to smokers within a few years

Peripheral Artery Disease
Risk reduced compared to smokers after quitting

Chronic Obstructive Lung Disease
Risk of death reduced compared to smokers after long term quitting

Lung Cancer
Risk as much as halved compared to smokers 10 years after quitting

Coronary Heart Disease
Risk halved compared to smokers 1 year after quitting; risk returns to that of nonsmokers 15 years after quitting

Ulcer
Risk reduced compared to smokers after quitting

Low-Birthweight Baby
Risk reduced for women who quit before pregnancy or during first trimester

Cervical Cancer
Risk reduced a few years after quitting

FIGURE 11.1

Benefits of Quitting Smoking

Source: Reprinted from U.S. Department of Health and Human Services, "The Health Benefits of Smoking Cessation: A Report of the Surgeon General 1990, at a Glance."

TABLE 11.5 ■ Sources of Caffeine

Product	Caffeine (mg)
Coffee (per 30 mL, about 1 oz.)	
(*Note:* 1 cup = 250 mL)	
Automatic percolated	12–24
Filtre drip	18–30
Instant regular	10–15
Average from ground beans	11–13
Instant decaffeinated	<1
Tea (per 30 mL, about 1 oz.)	
Weak	3–4
Strong	13–18
Decaffeinated tea	<0.01
Cola beverages (per 355 mL can)	28–64
Cocoa Products	
Dark chocolate bar (60 g, 2 oz.)	40–50
Milk chocolate bar (60 g, 2 oz.)	3–20
Baking chocolate (30 g, 1 oz.)	25–35
Chocolate milk (250 mL, 8 oz.)	2–8
Hot cocoa from mix (175 mL, 6 oz.)	5–30
Medications (1 tablet or capsule)	
Cold remedies	15–30
Headache relievers	30–32

Source: Health Canada, *Caffeine and You*, 1993.

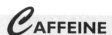

CAFFEINE

Caffeine is consumed as a natural part of coffee, tea, and chocolate. In its manufactured form, it is used as a food additive in cola beverages or as a component of certain

Caffeine: A stimulant found in coffee, tea, chocolate, and some soft drinks.

pharmaceutical preparations. For many people, it is part of their daily wake-up ritual.

Sources of Caffeine

Table 11.5 indicates the many sources of **caffeine.** On average, an estimated 60 percent of ingested caffeine is derived from coffee, 30 percent from tea, and 10 percent from cola beverages, chocolate, and drug preparations.

Levels of caffeine in food products vary, especially in those that are brewed, such as coffee and tea. The amount of caffeine that is transferred to the coffee or tea from the beans or leaves depends upon the temperature of the water, the time the water is in contact with the beans or leaves, and the brewing method employed.[35]

Caffeine and Your Health

Caffeine exhibits a number of biological effects resulting from its diuretic and stimulant properties. Some sensitive individuals experience side-effects such as insomnia, headaches, irritability, and nervousness. *Canada's Guidelines to Healthy Eating* advise consumers to limit caffeine.

Health Canada scientists reviewed the many studies dealing with caffeine and its potential effects on humans. They concluded that while these side-effects may occur, individuals do not face an increased risk of heart disease, hypertension, or adverse effects on pregnancy or on the foetus, provided that the total daily exposure to caffeine is moderated, and does not exceed 400–450 mg. Such moderation of caffeine intake is also important while lactating, as caffeine appears in breast milk.[36]

Products containing caffeine are used and enjoyed by many people throughout the world. The best way for consumers to avoid any adverse effects from caffeine is to recognize the many sources of this substance, to read product labels, and to moderate consumption of caffeine-containing products.

WHAT DO YOU THINK?

Do you consider caffeine a drug? Is the amount of caffeine you consume a concern, or has it ever been a concern? On an average day, how much caffeine do you think you consume? Do you think you could decrease the amount of caffeine you consume and not feel any ill effects?

How to Quit Smoking

Self-knowledge is the place to begin. By recognizing why you smoke, you can learn to replace reaching for a cigarette with other activities. Studies have found that there are six reasons why people smoke. Some people smoke for a single reason while others smoke for several. Read through these categories and see how many apply to you.

Stimulation In general, cigarettes seem to give you a physical lift. You think they help you wake up, get organized and stay alert during the day.

When you stop smoking, try a true pick-me-up such as a brisk walk or moderate exercise.

Handling Picking up a cigarette and watching the smoke as you exhale appears to satisfy you.

Toying with a pencil or doodling or playing with a coin are safe alternatives to lighting up.

Pleasure A pleasant, relaxing feeling seems to overcome you when you smoke a cigarette; smoking appears to ease your tension.

Moderate eating, physical exertion and/or social activities are healthy substitutes for the habit of smoking.

Relaxation When upset or angry, or to relieve the "blahs," you tend to reach for a cigarette believing it will make you feel better. Giving up cigarettes during the good times is easy enough for you. The slightest crisis, however, and you're back to smoking.

At the first sign of stress try taking several very deep, long, slow breaths before you react. Consider taking a leisurely walk or playing a strenuous game of racquet ball instead of reaching for a cigarette.

Craving Running out of cigarettes seems unbearable for you. Your desire for another cigarette begins the moment you put one out.

Quitting "cold turkey" is more effective than tapering off if you are this kind of smoker. Consider quitting when you have the flu or when you've lost your taste for cigarettes.

Habit Lighting a cigarette forgetting that one is already burning in the ashtray characterizes this type of smoker.

If you fall into this category, it's likely you actually derive little satisfaction from your habit. Asking yourself "Do I really want this cigarette?" every time you light one up might make you aware of the number you don't want.

Methods of Quitting

There are only two ways to kick the smoking habit: "cold turkey" and tapering off slowly. The choice is yours. Select that method which seems most comfortable for you.

"Cold Turkey" If you're a habitual smoker or one who craves the taste of tobacco, going "cold turkey" is likely the best way for you to quit smoking. On "quit" day you don't smoke a single cigarette. The same for the following day. And the next. And the next.

Sticking to your personal commitment to kick the smoking habit forever is easier if you have strategies to handle the gnawing urge to smoke. For example, if you are used to smoking when you drink coffee, switch to tea or juice. Or take a walk instead of a coffee break. If you smoke while watching television, take up knitting. If you miss something in your mouth, try replacing it with sugarless gum or mints.

Tapering OFF Slowly This method for giving up the cigarette habit involves reducing the number of cigarettes you smoke little by little each day until "quit" day when you stop smoking altogether.

It is recommended that you begin decreasing the number of cigarettes you smoke two weeks prior to "quit" day. During this time, you can learn to replace reaching for a cigarette with healthier activities and develop the confidence to control your smoking habit.

Begin by setting a quota of cigarettes you will smoke each day before "quit" day. Carry no more than that number of cigarettes with you. For example, if you are going to reduce your smoking by one cigarette a day until "quit" day and you currently smoke a pack a day, plan to carry only 19 cigarettes today, 18 cigarettes tomorrow, 17 cigarettes the next day and so forth. Ideally, by the time "quit" day arrives, you should be smoking about half as many cigarettes as you did at the beginning of your preparation period.

Whether you decide to go *"cold turkey"* or to *taper off,* you will have to expend some effort not only to quit smoking but to quit for good. If you should give in to your urge to smoke, don't think of yourself as a failure. Remember that you are human and only took a step backward. Decide then and there not to have another cigarette and try to stick with your commitment. Many people succeed only after several tries. If you would like more help, contact your local Unit of the Canadian Cancer Society and ask for the booklet "How to be a Happy Ex-Smoker".

Source: How To Quit Smoking, Canadian Cancer Society, 1987.

Managing Alcohol, Tobacco, and Caffeine

After reading this chapter, you probably recognize the threat of what many people consider to be recreational drugs. Assuming that your religion doesn't forbid it, there is nothing wrong with consuming moderate amounts of caffeine and alcohol. The concern lies in how these substances are used. As with the use of any substance that affects you in any way, you must understand the possible problems and options regarding use of alcohol, caffeine, or tobacco, and how it affects those around you.

Making Decisions for You

Societal pressure to drink is everywhere. It's not enough that you are bombarded with ads showing the appeal of alcohol. It also seems that most college social events feature alcohol. As you walk in the door, you're handed a beer. Because of the easy availability of alcohol especially after you turn 19 (or 18 in Quebec, Manitoba, or Alberta), you need to take extra time to decide how *you* want to behave in situations where alcohol is being served. Can you set a drinking limit per social event? Can you set a drinking limit per week? If enticed, how can you stick with your decisions?

Checklist for Change: Making Personal Choices

✓ Do you feel comfortable with how you currently use alcohol? Would you like to change any of your current drinking behaviours?

✓ Do you know the rules to follow for responsible drinking if you are either a party guest or host?

✓ Would you know how to access resources available to help yourself or others who might be experiencing a problem with alcohol?

✓ Are there any reasons why you should be concerned about the role of alcohol in your family?

✓ Have you established responsible drinking guidelines for yourself?

✓ Identify your smoking habits. Keep a daily journal and record when and where you smoked and whom you were with at the time. Maintain your diary for one or two weeks.

✓ Get support. Phone your local chapter of the American Cancer Society or community hospital to find out what programs are being offered and what support groups you can join.

✓ Develop strategies that will help you taper off.

✓ Set a quit date and announce it to family, friends, and roommates.

✓ Stop. A week before you quit, cut your cigarette consumption down to five cigarettes per day and smoke them in the late day or evening.

✓ Follow up by continuing to seek support from your support-group members. Increase your physical activity.

✓ If you fail to stop despite your best efforts, do not hit on yourself. Try again soon.

✓ Do you feel that your caffeine consumption is interfering with your life?

✓ Cut your caffeine consumption by one serving a day every few days until you have reached your goal.

✓ Mix caffeinated products with decaffeinated products, gradually increasing the proportion of the latter until the former is eliminated.

✓ Smokers may want to cut down on caffeine before giving up the nicotine habit.

✓ Find satisfying alternatives to coffee-associated behaviours.

Checklist for Change: Making Community Choices

✓ Have you prioritized the actions you can take to change the drinking environment on your campus?

✓ Do you act responsibly on your campus when you drink by not destroying property, hurting yourself or others, or drinking and driving?

✓ Do you voice your dissatisfactions to friends and others around you who display inappropriate behaviour when they are drinking?

✓ Have you become familiar with the policies and issues surrounding smoke-free environments on your campus and in your community?

✓ Are you aware of the influence that the media have on society? Have you thought of ways to counter the advertisements aimed at yourself and those you associate with?

✓ Do you take an active part in community organizations that are designed to help youth reduce their risky behaviours?

✓ Are you an active participant in community or nation-wide activities, such as Break Free, that encourage the adoption or maintenance of healthy behaviours?

✓ When you vote in local, provincial, or national elections, do you vote in support of legislation that supports healthy lifestyles (such as laws that ban the sale of cigarettes to those underage)?

✓ Do you support organizations in your community that are working to protect nonsmokers?

Critical Thinking

The health department at your school is organizing its annual health fair, and you are chairing the organizing committee. The fair is a popular event, and a large percentage of students turn out to participate. You are particularly interested, because as a first year student you learned from the free screenings offered that you had elevated blood pressure and high cholesterol. But you have run into a major glitch this year: the major corporate sponsors have withdrawn support due to economic conditions. Without corporate support, you can't hold the event. However, a major tobacco company has offered to fund the entire event. All they ask in return is the right to hand out free T-shirts to people leaving the fair. On the one hand, you feel that the event is valuable to students; certainly it alerted you to health problems. On the other hand, you think it is hypocritical for a tobacco company to be sponsoring a health event.

Using the DECIDE model described in Chapter 1, decide what you will recommend to your organizing committee. Remember to be creative in thinking about your options.

Summary

- Alcohol is a central nervous system depressant. While national consumption is declining, university students are under extreme pressure to consume alcohol.

- Alcohol's effect on the body is measured by the blood alcohol concentration (BAC), the ratio of alcohol to total blood volume. The higher the BAC, the greater the impaired judgement and coordination and drowsiness. Use during pregnancy can cause foetal alcohol effects (FAE) or foetal alcohol syndrome (FAS). Alcohol is also a causative factor in traffic accidents.

- Alcohol use becomes alcoholism when it interferes with school, work, or social and family relationships or entails violations of the law. Causes of alcoholism include biological and family factors and social and cultural factors. Alcoholism has far-reaching effects on families, especially on children.

- Most alcoholics do not admit to a problem until reaching a major life crisis or having their families intervene. Treatment options include detoxification at private medical facilities, therapy (family, individual, or group), and programs like Alcoholics Anonymous.

- The use of tobacco involves many social issues, including advertising targeted at youth and women, the largest-growing populations of smokers. Health care and lost productivity resulting from smoking cost the nation about $7.5 billion.

- Tobacco is available in smoking and smokeless forms, both containing addictive nicotine (a psychoactive substance). Smoking also delivers 4000 other chemicals to the lungs of smokers.

- Smokeless tobacco contains more nicotine than do cigarettes and dramatically increases risks for oral cancer and other oral problems.

- Quitting is complicated by the dual nature of smoking: smokers must kick a chemical addiction as well as a habit.

- Caffeine is a widely used central nervous system stimulant. No long-term ill-health effects have been proven, although caffeine may produce withdrawal symptoms for chronic users who try to quit.

Discussion Questions

1. When it comes to drinking alcohol, how much is too much? When you see a friend having "too many" drinks at a party, what actions do you normally take? What actions could you take?

2. What factors may cause someone to slip from being a social drinker to being an alcoholic? What effect does alcoholism have on an alcoholic's family?

3. Discuss the varied forms in which you can ingest tobacco. In each form, how do chemicals enter your system? What are the physiological effects of nicotine?

4. Discuss the varied risks of smokeless tobacco. Do you think that smokeless tobacco should be banned from major league baseball, as it was from the minor leagues?

5. Smokers often claim they have the right to smoke in public places. From what you have learned about side-stream smoke, how would you argue against a smoker's right to smoke in public?

6. After learning about the potential problems associated with caffeine use, have you considered altering the amount you consume?

Application Exercise

Reread the What Do You Think? scenario at the beginning of the chapter and answer the following questions.

1. What responsibility does the restaurant have in protecting the foetus from a known teratogen?

2. What responsibility does the mother have for protecting the foetus?

3. If you were the waiter/waitress, what would you do?

Health on the Net

Heart and Stroke Foundation of Canada
www.hsf.ca/

National Cancer Institute
www.cancer.ca/

World Health Organization: Cardiovascular Diseases Home Page
www.who.ch/programmes/ncd/cvd/cvd_home.htm

Cardiovascular Disease and Cancer

Reducing Your Risks

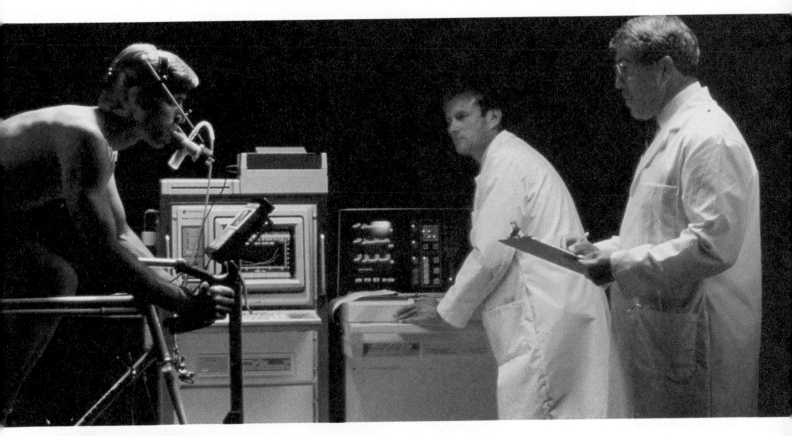

CHAPTER OBJECTIVES

◆ Describe the anatomy and physiology of the heart and the circulatory system.

◆ Review the various types of heart disease and their diagnoses and treatments.

◆ Identify the controllable risk factors for cardiovascular disease. Examine the risk factors you cannot control.

◆ Discuss the issues uniquely concerning women in relationship to cardiovascular disease.

◆ Discuss some of the new methods of diagnosis and treatment of cardiovascular disease.

◆ Define *cancer* and discuss how cancer develops.

◆ Discuss the probable causes of cancer, including biological causes, occupational and environmental causes, social and psychological causes, chemicals in foods, viral causes, medical causes, and combined causes.

◆ Understand and act in response to self-exams, medical exams, and symptoms related to different types of cancers.

◆ Discuss cancer detection and treatment, including radiation therapy, chemotherapy, and immunotherapy.

Thirty-two-year-old Michael is an avid exerciser. He runs 40 miles a week, lifts weights, and keeps his weight under control. His father died of a heart attack at the age of 43, and Michael does not intend to follow in his footsteps. Believing that a sedentary lifestyle and a high-fat diet are the major risk factors for heart disease, he has reduced his consumption of red meats and exercises aerobically every day. He tells his friends that he is "lean and mean" and extremely healthy. He has never had his blood pressure or cholesterol level checked and has never been to a doctor for any reason.

■ Is Michael correct in assuming that exercising and avoiding red meats will protect him from heart disease? Are there other things that he is doing that may put him at risk for a heart attack? Is heredity a risk factor in heart disease? As a responsible health consumer, what actions should Michael take to ensure that his risk is as low as he believes it is?

Despite many advances in medical technology, heart disease and cancer continue to be two of the leading causes of death in Canada. While absolute cures for these diseases do not exist, the actions you take today can have a significant impact on your ability to reduce the risks.

CIRCULATORY DISEASES

During the last century, slowly but surely, we consumed more and more protein-rich, high-fat, high-sugar, high-sodium, and high-calorie foods to the point that, today, over 23 percent of us are overweight and many of the rest of us are so out of shape that a simple trip up the stairs leaves us gasping for breath. Escalators and elevators, automobiles, and numerous other labour-saving devices have released us from much physical exertion. We sit on plump couches and flip through the TV channels by remote control rather than exerting ourselves to get up and change them by hand. We buy blowers to whisk our leaves away rather than get out the old rake. To compound the problem, millions of us continue to smoke and drink. It is no wonder that **circulatory diseases** are the leading cause

Circulatory diseases: Diseases of the heart and blood vessels.

Cardiovascular system: A complex system consisting of the heart and blood vessels that transports nutrients, oxygen, hormones, and enzymes throughout the body and regulates temperature, the water levels of cells, and the acidity levels of body components.

of death in Canada today, accounting for more than 38 percent of all deaths.

Death rates are, however, declining. From 1950 to 1993, the death rate for circulatory diseases fell by 52 percent for males and by 64 percent for females.[1]

How do health experts account for this decline? There are no simple answers. Advances in medical techniques, earlier and better diagnostic procedures and treatments, better emergency medical assistance programs, and training of ordinary citizens in cardiopulmonary resuscitation (CPR) have greatly aided victims of cardiovascular disease. Refinements in surgical techniques and improvements in heart transplants and artificial heart devices have enabled many to live longer lives. Educational programs have promoted public awareness of the role individual efforts, including diet and exercise, can play in risk reduction. Although recent studies show conflicting data on self-reported improvements in diet, obesity, exercise, and smoking behaviours, it is generally assumed that many people are making some positive changes in many areas. All these factors have contributed to increasing optimism about treating and preventing circulatory diseases.

You can reduce your risk for circulatory diseases by taking steps to change certain behaviours. For example, controlling high blood pressure and reducing your intake of saturated fats and cholesterol are two things you can do to lower your chances of heart attack. By maintaining your weight, decreasing your intake of sodium, exercising, and changing your lifestyle to reduce stress, you can lower your blood pressure. You can also monitor the levels of fat and cholesterol in your blood and adjust your diet to prevent your arteries from becoming clogged. By understanding how your cardiovascular system works, you will have a better chance of understanding your risks and of changing your behaviours to reduce them.

UNDERSTANDING YOUR CARDIOVASCULAR SYSTEM

The **cardiovascular system** is the network of elastic tubes through which blood flows as it carries oxygen and nutrients to all parts of the body. It includes the *heart, lungs, arteries, arterioles* (small arteries), and *capillaries* (minute blood vessels). It also includes *venules* (small veins) and *veins*, the blood vessels though which blood flows as it returns to the heart and lungs.[2]

Under normal circumstances, the human body contains approximately six litres of blood. This blood transports nutrients, oxygen, waste products, hormones, and enzymes throughout the body. It also regulates body temperature, cellular water levels, and acidity levels of body components, and aids in bodily defence against toxins and harmful microorganisms. An adequate blood supply is essential to health and well-being.

How does the heart ensure that blood is constantly recirculated to body parts? The four chambers of the heart work together to achieve this (see Figure 12.1). The two upper chambers of the heart, called **atria**, or auricles, are large collecting chambers that receive blood from the rest of the body. The two lower chambers, known as **ventricles**, pump the blood out again. Small valves regulate the steady, rhythmic flow of blood between chambers and prevent inappropriate backwash. The *tricuspid valve*, located between the right atrium and the right ventricle; the *pulmonary (pulmonic) valve*, between the right ventricle and the pulmonary artery; the *mitral valve*, between the left atrium and left ventricle; and the *aortic valve*, between the left ventricle and the aorta, permit blood to flow in only one direction.[3]

Heart activity depends on a complex interaction of biochemical, physical, and neurological signals. The following is a simplified version of the steps involved in heart function:

1. Deoxygenated blood enters the right atrium after having been circulated through the body.

2. From the right atrium, blood moves to the right ventricle and is pumped through the pulmonary artery to the lungs, where it receives oxygen.

3. Oxygenated blood from the lungs then returns to the left atrium of the heart.

4. Blood from the left atrium is forced into the left ventricle.

5. The left ventricle pumps blood through the aorta to all body parts.

Different types of blood vessels are required for different parts of this process. **Arteries** carry blood away from the heart—except for pulmonary arteries, which carry deoxygenated blood to the lungs, where it picks up oxygen and gives off carbon dioxide. As they branch off from the heart, the arteries divide into smaller blood vessels called

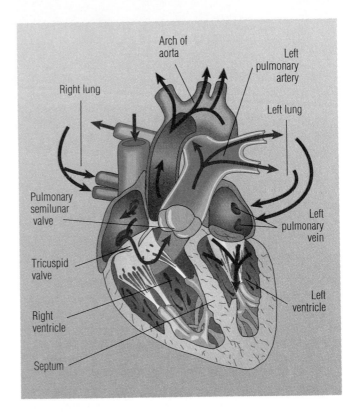

FIGURE 12.1

Anatomy of the Heart

arterioles, and then into even smaller blood vessels called **capillaries**. Capillaries have thin walls that permit the exchange of oxygen, carbon dioxide, nutrients, and waste products with body cells. The carbon dioxide and waste products are transported to the lungs and kidneys through **veins** and venules (small veins).

For the heart to function properly, the four chambers must beat in an organized manner. This is governed by an electrical impulse that directs the heart muscle to move when the impulse moves across it, which results in a sequential contraction of the four chambers. This signal starts in a small bundle of highly specialized cells, the **sinoatrial node (SA node)**, located in the right atrium. The SA node serves as a form of natural pacemaker for the heart.[4] People with damaged or nonfunctional natural pacemaker activity must often have a mechanical pacemaker inserted to insure the smooth passage of blood through the sequential phases of the heartbeat.

The average adult heart at rest beats 70 to 80 times per minute, although a well-conditioned heart may beat only 50 to 60 times per minute to achieve the same results. When overly stressed, a heart may beat over 200 times per minute, particularly in an individual who is overweight or out of shape. A healthy heart functions more efficiently and is less likely to suffer damage from overwork than is an unhealthy one.

What risk factors for heart disease do you currently have? What is your current resting heart rate? Do you know what your current cholesterol level is? Have you taken any action to reduce your fat intake or to improve your cardiovascular function? If not, why not? What actions can you take to improve your overall cardiovascular condition?

TYPES OF CARDIOVASCULAR DISEASES

Although most of us associate cardiovascular disease with heart attacks, there are actually a number of different types of cardiovascular system diseases. Current efforts are aimed at preventing and treating the most common forms of cardiovascular diseases:

- atherosclerosis (fatty plaque buildup in arteries)
- heart attack (myocardial infarction)
- chest pain (angina pectoris)
- irregular heartbeat (arrhythmia)
- congestive heart failure
- congenital and rheumatic heart disease
- stroke (cerebrovascular accident)

Methods of prevention and treatment of these diseases range from changes in diet and lifestyle to use of medications and surgery.

Atherosclerosis: A Major Culprit

Atherosclerosis is a general term for thickening and hardening of the arteries. Atherosclerosis is actually a type of **arteriosclerosis** and is characterized by deposits of fatty substances, cholesterol, cellular waste products, calcium, and *fibrin* (a clotting material in the blood) in the inner lining of an artery. The resulting buildup is referred to as **plaque**.[5]

Plaque may partially or totally block the blood's flow through an artery. Two things that can happen where plaque occurs are (1) bleeding (hemorrhage) into the plaque or (2) formation of a blood clot (thrombus) on the plaque's surface. If either of these occurs and an artery is blocked, the chances of a heart attack or stroke occurring are great.[6]

Atherosclerosis does not suddenly occur after a few months spent eating chocolate cheesecake and lounging on the couch. Evidence suggests that atherosclerotic plaque may actually begin to form while a person is still in the womb, and it becomes progressively worse as the years pass. Some individuals seem to be "plaque formers," while others exhibiting the same behaviour have much less buildup. In some people, their 20s seem to be a significant plaque-forming period; in others, plaque doesn't become a problem until their 50s or 60s.[7]

Did you realize that you may lay down significant deposits of atherosclerotic plaque during your 20s? What risk factors for plaque formation do you have right now? What is your cholesterol level? Have your parents been diagnosed with high cholesterol? What actions can you take now that may keep your risks for atherosclerosis low?

Atria: The two upper chambers of the heart, which receive blood.

Ventricles: The two lower chambers of the heart, which pump blood through the blood vessels.

Arteries: Vessels that carry blood away from the heart to other regions of the body.

Arterioles: Branches of the arteries.

Capillaries: Minute blood vessels that branch out from the arterioles; their thin walls allow for the exchange of oxygen, carbon dioxide, nutrients, and waste products with body cells.

Veins: Vessels that carry blood back to the heart from other regions of the body.

Sinoatrial node (SA node): Node serving as a form of natural pacemaker for the heart.

Atherosclerosis: A general term for thickening and hardening of the arteries.

Arteriosclerosis: Characterized by deposits of fatty substances, cholesterol, cellular waste products, calcium, and fibrin in the inner lining of an artery.

Plaque: Buildup of deposits in the arteries.

Myocardial infarction (MI): Heart attack.

Heart attack: A blockage of normal blood supply to an area in the heart.

Coronary thrombosis: A blood clot occurring in the coronary artery.

Collateral circulation: Adaptation of the heart to partial damage accomplished by rerouting needed blood through unused or underused blood vessels while the damaged heart muscle heals.

Exactly why some people are "atherosclerotic-prone" and others are not remains in question. There are several theories. Many scientists believe that the process of plaque buildup begins because the protective inner lining of the artery (*endothelium*) becomes damaged and that fats, cholesterol, and other substances in the blood are deposited in the damaged area, eventually obstructing blood flow. The three major causes of such damage are (1) dramatic fluctuations in blood pressure, (2) elevated levels of cholesterol and triglycerides in the blood, and (3) cigarette smoking. Cigarette smoke aggravates and speeds up the development of atherosclerosis particularly in the coronary arteries, the aorta, and the arteries of the legs.[8] We discuss each of these factors in detail in other sections of this chapter.

Heart Attack

Those of you raised on a weekly dose of TV doctor programs will recognize *Code Blue* as the term for a **myocardial infarction** (MI), or heart attack. However, you may not know exactly what a heart attack is. A **heart attack** involves a blockage of normal blood supply to an area of the heart. This condition is often brought on by a **coronary thrombosis**, or blood clot in the coronary artery. Coronary heart disease (CHD) and coronary artery disease (CAD) are general names for heart attack (and angina).

When blood does not flow readily, there is a corresponding decrease in oxygen flow. If the heart blockage is extremely minor, the otherwise healthy heart will adapt over time by utilizing small unused or underused blood vessels to reroute needed blood through other areas. This system, known as **collateral circulation**, is a form of self-preservation that allows a damaged heart muscle to heal.

When heart blockage is more severe, however, the body is unable to adapt on its own and outside lifesaving support is critical. The hour following a heart attack is believed to be the most critical period because over 40 percent of heart attack victims die within this time.

It is believed that normal nonatherosclerotic arteries can also go into spasm and cause circulatory impairment. Excessive calcium and potassium are among the suspected causes of these spasms.

Angina Pectoris

As a result of atherosclerosis and other circulatory impairments, the heart's oxygen supply is often reduced, a condition known as **ischemia**. Individuals with ischemia often suffer from varying degrees of **angina pectoris**, or chest pains. Many people experience short episodes of angina whenever they exert themselves physically. Symptoms may range from a slight feeling of indigestion to a feeling that the heart is being crushed. Generally, the more serious the oxygen deprivation, the more severe the pain. Although angina pectoris is not a heart attack, it does indicate underlying heart disease.

Ischemia: Reduced oxygen supply to the heart.

Angina pectoris: Severe chest pain occurring as a result of reduced oxygen flow to the heart.

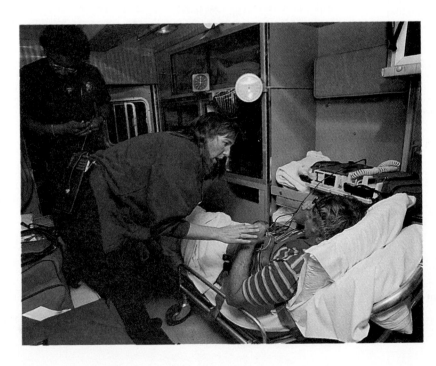

Because 40 percent of heart attack victims die within the first hour, immediate attention is vital to the patient's survival.

Currently, there are several methods of treating angina. In mild cases, rest is critical. The most common treatments for more severe cases involve using drugs that affect (1) the supply of blood to the heart muscle or (2) the heart's demand for oxygen. Pain and discomfort are often relieved with *nitroglycerin*, a drug used to relax (dilate) veins, thereby reducing the amount of blood returning to the heart and thus lessening its work load. Patients whose angina is caused by spasms of the coronary arteries are often given drugs called *calcium channel blockers*. These drugs prevent calcium atoms from passing through coronary arteries and causing heart contractions. They also appear to reduce blood pressure and to slow heart rates. **Beta blockers** are the other major type of drugs used to treat angina. The chemical action of beta blockers serves to control potential overactivity of the heart muscle.

Arrhythmias

An **arrhythmia** is an irregularity in heartbeat. It may be suspected, for instance, when a person complains of a racing heart in the absence of exercise or anxiety; *tachycardia* is the medical term for this abnormally fast heartbeat. On the other end of the continuum is *bradycardia,* or abnormally slow heartbeat. When a heart goes into **fibrillation**, it exhibits a totally sporadic, quivering pattern of beating resulting in extreme inefficiency in moving blood through the cardiovascular system. If untreated, this condition may be fatal. Not all arrhythmias are life-threatening. In many instances, excessive caffeine or nicotine consumption can trigger an arrhythmia episode. For the most part, in the

Beta blockers: Major type of drug used to treat angina, they control potential overactivity of the heart muscle.

Arrhythmia: An irregularity in heartbeat.

Fibrillation: A sporadic, quivering pattern of heartbeat resulting in extreme inefficiency in moving blood through the cardiovascular system.

Congenital heart disease: Heart disease that is present at birth.

Rheumatic heart disease: A heart disease caused by untreated streptococcal infection of the throat.

Stroke: A condition occurring when the brain is damaged by disrupted blood supply.

Thrombus: Blood clot.

Embolus: Blood clot that is forced through the circulatory system.

Aneurysm: A weakened blood vessel that may bulge under pressure and, in severe cases, burst.

Transient ischemic attacks (TIAs): Mild form of stroke; often an indicator of impending major stroke.

absence of other symptoms, arrhythmias are not serious. However, severe cases may require drug therapy or external electrical stimulus to prevent serious complications.

Congestive Heart Failure

When the heart muscle is damaged or overworked and lacks the strength to keep blood circulating normally through the body, its chambers are often taxed to the limit. Patients who have been afflicted with rheumatic fever, pneumonia, or other cardiovascular problems in the past often have weakened heart muscles. In addition, the walls of the heart and the blood vessels may be damaged from previous radiation or chemotherapy treatments for cancer. These weakened muscles respond poorly when stressed; blood flow out of the heart through the arteries is diminished, and the return flow of blood through the veins begins to back up, causing congestion in the tissues.[9] This pooling of blood causes enlargement of the heart and decreases the amount of blood that can be circulated. Blood begins to accumulate in other body areas, such as in the vessels in the legs and ankles or the lungs, causing swelling or difficulty in breathing. If untreated, congestive heart failure will result in death. Most cases respond well to treatment that includes *diuretics* (water pills) for relief of fluid accumulation; drugs, such as *digitalis*, that increase the pumping action of the heart; and drugs called *vasodilators* that expand blood vessels and decrease resistance, allowing blood to flow more easily and making the heart's work easier.

Congenital and Rheumatic Heart Disease

Approximately 1 out of every 125 children is born with some form of **congenital heart disease** (disease present at birth). These forms may range from slight murmurs caused by valve irregularities, which some children outgrow, to serious complications in heart function that can be corrected only with surgery. Their underlying causes are unknown but are believed to be related to hereditary factors; maternal diseases, such as German measles (rubella), occurring during foetal development; or chemical intake (particularly alcohol) by the mother during pregnancy. Because of advances in paediatric cardiology, the prognosis for children with congenital heart defects is better than ever before.

Rheumatic heart disease can cause similar heart problems in children. It is attributed to rheumatic fever, an inflammatory disease that may affect many connective tissues of the body, especially those of the heart, the joints, the brain, or the skin, and which is caused by an unresolved *streptococcal infection* of the throat (strep throat). In a small number of cases, this infection can lead to an immune response in which antibodies attack the heart as well as the bacteria.

Stroke

Like heart muscle, brain cells must have a continuous adequate supply of oxygen in order to survive. A **stroke** (also called a cerebrovascular accident) occurs when the blood supply to the brain is cut off. Strokes may be caused by a **thrombus** (blood clot), an **embolus** (a wandering clot), or an **aneurysm** (a weakening in a blood vessel that causes it to bulge and, in severe cases, burst). Figure 12.2 illustrates these blood vessel disorders.

When any of these events occurs, the result is the death of brain cells, which do not have the capacity to heal or regenerate. Strokes may cause speech impairments, memory loss, and loss of motor control. Although some strokes affect parts of the brain that regulate heart and lung function and kill within minutes, others are mild and cause only temporary dizziness or slight weakness or numbness. These mild forms of strokes are called **transient ischemic attacks (TIAs)** and are often indications of an impending major stroke. Knowing the warning signs or symptoms of stroke may help you or a loved one get medical attention earlier, when treatment may be more effective. Among the most common symptoms are:

- sudden weakness or numbness of the face, arm, or leg on one side of the body

- sudden dimness or loss of vision, particularly in only one eye

- loss of speech, or trouble talking or understanding speech

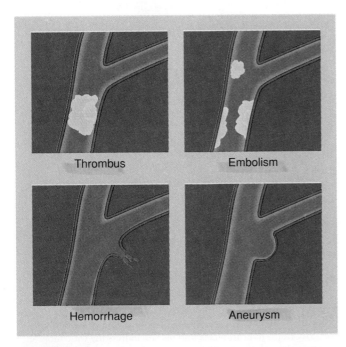

FIGURE 12.2

Common Blood Vessel Disorders

- sudden, severe headaches with no known cause

- unexplained dizziness, unsteadiness, or sudden falls, especially along with any of the previous symptoms

CONTROLLING YOUR RISKS FOR CIRCULATORY DISEASES

Our understanding of the role of stress management, sodium reduction, low-fat diets, and other preventive actions, coupled with better diagnostic aids, has allowed many people to avoid major circulatory episodes. Figure 12.3 summarizes known ways to reduce your risk for heart attack.

A knowledge of the factors that contribute to cardiovascular disease can lead to health-promoting lifestyle changes. Different risks can have a compounded effect when combined. For example, if you have high blood pressure, smoke cigarettes, have a high cholesterol level, and have a family history of heart disease, you run a much greater risk of having a heart attack than does someone with only one of these risks. To assess your own risks for heart disease, see the Rate Yourself box (page 292).

Risks You Can Control

Factors that increase the risk for cardiovascular disease fall into two categories: those that can be controlled and those that cannot. The following risk factors can be controlled. As you read about each factor, ask yourself whether it applies to you and note the steps you can take to reduce its influence.

Cigarette Smoking. During the 1980s, research showed the link between cigarette smoking and heart disease. The resulting public education and increase in tobacco costs led to a 35 percent drop in tobacco sales.[10] Generally, the more a person smokes, the greater the risk for heart attack or stroke. The risk for cardiovascular disease is 70 percent greater for smokers than for nonsmokers. Smokers who have a heart attack are more likely to die suddenly (within one hour) than are nonsmokers. Available evidence also indicates that chronic exposure to environmental tobacco smoke (*passive smoking*) increases the risk of heart disease by as much as 30 percent.[11] When the effects of smoking are combined with the effects of other risk factors, the danger is greater than the sum of the added effects.

Although we do not fully understand how cigarette smoking damages the heart, there are two plausible explanations. One theory states that nicotine increases heart rate, heart output, blood pressure, and oxygen use by heart muscles. Because the carbon monoxide in cigarette smoke displaces oxygen in heart tissue, the heart is forced to work harder to obtain sufficient oxygen. The other theory states that chemicals in smoke damage the lining of the coronary arteries, allowing cholesterol and plaque to accumulate more easily. This additional buildup constricts the vessels, increasing blood pressure and causing the heart to work harder.

Blood Fat and Cholesterol Levels. Excess fats in the body can contribute to circulatory disease. In fact, researchers are now discovering that high-fat diets are even more dangerous than previously thought. Fatty diets not only raise cholesterol levels slowly over time, but also can send the body's blood-clotting system into high gear and make the blood sludgy in just a few hours, increasing the risk for heart attack. Recent studies indicate that fatty foods apparently trigger production of factor VII, a blood-clotting substance. Switching to a low-fat diet promptly eliminates the risk of clotting.[12]

A fatty diet also increases the amount of cholesterol in the blood, contributing to atherosclerosis. In past years, cholesterol levels of between 200 and 250 milligrams per 100 millilitres of blood (mg/dL) were considered normal. Recent research indicates that levels between 180 and 200 mg/dL are more desirable for reducing the risk for circulatory diseases. Cholesterol comes in two varieties: **low-density lipoproteins (LDLs)** and **high-density lipoproteins (HDLs).** Scientists used to think that the critical question was whether a person had more of the "good" HDLs than the "bad" LDLs. But now according to scientists, what may really count is the HDL component LpA-I. The more of this protective protein a person has, it seems, the lower the risk for heart disease.[13] Reduction of salt intake and use of polyunsaturated fatty acids and n-3 fatty acids rich in seafood, as well as potassium, calcium, magnesium, and dietary fibre, aid in the prevention of circulatory disease.[14]

Triglycerides, the type of fat we normally consume, are also manufactured by our own bodies. As people get older or fatter or both, their triglyceride and cholesterol levels tend to rise. Although some heart patients have elevated triglyceride levels, a causal link between high triglyceride levels and heart disease has yet to be established. It may be that high triglyceride levels do not directly cause atherosclerosis but rather are among the abnormalities that speed its development.

Low-density lipoproteins (LDLs): Compounds that facilitate the transport of cholesterol in the blood to the body's cells.

High-density lipoproteins (HDLs): Compounds that facilitate the transport of cholesterol in the blood to the liver for metabolism and elimination from the body.

Triglycerides: The most common form of fat in the body; excess calories are converted into triglycerides and stored as body fat.

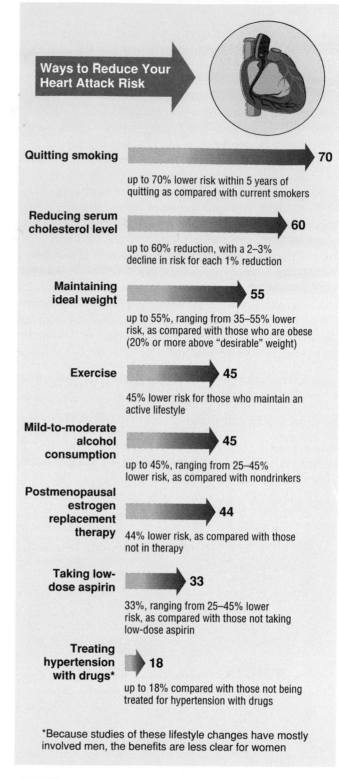

Ways to Reduce Your Heart Attack Risk

Quitting smoking — 70
up to 70% lower risk within 5 years of quitting as compared with current smokers

Reducing serum cholesterol level — 60
up to 60% reduction, with a 2–3% decline in risk for each 1% reduction

Maintaining ideal weight — 55
up to 55%, ranging from 35–55% lower risk, as compared with those who are obese (20% or more above "desirable" weight)

Exercise — 45
45% lower risk for those who maintain an active lifestyle

Mild-to-moderate alcohol consumption — 45
up to 45%, ranging from 25–45% lower risk, as compared with nondrinkers

Postmenopausal estrogen replacement therapy — 44
44% lower risk, as compared with those not in therapy

Taking low-dose aspirin — 33
33%, ranging from 25–45% lower risk, as compared with those not taking low-dose aspirin

Treating hypertension with drugs* — 18
up to 18% compared with those not being treated for hypertension with drugs

*Because studies of these lifestyle changes have mostly involved men, the benefits are less clear for women

FIGURE 12.3

Estimated Average Reduction in Risk for Heart Attack*
*Estimated risk reductions refer to the independent contribution of each risk factor to heart attack and do not address the wide range of known or hypothesized reactions among them.

Source: Adapted from information appearing in J. E. Mason, "Medical Progress: The Primary Prevention of Myocardial Infarction," *The New England Journal of Medicine* 326 (May 21, 1992): 1406–1416.

In general, LDL is more closely associated with cardiovascular risks than is total cholesterol. However, most authorities agree that by looking only at LDL, we ignore the positive effects of HDL. Perhaps the best method of evaluating risk is to examine the ratio of HDL to total cholesterol or the percentage of HDL in total cholesterol. If the percentage of HDL is less than 35, the risk increases dramatically.

The ratio of HDL to total cholesterol can be controlled either by lowering LDL levels or by raising HDL levels. The best way to lower LDL levels is to reduce your dietary intake of the major sources of saturated fat. However, medications can also be used.

High Blood Pressure. Sustained high blood pressure, or **hypertension,** that cannot be attributed to any specific cause is known as **essential hypertension.** Approximately 90 percent of all cases of high blood pressure fit this category. **Secondary hypertension** refers to high blood pressure caused by specific factors, such as kidney disease, obesity, or tumours of the adrenal glands. In general, the higher your blood pressure, the greater your risk for circulatory disease. High blood pressure is known as the "silent killer," because it usually has no symptoms. High blood pressure affects 16 percent of Canadians, and 33 percent of Canadians aged 55 to 64. Common forms of treatment are dietary changes (reducing salt and calorie intake), weight loss (when appropriate), the use of diuretics and other medications (only when prescribed by a physician), regular exercise, and the practice of relaxation techniques and effective coping and communication skills.

Blood pressure is measured in two parts and is expressed as two numbers separated by a slash—for example, 110/80, or 110 over 80. Both values are measured in *millimetres of mercury* (mm Hg). The first number refers to **systolic pressure,** or the pressure being applied to the walls of the arteries when the heart contracts, pumping blood to the rest of the body. The second value is **diastolic pressure,** or the pressure applied to the walls of the arteries during the heart's relaxation phase. During this phase, blood is reentering the chambers of the heart, preparing for the next heartbeat.

Normal blood pressure varies for different individuals depending on weight, physical condition, sex, and race. As a rule, men have a greater risk for high blood pressure than women have until age 55, when their risks become about equal. At age 75 and over, women are more likely victims of high blood pressure than are men.[15] For the average person, 110 over 80 is a normal blood pressure level. If your blood pressure exceeds 140 over 90, you probably need to take steps to lower it. See Table 12.1 for a summary of blood pressure values and what they mean.

Exercise. Inactivity is a definite risk factor for circulatory disease.[16] Moreover, physically inactive people also tend to be overweight and are more likely to smoke and to pay less attention to their overall health than are active people. The good news is that you don't have to be an exercise fanatic to reduce your risk. Even modest levels of low-intensity physical activity are beneficial if done regularly and long-term. Such activities include walking for pleasure, gardening, housework, and dancing.

Diet and Obesity. Like exercise, diet and obesity are believed to play a role in circulatory disease. Researchers are not certain whether high-fat, high-sugar, high-calorie diets are a direct risk for circulatory disease or whether they invite risk by causing obesity, which forces the heart to strain to push blood through the many kilometres of capillaries that supply each kilogram of fat. A heart that continuously has to move blood through an overabundance of vessels may become damaged. In fact, people who are overweight or obese are more likely to develop heart disease and stroke even if they have no other risk factors. Moreover, recent evidence indicates that how fat is distributed on the body may affect a person's risk. A waist/hip ratio greater than 1.0 for men or 0.8 for women indicates a significant increase in risk. This means that a man's waist measurement should not exceed his hip measurement, and a woman's waist measurement should not be more than 80 percent of her hip measurement.[17]

Diabetes. Diabetics, particularly those who have taken insulin for a number of years, appear to run an increased risk for the development of circulatory disease. In fact, circulatory disease is the leading cause of death among diabetic patients. Because overweight people have a higher risk for diabetes, distinguishing between the effects of the two conditions is difficult. Diabetics also tend to have elevated blood fat levels, increased atherosclerosis, and a tendency toward deterioration of small blood vessels, particularly in the eyes and extremities. Through a prescribed regimen of diet, exercise, and medication, diabetics can control much of their increased risk for heart disease.

Hypertension: Sustained elevated blood pressure.

Essential hypertension: Hypertension that cannot be attributed to any cause.

Secondary hypertension: Hypertension caused by specific factors, such as kidney disease, obesity, or tumours of the adrenal glands.

Systolic pressure: The upper number in the fraction that measures blood pressure, indicating pressure on the walls of the arteries when the heart contracts.

Diastolic pressure: The lower number in the fraction that measures blood pressure, indicating pressure on the walls of the arteries during the relaxation phase of heart activity.

Cardiac Risk Factor Index

Y ou can estimate your chance of suffering a heart attack or stroke by using this risk index. Remember, it's an estimate, not a diagnosis. Study each risk factor and its entire row. Choose the most appropriate description and circle the point number. For example, if your age is 25, circle 2 points. After checking out all 13 risk factors, total your score. Your score is an estimate of your risk.

Age	10–20 years	21–30 years	31–40 years	41–50 years	51–60 years	61 and over
	1	2	3	4	6	8
Heredity (parents' and siblings' cardiac health)	No family history of heart disease	One with heart disease after age 60	Two with heart disease after age 60	One with heart disease before age 60	Two with heart disease before age 60	Three with heart disease before age 60
	1	2	3	4	6	8
Weight	More than 2 kg below standard	–2 to +2 kg of standard weight	2 to 10 kg overweight	10 to 16 kg overweight	16 to 23 kg overweight	23 to 30 kg overweight
	0	1	2	3	5	7
Smoking	Nonsmoker	Occasional cigar or pipe; live or work with someone who smokes	10 cigarettes or fewer per day	11–20 cigarettes per day	21–30 cigarettes per day	31 cigarettes or more per day
	0	1	2	4	6	10
Exercise	Intensive job and recreational exertion	Moderate job and recreational exertion	Sedentary job and intensive recreation	Sedentary job and moderate recreation	Sedentary job and occasional recreation	Sedentary job; no special exercise
	0	1	2	4	6	8
Cholesterol level or fat % in diet	Cholesterol below 180 mg; diet contains no animal or solid fat	Cholesterol 181–205 mg; diet contains 10% animal or solid fat	Cholesterol 206–230 mg; diet contains 20% animal or solid fat	Cholesterol 231–255 mg; diet contains 30% animal or solid fat	Cholesterol 256–280 mg; diet contains 40% animal or solid fat	Cholesterol 281–300 mg; diet contains 50% animal or solid fat
	1	2	3	4	5	7
Sex and age	Female under age 40	Female age 40–50	Female under 50, male under 20	Male between 20–35	Male between 35–55	Male over 50
	1	2	4	5	6	7
Systolic blood pressure	Below 110	111–130	131–140	141–160	161–180	Above 180
	0	1	2	3	5	7

(continued)

Diastolic blood pressure	Below 80	80–85	86–90	91–95	96–100	Above 100
	0	1	2	4	7	9
Stress	No mental-emotional stress	Occasional mild stress	Frequent mild stress	Frequent moderate stress	Frequent high stress	Constant high stress
	0	1	2	3	4	5
Present heart disease symptoms	None	Occasional fast pulse and/or irregular rhythm	Frequent fast pulse and/or irregular rhythm	Dizziness on exertion	Occasional angina (chest pain)	Frequent angina (chest pain)
	0	2	4	6	8	10
Past personal history of heart disease	Completely benign	Heart disease symptoms; not physician-confirmed	History of heart disease symptoms; examined by physician	Mild heart disease; no present treatment	Heart disease under treatment	Hospitalized for heart disease
	0	2	4	6	8	10
Diabetes	No symptoms; negative family history	Positive family history of diabetes	Impaired glucose tolerance	Dietary control	Oral medication control	Insulin control
	0	1	3	5	7	9

If your total score is:

6–14 = Risk well below average

15–19 = Risk below average

20–25 = Risk generally average

26–32 = Risk moderately high

33–40 = Risk dangerous

41–56 = Risk very dangerous

57+ = Risk extreme

If your total score is "above average," work with your physician to reduce your risk factors.

_____

Source: Adapted by permission of St. Vincent Hospital & Medical Center, The Heart Institute, Portland, OR 97225.

Individual Response to Stress. Some scientists have noted a relationship between circulatory disease risk and a person's stress level, behaviour habits, and socioeconomic status. These factors may affect established risk factors. For example, people under stress may start smoking or smoke more than they otherwise would.[18] Other studies have challenged the apparent link between emotional stress and heart disease. Although it was once widely assumed that the Type A personality who suffered from high stress levels was a time bomb ticking toward a heart attack, this theory has not been proven clinically.

Recently, researcher-physician Robert S. Eliot demonstrated that approximately one out of five people has an extreme cardiovascular reaction to stressful stimulation. These people experience alarm and resistance so strongly that, when under stress, their bodies produce large amounts of stress chemicals, which in turn cause tremendous changes in the cardiovascular system, including remarkable increases in blood pressure. These people are called hot reactors. Although their blood pressure may be normal when they are not under stress—for example, in a doctor's office—it increases dramatically in response to even small amounts of everyday stress.

TABLE 12.1 ■ Blood Pressure Values and What They Mean to You

Classification	Systolic Reading	Diastolic Reading	Actions
Normal	Below 130	Below 85	Recheck in two years.
High normal	130–139	85–89	Recheck in one year.
Mild hypertension	140–159	90–99	Check in two months.
Moderate hypertension	160–179	100–109	See physician within a month.
Severe hypertension	180 or above	110 or above	See physician immediately.

Note: Systolic and diastolic values are based on an average of two or more readings taken at different times.

Source: Adapted from "Fifth Report of the Joint National Committee on Detection, Evaluation, and Treatment of High Blood Pressure," *Archives of Internal Medicine* 153 (January 25, 1993): 154–183 (published by the American Medical Association); and American Heart Association.

Cold reactors are those who are able to experience stress (even to live as Type As) without reacting with harmful cardiovascular responses. Cold reactors may internalize stress, but their self-talk and perceptions about the stressful events lead them to a non-response state in which their cardiovascular system remains virtually unaffected.[19] New research indicates that people who have an underlying predisposition toward a toxic core personality (in other words, who are chronically hostile and hateful) may be at greatest risk for a circulatory disease event.

Risks You Cannot Control

There are, unfortunately, some risk factors for circulatory disease that you cannot prevent or control. The most important are:

- *Heredity:* Having a family history of heart disease appears to increase risks significantly. Whether this is because of genetics or environment is an unresolved question.

- *Age:* Eighty percent of all fatal heart attacks occur in people over age 65. The risk for circulatory disease increases with age for both sexes.[20]

- *Sex:* Men are at much greater risk for circulatory disease until old age. Women under 35 have a fairly low risk unless they have high blood pressure, kidney problems, or diabetes. Using oral contraceptives while smoking also increases risk. Hormonal factors appear to reduce risk for women, although after menopause or after estrogen levels are otherwise reduced (e.g., hysterectomy), women's LDL levels tend to go up, increasing their risk for circulatory disease. (For a more detailed discussion of the sex factor, see the next section.)

- *Race:* Blacks are at 45 percent greater risk for high blood pressure and thus a greater risk for circulatory disease than are whites. In addition, blacks have a worse chance of surviving heart attacks.

*W*HAT DO YOU THINK?

Which do you think is your biggest circulatory disease risk factor right now? What is your second biggest risk factor? List four actions that you can take this week to reduce these two risk factors. Who can you get to help you in your attempt to change your health behaviours?

*W*OMEN AND CARDIOVASCULAR DISEASE

Heart disease is the number one killer of both men and women. In Canada, heart attacks kill about 9500 women a year; stroke takes another 8500 women's lives. That compares with about 5000 women who die annually from breast cancer. In fact, nearly twice as many women die of circulatory disease as of all cancers combined.[21]

While men do have more heart attacks and have them earlier in life, women have a much lower chance of surviving a heart attack. We understand the mechanisms that cause circulatory disease in men from years of male-oriented research. But only within the last decade have we

Cardiovascular Diseases Worldwide

Cardiovascular diseases kill more people than any other diseases annually, accounting for over 15 million deaths, or about 30 percent of the global total. Many more millions of people are disabled by them. Atherosclerotic disease is a lifelong process, with its initial stage in childhood and youth and with clinical manifestations in middle age or later. Its development is linked to unhealthy lifestyles (mainly tobacco use, unbalanced diet, and physical inactivity).

Cardiovascular diseases are emerging rapidly as a major public health concern in most developing countries. People in the developing world still suffer from heart ailments such as rheumatic heart disease, which is linked to an upper respiratory tract infection, and Chagas' heart disease, a parasite-related illness; both diseases are linked to low income, poverty, overcrowding, poor housing conditions, and inadequate health services.

WHO and ISFC started collaboration on rheumatic heart disease prevention in developing countries in 1984. UNESCO joined the program in 1992; that year also marked their joint collaboration on Chagas' disease prevention. In 1995 they began to promote healthy lifestyles and prevent the development of cardiovascular risk factors from early childhood onwards.

Source: World Health Organization, Cardiovascular Diseases, 1997, http://www.who.ch/press/1997/pr97-31.html.

---

moved toward a better understanding of how circulatory disease manifests itself in women.

Risk Factors in Women

Premenopausal women are unlikely candidates for heart attacks, except for those who suffer from diabetes, high blood pressure, or kidney disease, or who have a genetic predisposition to high cholesterol levels. Family history and smoking can also increase the risk for premenopausal women.

The Estrogen Element. Once her estrogen production drops with menopause, a woman's chances of developing circulatory disease rise rapidly. A 60-year-old woman has the same heart attack risk as a 50-year-old man. By her late 70s, a woman has the same heart attack risk as a man her age. To date, much of this changing risk has been attributed to the aging process, but some preliminary evidence indicates that hormones may play a bigger role than once thought. Recent results from Postmenopausal Estrogen/Progestin Interventions (PEPI), a longitudinal study of how various **hormone replacement therapies (HRT)** affect cardiovascular risks, indicate that HRT may reduce circulatory disease by as much as 12 to 25 percent. In this study, HRT seemed to reduce a woman's risk for circulatory disease by raising HDL cholesterol levels and lowering LDL cholesterol levels. Even when their total blood cholesterol levels are higher than men's, women may be at less risk because they typically have a higher percentage of HDL.[22]

But that's only part of the story. It's true that women aged 25 and over tend to have lower cholesterol levels than do men of the same age. But when they reach 45, things change. Most men's cholesterol levels become more stable, while both LDL and total cholesterol levels in women start to rise. And the gap widens further beyond age 55.[23]

Before age 45, women's total blood cholesterol levels average below 220 mg/dL. By the time she is 45 to 55, the average woman's blood cholesterol rises to between 223 and 246 mg/dL. Studies of men have shown that for every 1 percent drop in cholesterol, there is a 2 percent decrease in circulatory disease risk.[24] If this holds true for women, prevention efforts focussing on dietary interventions and exercise may significantly help postmenopausal women.

Symptoms in Postmenopausal Women

Postmenopausal women often do not display the same extreme symptoms of heart disease that men do. The first sign of heart disease in men is generally a myocardial infarction. In women, the first sign is usually uncomplicated

Hormone replacement therapies (HRT): Therapies that replace estrogen in postmenopausal women.

angina pectoris. Because chest discomfort rather than pain is the common manifestation of angina in women, and because angina has a much more favourable prognosis in women than in men, many physicians ignore the condition in their female patients or treat it too casually.

A heart attack also shows different signs in women than in men. In men, a heart attack usually manifests itself as crushing chest pain radiating to the arm. But in women, a heart attack can feel like severe abdominal pain or indigestion. If these symptoms are neglected, the outcome can be dire.

Neglect of Symptoms

Research has suggested three main reasons for the widespread neglect of the signs of heart disease in women: (1) physicians may often be gender-biased in their delivery of health care, tending to concentrate on women's reproductive organs rather than on the whole woman; (2) physicians tend to view male heart disease as a more severe problem because men have traditionally had a higher incidence of the disease; and (3) women decline major procedures more often than men do.

Although there is much debate about whether women have actually been ignored by past research concerning circulatory diseases, at least one study points out that the differences in treatment of suspected acute cardiac ischemia in men cannot be applied directly to women. More importantly, at least one study suggests that these differences may reflect overtreatment of men rather than undertreatment of women.[25]

*W*HAT DO YOU THINK?

How do men and women differ in their experiences of circulatory disease? Why do you think women's risks were largely ignored until fairly recently? What actions do you think individuals can take to help improve these situations for both men and women? What actions can communities and members of the medical community take?

Electrocardiogram (ECG): A record of the electrical activity of the heart measured during a stress test.

Angiography: A technique for examining blockages in heart arteries. A catheter is inserted into the arteries, a dye is injected, and an X-ray is taken to find the blocked areas. Also called cardiac catheterization.

Positron emission tomography (PET scan): Method for measuring heart activity by injecting a patient with a radioactive tracer that is scanned electronically to produce a three-dimensional image of the heart and arteries.

*N*EW WEAPONS AGAINST HEART DISEASE

The victim of a heart attack today has a variety of options that were not available a generation ago. Medications designed to strengthen heartbeat, control irregularities in rhythm, and relieve pain are widely prescribed. Triple and quadruple bypasses and angioplasty have become relatively commonplace procedures in hospitals throughout the nation.

Techniques of Diagnosing Heart Disease

Several techniques are used to diagnose heart disease, including electrocardiogram, angiography, and positron emission tomography scans. An **electrocardiogram (ECG)** is a record of the electrical activity of the heart measured during a stress test. Patients walk or run on treadmills while their hearts are monitored. A more accurate method of testing for heart disease is **angiography** (often referred to as *cardiac catheterization*) in which a needle-thin tube called a *catheter* is threaded through blocked heart arteries, a dye is injected, and an X-ray is taken to discover which areas are blocked. A more recent and even more effective method of measuring heart activity is **positron emission tomography**, also called a **PET scan**, which produces three-dimensional images of the heart as blood flows through it. During a PET scan, a patient receives an intravenous injection of a radioactive tracer. As the tracer decays, it emits positrons that are picked up by the scanner and transformed by a computer into colour images of the heart.

Newer tests that are now performed at many medical centers include:[26]

- *Radionuclide imaging* (includes such tests as thallium test, MUGA scan, and acute infarct scintigraphy). These tests involve injecting substances called radionuclides into the bloodstream. Computer-generated pictures can then show them in the heart. These tests can show how well the heart muscle is supplied with blood, how well the heart's chambers are functioning, and which part of the heart has been damaged by a heart attack.

- *Magnetic resonance imaging* (also called MRI or NMR). This test uses powerful magnets to look inside the body. Computer-generated pictures can show the heart muscle, identify damage from a heart attack, diagnose certain congenital heart defects, and evaluate disease of larger blood vessels such as the aorta.

- *Digital cardiac angiography* (also called DCA or DSA). This modified form of computer-aided imaging records pictures of the heart and its blood vessels.

Angioplasty Versus Bypass Surgery

During the 1980s, **coronary bypass surgery** seemed to be the ultimate technique for treating patients who had coronary blockages or who had suffered heart attacks. In coronary bypass surgery, a blood vessel taken from another site in the patient's body (usually the saphenous vein in the leg or the internal mammary artery) is implanted to transport blood by bypassing blocked arteries. Recently, experts have begun to question the effectiveness of bypass operations, particularly for elderly people.

A procedure called **angioplasty** (sometimes called balloon angioplasty) is associated with fewer risks and is believed by many experts to be more effective than bypass surgery in selected cardiovascular cases. This procedure is similar to angiography. A needle-thin catheter is threaded through blocked heart arteries. The catheter has a balloon at the tip, which is inflated to flatten fatty deposits against the artery walls, allowing blood to flow more freely. Angioplasty patients are generally awake but sedated during the procedure and spend only one or two days in the hospital after treatment. Most people can return to work within five days. Only about 1 percent of all angioplasty patients die during or soon after the procedure. However, there are some hazards in this procedure. In 3 to 7 percent of cases, the blood vessel that is stretched open by the balloon collapses spontaneously, and a bypass has to be done anyway. In addition, in about 30 percent of all angioplasty patients, the treated arteries become clogged again within six months. Some patients may undergo the procedure as many as three times within a five-year period. Some surgeons argue that given angioplasty's high rate of recurrence, bypass may be a more effective method of treatment.

New research suggests that in many instances, drug treatments may be just as effective in prolonging life as the invasive surgical techniques, but it is critical that doctors follow an aggressive drug treatment program and that patients comply with the doctors' drug orders.[27]

Research has indicated that the use of low-dose aspirin (325 milligrams daily or every other day) is beneficial to heart patients. However, a major problem associated with aspirin use is gastrointestinal intolerance, and this factor may outweigh its benefits for some people. Although the findings concerning the overall benefits of using aspirin to treat or prevent heart disease are inconclusive, the research seems promising thus far.[28]

Thrombolysis

Whenever a heart attack occurs, prompt action is the key factor in the patient's eventual prognosis. When a coronary artery gets blocked, the heart muscle doesn't die immediately, but time determines how much damage occurs. If a victim gets to an emergency room and is diagnosed

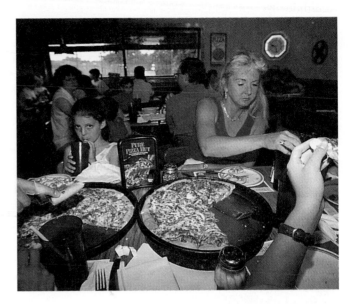

Controlling the amount and type of fat you eat is something you can do to lower your risk for cardiovascular disease.

fast enough, a form of reperfusion therapy called **thrombolysis** can sometimes be performed. Thrombolysis involves injecting an agent such as TPA (tissue plasminogen activator) to dissolve the clot and restore some blood flow, thereby reducing the amount of tissue that dies from ischemia.[29] These drugs must be used within one to three hours of a heart attack for best results.

*W*HAT DO YOU THINK?

With all the new diagnostic procedures, treatments, and differing philosophies about various prevention and intervention techniques, how can the typical health consumer ensure that he or she will get the best treatment when entering the health care system? Where can one go for information? Why might women, members of certain minority groups, and the elderly need a "health advocate" who can help them get through the system?

*A*N OVERVIEW OF CANCER

Approximately 60 700 Canadians will have died of cancer in 1997, which amounts to 166 cancer deaths each day.[30] Cancer caused by tobacco use will account for one-third of all cancer deaths. Cancers can be divided into three groups: those with good prognosis (breast, prostate, bladder, melanoma, body of the uterus, cervix, Hodgkin's disease, testis, and male bladder); those with fairly good prognosis (colorectal, non-Hodgkin's lymphoma, kidney, oral, larynx, and female bladder); and those with a poor prognosis (lung, stomach, adult leukemia, pancreas, ovary, brain, and multiple myeloma).[31]

Not everyone is equally at risk for all types of cancers. Cancer incidence and mortality vary greatly by age, sex, race, and socioeconomic status. Because cancer risk is strongly associated with lifestyle and behaviour, differences in ethnic and cultural groups can provide clues to factors involved in the development of cancer. Culturally influenced values and belief systems can also affect whether or not a person seeks care, participates in screenings, or follows recommended treatment options.

The cancer rate has been stable among women since 1987, and rising slightly for men, mainly due to an increase in prostate cancer. The number of deaths for both sexes has increased considerably because of the growing and aging population. Cancer tends to affect older Canadians; 72 percent of new cases and 81 percent of deaths involved people over 60.[32]

What Is Cancer?

Cancer is the name given to a large group of diseases characterized by the uncontrolled growth and spread of ab-

---

Coronary bypass surgery: A surgical technique whereby a blood vessel is implanted to bypass a clogged coronary artery.

Angioplasty: A technique in which a catheter with a balloon at the tip is inserted into a clogged artery; the balloon is inflated to flatten fatty deposits against artery walls, allowing blood to flow more freely.

Thrombolysis: Injection of an agent to dissolve clots and restore some blood flow, thereby reducing the amount of tissue that dies from ischemia.

Cancer: A large group of diseases characterized by the uncontrolled growth and spread of abnormal cells.

Neoplasm: A new growth of tissue that serves no physiological function resulting from uncontrolled, abnormal cellular development.

Tumour: A neoplasmic mass that grows more rapidly than surrounding tissues.

Malignant: Very dangerous or harmful; refers to a cancerous tumour.

Benign: Harmless; refers to a non-cancerous tumour.

Biopsy: Microscopic examination of tissue to determine if a cancer is present.

Metastasis: Process by which cancer spreads from one area to different areas of the body.

---

normal cells. It may seem hard to understand how normal, healthy cells become cancerous, but if you think of a cell as a small computer, programmed to operate in a particular fashion, the process will become clearer. Under normal conditions, healthy cells are protected by a powerful overseer, the immune system, as they perform their daily functions of growing, replicating, and repairing body organs. When something interrupts normal cell programming, however, uncontrolled growth and abnormal cellular development results in a new growth of tissue serving no physiologic function called a **neoplasm**. This neoplasmic mass often forms a clumping of cells known as a **tumour**.

Not all tumours are **malignant** (cancerous); in fact, most are **benign** (non-cancerous). Benign tumours are generally harmless unless they grow in such a fashion as to obstruct or crowd out normal tissues or organs. A benign tumour of the brain, for instance, is life-threatening when it grows in a manner that causes blood restriction and results in a stroke. The only way to determine whether a given tumour or mass is benign or malignant is through **biopsy,** or microscopic examination of cell development.

Benign and malignant tumours differ in several key ways. Benign tumours are generally composed of ordinary-looking cells enclosed in a fibrous shell or capsule that prevents their spreading to other body areas. Malignant tumours are usually not enclosed in a protective capsule and can therefore spread to other organs. This process, known as **metastasis**, makes some forms of cancer particularly aggressive in their ability to overcome bodily defences. By the time they are diagnosed, malignant tumours have frequently metastasized throughout the body, making treatment extremely difficult. Unlike benign tumours, which merely expand to take over a given space, malignant cells invade surrounding tissue, emitting clawlike protrusions that disrupt chemical processes within healthy cells. More specifically, malignant cells disturb the ribonucleic acid (RNA) and deoxyribonucleic acid (DNA) within the normal cells. Tampering with these substances, which control cellular metabolism and reproduction, produces **mutant cells** that differ in form, quality, and function from normal cells.

$\mathcal{W}$HAT CAUSES CANCER?

Although we can describe the process by which malignant cells spread throughout the body, we don't know for sure why this process occurs. We also do not know why some people have malignant cells in their bodies but never develop cancer. Scientists have proposed several theories for the cellular changes that produce cancer.

One theory of cancer development proposes that cancer results from some spontaneous error that occurs during cell reproduction. Perhaps cells that are overworked or aged are more likely to break down, causing genetic errors that result in mutant cells.

Another theory suggests that cancer is caused by some external agent or agents that enter a normal cell and initiate the cancerous process. Numerous environmental factors, such as radiation, chemicals, hormonal drugs, immunosuppressant drugs (drugs that suppress the normal activity of the immune system), and other toxins, are considered possible **carcinogens** (cancer-causing agents) (see Figure 12.4); perhaps the most common carcinogen is the tar in cigarettes. This theory of environmental carcinogens obviously has profound implications for our industrialized society. As in most disease-related situations, the greater the dose or the exposure to environmental hazards, the greater the risk of disease. People who are forced to work, live, and pass through areas that have high levels of environmental toxins may, in fact, be at greater risk for several types of cancers.

A third theory came out of research on certain viruses that are believed to cause tumours in animals. This research led to the discovery of **oncogenes**, suspected cancer-causing genes that are present on chromosomes. Although oncogenes are typically dormant, scientists theorize that certain conditions such as age, stress, and exposure to carcinogens, viruses, and radiation may activate these oncogenes. Once activated, they begin to grow and reproduce in an out-of-control manner.

There is still a great deal that remains unanswered about the oncogene theory of cancer development. Scientists are uncertain whether only people who develop cancer have oncogenes or whether we all have **proto-oncogenes**, genes that can become oncogenes under certain conditions. Many **oncologists** (physicians who specialize in the treatment of malignancies) believe that the oncogene theory may lead to a greater understanding of how individual cells function and may bring us closer to developing an effective treatment for cancerous cells.

Biological Factors

Some early cancer theorists believed that we inherit a genetic predisposition toward certain forms of cancer.[33] Recent research conducted by the University of Utah suggests that a gene for breast cancer exists. To date, however, the research in this area remains inconclusive. Although a rare form of eye cancer does appear to be passed genetically from mother to child, most cancers are not genetically linked. The complex interaction of hereditary predisposition, lifestyle, and environment on the development of cancer makes the likelihood of determining a single cause fairly remote.

Cancers of the breast, stomach, colon, prostate, uterus, ovaries, and lungs do appear to run in families. For example, a woman runs a much higher risk of having breast

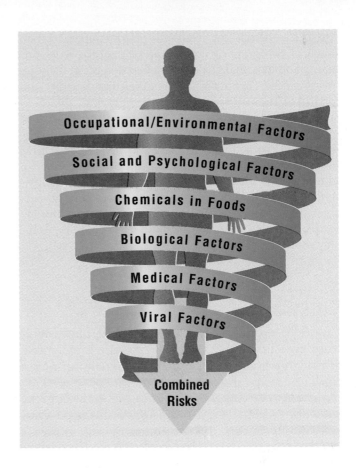

FIGURE 12.4

Suspected Causes of Cancer

cancer if her mother or sisters have had the disease. Hodgkin's disease and certain leukemias show similar familial patterns. Whether these familial patterns are attributable to genetic susceptibility or to the fact that people in the same families experience similar environmental risks remains uncertain.

Mutant cells: Cells that differ in form, quality, or function from normal cells.

Carcinogens: Cancer-causing agents.

Oncogenes: Suspected cancer-causing genes present on chromosomes.

Proto-oncogenes: Genes that can become oncogenes under certain conditions.

Oncologists: Physicians who specialize in the treatment of malignancies.

Sex also affects the likelihood of developing certain forms of cancer. For example, breast cancer occurs primarily among females, although men do occasionally get breast cancer. Obviously, factors other than heredity and familial relationships affect which sex develops a particular cancer. In the 1950s and 1960s, for example, women rarely contracted lung cancer. But with increases in the number of women who smoked and the length of time they had smoked, lung cancer became a leading cause of cancer deaths for Canadian women in the 1980s. Lifestyle is clearly a critical factor in the interaction of variables that predispose a person toward cancer. Although sex plays a role in certain cases, other variables are probably more significant.

Occupational/Environmental Factors

Various occupational hazards are known to cause cancer when exposure levels are high or exposure is prolonged. Overall, however, workplace hazards account for only a small percentage of all cancers. One of the most common occupational carcinogens is asbestos, a fibrous substance once widely used in the construction, insulation, and automobile industries. Nickel, chromate, and chemicals such as benzene, arsenic, and vinyl chloride have definitively been shown to be carcinogens for humans. Also, people who routinely work with certain dyes and radioactive substances may have increased risks for cancer. Working with coal tars, as in the mining profession, or working near inhalants, as in the auto-painting business, is also hazardous. Those who work with herbicides and pesticides also appear to be at higher risk, although the evidence is inconclusive to date for low-dose exposures.

Because people are sometimes forced to work near hazardous substances, it is imperative that worksites enact policies and procedures designed to minimize and/or eliminate toxic exposure to the above substances.

Ionizing radiation—radiation from X-rays, radon, cosmic rays, and ultraviolet radiation (primarily UV-B radiation)—is the only form of radiation proven to cause human cancer. (See the section on skin cancer.)

While reports about cancer case clusters in communities around nuclear power facilities have raised public concerns, studies show that clusters do not occur more often near nuclear power plants than they do by chance in wider geographical areas.[34]

Social and Psychological Factors

Although orthodox medical personnel are skeptical of overly simplistic prevention centres that focus on humour and laughter as the way to prevent cancer, we cannot rule out the possibility that negative emotional states contribute to disease development. People who are lonely, depressed, and lack social support have been shown to be more susceptible to cancer than are their mentally healthy counterparts. Similarly, people who are under chronic stress and have poor nutrition or sleep habits develop cancer at a slightly higher rate than does the general population. Experts believe that severe depression or prolonged stress may reduce the activity of the body's immune system, thereby wearing down bodily resistance to cancer. Although psychological factors may play a part in cancer development, exposure to substances such as tobacco and alcohol in our social environment are far more important.

Chemicals in Foods

Among the food additives suspected of causing cancer is *sodium nitrate,* a chemical used to preserve and give colour to red meat. Research indicates that the actual carcinogen is not sodium nitrate but nitrosamines, substances formed when the body digests the sodium nitrates. Sodium nitrate has not been banned, primarily because it kills the bacterium botulin, which is the cause of the highly virulent food-borne disease known as botulism. It should also be noted that the bacteria found in the human intestinal tract may contain more nitrates than a person could ever take in from eating cured meats or other nitrate-containing food products. Nonetheless, concern about the carcinogenic properties of nitrates has led to the introduction of meats that are nitrate-free or that contain reduced levels of the substance.

Much of the concern about chemicals in foods today centres on the possible harm caused by pesticide and herbicide residue left on foods by agricultural practices. While some of these chemicals cause cancer at high doses in experimental animals, the concentrations found in some foods are very low. Continued research regarding pesticide and herbicide use is essential for maximum food safety and the continuous monitoring of agricultural practices is necessary to ensure a safe food supply. Scientists and consumer groups stress the importance of a balance between chemical use and the production of quality food products.[35] Policies protecting consumer health and ensuring the continued improvement in food production through development of alternative, low-chemical pest and herbicide control and reduced environmental pollution should be the goal of prevention efforts.

Viral Factors

The chances of becoming infected with a "cancer virus" are very remote. Over the years, several forms of virus-induced cancers have been observed in laboratory animals and there is some indication that human beings display a similar tendency toward virally transmitted cancers. Evidence that the *herpes-related viruses* may be involved in the development of some forms of leukemia, Hodgkin's

Cancer and the Canadian Environment

Does the environment in an industrialized nation like Canada put us at risk of cancer? First, it's important to recognize that an estimated 80 percent of all cancers are caused by behavioural factors, and are therefore under human control.

Two of the leading risk factors associated with cancer are tobacco smoke and diet. Together they are responsible for about two-thirds of all new cancer cases. Tobacco smoke is the major cause of 80 to 90 percent of lung cancer cases. It is also an important cause of bladder and breast cancer. Diet-associated cancers include colon, rectum, breast, and stomach cancer. For example, high fat consumption is considered a risk factor for colon and possibly breast cancer.

Other well-established risk factors include work-related exposure, alcohol consumption, and radiation—including sunlight, drugs, and viruses.

Under the Canadian Environmental Protection Act (CEPA), carcinogens are considered toxic to human health. In theory, there is no "safe" level of exposure to a carcinogen. It is generally assumed, but has never been proven, that there is some chance of developing cancer at any level of exposure. In other words, contact between a single human cell and a carcinogen molecule may be enough to cause cancer. This does not mean that cancer is the inevitable or even the likely outcome of such an event.

Human cells have developed a range of defences to guard against all sorts of injuries, including those that lead to cancer. As a result, cancer usually occurs only after prolonged and continuous exposure to carcinogens. As exposure levels decrease, so does the risk of developing cancer.

For the average Canadian, the risk of developing cancer as a result of exposure to any particular pollutant in the environment is extremely small. People today are exposed to trace amounts of various chemicals in their air, water, and food. But the levels are generally far below those levels associated with harmful effects. In the workplace, however, exposure to much higher levels of chemicals can occur.

Source: Statistics Canada, "Cancer Incidence and Mortality, 1997," *Health Reports 1997*, 8, No. 4.

---

disease, cervical cancer, and Burkitt's lymphoma has surfaced in recent years. The *Epstein-Barr virus*, associated with mononucleosis, may also contribute to cancer development. Cervical cancer has also been linked to the *human papilloma virus*, the virus that causes genital warts.[36]

Although research is inconclusive, many scientists believe that selected viruses may help to provide an *opportunistic* environment for subsequent cancer development. It is likely that a combination of immunological bombardment by viral or chemical invaders and other risk factors substantially increases the risk of cancer.

Medical Factors

In some cases, medical treatment increases a person's risk for cancer. One famous example is the widespread use of the prescription drug *diethylstilbestrol (DES)* during the years 1940 to 1960 to control problems with bleeding during pregnancy and to reduce the risk of miscarriage. It was not until the 1970s that the dangers of this drug became apparent. Although DES caused few side-effects in the millions of women who took it, their daughters were found to have an increased risk for cancers of the reproductive organs.

Some scientists claim that the use of estrogen replacement therapy among postmenopausal women is dangerous because it increases the risks for uterine cancer. Others believe that because estrogen is critical to the prevention of osteoporosis and heart disease in aging women, its use should not be curtailed. Most medical professionals believe that properly administered estrogen therapy poses no substantially increased risks to most patients.

WHAT DO YOU THINK?

Based on what you've read and heard, what do you think causes most people to get cancer? Which risk factors do you think your family has? Which ones do you have, if any, that are different from your family's? What can you do about your personal risks?

TYPES OF CANCERS

As we said earlier, the term *cancer* refers not to a single disease but to hundreds of different diseases. However, four broad classifications of cancer are made according to the type of tissue from which the cancer arises.

Carcinomas. Epithelial tissues (tissues covering body surfaces and lining most body cavities) are the most common sites for cancers. Carcinoma of the breast, lung, intestines, skin, and mouth are examples. These cancers affect the outer layer of the skin and mouth as well as the mucous membranes. They metastasize through the circulatory or lymphatic system initially and form solid tumours.

Sarcomas. Sarcomas occur in the mesodermal, or middle, layers of tissue—for example, in bones, muscles, and general connective tissue. They metastasize primarily via the blood in the early stages of disease. These cancers are less common but generally more virulent than carcinomas. They also form solid tumours.

Lymphomas. Lymphomas develop in the lymphatic system—the infection-fighting regions of the body—and metastasize through the lymph system. Hodgkin's disease is one type of lymphoma. Lymphomas also form solid tumours.

Leukemia. Cancer of the blood-forming parts of the body, particularly the bone marrow and spleen, is called leukemia. A non-solid tumour, leukemia is characterized by an abnormal increase in the number of white blood cells.

The seriousness and general prognosis of a particular cancer are determined through careful diagnosis by trained oncologists. Once laboratory results and clinical observations have been made, cancers are rated by level and stage of development. Those diagnosed as "carcinoma in situ" are localized and are often curable. Cancers that are given higher level or stage ratings have spread farther and are less likely to be cured.

As Table 12.2 shows, the World Health Organization's research suggests that a majority of Canadian cancer cases could be prevented through lifestyle changes and improved screening practices.

Lung Cancer

Symptoms of lung cancer include a persistent cough, blood-streaked sputum, chest pain, and recurrent attacks of pneumonia or bronchitis. Treatment depends on the type and stage of the cancer. Surgery, radiation therapy, and chemotherapy are all treatment options. If the cancer is localized, surgery is usually the treatment of choice. If the cancer has spread, surgery is used in combination with radiation and chemotherapy. Unfortunately, despite advances in medical technology, survival rates for lung cancer have improved only slightly over the past decade. Just 13 percent of lung cancer patients live five or more years after diagnosis. These rates improve to 47 percent with early detection, but relatively few lung cancers are discovered in their early stages of development.[37]

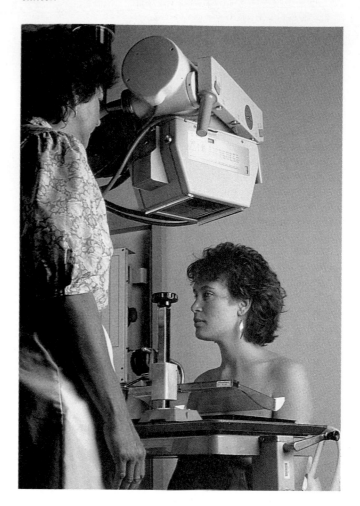

Mammography and other early detection techniques greatly increase a woman's chance of surviving breast cancer.

Prevention. Smokers, especially those who have smoked for over 20 years, and people who have been exposed to certain industrial substances such as arsenic and asbestos or to radiation from occupational, medical, or environmental sources are at the highest risk for lung cancer. Exposure to sidestream cigarette smoke increases the risk for nonsmokers. Some researchers have theorized that as many as 90 percent of all lung cancers could be avoided if people did not smoke. Substantial improvements in overall prognosis have been noted in smokers who quit at the first signs of precancerous cellular changes and allowed their bronchial linings to return to normal.

Breast Cancer

About 1 out of 10 women will develop breast cancer at some time in her life. Although this oft-repeated ratio has

TABLE 12.2 ■ Estimates of Preventable Cancer

According to research for the Cancer and Palliative Care Unit of the World Health Organization, a portion of cancer cases in Canada are potentially preventable, given current knowledge of risk factors. Lifestyle choices, such as smoking and diet, in particular, have been identified as the predominant determinants of human cancer.

The percentage of cancer cases that are potentially preventable was derived by comparing age-standardized cancer rates in Canada to those of countries where populations were largely Caucasian, and where cancer rates for different sites were lowest. It provides an indication of the effect that would be achievable if Canadians were to have the same lifestyle as people in the countries compared.

Cancer Site	Action	Percentage of Cancer Incidence Potentially Preventable
Lung	Eliminate smoking Reduce occupational exposure to carcinogens	60%
Prostate	Reduce fat consumption	78%
Breast	Reduce fat and increase vegetable consumption Reduce obesity (postmenopausal women) Screen women aged 50 to 69	
Colorectal	Reduce fat and increase vegetable consumption	77%
Lymphoma	Reduce exposure to herbicides and pesticides	86%
Bladder	Eliminate smoking and reduce dietary cholesterol Reduce occupational exposure to carcinogens	73%
Body of the uterus	Reduce obesity Benefit from the protective effect of oral contraceptives (women aged 20 to 54)	82%
Stomach	Reduce nitrite in cured meats and salt-preserved foods, and increase fruit and vegetable consumption	52%
Leukemia	Reduce exposure to radiation and benzene	70%
Oral	Eliminate smoking and reduce alcohol consumption Increase fruit and vegetable consumption	68%
Pancreas	Eliminate smoking Reduce sugar and increase vegetable consumption	64%
Melanoma of the skin	Reduce unprotected exposure to sunlight	77%
Kidney	Eliminate smoking Reduce fat consumption	67%
Brain	Reduce occupational exposure to carcinogens	70%
Ovary	Reduce fat consumption Benefit from the protective effect of oral contraceptives (women aged 20 to 54)	53%
Cervix	Eliminate smoking Encourage use of barrier contraceptives Screen women aged 20 to 69	62%

Source: Statistics Canada, *Canadian Social Trends,* Winter 1995, 6.

frightened many women, it represents a woman's lifetime risk. Thus, not until the age of 80 does a woman's risk of breast cancer rise to 1 in 10.[38] Here are the risks at earlier ages:

Age 50: 1 in 50

Age 60: 1 in 24

Age 70: 1 in 14

In 1997, approximately 18 000 women Canada will have been diagnosed with breast cancer for the first time. About 5000 women will die, making breast cancer the second leading cause of cancer death for women (after lung cancer).[39]

Warning signals of breast cancer include persistent breast changes such as a lump, thickening, swelling, dimpling, skin irritation, distortion, retraction or scaliness of the nipple, nipple discharge, pain, or tenderness. Risk factors for breast cancer may vary considerably.[40] Typically, risk factors include being over the age of 40, having a primary relative (a grandmother, mother, or sister) who had breast cancer, never having had children or never having breast-fed, having your first child after age 30, having had early menarche, having had a late age of menopause, and having a higher education and socioeconomic status. International variability in breast cancer incidence rates correlate with differences in diet, with more affluent societies having significantly higher cancer rates. However, it is important to note that a causal role for dietary factors has not been firmly established.[41]

Although risk factors are useful tools, they do not always adequately predict individual susceptibility. However, because of increased awareness, better diagnostic techniques, and improved treatments, breast cancer victims have a better chance of surviving today than they did in the past. A key factor in survival rests with individual recognition of early symptoms.[42]

Prevention. A recent study of the role of exercise in reducing the risk for breast cancer has generated excitement in the scientific community. Researchers speculated that exercise may protect women by altering the production of the ovarian hormones estrogen and progesterone during menstrual cycles.[43]

Regular self-examination (see Figure 12.5) and mammography offer the best hope for early detection of breast cancer. It is important to note that there is tremendous controversy over the cost-effectiveness and usefulness of getting a mammogram before the age of 40. However, many health professionals recommend that if you have any of the risk factors listed above, are prone to fibrous breasts, and are excessively worried about your own condition, a mammogram may be warranted. Consult with your physician if you are in doubt, as it is generally best to be a proactive health consumer.

Treatment. Today, women with breast cancer (and people with nearly any other type of cancer) have many decisions to make in determining the best treatment options available for them. Fortunately, there are services available to help you get the best information, even if you live in a fairly remote area of the country. The important thing to remember is that in most instances, taking the time to thoroughly check out your physician's track record and his or her philosophy on the best treatment is always a good idea. Often, cancer support groups can give you invaluable information and advice. Treatments range from the simple lumpectomy to radical mastectomy to various combinations of radiation or chemotherapy. Figure 12.6 reviews these options. Remember that it is always a good idea to seek more than one opinion before making a decision.

*W*HAT DO YOU THINK?

Why do you think there is such a big difference between mammography screening rates for varied ethnic groups? What actions could be taken to change such disparities? Why do you think so many women fail to be tested for breast cancer? Do you think men are better at seeking recommended screenings for cancers? Why or why not?

Colon and Rectum Cancers

Although colon and rectum cancers are a major cause of cancer deaths, many people are unaware of their potential risk. Bleeding from the rectum, blood in the stool, and changes in bowel habits are the major warning signals. People who are over the age of 40, who have a family history of colon and rectum cancer, a personal or family history of polyps (benign growths) in the colon or rectum, or inflammatory bowel problems such as colitis run an increased risk. Diets high in fats or low in fibre may also increase risk.[44]

Because colorectal cancer tends to spread slowly, the prognosis is quite good if it is caught in the early stages. Treatment often consists of radiation or surgery. Chemotherapy, although not used extensively in the past, is today a possibility. A permanent colostomy, the creation of an abdominal opening for the elimination of body wastes, is seldom required for people with colon cancer and even less frequently for those with rectum cancer.[45]

Prostate Cancer

Cancer of the prostate is the second leading cause of cancer deaths in males, killing an estimated 4000 men in 1997.[46] Most signs and symptoms of prostate cancer are nonspecific—that is, they mimic the signs of infection or enlarged prostate. Symptoms include weak or interrupted

How to Examine Your Breasts

Do you know that 95% of breast cancers are discovered first by women themselves? And that the earlier the breast cancer is detected, the better the chance for a complete cure? Of course, most lumps or changes are not cancer. But you can safeguard your health by making a habit of examining your breasts once a month – a day or two after your period or, if you're no longer menstruating, on any given day. And if you notice anything changed or unusual – a lump, thickening, or discharge – contact your doctor right away.

How to Look for Changes

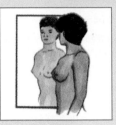

Step 1
Sit or stand in front of a mirror with your arms at your side. Turning slowly from side to side, check your breasts for
• changes in size or shape
• puckering or dimpling of the skin
• changes in size or position of one nipple compared to the other

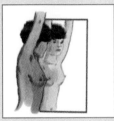

Step 2
Raise your arms above your head and repeat the examination in Step 1.

Step 3
Gently press each nipple with your fingertips to see if there is any discharge.

How to Feel for Changes

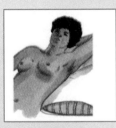

Step 1
Lie down and put a pillow or folded bath towel under your left shoulder. Then place your left hand under your head. (From now on you will be feeling for a lump or thickening in your breasts.)

Step 2
Imagine that your breast is divided into quarters.

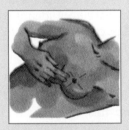

Step 3
With the fingers of your right hand held together, press firmly but gently, using small circular motions to feel the inner, upper quarter of your left breast. Start at your breastbone and work toward the nipple. Also examine the area around the nipple. Now do the same for the lower, inner portion of your breast.

Step 4
Next, bring your arm to your side and feel under your left armpit for swelling.

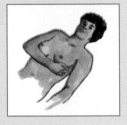

Step 5
With your arm still down, feel the upper, outer part of your breast, starting with your nipple and working outwards. Examine the lower, outer quarter in the same way.

Step 6
Now place the pillow under your right shoulder and repeat all the steps using your left hand to examine your right breast.

FIGURE 12.5

The illustration demonstrates breast self-examination—the ten-minute habit that could save your life.

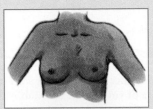

Lumpectomy
Performed when tumor is in earliest localized stages. Prognosis for recovery is better than 95 percent. Only tumor itself is removed. Some physicians may also remove normal tissue in surrounding area.

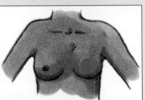

Simple mastectomy
Removal of breast and underlying tissue. Prognosis for full recovery better than 80 percent.

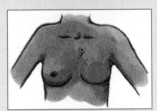

Modified radical mastectomy
Breast and lymph nodes in immediate area removed. Prognosis for full recovery dependent on level of spread.

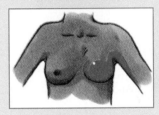

Radical mastectomy
Removal of breast, lymph nodes, pectoral muscles, all fat and underlying tissue. Prognosis for recovery may be as low as 60 percent dependent on level of spread.

FIGURE 12.6

The illustration depicts selected surgical procedures for diagnosed breast cancer. These surgeries are typically followed by radiation treatment and/or chemotherapy.

urine flow or difficulty starting or stopping the urine flow; the need to urinate frequently; pain or difficulty in urinating; blood in the urine; and pain in the lower back, pelvis, or upper thighs. Many males mistake these symptoms for other nonspecific conditions such as infections and delay treatment.

Fortunately, even with so many generalized symptoms, most prostate cancers are detected while they are still localized and tend to progress slowly. Prostate patients have an average five-year survival rate of 80 percent. Because the incidence of prostate cancer increases with age, every man over the age of 40 should have an annual prostate examination.[47]

Skin Cancer

Skin cancer may be one of the most underrated of all of the cancers, particularly among young people. Although

Reducing Your Risk for Skin Cancer

One of the best ways to reduce your risks for skin cancer is to become aware of your body. By establishing a personal base line of information and regular self-checks, you will be able to spot changes early.

- Stand in front of a large, well-lit mirror and look at your body from front to back and head to toe. Be careful to pay attention to hidden areas on the backs of your arms, between your fingers and toes, and on your genitals or buttocks. Use a hand-held mirror to examine hard-to-reach areas. Look for unusual growths or moles that bother you or that fit the symptoms of skin cancer.

- If you note potential areas of concern, consult a dermatologist. Many dermatologists will do baseline "mole mapping" to chart locations and sizes of moles for follow-up examinations.

- Check yourself at least once a month to note changes. Pay attention.

- Avoid sun exposure during high UV ray periods—particularly from 10 A.M. to 2 P.M.

- Wear protective hats, sunglasses that block harmful rays, and clothing that protects the arms and legs.

- Wear a sunscreen with an SPF of 17 or more.

- Be cautious in settings where reflective rays may cause considerable harm, such as when at a beach or lake, or when out in the snow.

- If you have sensitive, fair skin, use extra precautions. Cover up and pick the shady spots when outdoors. Remember, the fairer the hair and skin, the higher the SPF sunscreen you normally need—usually 17 to 30 or higher.

---

it is true that most people do not die of the common, highly curable *basal* or *squamous cell* skin cancers, many people do not know that another, highly virulent form of skin cancer known as **malignant melanoma** has become a major killer of young women. Rates for men over 50 are also increasing. Yet many people still bask unprotected on on beaches, apparently not making the connection between death from melanoma and sunlight overexposure. The perception that health and a well-tanned body go together couldn't be further from the truth. For more information on protecting yourself from skin cancer, see the Skills for Behaviour Change box.

Symptoms. Many people do not have any idea what to look for when considering skin cancer. Any unusual skin condition, especially a change in the size or colour of a mole or other darkly pigmented growth or spot, should be considered suspect. Scaliness, oozing, bleeding, the appearance of a bump or nodule, the spread of pigment beyond the border, change in sensation, itchiness, tenderness, and pain are all warning signs of the basal and squamous cell skin cancers. However, melanoma symptoms are slightly different. Often there is a sudden or progressive change in a mole's appearance from a small, mole-like growth to a large, ulcerated, and easily-prone-to-bleeding growth. A simple *ABCD* rule outlines the warning signals of melanoma: *A* is for asymmetry. One

> **Malignant melanoma:** A virulent cancer of the melanin (pigment-producing portion) of the skin.

half of the mole does not match the other half. *B* is for border irregularity. The edges are ragged, notched, or blurred. *C* is for colour. The pigmentation is not uniform. *D* is for diameter greater than 6 millimeters. Any or all of these symptoms should cause you to visit a physician.[48]

Testicular Cancer

Testicular cancer is currently one of the most common types of solid tumours found in males entering early adulthood. Those between the ages of 17 and 34 are at greatest risk. There has been a steady increase in tumour frequency over the past several years in this age group.

Although the exact cause of testicular cancer is unknown, several possible risk factors have been identified. Males with undescended testicles appear to be at greatest risk for the disease. In addition, some studies indicate that there may be a genetic influence.

In general, testicular tumours are first noticed as a painless enlargement of the testis or as an apparent thickening in testicular tissue. Because this enlargement is often painless, it is extremely important that all young males practise regular testicular self-examination (see Figure 12.7). If a suspicious lump or thickening is found, medical follow-up should be sought immediately.

Ovarian Cancer

Ovarian cancer is often silent, showing no obvious signs or symptoms until late in its development. The most common sign is enlargement of the abdomen (or a feeling of bloating) in women over the age of 40. Other symptoms

Follow the instructions in the diagram carefully and examine your testes immediately after your next hot bath or shower. Heat causes the testicles to descend and the scrotal skin to relax, making it easier to find unusual lumps.

Examine each testicle by placing the index and middle fingers of both hands on the underside of the testicle and the thumbs on the top. Gently roll the testicle between your thumb and fingers, feeling for small lumps.

Changes or anything abnormal will appear at the front or side of your testicle. Did you find any unusual lumps? Are there any unusual signs of any kind? Are there any markings or lumps at any site?

Keep in mind that not all lumps are a sign of testicular cancer. Unusual lumps at any location, however, should be checked by a physician. Early detection greatly increases your chances of a complete cure. Repeat the examination every month and record your findings.

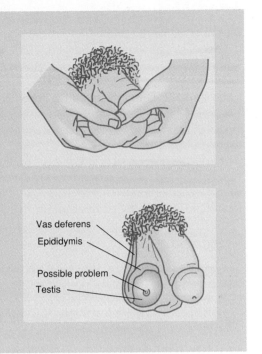

Vas deferens
Epididymis
Possible problem
Testis

FIGURE 12.7

Testicular Self-Exam

include vague digestive disturbances, such as gas and stomach aches that persist and cannot be explained.[49]

The risk for ovarian cancer increases with age, with the highest rates found in women in their 60s. Women who have never had children are twice as likely to develop ovarian cancer as are those who have. The main risk factor appears to be exposure to the reproductive hormone estrogen. Women who have multiple pregnancies or use oral contraceptives, which both inhibit estrogen, are at lower risk. In addition, having one or more primary relatives (mother, sisters, grandmothers) who have had the disease appears to increase individual risk. With the exception of Japan, the highest incidence rates are reported in the industrialized countries of the world.[50]

Prevention. A recent Yale University study indicates that diet may also play a role in ovarian cancer.[51] Researchers found that when comparing 450 Canadian women with newly diagnosed ovarian cancer with 564 demographically similar, healthy women, the women without ovarian cancer had a diet lower in saturated fat. Such results, particularly when combined with cardiovascular risks and other health risks, may provide yet another reason to hold the fat—or at least cut down on your overall intake.

The best way to protect yourself is with annual thorough pelvic examinations. Pap tests, although useful in detecting cervical cancer, do not reveal ovarian cancer.

Women over the age of 40 should have a cancer-related checkup every year. If you have any of the symptoms of ovarian cancer and they persist, see your doctor. If they continue to persist, get a second opinion.[52]

Uterine Cancer

Most uterine cancers develop in the body of the uterus, usually in the endometrium (lining). The rest develop in the cervix, located at the base of the uterus. The overall incidence of early-stage uterine cancer—that is, cervical cancer—has increased slightly in recent years in women under the age of 50. In contrast, invasive, later-stage forms of the disease appear to be decreasing. Much of this apparent trend may be due to more effective regular screenings of younger women using the **Pap test**, a procedure in which cells taken from the cervical region are examined for abnormal cellular activity. Although these tests are very effective for detecting early-stage cervical cancer, they are less effective for detecting cancers of the uterine lining

Pap test: A procedure in which cells taken from the cervical region are examined for abnormal cellular activity.

and are not effective at all for detecting cancers of the fallopian tubes or ovaries.[53]

Risk factors for cervical cancer include early age of first intercourse, multiple sex partners, cigarette smoking, and certain sexually transmitted diseases, such as the herpes virus and the human papilloma virus. For endometrial cancer, a history of infertility, failure to ovulate, obesity, and treatment with tamoxifen or unopposed estrogen therapy appear to be major risk factors.[54]

Early warning signs of uterine cancer include bleeding outside the normal menstrual period or after menopause or persistent unusual vaginal discharge. These symptoms should be checked by a physician immediately.[55]

Leukemia

Leukemia is a cancer of the blood-forming tissues that leads to proliferation of millions of immature white blood cells. These abnormal cells crowd out normal white blood cells (which fight infection), platelets (which control hemorrhaging), and red blood cells (which prevent anemia). As a result, symptoms such as fatigue, paleness, weight loss, easy bruising, repeated infections, nosebleeds, and other forms of hemorrhaging occur. In children, these symptoms can appear suddenly.[56]

Leukemia can be acute or chronic in nature and can strike both sexes and all age groups. Chronic leukemia can develop over several months and have few symptoms. Although many people believe that leukemia is a childhood disease, leukemia strikes many more adults than children.[57] Over the last 30 years, there has been a dramatic improvement in survival of patients with acute lymphocytic leukemia.

Oral Cancer

Cancer may develop in any part of the oral cavity. Most often it is found on the lips, the lining of the cheeks, the gums, and the floor of the mouth. The tongue, the pharynx, and the tonsils are other common sites. Tobacco use—smoking, chewing, or dipping—is the most common risk factor for oral cancer.

𝒲HAT DO YOU THINK?

What types of cancers do you think you and your friends are at greatest risk for right now? Do you practise regular breast or testicular self-exam? Would you be able to help your spouse or intimate partner with his or her exam?

𝓕ACING CANCER

While heart disease mortality rates have declined steadily over the past 50 years, cancer mortality rates have increased consistently in the same period. Many factors have contributed to the rise in cancer mortality—one being simply longer life expectancies—but the increase in the incidence of lung cancer is probably the most important reason. However, recent advancements in the diagnosis and treatment of many forms of cancer have reduced much of the fear and mystery that once surrounded this disease.

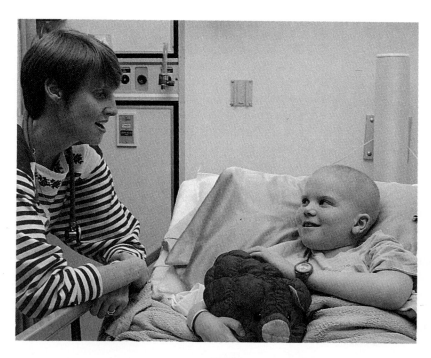

The treatment for childhood leukemia remains a difficult and disturbing experience for both children and parents even though survival rates have risen dramatically in recent years.

Cancer's Seven Warning Signals

1 Changes in bowel or bladder habits.

2 A sore that does not heal.

3 Unusual bleeding or discharge.

4 Thickening or lump in breast or elsewhere.

5 Indigestion or difficulty in swallowing.

6 Obvious change in a wart or mole.

7 Nagging cough or hoarseness.

If you have a warning signal,
see your doctor.

FIGURE 12.8

Cancer's Seven Warning Signals

Detecting Cancer

The earlier a person is diagnosed as having cancer, the better the prospect for survival. Various high-tech diagnostic techniques exist to detect cancer. These medical techniques, along with regular self-examinations and checkups, play an important role in the early detection and secondary prevention of cancer. Familiarize yourself with the Seven Warning Signals of cancer, as shown in Figure 12.8. If you notice any of these signals, and they don't appear to be related to anything else, you should see a doctor immediately. Make sure that appropriate diagnostic tests are completed whenever any warning signals appear. Also make a realistic assessment of your individual risk factors and try to avoid those you have some control over.

New Hope in Cancer Treatments

Although cancer treatments have changed dramatically over the last 20 years, surgery, in which the tumour and surrounding tissue are removed, is still common. Today's surgeons tend to remove less surrounding tissue than previously and to combine surgery with either **radiotherapy** (the use of radiation) or **chemotherapy** to kill cancerous cells.

Radiation works by destroying malignant cells or stopping cell growth. It is most effective in treating localized cancer masses. Unfortunately, in the process of destroying malignant cells, radiotherapy also destroys some healthy cells. In addition, in recent years, many scientists have come to suspect that radiotherapy may increase the risks

for other types of cancers. Despite these qualifications, radiation continues to be one of the most common and effective forms of treatment.

When cancer has spread throughout the body, it is necessary to use some form of chemotherapy. Currently, over 50 different anticancer drugs are in use, some of which have excellent records of success. A chemotherapeutic regimen including four anticancer drugs in combination with radiation therapy has resulted in remarkable survival rates for some cancers, including Hodgkin's disease. Ongoing research into new drug development will result in compounds that are less toxic to normal cells and more potent against tumour cells.[58] Current research indicates that some tumours may actually be resistant to certain forms of chemotherapy and that the treatment drugs do not reach the core of the tumour.[59] Scientists are currently working to circumvent resistance to chemotherapeutic drugs and to make tumour cells more vulnerable throughout treatment.

Whether used alone or in combination, radiotherapy and chemotherapy have possible side-effects, including extreme nausea, nutritional deficiencies, hair loss, and general fatigue. Long-term damage to the cardiovascular system and many other systems of the body can be significant. It is important that you discuss these matters fully with your doctors. The Building Communication Skills box offers advice on how to talk to your doctor about your cancer.

Other promising advances in the battle against cancer include:[60]

- A large clinical trial is under way to evaluate the usefulness of an estrogen-blocking drug called tamoxifen to treat women with some forms of breast cancer.

- **Immunotherapy** is a new technique designed to enhance the body's own disease fighting systems to help control cancer.

- New high-technology diagnostic imaging techniques have replaced exploratory surgery for some cancer patients. **Magnetic resonance imaging (MRI)** is one example of such technology. In MRI, a huge electromagnet is used to detect hidden tumours by mapping

Radiotherapy: The use of radiation to kill cancerous cells.

Chemotherapy: The use of drugs to kill cancerous cells.

Immunotherapy: A process that stimulates the body's own immune system to combat cancer cells.

Magnetic resonance imaging (MRI): A device that uses magnetic fields, radio waves, and computers to generate an image of internal tissues of the body for diagnostic purposes without the use of radiation.

Talking with Your Doctor about Cancer

Anytime there is the suspicion of cancer, the person involved is likely to react with great anxiety, fear, and anger. Emotional distress is sometimes so intense that the person involved is unable to serve as his or her own best advocate in making critical health-care decisions. If you find it difficult to know what to ask your doctor on a routine exam, imagine how hard it would be to discuss life or death options for yourself or a loved one. Having a list of important questions to ask when you appear at the doctor's office may help tremendously. Remember, your health-care provider should be your partner in making the best decisions for you. Actively challenging, questioning, and letting the physician know your wishes can make difficult decisions easier.

If the diagnosis is cancer, you may want to ask these questions:

- What kind of cancer do I have? What stage is it in? Based on my age and stage, what type of prognosis do I have?

- What are my treatment choices? Which do you recommend? Why?

- What are the expected benefits of each kind of treatment?

- What are the long- and short-term risks and possible side effects?

- Would a clinical trial be appropriate for me? (Clinical trials are research studies designed to answer specific questions and to find better ways to prevent or treat cancer. Often new cancer-fighting treatments are used.)

If surgery is recommended, you may want to ask these questions:

- What kind of operation will it be and how long will it take? What form of anesthesia will be used? How many similar procedures has this surgeon done in the last month? What is his or her success rate?

- How will I feel after surgery? If I have pain, how will you help me?

- Where will the scars be? What will they look like? Will they cause disability?

- Will I have any activity limitations after surgery? What kind of physical therapy, if any, will I have? When will I get back to normal activities?

If radiation is recommended, you may want to ask these questions:

- Why do you think this treatment is better than my other options?

- How long will I need to have treatments and what will the side effects be in the short and long term? What body organs/systems may be damaged?

- What can I do to take care of myself during therapy? Are there services available to help me?

- What is the long-term prognosis for people my age with my type of cancer using this treatment?

If chemotherapy is recommended, you may want to ask these questions:

- Why do you think this treatment is better than my other options?

- Which drug combinations pose the least risks and most benefits?

- What are the short- and long-term side effects on my body?

- What are my options?

Before beginning any form of cancer therapy, it is imperative that you be a vigilant and vocal consumer. Read and seek information from cancer support groups. Check the skills of your surgeon, your radiation therapist, and your doctor in terms of clinical work and interpersonal interactions. The time spent asking these questions and seeking information is well worth the effort.

---

the vibrations of the various atoms in the body on a computer screen. **Computerized axial tomography scanning (CAT scan)** uses X-rays to examine parts of the body. In both of these painless, non-invasive procedures, cross-section pictures can show a tumour's shape and location more accurately than can conventional X-rays.

Computerized axial tomography (CAT scan): A machine that uses radiation to view internal organs not normally visible on X-rays.

- A powerful enzyme inhibitor, TIMP-2, is showing promise for slowing the metastasis of tumour cells. A metastasis suppressor gene, NM23, has also been identified.

- *Neoadjuvant chemotherapy* (giving chemotherapy to shrink the cancer and then removing it surgically) has been tried against various types of cancers. This is a promising new treatment approach.

- *Prostatic ultrasound* (a rectal probe using ultrasonic waves to produce an image of the prostate) is currently being investigated as a potential means to increase the early detection of prostate cancer. Recently, prostatic ultrasound has been combined with a blood test for

prostate-specific antigen (PSA), an antigen found in prostate cancer patients. Although the reliability of PSA tests for screening has been questioned, it appears to show promise.

In addition, psychosocial and behavioural research has become increasingly important as health professionals seek the answers to questions concerning complex lifestyle factors that appear to influence risks for cancer as well as the survivability of patients with particular psychological and mental health profiles. Also, health care practitioners have become more aware of the psychological needs of patients and families and have begun to tailor treatment programs to meet the diverse needs of different people.

> **Prostate-specific antigen (PSA):** An antigen found in prostate cancer patients.

Life After Cancer

Heightened public awareness and an improved prognosis for cancer victims have made the cancer experience less threatening and isolating than it once was. Assistance for the cancer patient is more readily available than ever before. Cancer support groups, cancer information workshops, and low-cost medical consultation are just a few of the forms of assistance now offered in many communities. Increasing efforts in cancer research, improvements in diagnostic equipment, and advances in treatment provide hope for the future.

TAKING CHARGE

Managing Your Health

Although it is easy to read through a chapter like this and learn what we should be doing to keep ourselves healthy, few of us ever really think about what it takes to prevent serious illness. Relationships, financial worries, grades, time for fun, and other issues often take precedence over our long-term commitments to wellness.

Making Decisions for You

List the five things that matter to you most right now. Is appearance part of your list? Is being able to get through a day without feeling tired or unusually fatigued important? Are you motivated to change your health behaviours and take action to reduce your circulatory disease and cancer risks by exercising more, reducing stress, and eating properly? Was there anything about this chapter that helped you become more concerned about making a change now? Why is this important? What actions do you plan to take?

Checklist for Change: Making Personal Choices

✓ Determine your hereditary risks. If they are high, outline the steps that you can take to reduce your overall risk.

✓ Know about the normal circulatory disease risk changes that occur with age. Take the extra steps needed to minimize your risks as you age.

✓ If you smoke, quit. If you don't smoke, don't start.

✓ Find out what your cholesterol level is, including your HDL and LDL levels.

✓ Reduce saturated fat in your diet and take steps to reduce your triglyceride and cholesterol levels.

✓ Get out and exercise. Even a relaxing walk every day is a good risk reducer. Nobody says you have to run and exercise until you drop. Take it easy, but keep it up.

✓ Control your blood pressure. Monitor it regularly and see your doctor if you have high blood pressure.

✓ Lose weight if you are overweight. Obesity is a significant risk factor for both cardiovascular disease and cancer.

✓ Control your stress levels.

✓ Avoid excessive sunlight.

✓ Avoid excessive alcohol consumption.

✓ Do not use smokeless tobacco.

✓ Properly monitor estrogen use. While estrogen therapy does seem to lower women's risk for heart disease and osteoporosis, it should not be undertaken without careful discussion between a woman and her physician.

✓ Avoid occupational exposures to carcinogens. Exposure to several different industrial agents (nickel, chromate, asbestos, vinyl chloride, etc.) increases risk for various cancers.

✓ Eat your fruits and vegetables. Eat at least five servings of fruits and vegetables every day to reduce your risk for lung, colon, pancreatic, stomach, bladder, esophageal, mouth, and throat cancer.

(continued)

Checklist for Change: Making Community Choices

✓ Take a class in CPR. Your local Red Cross likely offers them; courses may be available on campus. Be prepared to offer bystander CPR.

✓ Consider becoming an Emergency Medical Technician (EMT). You don't have to make a career of it. But you could be prepared to save people in your dorm, your office building, and your community.

✓ Does your community have any major sources of carcinogens (toxic waste dumps, chemical factories, etc.)? What precautions are taken to ensure that any environmental risks are reduced?

✓ Does the Canadian Cancer Society have a local office at which you could volunteer some time?

✓ Does your community have cancer support groups that you could join if you were found to have cancer? Where would you find out about such support groups?

Critical Thinking

You've been good friends with one of your 30-something neighbours for some time. Recently, after spending a good deal of time working on a community project together, you start to date. After a few terrific dates, during which you really hit it off socially, you find out that your friend had cancer two years ago, and that there is a 50 percent chance the cancer will return within five years. You truly love this person, but wonder what to do. If you commit yourself to this relationship and the cancer returns, then what? You've always wanted to have children, but are concerned about what would happen if your partner died of cancer while the kids were young. On the other hand, there is a 50 percent chance that the cancer will not return.

Using the DECIDE model described in Chapter 1, decide whether or not you would continue the relationship. Does it make any difference to you whether the cancer survivor described is a male or female? Explain why.

Summary

◆ The cardiovascular system consists of the heart and circulatory system and is a carefully regulated, integrated network of vessels that supply the body with the nutrients and oxygen necessary to perform daily functions.

◆ Circulatory diseases combine to be the leading cause of death in Canada today.

◆ Risk factors for circulatory disease include cigarette smoking, high blood fat and cholesterol levels, high blood pressure, lack of exercise, high-fat diet, obesity, diabetes, and emotional stress. Some factors, such as age, sex, and heredity, are risk factors that are not under your control. Many of these factors have a compounded effect when combined.

◆ Women have a unique challenge in controlling their risk for circulatory diseases, particularly after menopause,

when estrogen levels are no longer sufficient to be protective.

◆ New methods developed for treating heart blockages include coronary bypass surgery and angioplasty.

◆ Cancer is a group of diseases characterized by uncontrolled growth and spread of abnormal cells.

◆ Early diagnosis of cancer affects your survival rate. Self-exams for breast, testicular, and skin cancer and knowledge of the Seven Warning Signals of cancer aid early diagnosis.

◆ New types of cancer treatments include various combinations of radiotherapy, chemotherapy, and immunotherapy.

Discussion Questions

1. List the different types of circulatory diseases. Compare and contrast their symptoms, risk factors, prevention, and treatment.

2. What are the major indicators that circulatory diseases poses a particularly significant risk to people your age? To the elderly? To people from particular racial or ethnic groups?

3. Discuss the role exercise, stress management, dietary changes, checkups, sodium reduction, and other factors can play in reducing your risk for circulatory diseases.

4. Discuss why age is such an important factor in women's risk for circulatory diseases. What can be done to lower women's risks in later life?

5. Describe some of the diagnostic and treatment alternatives for circulatory diseases. If you had a heart attack today, which treatment would you prefer? Explain why.

6. What is the difference between a benign and a malignant tumor?

7. List the likely causes of cancer. Do any of these causes put you at greater risk? What can you do to reduce this risk?

8. What are the symptoms of lung, breast, prostate, and testicular cancer? What can you do to increase your chances of surviving these cancers?

9. What could signal that you have cancer instead of a minor illness? How soon should you seek treatment for any of the seven warning signs?

Application Exercise

Reread the What Do You Think? scenario at the beginning of the chapter and answer the following questions:

1. Consider Michael's case in the chapter opener. Why do you think so many young Canadians deny their risk for circulatory diseases?

2. As a friend of Michael's, what advice might you give?

3. Think about people in your family who have significant circulatory disease risks. What could you do to help them become aware of their risks without preaching to them about their behaviours and turning them off?

4. What kinds of community support could people like Michael use?

Health on the Net

Heart and Stroke Foundation of Canada
www.hsf.ca/

National Cancer Institute
www.cancer.ca/

World Health Organization: Cardiovascular Diseases Home Page
www.who.ch/programmes/ncd/cvd/cvd_home.htm

13

Infectious and Noninfectious Conditions

Risks and Responsibilities

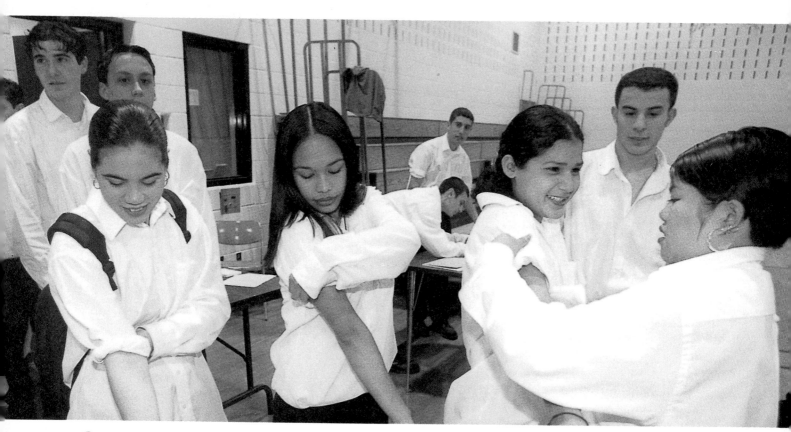

CHAPTER OBJECTIVES

◆ Discuss the risk factors for infectious diseases, including those you can control and those you cannot.

◆ Describe the most common pathogens.

◆ Discuss the immune system and explain the role of vaccinations in fighting disease.

◆ Discuss the various sexually transmitted diseases, their means of transmission, and actions that prevent the spread of STIs.

◆ Discuss the transmission, symptoms, treatment, and prevention of transmission of the HIV virus.

◆ Identify common respiratory disorders.

◆ Explain the common neurological disorders, including the varied types of headaches and seizure disorders.

◆ Describe the common gender disorders, risk factors for these conditions, their symptoms, and methods of their control or prevention.

◆ Discuss diseases of the digestive system, including their symptoms, prevention, and control.

◆ Discuss the varied musculoskeletal diseases and their effects on the body.

Gayle and Patrick have been seeing each other for a year. Their relationship has become sexually active. Both have had sexual involvement prior to this relationship. Gayle is concerned and goes to the Health Unit for a sexual health checkup. She learns she has a sexually transmitted infection. She can tell Patrick herself, the Health Unit staff can arrange a confidential meeting and tell Patrick for her, or she can ask her family doctor to talk with Patrick. She is afraid of Patrick's reaction and doesn't know if she is the carrier or became infected by Patrick.

- What do you think Gayle should do? What would you do?

Every moment of every day you are in constant contact with microscopic organisms that have the ability to make you sick. These disease-causing agents, or **pathogens**, are found in the air you breathe, in the foods you eat, and on nearly every person or object that you come into contact with. Although new varieties of pathogens arise all the time, scientific evidence indicates that pathogens have existed for at least as long as we have. There is fossil evidence that infections, cancer, heart disease, and a host of other ailments afflicted the earliest human beings. At times, infectious diseases wiped out whole groups of people through **epidemics** such as the Black Death, or bubonic plague, that wiped out more than half of the population of Europe and Asia in the 1300s and the influenza, tuberculosis, cholera, and other deadly epidemics of more recent centuries. In modern times, some infectious diseases have been conquered or contained by scientific advances such as vaccinations and pasteurization and by wholesale improvements in sanitation.[1] Still, worldwide, infectious diseases are the leading cause of premature death. Of about 52 million deaths from all causes in 1995, more than 17 million were due to infectious diseases, including about 9 million deaths in young children. Up to half the world's population of 5.72 billion are at risk of many endemic diseases. In addition, millions of people are developing cancers as a direct result of preventable infections by bacteria and viruses.[2]

We continue to be susceptible to a vast number of potentially threatening organisms and emerging diseases that defy conventional treatments. The more **virulent**, or aggressive, the organism, the higher the probability that it will overcome your body defences and cause disease. However, if your immune system is strong and your internal capacity to ward off disease is substantial, you will often be able to fight off even the most virulent attacker. Just because you inhale a flu virus does not mean that you will get the flu. Just because your hands are teeming with bacteria does not mean that you will get a bacterial disease. Several factors influence your susceptibility to diseases.

Infectious diseases in Canada are controlled through ongoing vigilance by public health networks operating at local, regional, and national levels. Clean food and water, immunizations, and an excellent health care system have maintained Canadians' health. Good nutrition is a factor in overall good health. Nutritional status has been found to have an effect on resistance to infectious diseases in certain population groups such as infants, young children, and the elderly. Nutritional status can also affect the course of an infectious disease, as has been shown with HIV-positive individuals.[3]

INFECTIOUS DISEASE RISK FACTORS

At one time, it was believed that most diseases were caused by a single factor, but today we recognize that most diseases are **multifactorial,** or caused by the interaction of several factors from inside and outside the person. For a disease to occur, the *host* must be *susceptible,* meaning that the immune system must be in a weakened condition; an *agent* capable of transmitting a disease must be present;

Pathogen: A disease-causing agent.

Epidemic: Disease outbreak that affects many people in a community or region at the same time.

Virulent: Said of organisms able to overcome host resistance and cause disease.

Multifactorial disease: Disease caused by interactions of several factors.

---

and the *environment* must be hospitable to the pathogen in terms of temperature, light, moisture, and other requirements. Other risk factors also apparently increase or decrease levels of susceptibility.

Risk Factors You Can't Control

Uncontrollable risk factors are those that increase your susceptibility and over which you may have little or no control. Some of the most common factors are:

Heredity. Perhaps the single greatest factor influencing your longevity is your parents' longevity. Being born into a family in which heart disease, cancer, or other illnesses are prevalent seems to increase your risk. Some people having a close relative who is a diabetic become diabetic themselves even though they take precautions, watch their weight, and exercise regularly. Still other diseases are caused by direct chromosomal inheritance. **Sickle cell anemia**, an inherited blood disease that primarily affects blacks, is often transmitted to the foetus if both parents carry the sickle cell trait.

Aging. Although we can do a great deal to lessen the effects of many negative aspects of the aging process, it is widely documented that after the age of 40 we become more vulnerable to most of the chronic diseases. Moreover, as we age, our immune systems respond less efficiently to invading organisms, increasing our risk for infection and illness. The same flu that produces an afternoon of nausea and diarrhea in a younger person may cause days of illness or even death in an older person. The very young are also at risk for many diseases, particularly if they are not vaccinated against them.

Environmental Conditions. Unsanitary conditions and the presence of drugs, chemicals, and hazardous pollutants and wastes in our food and water probably have a great effect on our immune systems. That **immunological competence**—the body's ability to defend itself against pathogens—is weakened in such situations has been well documented.[4]

Risk Factors You Can Control

Although our degree of control over risk factors for disease may vary according to our socioeconomic condition, cultural upbringing, geographic location, and a host of other variables, we all have some degree of personal control over certain risk factors for disease. Too much stress, inadequate nutrition, a low physical fitness level, lack of sleep, misuse or abuse of legal and illegal substances, poor personal hygiene, high-risk behaviours, and other variables significantly increase the risk for a number of diseases. These variables are discussed individually in various chapters of this text.

*T*HE PATHOGENS: ROUTES OF INVASION

Pathogens enter the body in several ways. They may be transmitted by direct contact between infected persons, such as during sexual relations, kissing, or touching, or by indirect contact, such as by touching an object the infected person has had contact with. The hands are probably the greatest source of transmission. You may also **autoinoculate** yourself, or transmit a pathogen from one part of your body to another. For example, you may touch a sore on your lip that is teeming with viral herpes and then transmit the virus to your eye when you subsequently scratch your itchy eyelid.

Pathogens are also transmitted by *airborne contact*, either through inhaling the droplet spray from a sneeze or through breathing in air that carries a particular pathogen. You may become the victim of *food-borne infection* if you eat something contaminated by microorganisms. The *E. coli* bacteria and other virulent pathogens are responsible for a variety of *emerging* diseases that pose significant threats to humans. Examples of these are found in Table 13.1.

Your "best friend" may be the source of *animal-borne pathogens*. Dogs as well as cats, livestock, and wild animals can spread numerous diseases through their bites or faeces or by carrying infected insects into your living areas. For example, ticks in some regions carry Lyme disease. *Water-borne* diseases are transmitted directly from drinking water and indirectly from foods washed or sprayed with water containing their pathogens. These pathogens can also invade your body if you wade or swim in contaminated streams, lakes, and reservoirs. What are the most common pathogens and how can you best protect yourself against them?

Bacteria

Bacteria are single-celled organisms that are plantlike in nature but lack chlorophyll (the pigment that gives plants their green colouring). There are three major types of bacteria: cocci, bacilli, and spirilla. Bacteria may be viewed under a standard light microscope.

TABLE 13.1 ■ Emerging Diseases: Challenges to Public Health

Disease/Cause Agent	Description
Ebola virus	A deadly disease concentrated in portions of Africa. Ebola can be transferred only by direct contact with infected blood, organs, secretions, semen, or contaminated needles. Transmission is enhanced by unsanitary, overcrowded conditions and poor preventive practices.
Dengue:	More than 200 000 cases in Latin America alone during 1994, of which 5000 were dengue hemorrhagic fever (DHF), a severe form of the disease that causes high mortality. It is the first time that dengue has been reported in some Latin America and Caribbean countries in half a century.
E. coli bacteria	Illness caused by ingesting undercooked meats tainted by *Escherichia coli* bacteria.
Flesh-eating strep	A rare disease caused by a strain of Group A Strep bacterium that produces materials that dissolve tissue. Early diagnosis and treatment with antibiotics arrests the disease.
Cholera	A bacterial disease affecting the intestinal tract of individuals who eat or drink food or water contaminated by faecal waste of an infected person. Although still rare, recent outbreaks in developing countries pose a potential threat to North Americans as well because of increased international travel.
Tuberculosis	A pulmonary disease once thought to be almost eliminated from North America. Depressed social conditions and improper use of antibiotics have revived this airborne disease that is particularly threatening to people with weakened immune systems. Strict adherence to drug therapy for several months can cure the condition.

Although there are several thousand species of bacteria, only approximately 100 cause diseases in humans. In many cases, it is not the bacteria themselves that cause disease but rather the poisonous substances, called **toxins**, that they produce. Some of these toxins are extremely powerful. Bacterial infections can take many forms. The following are the most common.

Staphylococcal Infections. One of the most common forms of bacterial infection is the staph infection. **Staphylococci** are normally present on our skin at all times and usually cause few problems. But when there is a cut or break in the **epidermis**, or outer layer of the skin, staphylococci may enter and cause a localized infection. If you have ever suffered from acne, boils, styes (infections of the eyelids), or infected wounds, you have probably had a staph infection.

At least one staph-caused disorder, **toxic shock syndrome**, is potentially fatal. Media reports in the early 1980s indicated that the disorder was exclusive to menstruating women, particularly those who used high-absorbency tampons and left them inserted for prolonged periods of time. Although most cases of toxic shock syndrome have occurred in menstruating women, the disease was first reported in 1978 in a group of children and continues to be reported in men, children, and nonmenstruating women. Most cases that are not related to menstruation occur in patients recovering from wounds, surgery, and similar incidents. Although tampons are strongly implicated, the actual mechanisms that produce this disease remain uncertain.

To reduce the likelihood of contracting toxic shock syndrome, take the following precautions: (1) avoid

Sickle cell anemia: Genetic disease commonly found among African-Americans; results in organ damage and premature death.

Immunological competence: Ability of the immune system to defend the body from pathogens.

Autoinoculation: Transmission of a pathogen from one part of your body to another.

Bacteria: Single-celled organisms that may be disease-causing.

Toxins: Poisonous substances produced by certain microorganisms that cause various diseases.

Staphylococci: Round, gram-positive bacteria, usually found in clusters.

Epidermis: The outermost layer of the skin.

Toxic shock syndrome: A potentially life-threatening bacterial infection that is most common in menstruating women.

superabsorbent tampons except during the heaviest menstrual flow; (2) change tampons at least every four hours; and (3) use napkins at night instead of tampons. Call your doctor immediately if you have any of the following symptoms during menstruation: high fever, headache, vomiting, diarrhea and the chills, stomach pains, or shocklike symptoms such as faintness, rapid pulse, pallor (which can be caused by a drop in blood pressure), or a sunburnlike rash, particularly on fingers and toes.

Streptococcal Infections. Another common form of bacterial infection is caused by microorganisms called **streptococci**. A "strep throat" (severe sore throat characterized by white or yellow pustules at the back of the throat) is the typical streptococcal problem. Scarlet fever (characterized by acute fever, sore throat, and rash) and rheumatic fever (said to "lick the joints and bite the heart") are serious streptococcal infections.

Pneumonia. In the late nineteenth century and early twentieth century, **pneumonia** was one of the leading causes of death in North America. This disease is characterized by chronic cough, chest pain, chills, high fever, fluid accumulation, and eventual respiratory failure. One of the most common forms of pneumonia is caused by bacterial infection and responds readily to antibiotic treatment. Other forms are caused by the presence of viruses, chemicals, or other substances in the lungs. In these types of pneumonia, treatment may be more difficult.

Legionnaire's Disease. This bacterial disorder gained widespread publicity in 1976, when several Legionnaires at the American Legion convention in Philadelphia contracted the disease and died before the invading organism was isolated and effective treatment devised. The symptoms are similar to those for pneumonia, which sometimes makes identification difficult. In people whose resistance is lowered, particularly the elderly, delayed identification can have serious consequences. If they are misdiagnosed as suffering from pneumonia, they may be given **penicillin**, which is ineffective as a treatment for Legionnaire's disease, instead of the required erythromycin.

Streptococci: Round bacteria, usually found in chain formation.

Pneumonia: Bacterially caused disease of the lungs.

Penicillin: Antibiotic used to fight a variety of bacterially caused ailments.

Tuberculosis (TB): A disease caused by bacterial infiltration of the respiratory system.

Periodontal diseases: Diseases of the tissue around the teeth.

Viruses: Minute parasitic microbes that live inside another cell.

Tuberculosis. One of the leading fatal diseases in Europe and North America in the early 1900s, **tuberculosis (TB)** was largely controlled by the mid-1900s through improved sanitation, isolation of infected persons, and treatment with drugs such as rifampin or Isoniazid.

However, Switzerland, Italy, and the United States are all experiencing a resurgence of new cases. Several factors are contributing to this, including the phasing-out of TB surveillance and control programs, the emergence of multiple-drug-resistant TB (MAR-TB), large-scale migration, social and natural disasters, and infection with the human immunodeficiency virus (HIV).

The risk of developing clinical TB in tuberculin-positive individuals is very high in HIV-seropositive patients.[5] In Canada, 2000 new cases of TB are reported each year, and this figure has remained constant since 1987.[6]

Tuberculosis is caused by bacterial infiltration of the respiratory system. It is transmitted from person to person by the breathing of air infected by coughing or sneezing over the course of several hours for as long as six months. Many people infected with TB are contagious without actually showing any symptoms themselves. Symptoms include persistent coughing, weight loss, fever, and spitting up blood. Fortunately, the average healthy person is not at high risk; however, those who may be fighting other diseases, such as some of the HIV-related diseases, may be at increased risk. A quick test can usually detect TB. If you do have it, you can usually be treated and made noncontagious within two weeks. You can often be cured within six months.

Periodontal Diseases. Diseases of the tissue around the teeth, called **periodontal diseases**, affect three out of four adults over 35. Improper home tooth care, including lack of flossing and poor brushing habits, and the failure to obtain professional dental care regularly lead to increased bacterial growth, caries (tooth decay), and gum infections. If left untreated, permanent tooth loss may result.

---

*W*HAT DO YOU THINK?

Why do you think we are experiencing increases in many infectious diseases today? Why are some bacterial agents becoming more resistant to current treatment regimens? What can be done to reduce the spread of infectious diseases such as tuberculosis? What can you do to reduce your own risks?

Viruses

Viruses are the smallest of the pathogens, being approximately 1/500 the size of bacteria. Because of their tiny size, they are visible only under an electron microscope and were therefore not identified until this century. At present, over 150 viruses are known to cause diseases in humans.

Essentially, a virus consists of a protein structure that contains either *ribonucleic acid (RNA)* or *deoxyribonucleic acid (DNA)*. It is incapable of carrying out the normal cell functions of respiration and metabolism. It cannot reproduce on its own and can only exist in a parasitic relationship with the cell it invades.

Treatment of viral diseases is difficult because many viruses can withstand heat, formaldehyde, and large doses of radiation with little effect on their structure. In addition, some viruses may have **incubation periods** (the length of time required to develop fully and therefore to cause symptoms in their hosts) that are measured in years rather than hours or days. Termed **slow-acting viruses**, these viruses infect the host and remain in a semidormant state for years, causing a slowly developing illness. HIV is the most recent deadly example of a slow-acting virus.

Drug treatment for viral infections is limited. Drugs powerful enough to kill viruses also kill the host cells, although there are some drugs available that block stages in viral reproduction without damaging the host cells.

We have another form of virus protection within our own bodies. When exposed to certain viruses, the body begins to produce a protein substance known as **interferon**. Interferon does not destroy the invading microorganisms but sets up a protective mechanism to aid healthy cells in their struggle against the invaders. Although interferon research is promising, it should be noted that not all viruses stimulate interferon production.

The Common Cold. Caused by any number of viruses (some experts claim there may be over 100 different viruses responsible for the common cold), colds are **endemic** (always present to some degree) among peoples throughout the world. Current research indicates that otherwise healthy people carry cold viruses in their noses and throats most of the time. These viruses are held in check until the host's resistance is lowered. In the true sense of the word, it is possible to "catch" a cold—from the airborne droplets of another person's sneeze or from skin-to-skin or mucous membrane contact—though recent studies indicate that the hands may be the greatest avenue of cold and other viral transmission.

The best rule of thumb for treating the common cold is to keep your resistance level high. Sound nutrition, adequate rest, stress reduction, and regular exercise appear to be your best bets in helping you fight off infection. Also, avoiding people with newly developed colds (colds appear to be most contagious during the first 24 hours of onset) is advisable. Once you contract a cold, bed rest, plenty of fluids, and aspirin for relief of pain and discomfort are the tried-and-true remedies for adults. Children should not be given aspirin for colds or the flu because of the possibility that this may lead to a potentially fatal disease known as Reye's syndrome. Several over-the-counter preparations have proved effective for alleviating certain cold symptoms.

Influenza. In otherwise healthy people, **influenza**, or flu, is usually not serious. Symptoms, including aches and pains, nausea, diarrhea, fever, and coldlike ailments, generally pass very quickly. (See Figure 13.1 for a comparison of cold and flu symptoms.) However, in combination with other disorders, or among the elderly (people over the age of 65), those with respiratory or heart disease, or

Incubation period: The time between exposure to a disease and the appearance of the symptoms.

Slow-acting viruses: Viruses having long incubation periods and causing slowly progressive symptoms.

Interferon: A protein substance produced by the body that aids the immune system by protecting healthy cells.

Endemic: Describing a disease that is always present to some degree.

Influenza: A common viral disease of the respiratory tract.

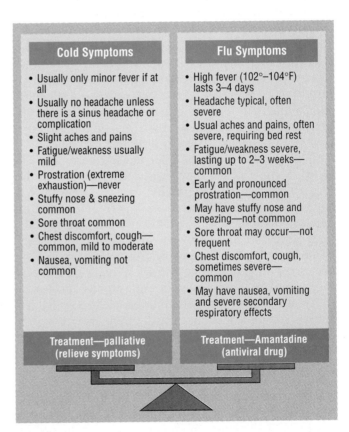

FIGURE 13.1

Cold or flu? Weighing your symptoms may answer your questions.

Source: Adapted from *National Institutes of Health Bulletin* and H. Sheldon, *Introduction to Human Diseases* (Philadelphia: W. B. Saunders, 1992).

TABLE 13.2 ■ Forms of Hepatitis: A Comparison

Disease	Incubation Period	Acute Infectious (% symptomatic)	Outcome
Hepatitis B	45–180 days	<10% of childhood infections 50% of adult infections	1% develop fulminant hepatitis. 1–10% of adults become chronic carriers. >90% perinatal or early childhood infections become carriers.
Hepatitis A	15–45 days	<10% of childhood infections 50% of adult infections	No chronic carriers
Hepatitis C	14–168 days	More often asymptomatic	50% become chronic carriers

Source: Canadian Communicable Diseases Report, Supplement 21S4, November 1995.

the very young (children under the age of 5), the flu can be very serious.

To date, three major varieties of flu virus have been discovered, with many different strains existing within each variety. The "A" form of the virus is generally the most virulent, followed by the "B" and "C" varieties. Although if you contract one form of influenza you may develop immunity to it, you will not necessarily be immune to other forms of the disease. There is little that can be done to treat flu patients once the infection has become established. Some vaccines have proved effective preventives for certain strains of flu virus, but they are totally ineffective against others. Flu vaccination is recommended for adults and children with chronic and pulmonary disorders, people of any age who are residents of nursing homes, people 65 years of age or over, and people with diabetes and other metabolic diseases. In many juridictions, vaccination for these most vulnerable groups can be at no cost to the person. Vaccination for people in essential services is recommended, but usually the person bears the cost. Because flu shots take anywhere from two to three weeks to become effective, you should get these shots in the fall, before the flu season begins.

Infectious Mononucleosis. This affliction of university-aged people is often jokingly referred to as the "kissing disease." The symptoms of mononucleosis, or "mono," include sore throat, fever, headache, nausea, chills, and a pervasive weakness or tiredness in the initial stages. As the disease progresses, lymph nodes may become increasingly enlarged, and jaundice, spleen enlargement, aching joints, and body rashes may occur.

Theories on the transmission and treatment of mononucleosis are highly controversial. Caused by the *Epstein-*

Barr virus, mononucleosis is readily detected through a *monospot test,* a blood test that measures the percentage of specific forms of white blood cells. Because many viruses are spread by transmission of body fluids, many people once believed that young people passed the disease on by kissing. Although this is still considered a possible cause, mononucleosis is not believed to be highly contagious. It does not appear to be easily contracted through normal, everyday personal contact. Multiple cases among family members are rare, as are cases between intimate partners.

Treatment of mononucleosis is often a lengthy process that involves bed rest, balanced nutrition, and medications to control the symptoms of the disease. Gradually, the body develops a form of immunity to the disease and the person returns to normal activity levels.

Hepatitis. One of the most highly publicized viral diseases is **hepatitis.** The hepatitis incidence has been rising in Canada, and educational programs have been initiated in the hope of preventing new outbreaks. Hepatitis is generally defined as a virally caused inflammation of the liver, characterized by symptoms that include fever, headache, nausea, loss of appetite, skin rashes, pain in the upper right abdomen, dark yellow (with a brownish tinge) urine, and the possibility of jaundice (the "disease your friends diagnose" because of the yellowing of the whites of the eyes and the skin).

Treatment of all the forms of viral hepatitis (see Table 13.2) is somewhat limited. A proper diet, bed rest, and antibiotics to combat bacterial invaders that may cause additional problems are recommended. Vaccines for hepatitis are available, although costs are high for the series of injections. Many provinces are beginning to require vaccinations against hepatitis B for health care workers and others who may be exposed to blood-borne pathogens.

Mumps. Until 1968, mumps was a common viral disorder among children. That year a vaccine become available and the disease seemed to be largely under control, with reported cases declining from 80 per 100 000 people in 1968 to less than 1.2 per 100 000 people in 1995. Approximately one-half of all mumps infections are not apparent because they produce only minor symptoms. Typically, there is an incubation period of 16 to 18 days, followed by symptoms caused by the lodging of the virus in the glands of the neck. The most common symptom is the swelling of the parotid (salivary) glands. One of the greatest dangers associated with mumps is the potential for sterility in men who contract the disease in young adulthood. Also, some victims suffer hearing loss.

Chicken Pox. Caused by the *herpes zoster varicella* virus, chicken pox produces the characteristic symptoms of fever and tiredness 13 to 17 days after exposure, followed by skin eruptions that itch, blister, and produce a clear fluid. The virus is present in these blisters for approximately one week. Symptoms are generally mild, and immunity to subsequent infection appears to be lifelong. Although a vaccine for chicken pox has been developed, it has not been approved in Canada at this time. Many children still contract the disease. Scientists believe that after the initial infection, the virus goes into permanent hibernation and, for most people, there are no further complications. For a small segment of the population, however, the zoster virus may become reactivated. Blisters will develop, usually on only one side of the body and tending to stop abruptly at the midline. Cases in which the disease covers both sides of the body are far more serious. This disease, known as shingles, affects over 5 percent of the population each year. More than half the sufferers are over 50 years of age.

Measles. Technically referred to as rubeola, **measles** is a viral disorder that often affects young children. Symptoms, appearing about ten days after exposure, include an itchy rash and a high fever. **Rubella** (German measles), is a milder viral infection that is believed to be transmitted by inhalation, after which it multiplies in the upper respiratory tract and passes into the bloodstream. It causes a rash, especially on the upper extremities. It is not generally a serious health threat and usually runs its course in three to four days. The major exceptions to this rule are among newborns and pregnant women. Rubella can damage a foetus, particularly during the first trimester, creating a condition known as congenital rubella, in which the infant may be born blind, deaf, retarded, or with heart defects. Immunization has greatly reduced the incidence of both measles and German measles. Infections in children not immunized against measles can lead to fever-induced problems such as rheumatic heart disease, kidney damage, and neurological disorders.

Other Pathogens

Fungi. Hundreds of species of **fungi**, multi- or unicellular primitive plants, inhabit our environment and serve useful functions. Mouldy breads, cheeses, and mushrooms used for domestic purposes pose no harm to humans. But some species of fungi can produce infections. Candidiasis (a vaginal yeast infection), athlete's foot, ringworm, and jock itch are examples of fungal diseases. Keeping the affected area clean and dry plus treatment with appropriate medications will generally bring prompt relief from these infections.

Protozoa. **Protozoa** are microscopic, single-celled organisms that are generally associated with tropical diseases such as African sleeping sickness and malaria. Although these pathogens are prevalent in the developing countries of the world, they are largely controlled in Canada. The most common protozoan disease in North America is trichomoniasis, an infection discussed further in the sexually transmitted diseases section of this chapter. A common water-borne protozoan disease in many regions of the country is giardiasis, sometimes called "beaver feaver." Persons who drink or are exposed to the *giardia* pathogen may suffer symptoms of intestinal pain and discomfort weeks after infection. Protection of water supplies is the key to prevention.

Parasitic Worms. Parasitic worms are the largest of the pathogens. Ranging in size from the relatively small pinworms typically found in children to the relatively large tapeworms found in all forms of warm-blooded animals, most parasitic worms are more a nuisance than a threat. Of special note today are the new forms of worm infestations commonly associated with eating raw fish in Japanese sushi restaurants. Cooking fish and other foods to temperatures sufficient to kill the worms or their eggs is an effective means of prevention.

Hepatitis: A virally caused disease in which the liver becomes inflamed, producing such symptoms as fever, headache, and jaundice.

Measles: A viral disease that produces symptoms including an itchy rash and a high fever.

Rubella (German measles): A milder form of measles that causes a rash and mild fever in children and may cause damage to a foetus or a newborn baby.

Fungi: A group of plants that lack chlorophyll and do not produce flowers or seeds; several microscopic varieties are pathogenic.

Protozoa: Microscopic, single-celled organisms.

Rickettsia. Once believed to be closely related to viruses, **rickettsia** are now considered to be bacteria-like organisms. They produce toxins and multiply within small blood vessels, causing vascular blockage and tissue death. Rickettsia require an insect vector (carrier) for transmission to humans. Two common forms of human rickettsia disease are Rocky Mountain spotted fever, carried by a tick, and typhus, carried by a louse, flea, or tick. Both diseases can be life-threatening. They produce similar symptoms, including high fever, weakness, rash, and coma. You do not actually have to be bitten by a vector to contract these diseases. Because the vectors themselves harbour the developing rickettsia in their intestinal tracts, insect excrement deposited on the skin and entering the body through abrasions and scratches may be a common source of infection.

YOUR BODY'S DEFENCES: KEEPING YOU WELL

Although all of the pathogens described in the preceding section pose a threat if they take hold in your body, the chances that they will take hold are actually quite small. To do so, they must overcome a number of effective barriers, many of which were established in your body before you were born.

Physical and Chemical Defences

Perhaps our single most critical early defence system is the skin. Layered to provide an intricate web of barriers, the skin allows few pathogens to enter. **Enzymes**, complex proteins manufactured by the body that appear in body secretions such as sweat, provide additional protection, destroying microorganisms on skin surfaces by producing inhospitable pH levels. Normal body pH is 7.0, but enzymatic or biochemical changes may cause the body chemistry to become more acidic (pH of less than 7.0), or more alkaline (pH of more than 7.0). In either case, microorganisms that flourish at a selected pH will be weakened or destroyed as these changes occur. A third protection is our frequent slight elevations in body temperature, which create an inhospitable environment for

Rickettsia: A small form of bacteria that live inside other living cells.

Enzymes: Organic substances that cause bodily changes and destruction of microorganisms.

Antigen: Substance capable of triggering an immune response.

many pathogens. Only when there are cracks or breaks in the skin can pathogens gain easy access to the body.

The linings of the body provide yet another protection against pathogens. Mucous membranes in the respiratory tract and other linings of the body trap and engulf invading organisms. *Cilia*, hairlike projections in the lungs and respiratory tract, sweep unwanted invaders toward body openings, where they are expelled. Tears, nasal secretions, ear wax, and other secretions found at body entrances contain enzymes designed to destroy or neutralize invading pathogens. Finally, any invading organism that manages to breach these initial lines of defence faces a formidable specialized network of defences thrown up by the immune system.

The Immune System: Your Body Fights Back

Immunity is a condition of being able to resist a particular disease by counteracting the substance that produces the disease. Any substance capable of triggering an immune response is called an **antigen.** An antigen can be a virus, a bacterium, a fungus, a parasite, or a tissue or cell from another individual. When invaded by an antigen, the body responds by forming substances called **antibodies** that are matched to the specific antigen much as a key is matched to a lock. Antibodies belong to a mass of large molecules known as immunoglobulins, a group of nine chemically distinct protein substances, each of which plays a role in neutralizing, setting up for destruction, or actually destroying antigens. Once an antigen breaches the body's initial defences, the body begins a careful process of antigen analysis. It considers the size and shape of the invader, verifies that the antigen is not part of the body itself, and then begins to produce a specific antibody to destroy or weaken the antigen. This process, which is much more complex than described here, is part of a system called *humoral immune responses.* Humoral immunity is the body's major defence against many bacteria and bacterial toxins.

Cell-mediated immunity is characterized by the formation of a population of lymphocytes that can attack and destroy the foreign invader. These lymphocytes constitute the body's main defence against viruses, fungi, parasites, and some bacteria. Key players in this immune response are specialized groups of white blood cells known as *macrophages* (a type of phagocytic, or cell-eating, cell) and *lymphocytes,* other white blood cells in the blood, lymph nodes, bone marrow, and certain glands.

Two forms of lymphocytes in particular, the *B-lymphocytes* (B-cells) and *T-lymphocytes* (T-cells), are involved in the immune response. There are different types of B-cells, named according to the area of the body in which they develop. Most are manufactured in the soft tissue of the hollow shafts of the long bones. T-cells, in contrast, develop and multiply in the thymus, a multilobed organ that lies behind the breastbone. T-cells assist your immune system in several ways. *Regulatory T-cells* help direct the activities of the immune system and assist other cells, particularly B-cells, to produce antibodies. Dubbed "helper Ts," these cells are essential for activating B-cells, other T-cells, and macrophages. Another form of T-cell, known as the "killer Ts" or "cytotoxic Ts," directly attacks infected or malignant cells. Killer Ts enable the body to rid itself of cells that have been infected by viruses or transformed by cancer; they are also responsible for the rejection of tissue and organ grafts. The third type of T-cells, "suppressor Ts," turns off or suppresses the activity of B-cells, killer Ts, and macrophages. Suppressor Ts circulate in the bloodstream and lymphatic system, neutralizing or destroying antigens, enhancing the effects of the immune response, and helping to return the activated immune system to normal levels. After a successful attack on a pathogen, some of the attacker T- and B-cells are preserved as *memory T- and B-cells,* enabling the body to quickly recognize and respond to subsequent attacks by the same kind of organism at a later time. Thus macrophages, T- and B-cells, and antibodies are the key factors in mounting an immune response.

Once people have survived certain infectious diseases, they become immune to those diseases, meaning that in all probability they will not develop them again. Upon subsequent attack by the disease-causing microorganism, their memory T- and B-cells are quickly activated to come to their defence. Immunization works on the same principle. Vaccines containing an attenuated (weakened) or killed version of the disease-causing microorganism or containing an antigen that is similar to but not as dangerous as the disease antigen are administered to stimulate the person's immune system to produce antibodies against future attacks—without actually causing the disease.

Autoimmune Diseases. Although white blood cells and the antigen-antibody response generally work in our favour by neutralizing or destroying harmful antigens, the body sometimes makes a mistake and targets its own tissue as the enemy, builds up antibodies against that tissue, and attempts to destroy it. This is known as autoimmune disease (*auto* means "self"). Common examples of this type of disease are rheumatoid arthritis, lupus erythematosus, and myasthenia gravis.

In some cases, the antigen-antibody response completely fails to function. The result is a form of *immune deficiency syndrome.* Perhaps the most dramatic case of this syndrome was the "bubble boy," a youngster who died in 1984 after living his short life inside a sealed-off environment designed to protect him from all antigens. A much more common immune system disorder is *acquired immune deficiency syndrome* (AIDS), which we will discuss later in this chapter.

Fever

If an infection is localized, pus formation, redness, swelling, and irritation often occur. These symptoms indicate that the invading organisms are being fought systematically. Another indication is the development of a fever, or a rise in body temperature above the norm of 37°C. Fever is frequently caused by toxins secreted by pathogens that interfere with the control of body temperature. Although this elevated temperature is often harmful to the body, it is also believed to act as a form of protection. Elevations of body temperature by even one or two degrees provide an environment that destroys some types of disease-causing organisms. Also, as body temperature rises, the body is stimulated to produce more white blood cells which destroy more invaders.

Pain

Although pain is not usually thought of as a defence mechanism, it plays a valuable role in the body's response to invasion. Pain is generally a response to injury. Pain may be either direct, caused by the stimulation of nerve endings in an affected area, or referred, meaning it is present in one place while the source is elsewhere. An example of referred pain is the pain in the arm or jaw often experienced by someone having a heart attack. Regardless of the cause of pain, most pain responses are accompanied by inflammation. Pain tends to be the earliest sign that an injury has occurred and often causes the person to slow down or stop the activity that was aggravating the injury, thereby protecting against further damage. Because it is often one of the first warnings of disease, persistent pain should not be overlooked or masked with short-term pain relievers.

Vaccines: Bolstering Your Immunity

Our natural defence mechanisms are our strongest allies in the battle against disease, being with us from birth until death. There are periods in our life, however, when either invading organisms are too strong or our own natural immunity is too weak to protect us from catching a given disease. It is at such times that we need outside assistance in developing immunity to an invading organism. Such assistance is generally provided in the form of a **vaccination.** Vaccines are given orally or by injection, and this form of artificial immunity is termed *acquired immunity,* in contrast to *natural immunity,* which a mother passes to her foetus via their shared blood supply.

Antibodies: Substances produced by the body that are individually matched to specific antigens.

Vaccination: Inoculation with killed or weakened pathogens or similar, less dangerous antigens in order to prevent or lessen the effects of some disease.

Today, depending on the virulence of the organism, vaccines containing live, weakened, or dead organisms are given to people for a variety of diseases. In some instances, if a person is already weakened by other diseases, vaccination may provoke an actual case of the disease. This was what happened with the smallpox vaccinations administered routinely in the 1960s. It was believed that the risk of contracting smallpox from the vaccine was actually greater than was the chance of contracting the disease in an environment where it had essentially been eradicated. For this reason, routine smallpox inoculations were eliminated in the late 1960s. Currently recommended childhood vaccinations are shown in Table 13.3.

SEXUALLY TRANSMITTED INFECTIONS

There are more than 20 different types of **sexually transmitted infections** (**STIs**, also called STDs, or sexually transmitted diseases). These infections were once referred to as venereal diseases, but the newer classification is believed to be broader in scope and more reflective of the numbers and types of these communicable diseases. At the present rate of infection, it is expected that the incidence of STIs will double by the year 2000, with more virulent, antibiotic-resistant, and untreatable strains appearing regularly.

In many victims, the early symptoms of an STI are not serious. They may range from mild discomfort to annoying itching or discharge. (See Figure 13.2 for signs that may indicate the presence of an STI.) Left untreated, however, some of these diseases can have grave consequences, such as sterility, blindness, central nervous system destruction, disfigurement, and even death. Infants born to mothers carrying the organisms for these diseases are at risk for a variety of health problems.

As with many of the communicable diseases, much of the pain, suffering, and anguish associated with STIs could be eliminated or substantially reduced through education, responsible action, and prompt treatment when symptoms first occur. Overcoming the tendency to pass moral judgements on victims would certainly lower the barriers to treatment. Being prepared to deal with the pressure to engage in sexual activity can also be helpful.

Possible Causes: Why Me?

Sexually transmitted infections affect people of both sexes and of all socioeconomic levels, ages, ethnic groups, and regions of the world. Several reasons have been proposed to explain the present high rates of STIs. The first relates to the moral and social stigma associated with these diseases. Shame and embarrassment often keep infected people from seeking treatment. Unfortunately, these people usually continue to be sexually active, thereby infecting unsuspecting partners. People who are uncomfortable discussing sexual issues may also be less likely to use and/or ask their partners to use condoms as a means of protection against STIs and/or pregnancy.

TABLE 13.3 ▪ Recommended Childhood Immunization Schedule

Age	Immunization Against:
2 months	Diphtheria, pertussis, tetanus, poliomyelitis, haemophilus influenzae b[1]
4 months	Diphtheria, pertussis, tetanus, poliomyelitis, haemophilus influenzae b
6 months	Diphtheria, pertussis, tetanus, polioymyelitis,[2] haemophilus influenzae b
12 months	Measles, mumps, rubella[3]
18 months	Diphtheria, pertussis, tetanus, poliomyelitis, haemophilus influenzae b
4–6 years	Diphtheria, pertussis, tetanus, poliomyelitis
9–13 years	Hepatitis B[4]
14–16 years	Diphtheria, tetanus, poliomyelitis

Notes:

1. Haemophilus influenzae b requires a series of immunizations. The exact number and timing of each may vary with the brand of vaccine used.

2. If oral polio virus vaccine is used exclusively in a series of immunizations, this dose may be omitted.

3. A second dose of MMR vaccine is recommended for children and youth. It may be administered any time after a minimum one-month waiting period; provincial schedules differ.

4. Hepatitis B requires a series of immunizations. In some jurisdictions, they may be administered at a younger age.

Source: Adapted from *Canadian Immunization Guide*, 4th ed., Minister of Supply and Services Canada, 1993.

Another reason proposed for the STI epidemic is our casual attitude about sex. Bombarded by media hype that glamourizes easy sex, many people take sexual partners without considering the consequences. Others are pressured into sexual relationships they don't really want. Generally, the more sexual partners a person has, the greater the risk for contracting an STI. Evaluate your attitude about STIs by taking the Rate Yourself box self-assessment.

Ignorance about the infections themselves and an inability to recognize actual symptoms or to acknowledge that a person may be asymptomatic yet still have the disease are also factors behind the STI epidemic. A person who is infected but asymptomatic may unknowingly spread an STI to an unsuspecting partner, who may then ignore or misinterpret any symptoms that do appear. By the time either partner seeks medical help, he or she may have infected several others.

Modes of Transmission

Sexually transmitted infections are generally spread through some form of intimate sexual contact. Sexual intercourse and anal intercourse, oral-genital contact, and hand-genital contact are (in decreasing order of likelihood) the most common modes of transmission. More rarely, pathogens for STIs are transmitted mouth to mouth or, even more infrequently, through contact with fluids from body sores. While each STI is a different disease caused by a different pathogen, all STI pathogens prefer dark, moist places, especially the mucous membranes lining the reproductive organs. The majority of these organisms are susceptible to light, excess heat, cold, and dryness, and many die quickly on exposure to air. (The toilet seat is not a likely breeding ground for most bacterial or viral STIs!) Although most STIs are passed on by sexual contact, other kinds of close contact, such as sleeping on the sheets used by someone who has pubic lice, may also cause you to get an STI. One method of preventing the spread of STIs is to always use a condom during all sexual intercourse. To fully protect yourself, follow these basic rules:

- Decide ahead of time that you will not have sex without using a condom. Make sure that you have one with you.

- Never reuse a condom.

- Use only latex condoms.

- Store condoms in a cool, dry place—not in the glove compartment of your car or in your wallet.

- If a condom appears brittle or sticky, get rid of it.

- Put the condom on (correctly) before having any contact between genitals.

- Use condoms for oral sex as well; use a dental dam for oral sex with a female.

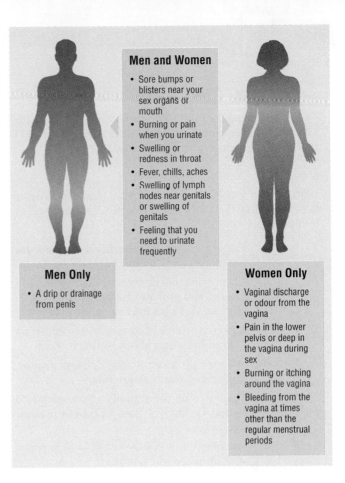

Men and Women
- Sore bumps or blisters near your sex organs or mouth
- Burning or pain when you urinate
- Swelling or redness in throat
- Fever, chills, aches
- Swelling of lymph nodes near genitals or swelling of genitals
- Feeling that you need to urinate frequently

Men Only
- A drip or drainage from penis

Women Only
- Vaginal discharge or odour from the vagina
- Pain in the lower pelvis or deep in the vagina during sex
- Burning or itching around the vagina
- Bleeding from the vagina at times other than the regular menstrual periods

FIGURE 13.2

The illustration lists signs or symptoms that may mean you have an STI.

- Apply a water-based lubricant containing spermicide to the condom for additional protection.

- If the condom breaks, tears, or becomes dislodged, wash the genitals thoroughly with soap and water, apply a spermicide to the area, and put on another condom before additional contact. It only takes a fraction of a second to become infected with disease-laden body fluids or to infect someone else if you are a carrier.

- Hold the condom in place during withdrawal to make sure it doesn't come off.

Like other communicable diseases, STIs have both pathogen-specific incubation periods and periods of time during which transmission is most likely, called periods of

Sexually transmitted infections (STIs): Infectious diseases transmitted via some form of intimate, usually sexual, contact.

STI Attitude and Belief Scale

The following quiz will help you evaluate whether your beliefs and attitudes about STIs lead you to take risks that may heighten your risk for contracting an STI.

Directions

Indicate that you believe the following items are true or false by circling the T or the F. Then consult the answer key that follows.

T F 1. You can usually tell whether someone is infected with an STI, especially HIV infection.

T F 2. Chances are that if you haven't caught an STI by now, you probably have a natural immunity and won't get infected in the future.

T F 3. A person who is successfully treated for an STI needn't worry about getting it again.

T F 4. So long as you keep yourself fit and healthy, you needn't worry about STIs.

T F 5. The best way for sexually active people to protect themselves from STIs is to practise safer sex.

T F 6. The only way to catch an STI is to have sex with someone who has one.

T F 7. Talking about STIs with a partner is so embarrassing that you're best off not raising the subject and hoping the other person will.

T F 8. STIs are mostly a problem for people who are promiscuous.

T F 9. You don't need to worry about contracting an STI so long as you wash yourself thoroughly with soap and hot water immediately after sex.

T F 10. You don't need to worry about AIDS if no one you know has ever come down with it.

T F 11. When it comes to STIs, it's all in the cards. Either you're lucky or you're not.

T F 12. The time to worry about STIs is when you come down with one.

T F 13. As long as you avoid risky sexual practices, such as anal intercourse, you're pretty safe from STIs.

T F 14. The time to talk about safer sex is before any sexual contact occurs.

T F 15. A person needn't be concerned about an STI if the symptoms clear up on their own in a few weeks.

Scoring Key

1. *False.* While some STIs have telltale signs, such as the appearance of sores or blisters on the genitals or disagreeable genital odours, others do not. Several STIs, such as chlamydia, gonorrhea (especially in women), internal genital warts, and even HIV infection in its early stages, cause few if any obvious signs or symptoms. You often cannot tell whether your partner is infected with an STI. Many of the nicest-looking and best-groomed people carry STIs, often unknowingly. The only way to know whether a person is infected with HIV is by means of an HIV-antibody test.

2. *False.* If you practise unprotected sex and have not contracted an STI to this point, count your blessings. The thing about good luck is that it eventually runs out.

3. *False.* Sorry. Successful treatment does not render immunity against reinfection. You still need to take precautions to avoid reinfection, even if you have had an STI in the past and were successfully treated. If you answered true to this item, you're not alone. About one in five respondents in a recent survey of more than 5500 college students across Canada believed that a person who gets an STI cannot get it again.

4. *False.* Even people in prime physical condition can be felled by the tiniest of microbes that cause STIs. Physical fitness is no protection against these microscopic invaders.

5. *True.* If you are sexually active, practising safer sex is the best protection against contracting an STI.

6. *False.* STIs can also be transmitted through nonsexual means, such as by sharing contaminated needles or, in some cases, through contact with disease-causing organisms on towels and bedsheets or even toilet seats.

7. *False.* Because of the social stigma attached to STIs, it's understandable that you may feel embarrassed raising the subject with your partner. But don't let embarrassment prevent you from taking steps to protect your own and your partner's welfare.

8. *False.* While it stands to reason that people who are sexually active with numerous partners stand a greater chance that one of their sexual partners carries an STI, all it takes is one infected partner to pass along an STI to you, even if he or she is the only partner you've had or even if the two of you only had sex once. STIs are a potential problem for anyone who is sexually active.

9. *False.* While washing your genitals immediately after sex may have some limited protective value, it is no substitute for practising safer sex.

(continued)

10. *False.* You can never know whether you may be the first among your friends and acquaintances to become infected. Moreover, symptoms of HIV infection may not appear for years after initial infection with the virus, so you may have sexual contacts with people who are infected but don't know it and who are capable of passing along the virus to you. You in turn may then pass it along to others, whether or not you are aware of any symptoms.

11. *False.* Nonsense. While luck may play a part in determining whether you have a sexual contact with an infected partner, you can significantly reduce your risk of contracting an STI.

12. *False.* The time to start thinking about STIs (thinking helps, but worrying only makes you more anxious than you need be) is now, not after you have contracted an infection. Some STIs, like herpes and AIDS, cannot be cured. The only real protection you have against them is prevention.

13. *False.* Any sexual contact between the genitals, or between the genitals and the anus, or between the mouth and genitals, is risky if one of the partners is infected with an STI.

14. *True.* Unfortunately, too many couples wait until they have commenced sexual relations to "have a talk." By then it may already be too late to prevent the transmission of an STI. The time to talk is before any intimate sexual contact occurs.

15. *False.* Several STIs, notably syphilis, HIV infection, and herpes, may produce initial symptoms that clear up in a few weeks. But while the early symptoms may subside, the infection is still at work within the body and requires medical attention. Also, as noted previously, the infected person is capable of passing along the infection to others, regardless of whether noticeable symptoms were ever present.

Interpreting Your Score

First, add up the number of items you got right. The higher your score, the lower your risk. The lower your score, the greater your risk. A score of 13 correct or better may indicate that your attitudes toward STIs would probably decrease your risk of contracting them. Yet even one wrong response on this test may increase your risk of contracting an STI. You should also recognize that attitudes have little effect on behaviour unless they are carried into action. Knowledge alone isn't sufficient to protect yourself from STIs. You need to ask yourself how you are going to put knowledge into action by changing your behaviour to reduce your chances of contracting an STI.

Source: Adapted from Jeffrey S. Nevid with Fern Gotfried, *Choices: Sex in the Age of STDs,* 10–13. © 1995 by Allyn & Bacon. Reprinted by permission.

communicability. Although there are more than 20 different types of sexually transmitted infections, we will discuss only those STIs that are most likely to pose a risk for the average adult.

Chlamydia

Since 1991, **chlamydia** has been the most common STI in Canada. The Laboratory Centre for Disease Control estimates that in 1993 there were 44 296 cases of genital chlamydia. Figures suggest a recent, relative decrease.[7]

The name of the disease is derived from the Greek verb *chlamys,* meaning to "to cloak," because, unlike most bacteria, chlamydia can only live and grow inside other cells. Although many people classify chlamydia as either *nonspecific* or *nongonococcal urethritis (NGU),* a person may have NGU without having the organism for chlamydia. In over half of the cases of NGU (infections of the urethra and surrounding tissues that are not caused by gonococcal bacteria), however, *Chlamydia trachomatis,* the bacte-

rial organism that causes chlamydia, is present. For this reason, the two disease terms tend to be used interchangeably, even though NGU may be caused by other organisms.

In males, early symptoms may include painful and difficult urination, frequent urination, and a watery, puslike discharge from the penis. Symptoms in females may include a yellowish discharge, spotting between periods, and occasional spotting after intercourse. Unfortunately, many chlamydia victims display no symptoms and therefore do not seek help until the disease has done secondary damage. Females are especially prone to be asymptomatic; over 70 percent do not realize they have the disease until secondary damage occurs.

Chlamydia: Bacterially caused STI of the urogenital tract.

TABLE 13.4 ▪ Screening for STIs

Screening to detect asymptomatic STI infection is divided into 3 categories:

- **Case Finding:** A patient-based strategy in individuals with an increased likelihood of one or more STIs, e.g., sexual contacts to gonorrhea
- **Focussed Screening:** A group-based strategy in subpopulations with high STI prevalence rates, e.g., street youth, core groups, adolescents, and those with a history of STI
- **General Screening:** A population-based strategy in certain members of the general public who are not considered to be at increased risk for STI but in whom serious consequences may occur if infected, e.g., syphilis and HIV testing in pregnancy

	Case Finding	Focussed Screening	General Screening
Procedures			
Sexual history	x	x	x
Physical examination			
External genital	x	x	x
Internal genital	Adults, adolescents	Adults, adolescents	—
Targeted extragenital	x	x	x
Laboratory tests			
Neisseria gonorrhoeae	x	x	—
Chlamydia trachomatis	x	x	—
Treponema pallidum	x	x	x
Pap smear	Adults, adolescents	Adults, adolescents	
Hepatitis B (HBV)	Optional	Optional	x
HIV	x	x	x

Source: Adapted from "Screening for Sexually Transmitted Disease: Canadian STD Guidelines," *Canada Communicable Disease Report,* Supplement 21S4, November 1995.

The secondary damage resulting from chlamydia is serious in both sexes. Male victims can suffer damage to the prostate gland, seminal vesicles, and bulbourethral glands as well as arthritislike symptoms and damage to the blood vessels and heart. In females, secondary damage from chlamydia may include inflammation that damages the cervix or fallopian tubes, causing sterility, and damage to the inner pelvic structure, leading to pelvic inflammatory disease (PID). If an infected woman becomes pregnant, she has a high risk for miscarriages and stillbirths. Chlamydia may also be responsible for one type of **conjunctivitis**, an eye infection that affects not only adults but also infants, who can contract the disease from an infected mother during delivery. Untreated conjunctivitis can cause blindness.

Chlamydia can be controlled through responsible sexual behaviour and familiarity with the early symptoms of the disease. If detected early enough, chlamydia is easily treatable with antibiotics such as tetracycline, doxycycline, or erythromycin. In most cases, treatment is successfully completed in two to three weeks. Unfortunately, chlamydia checks are not a routine part of many STI testing procedures. You may have to request a chlamydia check specifically before one is performed on you.

🖋 WHAT DO YOU THINK?

Why do you think that even though many university students have heard about the risks of STIs and HIV disease, they remain apathetic, fail to use condoms, and in general, act irresponsibly? What actions do you think could be taken to make you and your friends engage in self-protecting behaviours?

Pelvic Inflammatory Disease (PID)

Pelvic inflammatory disease (PID) is actually not one disease but a term used to describe a number of infections of the uterus, fallopian tubes, and ovaries. Although PID is often the result of an untreated sexually transmitted infection, especially chlamydia or gonorrhea, it is not actually an STI. Nonsexual causes of PID are also common, including excessive vaginal douching, cigarette smoking, and substance abuse.

Symptoms may include acute inflammation of the pelvic cavity, severe pain in the lower abdomen, menstrual irregularities, fever, nausea, painful intercourse, tubal pregnancies, and severe depression.[8] The major consequences of untreated PID are infertility, ectopic pregnancy, chronic pelvic pain, and recurrent upper genital infections. Risk factors include young age at first sexual intercourse, multiple sex partners, high frequency of sexual intercourse, and change of sexual partners within the last 30 days.[9] Regular gynecological examinations and early treatment for STI symptoms reduce risk.

Gonorrhea

The national rate of reported cases of **gonorrhea** has declined steadily since 1981. There were 5500 cases of gonorrhea reported in 1995 compared to 56,330 in 1981; this represents a tenfold drop in the number of cases reported over the 14-year period. Over the same period, the rate of infection fell twelvefold from 226.2 cases per 100 000 population in 1981 to 18.6 cases per 100 000 in 1995. The rate of infection has decreased 62 percent from 1990 to 1995, from 49.7 cases per 100 000 in 1990 to 18.6 cases per 100 000 in 1995. Presently, the majority of endemic gonococcal infections is thought to reside within core groups: a small subset of the population whose members frequently acquire new sexual partners. More research needs to be conducted to assess and describe core groups within a Canadian context; appropriate prevention and control strategies, aimed at reducing or ideally eliminating indigenous gonococcal infections, can then be implemented.[10]

Caused by the bacterial pathogen, *Neisseria gonorrhoea,* this disease primarily infects the linings of the urethra, genital tract, pharynx, and rectum. It may be spread to the eyes or other body regions via the hands or body fluids.

In males, a typical symptom is a white milky discharge from the penis accompanied by painful, burning urination two to nine days after contact. This is usually enough to send most men to their physician for treatment. Only about 20 percent of all males with gonorrhea are asymptomatic.

In females, the situation is just the opposite. Only about 20 percent of all females experience any form of discharge, and few develop a burning sensation upon urinating until much later in the course of the disease (if ever). The organism can remain in the woman's vagina, cervix, uterus, or fallopian tubes for long periods with no apparent symptoms other than an occasional slight fever. Thus a woman can be unaware that she has been infected and that she may be infecting her sexual partners.

Upon diagnosis, an antibiotic regimen using penicillin, tetracycline, spectiomycin, ceftriaxone, or other drugs is begun. A penicillin-resistant form of gonorrhea may require a particularly strong combination of antibiotics. Treatment is generally completely effective within a short period of time if the disease is detected early.

If the disease goes undetected in a woman, it can spread throughout the genital-urinary tract to the fallopian tubes and ovaries, causing sterility, or at the very least, severe inflammation and pelvic inflammatory disease symptoms. If an infected woman becomes pregnant, the disease can cause conjunctivitis in her infant. To prevent this, physicians routinely administer silver nitrate or penicillin preparations to the eyes of newborn babies.

Untreated gonorrhea in the male may spread to the prostate, testicles, urinary tract, kidney, and bladder. Blockage of the vasa deferentia due to scar tissue formation may cause sterility. In some cases, the penis develops a painful curvature during erection.

Syphilis

Syphilis, the other well-known sexually transmitted infection, is also caused by a bacterial organism, the spirochete known as *Treponema pallidum.* Because it is extremely delicate and dies readily upon exposure to air, dryness, or cold, the organism is generally transferred only through direct sexual contact. Typically, this means contact between sexual organs during intercourse, but in rare instances, the organism enters the body through a break in the skin, through deep kissing in which body fluids are exchanged, or through some other transmission of body fluids.

Syphilis is called the "great imitator" because its symptoms resemble those of several other diseases. Only an astute physician who has reason to suspect the presence of the disease will order the appropriate tests for a diagnosis. Unlike most of the other STIs, syphilis generally progresses through several distinct stages.

Primary Syphilis. The first stage of syphilis, particularly for males, is often characterized by the development of a sore known as a **chancre** (pronounced "shank-er"),

---

Conjunctivitis: Serious inflammation of the eye caused by any number of pathogens or irritants; can be caused by STIs such as chlamydia.

Pelvic inflammatory disease (PID): Term used to describe various infections of the female reproductive tract.

Gonorrhea: Second most common STI in Canada; if untreated, may cause sterility.

Syphilis: One of the most widespread STIs; characterized by distinct phases and potentially serious results.

Chancre: Sore often found at the site of syphilis infection.

located most frequently at the site of the initial infection. This chancre is usually about the size of a dime and is painless, but it is oozing with bacteria, ready to spread to an unsuspecting partner. Usually the chancre appears between three to four weeks after contact.

In males, the site of the chancre tends to be the penis or scrotum because this is the site where the organism first makes entry into the body. But, if the disease was contracted through oral sex, the sore can appear in the mouth, throat, or other "first contact" area. In females, the site of infection is often internal, on the vaginal wall or high on the cervix. Because the chancre is not readily apparent, the likelihood of detection is not great. In both males and females, the chancre will completely disappear in three to six weeks.

Secondary Syphilis. From a month to a year after the chancre disappears, secondary symptoms may appear, including a rash or white patches on the skin or on the mucous membranes of the mouth, throat, or genitals. Hair loss may occur, lymph nodes may become enlarged, and the victim may run a slight fever or develop a headache. In rare cases, sores develop around the mouth or genitals. As during the active chancre phase, these sores contain infectious bacteria, and contact with them may spread the disease. In some people, symptoms follow a textbook pattern; in others, there are no symptoms at all. In a few cases, there may be arthritic pain in the joints. Because symptoms vary so much and because the symptoms that do appear are so far removed from previous sexual experience that the victim seldom connects the two, the disease often goes undetected even at this second stage. Symptoms may persist for a few weeks or months and then disappear, leaving the victim thinking that all is well.

Latent Syphilis. The syphilis spirochetes begin to invade body organs after the secondary stage. There may be periodic reappearance of previous symptoms, including the presence of infectious lesions, for between two and four years after the secondary period. After this period, the disease is rarely transmitted to others, except during pregnancy, when it can be passed on to the foetus. The child will then be born with congenital syphilis, which can cause death or severe birth defects such as blindness, deafness, or disfigurement. Because in most cases the foetus does not become infected until after the first trimester,

treatment of the mother during this period will usually prevent infection of the foetus.

In some instances, a child born to an infected mother will show no apparent signs of the disease at birth but, within several weeks, will develop body rashes, a runny nose, and symptoms of paralysis. *Congenital syphilis* is usually detected before it progresses much farther. But sometimes the child's immune system will ward off the invading organism, and further symptoms may not surface until the teenage years.

In addition to causing congenital syphilis, latent syphilis, if untreated, will continue to progress, infecting more and more organs until the disease reaches its final stage, late syphilis.

Late Syphilis. Most of the horror stories concerning syphilis involve the late stages of the disease. Years after syphilis has entered the body and progressed through the various organs, its net effects become clearly evident. Late-stage syphilis indications may include heart damage, central nervous system damage, blindness, deafness, paralysis, premature senility, and, ultimately, insanity.

Treatment for Syphilis. Treatment for syphilis resembles that for gonorrhea. Because the organism is bacterial, it is treated with antibiotics, usually penicillin, benzathine penicillin G, or doxycycline. Blood tests are administered to determine the exact nature of the invading organism, and the doses of antibiotics are much stronger than those taken by the typical gonorrhea patient. The major obstacle to treatment is misdiagnosis of this "imitator" disease.

Pubic Lice

Often called "crabs," pubic lice are more annoying than dangerous. **Pubic lice** are small parasites that are usually transmitted during sexual contact. They prefer the dark, moist regions of the body and, during sex, move easily from partner to partner. Although sexual contact is the most common mode of transmission, you can become infested with pubic lice from lying on sheets that an infected person has slept on. Sleeping in hotel and dormitory rooms in which blankets and sheets are not washed regularly or sitting on toilet seats where the nits or larvae have been dropped and lie in wait for a new carrier may put you at risk.

Venereal Warts

Venereal warts (also known as genital warts or condylomas) are caused by a small group of viruses known as *human papilloma viruses* (HPVs). A person becomes infected when an HPV penetrates the skin and mucous membranes of the genitals or anus through sexual contact. The virus appears to be relatively easy to catch. The typical incubation period is from six to eight weeks after

---

Pubic lice: Parasites that can inhabit various body areas, especially the genitals; also called "crabs."

Venereal warts: Warts that appear in the genital area or the anus; caused by the human papilloma viruses (HPVs).

---

contact. Many people have no apparent symptoms, particularly if the warts are located inside the reproductive tract. Others may develop a series of itchy bumps on the genitals, which may range in size from a small pinhead to large cauliflowerlike growths that can obstruct normal urinary or reproductive activity. On dry skin (such as on the shaft of the penis), the warts are commonly small, hard, and yellowish-gray, resembling warts that appear on other parts of the body. Venereal warts are of two different types: (1) *full-blown genital warts* that are noticeable as tiny bumps or growths, and (2) the much more prevalent *flat warts* that are not usually visible to the naked eye.

Risks of Venereal Warts.
Many venereal warts will eventually disappear on their own. Others will grow and generate unsightly flaps of irregular flesh on the external genitalia. The greatest threat from venereal warts may lie in the apparent relationship between them and a tendency for *dysplasia,* or changes in cells that may lead to a precancerous condition. Exactly how HPV infection leads to cervical cancer is uncertain. What is known is that within five years after infection, 30 percent of all HPV cases will progress to the precancerous stage. Of those cases that become precancerous and are left untreated, 70 percent will eventually result in actual cancer. In addition, venereal warts may pose a threat to a pregnant woman's unborn foetus if the foetus is exposed to the virus during birth. caesarean deliveries may be considered in serious cases.

Treatment for Venereal Warts.
Treatment for venereal warts may take several forms:

1. Warts are painted with a medication called podophyllin during a visit to the doctor's office. The podophyllin is washed off after about four hours, and a few days later the warts begin to dry up and fall off. Sometimes more than one trip to the doctor is necessary. This procedure is relatively painless.

2. Warts may be removed by *cryosurgery,* a procedure in which an instrument treated with liquid nitrogen is held to the affected area, "freezing" the tissue. Within a few days, the warts fall off.

3. Depending on size and location, some warts are removed by *simple excision.*

4. For larger warts, *laser surgery* is often used. This is a major procedure that generally requires general anesthesia. The frequency of laser use for wart removal is currently being questioned by many health experts. (Precautions must also be taken during this procedure to shield medical staff from infection by viral spray.)

5. Creams containing 5-Fluoracil (an anticancer drug) are being used to prevent further precancerous cell development.

6. For warts located externally, injections of interferon are sometimes given to keep the virus from spreading to healthy tissue. This treatment shows promise, but it is expensive and, in large doses, may cause flulike symptoms.

Prevention is clearly a better approach. What is true about protecting yourself from HIV infection is also true about protecting yourself from genital warts and other STIs (see the section on AIDS prevention later in this chapter).

Candidiasis (Moniliasis)

Unlike many of the other sexually transmitted infections, which are caused by pathogens that come from outside the body, the yeastlike fungus caused by the *Candida albicans* organism normally inhabits the vaginal tract in most women. Only under certain conditions will these organisms multiply to abnormal quantities and begin to cause problems.

The likelihood of **candidiasis** (also known as moniliasis) is greatest if a woman has diabetes, if her immune system is overtaxed or malfunctioning, if she is taking birth control pills or other hormones, or if she is taking broad-spectrum antibiotics. All of the above factors decrease the acidity of the vagina, making conditions more favourable for the development of a yeastlike infection.

Symptoms of candidiasis include severe vaginal itching, a white cheesy discharge, swelling of the vaginal tissue due to irritation, and a burning sensation. These symptoms are often collectively called **vaginitis**. When this microbe infects the mouth, whitish patches form, and the condition is referred to as thrush. This monilial infection also occurs in males and is easily transmitted between sexual partners.

Antifungal drugs applied on the surface or by suppository usually cure the disease in just a few days. For approximately one out of ten women, however, nothing seems to work, and the organism returns again and again. In patients with this chronically recurring infection, symptoms are often aggravated by contact of the vagina with soaps, douches, perfumed toilet paper, chlorinated water, and spermicides. Tight-fitting jeans and pantyhose can provide the combination of moisture and irritant the organism thrives on.

Candidiasis: Yeastlike fungal disease often transmitted sexually.

Vaginitis: Set of symptoms characterized by vaginal itching, swelling, and burning.

Trichomoniasis

Unlike many of the other STIs, **trichomoniasis** is caused by a protozoan. Although many men and women have this organism present, most remain free of symptoms until their bodily defences are weakened. Both men and women may transmit the disease, but women are the more likely candidates for infection. The "trich" infection may cause a foamy, yellowish discharge with an unpleasant odour that may be accompanied by a burning sensation, itching, and painful urination. These symptoms are most likely to occur during or shortly after menstruation, but they can appear at any time or be absent altogether in an infected woman. Although usually transmitted by sexual contact, the "trich" organism may be easily spread by toilet seats, wet towels, or other items that have discharged fluids on them. You can also contract trichomoniasis by sitting naked on the bench of the dressing room of your local health spa or locker room. Treatment includes oral metronidazole, usually given to both sexual partners to avoid the possible "ping-pong" effect of repeated cross-infection so typical of the STIs.

General Urinary Tract Infections

Although *general urinary tract infections (UTIs)* can be caused by various factors, some forms are sexually transmitted. Any time invading organisms enter the genital area, there is a risk that they may travel up the urethra and enter the bladder. Similarly, organisms normally living in the rectum, urethra, or bladder may travel to the sexual organs and eventually be transmitted to another person.

You can also get a UTI through autoinoculation (transmission to yourself by yourself). This frequently occurs during the simple task of wiping yourself after defecating. Wiping from the anus forward may transmit organisms found in faeces to the vaginal opening or to the urethra. Contact between the hands and the urethra and between the urethra and other objects are also common means of autoinoculation of bacterial and viral pathogens. Women, with their shorter urethras, are more likely to contract UTIs. Treatment depends on the nature and type of pathogen.

Trichomoniasis: Protozoan infection characterized by foamy, yellowish discharge and unpleasant odour.

Genital herpes: STI caused by herpes simplex virus type 2.

Acquired immune deficiency syndrome (AIDS): Extremely virulent sexually transmitted disease that renders the immune system inoperative.

Human immunodeficiency virus (HIV): The slow-acting virus that causes AIDS.

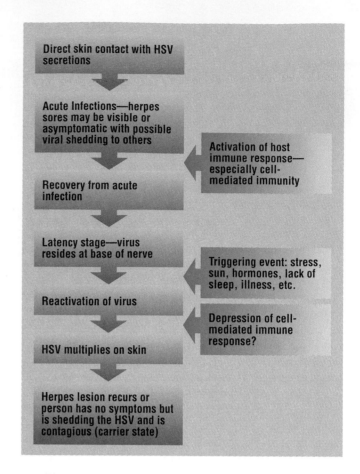

FIGURE 13.3

The Herpes Cycle
Source: Adapted by permission of J. B. Lippincott from "Sexually Transmitted Diseases in the 1990's," *STD Bulletin* 11 (1992): 4.

Herpes

Herpes is a general term for a family of diseases characterized by sores or eruptions on the skin. Herpes infections range from mildly uncomfortable to extremely serious. One subcategory, *herpes simplex,* is caused by a virus. Herpes simplex virus type 1 (HSV-1) causes the cold sores and fever blisters that most of us have been afflicted with at one time or another. The herpes simplex virus (HSV) is one of the most common disease agents in Canada; in 1994, over 14 000 cases were identified in laboratory tests, and many more undoubtedly went unreported.[11]

Genital herpes, caused by *herpes simplex virus type 2 (HSV-2),* is one of the most widespread STIs in the world. Typically, genital herpes is characterized by distinct phases. First, the herpes virus must gain entrance to the body, which it usually does through the mucous membranes of the genital area. Once these organisms invade, the victim will experience the *prodromal* (precursor) phase of the disease, which is characterized by a burning sensation and redness at the site of the infection. This phase is typically followed by the formation of a small blister filled with a clear fluid containing the virus. If you pick at this blister or otherwise spread this clear fluid by your hands, you can autoinoculate other body parts. Particularly dangerous is the possibility of spreading the infection to your eyes this way because a herpes lesion on the eye may cause blindness.

Over a period of days, this unsightly blister will crust, dry, disappear, and the virus will travel to the base of an affected nerve supplying the area and become dormant. Only when the victim becomes overly stressed, when diet is inadequate, when the immune system is overworked, or when there is excessive exposure to sunlight or other stressors will the virus reactivate (at the same site every time) and begin the blistering cycle all over again. This cyclical recurrence can be painful, unsightly, and, most important, highly contagious. Fluids from these blisters may readily be transmitted to sexual partners. Through oral sex, herpes simplex type 2 may be transmitted to the mouth. Symptoms are similar to those of herpes simplex type 1. Figure 13.3 summarizes the herpes cycle.

Genital herpes is especially serious in pregnant women because of the danger of infecting the baby as it passes through the vagina during birth. For that reason, many physicians recommend caesarean deliveries for infected women. Additionally, women who have a history of genital herpes also appear to have a greater risk of developing cervical cancer.

Although there is no cure for herpes at present, certain drugs have shown some success in reducing symptoms. Unfortunately, they only seem to work if the disease is confirmed during the first few hours after contact. As you may guess, this is rather rare. The effectiveness of other treatments, such as L-lysine, is largely unsubstantiated to date. Although lip balms and cold-sore medications may provide temporary anesthetic relief, it is useful to remember that rubbing anything on a herpes blister may spread herpes-laden fluids to other tissues or, via the hands, to other body parts.

Preventing Herpes.   If you are worried about contracting herpes, there are several precautions that you should take:

■ Avoid any form of kissing if you notice a sore or blister on your partner's mouth. Kiss no one, not even a peck on the cheek, if you know that you have a herpes lesion. Allow a bit of time after the sores go away before you start kissing again.

■ Be extremely cautious if you have casual sexual affairs. Not every partner will feel obligated to tell you that he or she may have a problem. Protecting against risk is up to you.

■ Wash your hands immediately with soap and water after any form of sexual contact.

Women carry not only the burden of their own health, but frequently that of a child infected before birth or at the time of delivery.

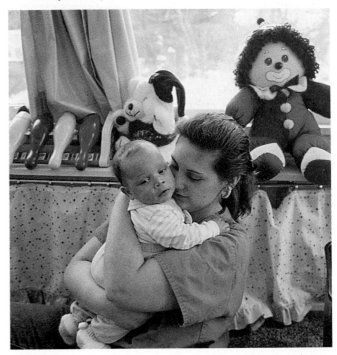

■ If you have herpes, reduce the risk of a herpes episode by avoiding excessive stress, sunlight, or whatever else appears to trigger a herpes outbreak in you.

■ If you have questionable sores or lesions, seek medical help at once. Do not be afraid to name your contacts.

■ Since the herpes organism dies quickly upon exposure to air, toilet seats, soap, and similar sources are not likely means of transmission.

■ If you have herpes, be responsible in your sexual contacts with others. If you have herpes lesions that might put your partner at risk, let that person know. Although it is not necessary to announce openly a herpes problem, use common sense in determining the appropriate time and place for a candid herpes discussion with your partner.

*A*CQUIRED IMMUNE DEFICIENCY SYNDROME (AIDS)

Since 1982, when the first case of **acquired immune deficiency syndrome (AIDS)** was diagnosed, the numbers of AIDS-diagnosed individuals and of persons infected with **human immunodeficiency virus (HIV)** have skyrocketed, both in North America and worldwide. Few regions of the world have been spared. In 1994, the World Health Organization estimated that more than 4.5 million AIDS cases had occurred since the late 1970s and that 18 million adults and 1.5 million children had been infected with HIV. Countries in southern and central Africa and South Asia accounted for three-quarters of these infections.[12]

In Canada, there were 380 AIDS cases per million people in 1994. AIDS is a much more common disease in the United States, where there were 1542 AIDS cases per million people in the same year—the highest rate in the developed world. Moreover, the distribution of cases by risk factor is different in the United States, with a much larger proportion of cases in that country contracted through injected drug use. Figure 13.4 compares rates of AIDS in developed countries; Figure 13.5 shows global prevalence of the disease. The Focus on Canada box gives a more detailed picture of AIDS in Canada.

*W*HAT DO YOU THINK?

Why do you think HIV infection is increasing among some groups? What actions can we take to reduce the spread of HIV/AIDS? Why is the global HIV/AIDS epidemic of concern to Canadians?

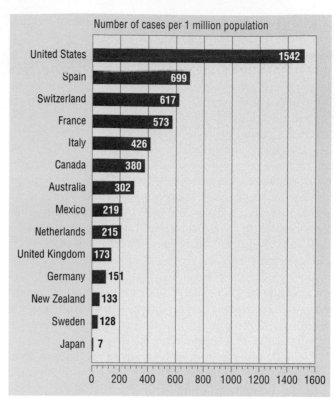

FIGURE 13.4

Rates of AIDS Cases for Selected Countries, 1994

Source: Health Canada, Division of HIV/AIDS Epidemiology, Laboratory Centre for Disease Control, *Quarterly Surveillance Update: AIDS in Canada,* January 1995.

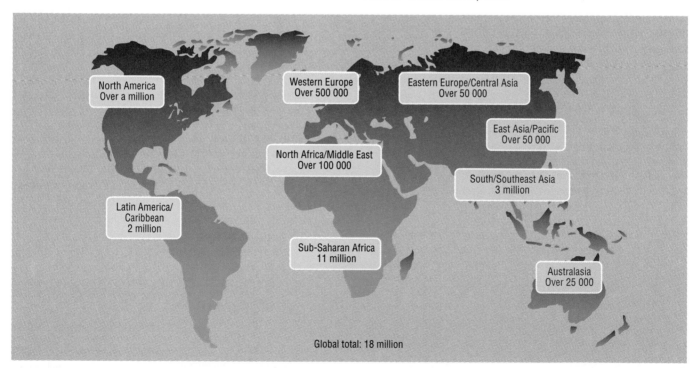

FIGURE 13.5

Estimated Distribution of Total Adult HIV, Late 1970s/Early 1980s to Late 1994

Source: World Health Organization, *Weekly Epidemiological Record,* 70, No. 2, January 13, 1995.

AIDS in Canada

How widespread is AIDS in Canada? The answer depends partly on the definition of AIDS—that is, the criteria used by a physician to establish a diagnosis of AIDS. The Canadian definition of an AIDS case for surveillance purposes was established on the basis of objective, internationally recognized case criteria, established shortly after the epidemic began. The criteria were widened in 1987 to include presumptive diagnoses of indicator diseases, and two recently defined syndromes, HIV encephalopathy and HIV wasting syndrome. In July 1993, the Canadian criteria were widened again, this time to include pulmonary tuberculosis, recurrent bacterial pneumonia, and invasive cervical cancer. This revision was consistent with changes made in all European countries, Australia, and New Zealand, but was somewhat different from revised U.S. criteria. Health Canada defines an AIDS case as a person with a disease characterized by: at least one indicator disease diagnosed definitively, and an HIV-positive test result or absence of specific causes for underlying immunodeficiency.

As of March 31, 1997, a cumulative total of 14 836 cases of AIDS in Canada had been reported to the Bureau of HIV/AIDS and STD, including 159 in children under 15 years old. Adjusting for reporting delay patterns and underreporting, the cumulative total from the beginning of the epidemic to the end of 1996 is estimated to be more than 20 000. Most recent reports indicate a notable decrease in the annual incidence of AIDS cases starting about 1996.

A decreasing trend of reported AIDS cases is apparent among men who have sex with men (77.7 percent of all cases before 1990, 68.6 percent between 1990 and 1995, and 62.2 percent in 1996). There is a marked increase in cases attributed to intravenous drug use (1.5 percent before 1990, 4.9 percent between 1990 and 1995, and 10.3 percent in 1996). Heterosexual transmission is increasing (2.2 percent before 1990, 5.6 percent between 1990 and 1995, and 9.2 percent in 1996). AIDS cases in women have also increased (6.2 percent before 1990, 6.9 percent between 1990 and 1995, and 9.5 percent in 1996). In women, a rising proportion of AIDS cases is attributed to intravenous drug use (25% in 1996). However, heterosexual contact accounts for 63 percent of AIDS cases among adult women.

Since the beginning of the AIDS epidemic, there has been a change in the number of cases resulting from blood transfusions: initially the number was increasing, then there was a dramatic decline.

A cumulative total of 10 837 deaths were reported up to March 31, 1997. This represents 72.8 percent of all reported cases. For men aged 20 to 44 in 1993, AIDS was the third leading cause of death, with only suicide and motor vehicle accidents causing more deaths.

The numbers of AIDS deaths for 1996 had declined by 20 to 30 percent compared with 1993. What accounts for this decline? One factor is that individuals infected with HIV receive newer and more effective treatment, including protective measures. These recent advances in treatment delay the onset of AIDS by slowing the progression from HIV infection to AIDS. Thus, better survival may result from improved management. However, the accuracy of trend analysis may be limited if "reporter fatigue" and staffing changes are leading to some health care personnel not reporting deaths or delaying in reporting.

The data on the distribution of the AIDS cases more recently diagnosed nationally is evidence that there continue to be several epidemics at different stages occurring in different subpopulations in Canada. There is a trend of increasing AIDS cases in women, who appear to be acquiring the infection primarily through intravenous drug use and heterosexual contact with HIV-infected individuals.

Sources: Health Canada, *Annual Report on AIDS in Canada,* December 1996, Cat. No. H43-53/29 - 1996E; Health Canada, Division of HIV/AIDS Surveillance, Bureau of HIV/AIDS and STD, LCDC, HPB, *AIDS in Canada: Quarterly Surveillance Update,* May 1997; *HIV/AIDS EPI Update,* January 1996; *HIV and AIDS Among Women in Canada;* Health Canada Division, of HIV/AIDS Epidemiology, Laboratory Centre for Disease Control, *Quarterly Surveillance Update: AIDS in Canada,* January 1995; Health Canada, Division of HIV/AIDS Surveillance, Bureau of HIV/AIDS and STD, *Quarterly Surveillance Update,* May 1997; Statistics Canada, "15 Years of AIDS in Canada," *Canadian Social Trends,* Summer 1996, 11–00.

How HIV Is Transmitted

HIV typically enters one person's body when another person's infected body fluids (semen, vaginal secretions, blood, etc.) gain entry through a breach in body defences. Mucous membranes of the genital organs and the anus provide the easiest route of entry. If there is a break in the mucous membranes (as can occur during sexual intercourse, particularly anal intercourse), the virus enters and begins to multiply.

After initial infection, the HIV typically begins to multiply rapidly in the body, invading the bloodstream and cerebrospinal fluid. It progressively destroys helper T-lymphocytes, weakening the body's resistance to disease. The virus also changes the genetic structure of the cells it attacks. In response to this invasion, the body quickly begins to produce antibodies.

Despite some rather hysterical myths, HIV is not a highly contagious virus. Countless studies of people living

Communicating with Your Partner About STIs

The more people know about sexually transmitted infections and the more they internalize personal susceptibility, the greater the chance that they will adopt safer behaviours. Yet, despite large-scale public awareness and education programs, infection continues. Many medical, education, and youth officials feel that the major obstacle to preventing STIs among young people is the discomfort most feel about discussing personal needs and feelings regarding these infection and practising safer sex behaviours. For many young people, discussing STI status and safer sex practices, such as condom use, can be uncomfortable. Some fear that raising the issue suggests lack of trust in the partner; others worry that safer behaviours will ruin their sexual enjoyment; and still others fail to recognize their personal vulnerability. As a result, a great many put themselves at risk for infection rather than hurt the other person's feelings. Therefore, a major goal in the fight against STIs is to improve one-on-one communication between young people considering sexual intimacy. The following tips can help open the lines of communication.

- *Remember that you have a responsibility to your partner to disclose your status.* You also have a responsibility to yourself to do what needs to be done to stay healthy. Do not be afraid to ask your partner's STI status. If either person's status is unknown, suggest going through the testing together as a means of sharing something important with each other.

- *Be direct, honest, and determined in talking about sex before you become involved.* Do not act silly or evasive. Get to the point, ask clear questions, and do not be put off receiving a response. Remember, a person who does not care enough to talk about sex probably does not care enough to take responsibility for his or her actions.

- *Discuss the issues without sounding defensive or accusatory.* Develop a personal comfort level with the subject prior to raising the issue with your partner. Be prepared with complete information and articulate your feelings clearly. Reassure your partner that your reasons for desiring abstinence or safer sex arise from respect and not distrust. Sharing feelings is easier in a calm, suspicion-free environment in which both people feel comfortable.

- *Encourage your partner to be honest and to share feelings.* This will not happen overnight. If you have never had a serious conversation with this person before you get into an intimate situation, you cannot expect honesty and openness when the lights go out.

- *Analyze your own beliefs and values ahead of time.* The worst thing you can do is to get yourself into an awkward situation before you have had time to think about what is important to you and what you believe in. Know where you will draw the line on certain actions, and be very clear with your partner about what you expect. If you believe that using a condom is necessary, make sure you communicate this to your partner.

- *Decide what you will do if your partner does not agree with you.* Anticipate your partner's potential objections or excuses and prepare your responses accordingly.

- *Ask questions about past history.* Although it may seem as though you are prying into another person's business, your own health future depends upon knowing basic information about your partner's past. An idea of your partner's past sexual practices and use of injected drugs is very valuable. Again, it is important to let your partner know why you are concerned and that you are not inquiring due to jealousy or other ulterior motives.

- *Ask about the significance of monogamy in your partner's relationships.* A basic question to ask before becoming involved in a regular sexual relationship is: "How important is a committed relationship to you?" You will need to decide early how important this relationship is to you and how much you are willing to work at arriving at an acceptable compromise on lifestyle.

in households with a person with HIV/AIDS have turned up no documented cases of HIV infection due to casual contact. Other investigations provide overwhelming evidence that insect bites do not transmit the HIV virus. The virus is actually quite selective in the way it transmits itself from person to person.

Engaging in High-Risk Behaviours. HIV is not a disease of certain groups. People are not predestined to get the disease because they belong to a group or associate with a group. Thus, HIV is not a gay disease, or a disease of minority groups, or Haitians, or any other class of people. It is a disease of certain high-risk behaviours. If you

engage in the behaviour, you increase your risk for the disease. If you don't engage in the behaviour, your risk is minimal. Promiscuous sex—in males and females of all ages, races, ethnic groups, sexual orientations, and socioeconomic conditions—is the greatest threat. Anyone at any time who engages in unprotected sex with a person who has engaged in high-risk behaviours is at risk. A celibate or monogamous gay man or a drug-injecting woman who never shares her needles is at very low risk for HIV. But a person who has had sex with anyone who's ever had sex with an injecting drug user could be infected. You can't tell by looking at someone; you can't tell by questioning, unless the person has been tested recently and is HIV-

Reducing Your Risks for HIV Disease

HIV disease is not uncontrollable. HIV cannot, like cold or flu viruses, be caught casually. The transmission of HIV depends upon specific behaviours. Therefore, HIV infection can be prevented by following safe practices. The following list offers ways to reduce your risk for infection and limit the impact of the disease.

- Avoid casual sexual partners. Ideally, only have sex if you are in a long-term mutually monogamous relationship with someone who is equally committed to the relationship and whose HIV status is negative.

- Avoid unprotected intimate sexual activity involving the exchange of blood, semen, or vaginal secretions with people whose present or past behaviours put them at risk for infection. Do not be afraid to ask intimate questions about your partner's sexual past. You expose yourself to your partner's history whenever you choose to have sexual relations. Postpone sexual involvement until you are assured that he or she is not infected.

- All sexually active adults who are not in a lifelong monogamous relationship should practise safer sex by using latex condoms. Remember, however, that condoms still do not provide 100 percent safety.

- Never share injecting needles with anyone for any reason.

- Never share any devices through which the exchange of blood could occur, including needles, razors, tattoo instruments, any body-piercing instruments, and any other sharp objects.

- Avoid injury to body tissue during sexual activity. HIV can enter the bloodstream through microscopic tears in anal or vaginal tissues.

- Avoid unprotected oral sex or any sexual activity in which semen, blood, or vaginal secretions could penetrate mucous membranes through breaks in the membrane. Always use a condom or a dental dam during oral sex.

- Avoid using drugs that may dull your senses and affect your ability to make decisions about responsible precautions with potential sex partners.

- Wash your hands before and after sexual encounters. Urinate after sexual relations and, if possible, wash your genitals.

- Although total abstinence is the only absolute means of preventing the sexual transmission of HIV, abstinence can be a difficult choice to make. If you are in doubt about the potential risks of having sex, consider other means of intimacy, at least until you can assure your safety. Enjoyable and safer alternatives include massage, dry kissing, hugging, holding and touching, and masturbation (alone or with a partner).

- When receiving care from medical professionals such as dentists or doctors, make sure they take appropriate precautions to prevent potential transmission, including washing their hands and wearing gloves and masks. Be sure that all equipment used for treatment is properly sterilized.

- If you are worried about your own HIV status, have yourself tested rather than risk infecting others inadvertently.

- If you are a woman and HIV-positive, you should take the steps necessary to ensure that you do not become pregnant.

- If you suspect that you may be infected or if you test positive for HIV antibodies, *do not* donate blood, semen, or body organs.

---

negative. So, what should you do? The Building Communication Skills box offers some direct advice.

Of course, the best answer is abstinence. If you don't exchange body fluids, you won't get the disease. As a second line of defence, if you decide to be intimate, the next best option is to use a condom. The following activities are high-risk behaviours.

Exchange of Body Fluids. The exchange of HIV-infected body fluids during sexual intercourse is the greatest risk factor. Substantial research evidence indicates that blood, semen, and vaginal, cervical, and anal secretions are the major fluids of concern. Although the virus was found in one person's saliva (out of 71 people in a study population), most health officials state that saliva is not a high-risk body fluid. But the fact that the virus has been found in saliva does provide a good rationale for using caution when engaging in deep, wet kissing.

Initially, public health officials also included breast milk in the list of high-risk fluids because a small number of infants apparently contracted HIV while breast-feeding. Subsequent research has indicated that HIV transmission could have been caused by bleeding nipples rather than actual consumption of breast milk. Infection through contact with faeces and urine is believed to be highly unlikely though technically possible.

Receiving a Blood Transfusion Prior to 1986. A small group of people became infected with HIV as a result of having received a blood transfusion before 1986, when the Canadian Red Cross implemented a stringent testing program for all donated blood. Today, because of these massive screening efforts, the risk of receiving HIV-infected blood is almost nonexistent.

Injecting Drugs. Another source of infection is sharing or using HIV-contaminated needles. While illegal drug users are the people we usually think of as being in this category, it is important to remember that others may also share needles—for example, diabetics who inject insulin. People who share needles and also engage in sexual activities with members of high-risk groups, such as those who exchange sex for drugs, increase their risks dramatically. Essentially any needle prick with an HIV-contaminated needle offers the risk of infection. Thus, tattooing, body piercing, and any practice using unsterilized needles presents a potential risk.

Mother-to-Infant Transmission (Perinatal). Infants may contract AIDS from their infected mothers while in the womb or while passing through the vaginal tract during delivery.

Symptoms of the Disease

A person may go for months or years after infection by HIV before any significant symptoms appear. The incubation time varies greatly from person to person. Children have shorter incubation periods than do adults. Newborns and infants are particularly vulnerable to AIDS because human beings do not become fully immunocompetent (that is, their immune system is not fully developed) until they are 6 to 15 months old. New information suggests that some very young children show the "adult" progression of the disease. In adults, the average length of time it takes the virus to cause the slow, degenerative changes in the immune system that result in the onset of

AIDS is eight to ten years. During this time, the person may experience a large number of opportunistic infections (infections that gain a foothold when the immune system is not functioning effectively). Colds, sore throats, fever, tiredness, nausea, night sweats, and other generally non-life-threatening conditions commonly appear.

Testing for HIV Antibodies

Once antibodies have begun to form in reaction to the presence of HIV, a blood test known as the **ELISA** test may detect their presence. If sufficient antibodies are present, the ELISA test will be positive. When a person who previously tested *negative* (no HIV antibodies present) has a subsequent test that is *positive,* seroconversion is said to have occurred. In such a situation, the person would typically take another ELISA test, followed by a more expensive, more precise test known as the **Western blot** to confirm the presence of HIV antibodies.

Although the ELISA is viewed as quite accurate, it is a conservative test in that it errs on the side of caution, meaning it produces a large number of *false positive results.* It was deliberately designed to do this because it was intended as a test for screening the nation's blood supply. There have also been instances of *false negative results.* Some health professionals believe that there are chronic carriers of HIV who, for unknown reasons, continually show false negative results on both the ELISA and the Western blot test. This, of course, raises serious concerns about risks for these people's sexual partners. It should be noted that these tests are not AIDS tests per se. Rather, they detect antibodies for the disease, indicating the presence of the HIV in the person's system. Whether or not the person will develop AIDS depends to some extent on

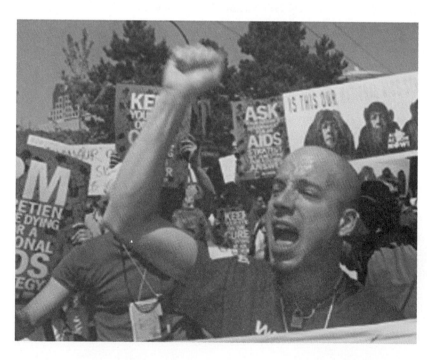

Numerous demonstrations by gay activists have successfully called attention to the need for AIDS research and treatment programs.

the strength of the immune system. However, the vast majority of all infected people do develop some form of the disease.

Treatment in the 1990s

Although the list of possible anti-HIV agents has grown considerably in the last five years, many would-be cures remain on the unapproved list for human testing. Of those that have gained approval, *Zidovudine (AZT)*, an anti-cancer drug known to delay the progress of the immunodeficiency that leads to AIDS, has had promising results. AZT also decreases the frequency of opportunistic infections and mental dysfunction. Clinical benefits may be apparent within six weeks of therapy, and continued treatment appears to prolong survival. But not all HIV-infected individuals can tolerate AZT treatments. Extreme nausea, headache, anemia, insomnia, and other side-effects have forced many patients to seek alternative treatments.[13] Moreover, AZT is very expensive.

Newer forms of treatment include *ddI (29,39-dideoxyinosine)*, a drug that blocks HIV reproduction with fewer side-effects than seen with AZT; and *ddA (29,39-dideoxyadenosine)* and *ddC (29,39-dideoxycytidine)*, chemicals that also fight HIV reproduction. *Pentamidine,* in both the injectable and the aerosol form, has been used to treat *pneumocystis carinii* pneumonia, the type of pneumonia that frequently attacks HIV-infected persons. The injected form of Pentamidine causes severe pain and other adverse effects, while the newer aerosol version is said to be less toxic.[14] In addition to these antiviral treatments, scientists are experimenting with immunomodulators, which regenerate or revitalize a failing immune system.[15]

The Canadian HIV Trials Network, established in 1990 by the University of British Columbia and located at St. Paul's Hospital in Vancouver, has significantly improved access of Canadians living with HIV/AIDS and their physicians to clinical trial drugs for the treatment of HIV infection and AIDS.

Preventing HIV Infection

Although scientists have been searching for over a decade for a vaccine to protect people from HIV infection, they have had no success so far. The only effective prevention strategies known all closely relate to the means by which people contract HIV.

HIV infection and AIDS are not uncontrollable conditions. You can reduce your risks by the choices you make in sexual behaviours and the responsibilities you take for your health and for that of your loved ones. The Skills for Behaviour Change box presents ways to reduce your risk for contracting HIV.

Because the status of your immune system is an important factor in whether or not you are susceptible to any of the STIs, it is important that you do everything possible to protect yourself. Adequate nutrition, sleep, stress management, vaccinations, and other preventive maintenance activities can do a great deal to ensure your long-term health.

NONINFECTIOUS DISEASES

Typically, when we think of the major ailments and diseases affecting people today, we think of "killer" diseases such as cancer and heart disease. But although these diseases capture much of the media attention, other forms of chronic disease often cause substantial pain, suffering, and disability. Fortunately, the majority of these diseases can be prevented or their onset delayed.

To prevent the development of certain noninfectious and chronic diseases, we must identify the major common characteristics of these diseases. They are not transmitted by any pathogen or by any form of personal contact. They usually develop over a long period of time, and they cause progressive damage to human tissues. Although these conditions normally do not result in death, they do lead to illness and suffering for many people. Lifestyle and personal health habits appear to be major contributing factors to the general increase observed in the incidence of chronic diseases in Canada in recent years. Education, reasonable changes in lifestyle behaviours, and public health efforts aimed at prevention and control could minimize the effects of many of these diseases.

RESPIRATORY DISORDERS

Allergy-Induced Problems

An **allergy** occurs as a part of the body's attempt to defend itself against a specific *antigen* or *allergen* by producing specific *antibodies*. When foreign pathogens such as bacteria or viruses invade the body, the body responds by producing antibodies to destroy these invading antigens. Under normal conditions, the production of antibodies is a positive element in the body's defence system. However,

---

ELISA: Blood test that detects presence of antibodies to HIV virus.

Western blot: More precise test than the ELISA to confirm presence of HIV antibodies

Allergy: Hypersensitive reaction to a specific antigen or allergen in the environment in which the body produces excessive antibodies to that antigen or allergen.

for unknown reasons, in some people the body overreacts by developing an overly elaborate protective mechanism against relatively harmless allergens or antigens. The resultant *hypersensitivity reaction* to specific allergens or antigens in the environment is fairly common, as anyone who has awakened with a runny nose or itchy eyes will testify. Most commonly, these hypersensitivity, or allergic, responses occur as a reaction to environmental antigens such as moulds, animal dander (hair and dead skin), pollen, ragweed, or dust. Once excessive antibodies to these antigens are produced, they trigger the release of **histamines**, chemical substances that dilate blood vessels, increase mucous secretions, cause tissues to swell, and produce other allergylike symptoms (see Figure 13.6).

Although many people think of allergies as childhood diseases, in reality allergies tend to become progressively worse with time and with increased exposure to allergens. In these circumstances, allergic responses become chronic in nature, and treatment becomes difficult. Many people take allergy shots to reduce the severity of their symptoms with some success. In most cases, once the offending antigen has disappeared, allergy-prone people suffer few symptoms. Although allergies can cause numerous problems, one of the most significant effects is on the immune system.

Hay Fever

Perhaps the best example of a chronic respiratory disease is **hay fever.** Usually considered to be a seasonally related disease (most prevalent when ragweed and flowers are blooming), hay fever is common throughout the world. Hay fever attacks, which are characterized by sneezing and itchy, watery eyes and nose, cause a great deal of misery for countless people. Hay fever appears to run in families, and research indicates that lifestyle is not as great a factor in developing hay fever as it is in other chronic diseases. Instead, an overzealous immune system and an exposure to environmental allergens including pet dander, dust, pollen from various plants, and other substances appear to be the critical factors that determine vulnerability. For some people, a change in setting may help; for others, medical assistance in the form of injections or antihistamines may provide the only possibility of relief.

Asthma

Unfortunately for many hay fever sufferers, their condition is often complicated by the development of another chronic respiratory disease, **asthma.** Asthma is characterized by attacks of wheezing, difficulty in breathing, shortness of breath, and coughing spasms. Although most asthma attacks are mild, they can trigger bronchospasms (contractions of the bronchial tubes in the lungs) of such a severe nature that, unless treatment is rapid, death may occur. Between attacks, most people have few symptoms.

In the majority of cases, asthma occurs in children under the age of ten, afflicting males nearly twice as often as females. Although many children outgrow the condition, a number of them suffer recurrences as adults.

Although exposure to allergens such as dust, pollen, and animal dander may trigger many asthmatic episodes, emotional factors and excessive anxiety or stress can also trigger an attack. *Exercise-induced asthma (EIA)* is a type of asthma that has gained increasing attention. Friends who bow out of a long run or a tennis game by claiming to be allergic to exercise may not be joking.

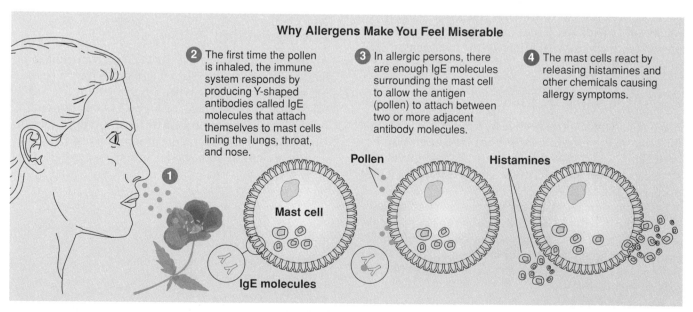

Why Allergens Make You Feel Miserable

2 The first time the pollen is inhaled, the immune system responds by producing Y-shaped antibodies called IgE molecules that attach themselves to mast cells lining the lungs, throat, and nose.

3 In allergic persons, there are enough IgE molecules surrounding the mast cell to allow the antigen (pollen) to attach between two or more adjacent antibody molecules.

4 The mast cells react by releasing histamines and other chemicals causing allergy symptoms.

Pollen

Histamines

Mast cell

IgE molecules

FIGURE 13.6

Steps of an Allergy Response

Relaxation techniques appear to help some asthma sufferers. Drugs may be necessary for serious cases. Doctors warn against using over-the-counter inhalers because the medication in them wears off quickly, raises the pulse rate, and stresses the heart. New prescription drugs such as Seldane, inhalers containing albuterol, and Cromolyn, appear to work better than OTC products and without serious side-effects. Determining the specific allergen that provokes asthma attacks and taking steps to reduce your exposure, avoiding triggers such as exercise or stress, and finding the most effective medications are big steps in asthma prevention and control.

Emphysema

Emphysema involves the gradual destruction of the **alveoli** (tiny air sacs) of the lungs. As the alveoli are destroyed, the affected person finds it more and more difficult to exhale. The victim typically struggles to take in a fresh supply of air before the air held in the lungs has been expended. The chest cavity gradually begins to expand, producing the barrel-shaped chest characteristic of the chronic emphysema victim.

The exact cause of emphysema is uncertain. There is, however, a strong relationship between the development of emphysema and long-term cigarette smoking and exposure to air pollution. Victims of emphysema often suffer discomfort over a period of many years. What we all take for granted—the easy, rhythmic flow of air in and out of our lungs—becomes a continuous struggle for people with emphysema. Inadequate oxygen supply, combined with the stress of overexertion on the heart, eventually takes its toll on the cardiovascular system and leads to premature death. Unfortunately, there is little that can be done to reverse the effects of the disease.

Chronic Bronchitis

Although often dismissed as "smoker's cough" or a bad case of the common cold, **chronic bronchitis** may be a serious, if not life-threatening, respiratory disorder. In this ailment, the bronchial tubes become so inflamed and swollen that normal respiratory function is impaired. Symptoms of chronic bronchitis include a productive cough and shortness of breath that persist for several weeks over the course of the year. Cigarette smoking is the major risk factor for this disease, although fumes, dust, and particulate matter in the air are also contributing factors. Victims of chronic bronchitis must often use respiratory devices similar to those used by emphysema patients. They must also avoid those factors, such as cigarettes, that contributed to the development of bronchitis. Bronchitis coupled with a severe cold may be serious enough to warrant immediate medical attention.

𝒩EUROLOGICAL DISORDERS

Headaches

Almost all of us have experienced the agony of at least one major headache in our lives, whether it be of the mild, throbbing variety or the severe, pounding ache that makes us nauseated or dizzy. Not all headaches are equal; more important, it's possible that not all headaches have the same cause, although some headache experts suggest that all serious headaches share the same basic causes but fall along a spectrum, with ordinary tension headaches at one end and full-blown migraines at the other.[16] Headaches may result from dilated blood vessels within the brain, underlying organic problems, or excessive stress and anxiety. The following are the most common forms of headaches and the most effective methods of treatment.

Tension Headache. Tension headaches are generally caused by muscle contractions or tension in the neck or head. This tension may be caused by actual strain placed on neck or head muscles due to overuse, static positions held for long periods of time, or tension triggered by stress. Recent research indicates that tension headaches may be a product of a more "generic mechanism" in which chemicals deep inside the brain may cause the muscular tension, pain, and suffering often associated with an attack. Triggers for this chemical assault may be red wine, lack of sleep, fasting, menstruation, or other factors, and the same symptoms (sensitivity to light and sound, nausea, and/or throbbing pain) may be characteristic of different types of headaches. Symptoms may vary in intensity and duration. Relaxation, hot water treatment, and massage have surfaced as the new "holistic treatments,"

Histamines: Chemical substances that dilate blood vessels, increase mucous secretions, and produce other allergy-like symptoms.

Hay fever: A chronic respiratory disorder that is most prevalent when ragweed and flowers bloom.

Asthma: A chronic respiratory disease characterized by attacks of wheezing, shortness of breath, and coughing spasms.

Emphysema: A respiratory disease in which the alveoli become distended or ruptured and are no longer functional.

Alveoli: Tiny air sacs of the lungs.

Chronic bronchitis: A serious respiratory disorder in which the bronchial tubes become so inflamed and swollen that respiratory function is impaired.

while aspirin, Tylenol, Aleve, and Advil are the old standby forms of pain relief. Although such painkillers may bring temporary relief of symptoms, it is believed that, over time, the drugs may dull the brain's own pain-killing weapons and result in more headaches rather than fewer.

Migraine Headache. If you've ever experienced pulsating pain on one side of the head in combination with dizzy spells, nausea, and a severe intolerance for light and noise, you are probably one of those who suffer from **migraine.** Many migraine victims suffer excruciatingly painful, recurring headaches that last for minutes, hours, or even days and possibly some temporary visual impairment. While past research focussed on an unusual alternating dilation and constriction of blood vessels in the brain as a possible cause of migraine attacks, more recent thinking questions this theory. Today, many believe that the key to identifying the origin of migraines lies in the cortex of the brain.[17] Other doctors believe that pain signals start deep in the brain in areas normally rich in the painkilling chemical serotonin.[18]

When true migraines occur, relaxation is only minimally effective as a treatment. Often, strong pain-relieving drugs prescribed by a physician are necessary.

Secondary Headaches. Secondary headaches arise as a result of some other underlying condition. A good example is a person with a severe sinus blockage that causes pressure in the sinus cavity. This pressure may induce a headache. Hypertension, allergies, low blood sugar, diseases of the spine, the common cold, poorly fitted dentures, problems with eyesight, and other types of pain or injury can trigger this condition. Relaxation and pain relievers such as aspirin are of little help in treating secondary headaches. Rather, medications or other therapies designed to relieve the underlying organic cause of the headache must be included in the treatment regimen.

Psychological Headaches. With this type of headache, the "it's all in your head" diagnosis may, in fact, be correct. Rather than having a physical cause, psychological headaches stem from anxiety states, depression, and other emotional factors. Psychological headaches result from the stress of severe emotional disturbances, particularly depression. Unlike in tension headaches, no muscles or blood vessels appear to be involved, thereby making relaxation and painkillers virtually worthless as treatment. Only therapy designed to treat the underlying depression or emotional problem appears to be effective in reducing the headache.

Seizure Disorders

The word **epilepsy** is derived from the Greek *epilepsia,* meaning "seizure." Reports of epilepsy appeared in Greek medical records as early as in 300 B.C. Ancient peoples interpreted seizures as invasions of the body by evil spirits or as punishments by the gods. Although much of the mys-

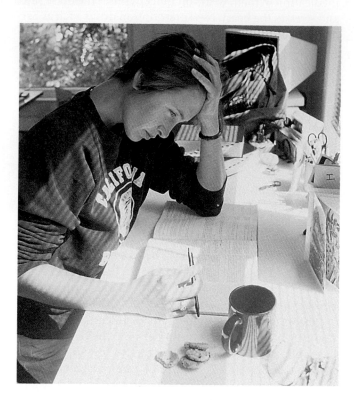

Tension headaches are triggered by many factors, including lack of sleep, stress, and strain on head and neck muscles.

tery surrounding epileptic seizures has been solved in recent years, the stigma and lack of understanding remain.

These disorders are generally caused by abnormal electrical activity in the brain and are characterized by loss of control of muscular activity and unconsciousness. Symptoms vary widely from person to person.

There are several forms of seizure disorders, the most common of which are:

1. *Grand mal, or major motor seizure:* These seizures are often preceded by a shrill cry or a seizure aura (body sensations such as ringing in the ears or a specific smell or taste that occurs prior to a seizure). Convulsions and loss of consciousness generally occur and may last from 30 seconds to several minutes or more. Keeping track of the length of time elapsed is one aspect of first aid.

2. *Petit mal, or minor seizure:* These seizures involve no convulsions. Rather, a minor loss of consciousness that may go unnoticed occurs. Minor twitching of muscles may take place, usually for a shorter time than the duration of grand mal convulsions.

3. *Psychomotor seizure:* These seizures involve both mental processes and muscular activity. Symptoms may include mental confusion and a listless state characterized by such activities as lip smacking, chewing, and repetitive movements.

4. *Jacksonian seizure:* This is a progressive seizure that often begins in one part of the body, such as the fingers, and moves to other parts, such as the hand or arm. Usually only one side of the body is affected.

In the majority of cases, people afflicted with seizure disorders can lead normal, seizure-free lives when under medical supervision. Epilepsy is seldom fatal. The greatest risk for epileptics whose seizures are uncontrolled is motor vehicle or other accidents. Public ignorance about these disorders is one of the most serious obstacles confronting victims of seizure disorders. Improvements in medication and surgical interventions to reduce some causes of seizures are among the most promising treatments today.

*W*HAT DO YOU THINK?

Do you suffer from recurrent headaches or other neurological problems? What do you think are the major causes of your problems? What actions might you take to reduce your risks and/or symptoms?

*S*EX-RELATED DISORDERS

Fibrocystic Breast Condition

Fibrocystic breast condition is a common, noncancerous problem among women in Canada. Symptoms range in severity from a small palpable lump to large masses of irregular tissue found in both breasts. The underlying causes of the condition are unknown. Although some experts believe it to be related to hormonal changes that occur during the normal menstrual cycle, many women report that their conditions neither worsen nor improve during their cycles. In fact, in most cases, the condition appears to run in families and to become progressively worse with age, irrespective of pregnancy or other hormonal disruptions. Although the majority of these cyst formations consists of fibrous tissue, some are filled with fluid. Treatment often involves removal of fluid from the affected area or surgical removal of the cyst itself.

Premenstrual Syndrome (PMS)

Premenstrual syndrome (PMS), a condition describing a series of characteristic symptoms that occur prior to menstruation in some women, is characterized by as many as 150 possible physical and emotional symptoms that vary from person to person and from month to month. These symptoms usually appear a week to ten days preceding the menstrual period and include depression, tension, irritability, headaches, tender breasts, bloated abdomen, backache, abdominal cramps, acne, fluid retention, diarrhea, and fatigue. It is believed that women who have PMS develop a predictable pattern of symptoms during the menstrual cycle and that the severity of their symptoms may be influenced by external factors, such as stress.

Women usually experience PMS for the first time after the age of 20, and it may remain a regular part of their reproductive life unless they seek treatment. For many women, the first day of their period brings immediate relief. For others, the depressive symptoms persist all month and are only heightened prior to the menstrual period.

Most authorities believe that the most plausible cause of PMS is a hormonal imbalance related to the rise in estrogen levels preceding the menstrual period. This theory is substantiated by the fact that women with PMS who are given prescriptions for progesterone often experience relief of symptoms. Critics of this theory argue that controlled research has not yet been conducted on the effects of progesterone on PMS.

Common treatments for PMS include hormonal therapy in addition to drugs and behaviours designed to relieve the symptoms. These include aspirin for pain, diuretics for fluid buildup, decreases in caffeine and salt intake, increases in complex carbohydrate intake, stress reduction techniques, and exercise.

Endometriosis

Whether the incidence of **endometriosis** is on the rise or whether the disorder is simply attracting more attention is difficult to determine. Victims of endometriosis tend to be women between the ages of 20 and 40. Symptoms include severe cramping during and between menstrual cycles, irregular periods, unusually heavy or light menstrual flow, abdominal bloating, fatigue, painful bowel movements with periods, painful intercourse, constipation, diarrhea, menstrual pain, infertility, and low back pain. What is this disease? What causes it? What are the common methods of treatment?

Although much remains unknown about the causes of endometriosis, we do know that the disease is characterized

Migraine: A condition characterized by localized headaches that result from alternating dilation and constriction of blood vessels.

Epilepsy: A neurological disorder caused by abnormal electrical brain activity; can be accompanied by altered consciousness or convulsions.

Fibrocystic breast condition: A common, noncancerous condition in which a woman's breasts contain fibrous or fluid-filled cysts.

Premenstrual syndrome (PMS): A series of physical and emotional symptoms that may occur in women prior to their menstrual periods.

Endometriosis: Abnormal development of endometrial tissue outside the uterus resulting in serious side-effects.

by the abnormal growth and development of endometrial tissue (the tissue lining the uterus) in regions of the body other than the uterus. Among the most widely accepted theories concerning the causes of endometriosis are the transmission of endometrial tissue to other regions of the body during surgery or through the birthing process; the movement of menstrual fluid backward through the fallopian tubes during menstruation; and abnormal cell migration through body-fluid movement. Women with cycles shorter than 27 days and those with flows lasting over a week are at increased risk. The more aerobic exercise a woman engages in and the earlier she starts, the less likely she is to develop endometriosis.

Treatment of endometriosis ranges from bed rest and reduction in stressful activities to **hysterectomy** (the removal of the uterus) and/or the removal of one or both ovaries and the fallopian tubes. In some areas, where the rate of hysterectomy is high, physicians have been criticized for overreliance on this procedure. More conservative treatments that involve dilation and curettage, surgically scraping endometrial tissue off the fallopian tubes and other reproductive organs, and combinations of hormone therapy have become more acceptable. Hormonal treatments include gonadotropin-releasing hormone (GnRH) analogues, various synthetic progesterone-like drugs (Provera), and oral contraceptives.

*W*HAT DO YOU THINK?

Which of the preceding health problems do you think causes the most problems for women in Canada? Are these problems related to stigma associated with the condition, related to the condition's physiological effects, or psychological in nature? What actions should be taken to increase awareness and understanding of these conditions?

*D*IGESTION-RELATED DISORDERS

Diabetes

In healthy people, the *pancreas,* a powerful enzyme-producing organ, produces the hormone **insulin** in sufficient quantities to allow the body to use or store glucose (blood sugar). When this organ fails to produce enough insulin to regulate sugar metabolism or when the body fails to use insulin effectively, a disease known as **diabetes** occurs. Diabetics exhibit **hyperglycemia**, or elevated blood sugar levels, and high glucose levels in their urine. Other symptoms include excessive thirst, frequent urination, hunger, tendency to tire easily, wounds that heal slowly, numbness or tingling in the extremities, changes in vision,

skin eruptions, and, in women, a tendency toward vaginal yeast infections.

Many diabetics remain ignorant of their condition until they begin to show overt symptoms. How does a person become diabetic? The more serious form, known as type 1 (insulin-dependent) diabetes or diabetes mellitus, usually begins early in life. Type 1 diabetics typically must depend on insulin injections or oral medications for the rest of their lives because insulin is not present in their bodies. Adult-onset (non-insulin-dependent), or type 2 diabetes, in which insulin production is deficient, tends to develop in later life. These diabetics can often control the symptoms of their disease, with minimal medical intervention, through a regimen of proper diet, weight control, and exercise. They may be able to avoid oral medications or insulin indefinitely.

Diabetes tends to run in families, and a tendency toward being overweight, coupled with inactivity, dramatically increases a person's risk. Older persons and mothers of babies weighing over 4 kilograms also run an increased risk. Approximately 80 percent of all patients are overweight at the time of diagnosis. Weight loss and exercise are important factors in lowering blood sugar and improving the efficiency of cellular use of insulin. Both can help to prevent overwork of the pancreas and the development of diabetes. People who develop diabetes today have a much better prognosis than did those who developed diabetes just 20 years ago.

Most physicians attempt to control diabetes with a variety of insulin-related drugs. Most of these drugs are taken orally, although self-administered hypodermic injections are prescribed when other treatments are inadequate. Recent breakthroughs in individual monitoring and the implanting of insulin monitors and insulin infusion pumps that regulate insulin intake "on demand" have provided many diabetics with the opportunity to lead normal lives. Other diabetics have found that they can help to control their diabetes by eating foods that are rich in complex carbohydrates, low in sodium, and high in fibre; by losing weight; and by getting regular exercise.

Colitis and Irritable Bowel Syndrome (IBS)

Ulcerative colitis is a disease of the large intestine in which the mucous membranes of the intestinal walls become inflamed. Victims with severe cases may have as many as 20 bouts of bloody diarrhea a day. Colitis can also produce severe stomach cramps, weight loss, nausea, sweating, and fever. What causes colitis? Although some experts believe that it occurs more frequently in people with high stress levels, this theory is controversial. Hypersensitivity reactions, particularly to milk and certain foods, have also been considered as a possible cause. It is difficult to determine the cause of colitis because the disease goes into unexplained remission and then recurs without apparent reason. This pattern often continues over periods of years and may be related to the later development of colorectal cancer. Because the cause of colitis remains unknown, treatment focusses exclusively on relieving the symptoms. Increasing fibre intake and taking anti-inflammatory drugs, steroids, and other medications designed to reduce inflammation and soothe irritated intestinal walls have been effective in relieving symptoms.

Many people develop a condition related to colitis known as **irritable bowel syndrome (IBS)**, in which nausea, pain, gas, diarrhea attacks, or cramps occur after eating certain foods or when a person is under unusual stress. IBS symptoms commonly begin in early adulthood. Symptoms may vary from week to week and can fade for long periods of time only to return. The cause of IBS is unknown, but researchers suspect that people with IBS have digestive systems that are overly sensitive to what they eat and drink, to stress, and to certain hormonal changes. They may also be more sensitive to pain signals from the stomach. Stress management, relaxation techniques, regular activity, and diet can bring IBS under control in the vast majority of cases.

Diverticulosis

Diverticulosis occurs when the walls of the intestine become weakened for undetermined reasons and small pea-sized bulges develop. These bulges often fill with faeces and, over time, become irritated and infected, causing pain and discomfort. If this irritation persists, bleeding and chronic obstruction may occur, either of which can be life-threatening. If you have a persistent pain in the lower abdominal region, seek medical attention at once.

Peptic Ulcers

An ulcer is a lesion or wound that forms in body tissue as a result of some form of irritant. A **peptic ulcer** is a chronic ulcer that occurs in the lining of the stomach or the section of the small intestine known as the *duodenum*. It had long been thought to be caused by the erosive effect of digestive juices on these tissues.

Researchers have recently concluded that a common bacteria, *Helicobacter pylori*, may be the cause of most ulcers, and called for the use of powerful antibiotics to treat the disorder. This is a dramatic departure from the typical treatment using acid-reducing drugs known as H2 blockers, such as cimetidine (Tagamet) or ranitidine (Zantec). The new treatment recommends a two-week course of antibiotics. H2 blockers will still be used in ulcer cases in which excess stomach acid or overuse of drugs such as aspirin and ibuprofen have caused an irritation. The good news is that ulcers treated with germ-killing drugs appear less likely to recur.

Ulcers appear to run in families and to be more prevalent in people who are highly stressed over long periods of time and who consume high-fat foods or excessive amounts of alcohol. People with ulcers should avoid high-fat foods, alcohol, and substances such as aspirin that may irritate organ linings or cause increased secretion of stomach acids and thereby exacerbate this condition. In some cases, surgery has been necessary to relieve persistent symptoms.

Gallbladder Disease

Gallbladder disease, also known as *cholecystitis*, occurs when the gallbladder has been repeatedly irritated by chemicals, infection, or overuse, thus reducing its ability to release bile used for the digestion of fats. Usually, gallstones, consisting of calcium, cholesterol, and other minerals, form in the gallbladder itself. When the patient eats foods that are high in fats, the gallbladder contracts to release bile; these contractions cause pressure on the stone formations. One of the characteristic symptoms of gallbladder disease is acute pain in the upper right portion of the abdomen after eating fatty foods. This pain, which can last several hours, may feel like a heart attack or an ulcer attack and is often accompanied by nausea.

Not all gallstones cause acute pain. In fact, small stones that pass through one of the bile ducts and become lodged may be more painful than gallstones that are the size of golf balls. Many people find out that they have gallstones only after undergoing ultrasound and diagnostic X-rays to rule out other conditions. The absence of symptoms is significant because gallstones are considered to be a predisposing factor for gallbladder cancer.

Hysterectomy: Surgical removal of the uterus.

Insulin: A hormone produced by the pancreas; required by the body for the metabolism of carbohydrates.

Diabetes: A disease in which the pancreas fails to produce enough insulin or the body fails to use insulin effectively.

Hyperglycemia: Elevated blood sugar levels.

Ulcerative colitis: An inflammatory disorder that affects the mucous membranes of the large intestine, producing bloody diarrhea.

Irritable bowel syndrome (IBS): Nausea, pain, gas, or diarrhea caused by certain foods or stress.

Diverticulosis: A condition in which bulges form in the walls of the intestine; results in irritation and infection of the intestine.

Peptic ulcer: Damage to the stomach or intestinal lining, usually caused by digestive juices.

Current treatment of gallbladder disease usually involves medication to reduce irritation, restriction of fat consumption, and surgery to remove the gallstones. New medications designed to dissolve small gallstones are currently being used with some patients. In addition, some doctors use a technique known as lithotripsy, in which a series of noninvasive shock waves break up small stones. Lasers and laparoscopic surgery now reduce the risks associated with large surgical incisions.

*W*HAT DO YOU THINK?

What role does improved diet have in reducing your risks for and symptoms of the above diseases? Are you or any of your family members at risk for these problems? What actions can you take today that will begin to reduce your risks?

*M*USCULOSKELETAL DISEASES

Most of us will encounter some form of chronic musculoskeletal disease during our lifetime. Some form of arthritis will afflict half of those over 65; low back pain hits most of us at some point in our life. While these diseases are found throughout the world, the cures differ in different places. The Global Perspectives box looks at one alternative cure.

Arthritis

Ontario Health Survey (OHS) and the 1987 Canadian Health and Activity Limitation Survey found that 20.6 percent of the population aged 16 and older reported arthritis, rheumatism, or back or limb and joint disorders. In the Ontario Health Survey, 18.5 percent of the population aged 16 and older reported **arthritis**, and 15.2 percent reported this as a long-term chronic health problem. The prevalence of any arthritis increased with age, from 6.3 percent in the 16–74 age group to 51.2 percent in those aged 75 and over, and the overall prevalence was 21.1 percent for women and 15.7 percent for men.[19]

Arthritis: Painful inflammatory disease of the joints.

Osteoarthritis: A progressive deterioration of bones and joints that has been associated with the "wear and tear" theory of aging.

Rheumatoid arthritis: A serious inflammatory joint disease.

Lupus: A disease in which the immune system attacks the body, producing antibodies that destroy or injure organs such as the kidneys, brain, and heart.

Osteoarthritis is a progressive deterioration of bones and joints that has been associated with the "wear and tear" theory of aging. More recent research indicates that as joints are used, they release enzymes that digest cartilage while other cells in the cartilage try to repair the damage. When the enzymatic breakdown overpowers cellular repair, the pain and swelling characteristic of arthritis may occur. Weather extremes, excessive strain, and injury often lead to osteoarthritis flare-ups. But a specific precipitating event does not seem to be necessary.

Although age and injury are undoubtedly factors in the development of osteoarthritis, heredity, abnormal use of the joint, diet, abnormalities in joint structure, and impaired blood supply to the joint may also contribute. Osteoarthritis of the hands seems to have a particularly strong genetic component. Extreme disability as a result of osteoarthritis is rare. However, when joints become so distorted that they impair activity, surgical intervention is often necessary. Joint replacement and bone fusion are common surgical repair techniques. For most people, anti-inflammatory drugs and pain relievers such as aspirin and cortisone-related agents ease discomfort. In some sufferers, applications of heat, mild exercise, and massage may also relieve the pain.

Rheumatoid arthritis is similar to, but far more serious than, osteoarthritis. Rheumatoid arthritis is an inflammatory joint disease that can occur at any age, but most commonly appears between the ages of 20 and 45. It is three times more common among women than among men during early adulthood but equally common among men and women in the over-70 age group. Symptoms may be gradually progressive or sporadic, with occasional unexplained remissions.

Rheumatoid arthritis typically attacks the synovial membrane, which produces the lubricating fluids for the joints. Advanced rheumatoid arthritis often involves destruction of the bony ends of joints. The remedy for this condition is typically bone fusion, which leaves the joint immobile. In some instances, joint replacement may be a viable alternative.

Although the exact cause of this form of arthritis is unknown, some experts theorize that it is an autoimmune disorder, in which the body responds as if its own cells were the enemy, eventually destroying the affected body parts. Other theorists believe that rheumatoid arthritis is caused by some form of invading microorganism that takes over the joint. Certain toxic chemicals and stress have also been mentioned as possible causes.

Regardless of the cause, treatment of rheumatoid arthritis is similar to that for osteoarthritis. Emphasis is placed on pain relief and attempts to improve the functional mobility of the patient. In some instances, immunosuppressant drugs are given to reduce the inflammatory response.

Fibromyalgia is a chronic, painful rheumatological-like disorder. Symptoms include widespread pain; stiffness and numerous tender points; weakness; swelling; and neurovascular complaints including coldness, numbness, tingling, mottled skin, headaches, auditory sensitivity, irritable bowel syndrome, sleep disorders, depression, and dysmenorrhea. The cause of fibromyalgia remains a mystery, with many theories under investigation. Acute sleep disturbances, muscular irregularities, and forms of psychopathological disturbance have been considered as possible culprits. What is known is that the disease primarily affects women (particularly in their 30s and 40s), that the disease causes more chronic pain and debilitation than other muscloskeletal disorders, and that significant research must be conducted before an effective, long-term treatment will be available.

Systemic Lupus Erythematosus (SLE)

Lupus is a disease in which the immune system attacks the body, producing antibodies that destroy or injure organs such as the kidneys, brain, and heart. The symptoms vary from mild to severe and may disappear for periods of time. A butterfly-shaped rash covering the bridge of the nose and both cheeks is common. Nearly all SLE sufferers have aching joints and muscles, and 60 percent of them develop redness and swelling that moves from joint to joint. Extensive research has not yet found a cure for this sometimes fatal disease.

Low Back Pain

Most people will experience low back pain at some point during their lifetimes. Although some of these low back pain (LBP) episodes may result from muscular damage and be short-lived and acute, others may involve dislocations, fractures, or other problems with spinal vertebrae or discs and be chronic or require surgery. Low back pain is epidemic throughout the world.

Risk Factors for Low Back Pain. Health experts believe that the following factors contribute to LBP:

- age
- body types
- posture
- strength and fitness
- psychological factors
- occupational risks

Preventing Back Pain and Injury. Almost 90 percent of all back problems occur in the lumbar spine region (lower back). Consciously protecting this region of the body from blows, excessive strain, or sharp twists when muscles are not warmed up is essential. You can avoid many problems by consciously attempting to maintain good posture.

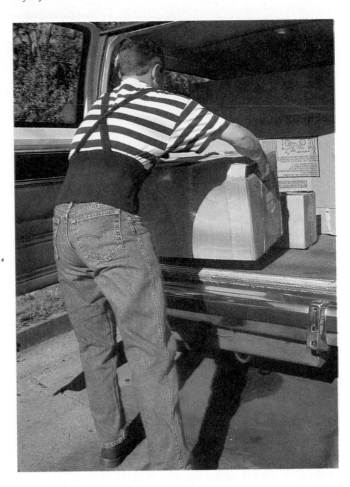

Taking precautions, such as wearing a protective belt when moving heavy objects, can help you avoid back injury.

In addition, exercise, particularly exercise that strengthens the abdominal muscles and stretches the back muscles, is important. New research indicates that many traditional surgical and medicinal treatments for back injury may be less effective than most practitioners currently think.[20] If you injure your back, be sure to consult with at least two different experts in rehabilitation and therapy to determine your best options. Consult an exercise physiologist, biomechanist, physical therapist, or physician specializing in bone and joint injuries for recommended exercises.

*O*THER MALADIES

During the last decade, numerous afflictions have surfaced that seem to be products of our times. Some of these health problems relate to specific groups of people, some are due to technological advances, and some are unexplainable. Still other diseases have been present for

Western Problems, Eastern Cures

Certainly the best "cure" for backache and other chronic musculoskeletal disorders is prevention. But for those suffering already, Western and Eastern science offer very different views of how to solve the problem. In Canada, you may take pain relievers for temporary relief, visit an M.D. or chiropractor, and do physical therapy. If your back hurts in China, you may visit an acupuncturist.

Originating in China over 2000 years ago, acupuncture is based on the idea that the body has 14 well-defined pathways (called meridians) of energy. These pathways convey the body's life force, known as *qi* (pronounced *chee*). According to Chinese medical theory, pain and illness occur when *qi* builds up or diminishes. To adjust its flow, acupuncturists insert stainless-steel needles into one or more of the nearly 2000 acupuncture points on the skin. The needles, which cause little if any sensation, stay in place for 10 to 45 minutes.

Recently, acupuncture has gained more acceptance in North America. Many patients suffer from untraceable or intractable pain in the back, head, neck, and other areas.

They report milder symptoms and often lasting relief after acupuncture.

At the Boston Veterans Affairs Medical Center and the neurology department of the Boston University School of Medicine, Margaret Naeser has used acupuncture needles and low-energy lasers to stimulate acupuncture points on stroke patients, helping them regain partial mobility and strength in their hands, arms, and legs. For the 60 percent of patients who benefited, the progress was significant; many were long-time stroke survivors who had plateaued in their recoveries and were no longer expected to gain motor improvement.

In Asia, acupuncture is used for a wide spectrum of problems: pain, menstrual disorders, digestive problems, infertility, even schizophrenia and depression.

Source: Adapted by permission of the author from Madeline Drexler, "Healing Needles," *Boston Globe Magazine,* September 11, 1994, 10–11.

---

many years and continue to cause severe disability (see Table 13.5). Among conditions that have received attention in recent years are chronic fatigue syndrome and disorders related to the use of video display terminals.

Chronic Fatigue Syndrome (CFS)

In the late 1980s, a characteristic set of symptoms including chronic fatigue, headaches, fever, sore throat, enlarged lymph nodes, depression, poor memory, general weakness, nausea, and symptoms remarkably similar to mononucleosis were noted. Researchers initially believed that they were really talking about a series of symptoms caused by the same virus as mononucleosis, the Epstein-Barr virus. In some instances, the symptoms were so severe that patients required hospitalization. Since those initial studies, however, researchers have all but ruled out the possibility of a mysterious form of the Epstein-Barr virus. Despite extensive testing, no viral cause has been found to date. Today, in the absence of a known pathogen, many researchers believe that the illness, now commonly referred to as chronic fatigue syndrome (CFS), may have strong psychosocial roots.

The diagnosis of chronic fatigue syndrome depends on two major criteria and eight or more minor criteria. The major criteria are debilitating fatigue that persists for at least six months and the absence of diagnoses of other illnesses that could cause the symptoms. Minor criteria include headaches, fever, sore throat, painful lymph nodes, weakness, fatigue after exercise, sleep problems, and rapid onset of these symptoms. Because an exact cause is not apparent, treatment of CFS focusses on improved nutrition, rest, counselling for depression, judicious exercise, and development of a strong support network.

Job-Related Disorders

During the last decade, a new potential health risk for computer users has been the topic of growing debate. Adverse health effects have been noted in people who work at computer video display terminals (VDTs) for several hours per day. Many university students are regular high-volume users of VDTs and therefore at risk.

Most of these problems relate to eyestrain and discomfort in the low back, neck, shoulders, and wrists. Questions about the danger posed by radiation from the electrical fields produced within the circuits of the VDT

TABLE 13.5 ▪ Other Modern Afflictions

Disease	Description	Treatment
Parkinson's disease	Disease affecting mostly people over the age of 55. Symptoms include tremors, rigidity, slowed movement, loss of autonomic movements, and difficulty walking.	Unknown cause makes prevention difficult. Tranquillizers are useful in controlling nerve responses.
Multiple sclerosis	Disease that affects women more than men. Precise cause uncertain. Symptoms include vision problems, tingling and numbness in extremities, chronic fatigue, and neurological impairments.	Medication to control symptoms and slow progression of the disease. Stress management may be helpful.
Cystic fibrosis	Inherited disease occurring in 1 out of every 1600 births. Characterized by pooling of large amounts of mucus in lungs, digestive disturbances, and excessive sodium excretion. Results in premature death.	Most treatments are geared toward relief of symptoms. Antibiotics are administered for infection. Recent strides in genetic research suggest better treatments and potential cure in the near future.
Sickle cell disease	Inherited disease affecting mostly blacks. Disease affects hemoglobin, forming sickle-shaped red blood cells that interfere with oxygenation. Results in severe pain, anemia, and premature death.	Reduce stress and attend to minor infections immediately. Seek genetic counselling.
Cerebral palsy	Disorder characterized by the loss of voluntary control over motor functioning. Believed to be caused by a lack of oxygen to the brain at birth, brain disorders or an accident before or after birth, poisoning, or brain infections.	Follow preventive actions to reduce accident risks; improved neonatal and birthing techniques.
Graves' disease	Thyroid disorder characterized by swelling of the eyes, staring gaze, and retraction of the eyelid. Can result in loss of sight. The cause is unknown and it can occur at any age.	Medication may help control symptoms. Radioactive iodine supplements also may be administered.

and about the potential effects on pregnant women and their foetuses remain unanswered.

Carpal tunnel syndrome is a common occupational injury in which the median nerve in the wrist becomes irritated, causing numbness, tingling, and pain in the fingers and hands. This condition is worsened by the repetitive typing motions made by computer users and is often classified as one of the common repetitive motion injuries. For those who must work on a computer for hours at a time, day after day, experts recommend regular breaks. Remove your hands from the keyboard to exercise them about every 20 minutes; stretch other body parts such as the neck and shoulders periodically. Attention to the design, height, and support of your chair and a keyboard placed at a comfortable angle and height can save countless hours of suffering.

> **Carpal tunnel syndrome:** A common occupational injury in which the median nerve in the wrist becomes irritated, causing numbness, tingling, and pain in the fingers and hands.

Managing Your Disease Risks

Infectious diseases pose serious challenges throughout the world. In particular, sexually transmitted diseases, including HIV infection, present an increasing health risk to young people. All infectious diseases can be prevented by practising safe and responsible behaviours. In addition, many noninfectious diseases can be prevented or their onset delayed by following positive personal health habits.

Making Decisions for You

Protecting yourself from infectious diseases is not always easy. Because most pathogens are microscopic, exposure to one can occur without your knowledge. Therefore, you need to be aware of your risks. What can you do to improve your own awareness of your potential exposure to disease-causing pathogens?

What are some actions you can take to reduce your risk of contracting a sexually transmitted disease? What steps could you take right now to ensure the sexual health of your partners? Finally, if you thought you had been exposed to HIV, would you seek testing?

Checklist for Change: Making Personal Choices

✓ Be aware of factors that can threaten your health status.

✓ Know your disease and immunization history.

✓ Take the proper precautions to protect yourself from exposure to infectious pathogens.

✓ Know the health status of your intimate partners.

✓ Communicate openly and honestly with your partners about your feelings regarding sexual intimacy.

✓ If you have a condition that can be spread through casual contact, remember to wash your hands frequently.

✓ Avoid travelling to places where outbreaks of infectious diseases have not been controlled.

✓ Maintain a healthy routine of sleep, nutrition, and exercise.

✓ Cook foods at their appropriate temperatures.

✓ Respect the symptoms that indicate a possible infection and seek treatment immediately.

✓ Recognize your responsibility for the health of others.

✓ Behave in sexually responsible ways.

✓ Limit your sexual partners.

✓ Avoid using alcohol or other drugs during intimate sexual encounters.

✓ Assess your level of risk for acquiring an STI, including HIV infection.

✓ Respect the rights and needs of individuals affected by an infectious disease.

✓ Adopt personal health habits that will help prevent a chronic disease.

✓ Identify actions you can take today to reduce your own risks for the diseases and disorders discussed in this chapter.

Checklist for Change: Making Community Choices

✓ Does your student health service offer testing for all STIs, including HIV?

✓ Do you support government spending for HIV research and health promotion (education)?

✓ Does your local school system offer a sex education curriculum including discussion about how to stop the spread of the HIV virus?

✓ If you worked for a government agency charged with helping people improve their personal health habits, what approaches would you take?

✓ Have you done anything to support campaigns raising money for research into chronic illnesses?

✓ What role should businesses play in improving employee health? Should the federal government provide tax credits to help businesses buy proper equipment?

Critical Thinking

You have been in a relationship for several months that has grown from a nice friendship to a state of passionate sexual intimacy. During this time, a close and trusting bond has also developed. You have remained monogamous and believe that your partner has as well, although you have never discussed it. Nor has any discussion arisen about each other's sexual history or HIV status. You have been involved in sexual relationships in the past and have never been tested for HIV antibodies, and you're quite certain your partner is experienced as well. You trust your partner but recognize that, without complete information, you are both at risk for HIV infection. You want to take some precautionary steps but worry about insulting your partner's feelings.

Use the DECIDE model described in Chapter 1 to decide what you would do in this situation. Develop several different strategies and approaches for reaching the desired result.

Summary

- The major uncontrollable risk factors for contracting infectious diseases are heredity, age, and environmental conditions. The major controllable risk factors are stress, nutrition, fitness level, sleep, hygiene, avoidance of high-risk behaviours, and drug use.

- The major pathogens are bacteria, viruses, fungi, protozoa, rickettsia, and parasitic worms.

- Your body uses a number of defence systems to keep pathogens from invading. The skin is our major protection, helped by enzymes. The immune system creates antibodies to destroy antigens. In addition, fever and pain play a role in defending the body. Vaccines bolster the body's immune system against specific diseases.

- Sexually transmitted diseases are spread through intercourse, oral sex, anal sex, hand-genital contact, and sometimes through mouth-to-mouth contact. Major STIs include chlamydia, pelvic inflammatory disease, gonorrhea, syphilis, pubic lice, venereal warts, candidiasis, trichomoniasis, and herpes.

- Acquired immune deficiency syndrome (AIDS) is caused by the human immunodeficiency virus (HIV). HIV is not confined to certain high-risk groups. Your risk for HIV infection can be cut by deciding not to engage in risky sexual activities.

- Headaches may be caused by a variety of factors, the most common of which are tension, dilation and/or contraction of blood vessels in the brain, chemical influences on muscles and vessels that cause inflammation and pain, and underlying physiological and psychological disorders.

- Several modern maladies affect only women. Fibrocystic breast condition is a common, noncancerous buildup of irregular tissue. Premenstrual syndrome (PMS) is the name given to a wide variety of symptoms that appear to be related to the menstrual cycle. Endometriosis is the buildup of endometrial tissue in regions of the body other than the uterus.

- Pathogens, problems in enzyme or hormone production, anxiety or stress, functional abnormalities, and other problems are often listed as probable causes of digestive disorders.

- Musculoskeletal diseases such as arthritis, lower back pain, repetitive motion injuries, and other problems cause significant pain and disability in millions of people.

Discussion Questions

1. What is a pathogen? What are the similarities and differences between pathogens and antigens? What are the risk factors that can threaten your health? What factors are controllable?

2. What is the difference between natural and acquired immunity?

3. Identify five sexually transmitted diseases. What are their symptoms? How do they develop? What are their potential long-term risks?

5. Why might it be inappropriate to identify groups as at high risk for HIV infection? Why might HIV infection be better referred to as a sexually transmissible disease than as a sexually transmitted disease?

6. What are some of the major noninfectious chronic diseases affecting Canadians today? What are the common risk factors?

7. List the common respiratory diseases affecting Canadians. Which of these diseases have a genetic basis? An environmental basis? An individual basis?

8. Compare and contrast the different types of headaches, including their symptoms and treatments.

9. Do you believe that PMS is a disorder or disease or simply a catchall name for many naturally occurring events in the menstrual cycle?

10. What are the medical risks of fibrocystic breast condition and endometriosis? How can they be treated?

11. Describe the symptoms and treatment of diabetes.

12. How can you tell whether your stomach is reacting to final exams or telling you you have a serious medical condition?

Application Exercise

Reread the What Do You Think? scenario at the beginning of this chapter and answer the following questions:

1. What was your initial reaction to the scenario?

2. What are some other legal issues that could arise or that already exist regarding all infectious diseases, including

STIs? Why do the rights of all the individuals involved in relationships need to be considered?

3. What services exist on your campus for people living with HIV infection or AIDS? What services focus on informing people about sexually transmitted diseases?

Health on the Net

Canadian Infectious Disease Society
www.ualberta.ca/~mmid/cids/

Laboratory Centre for Disease Control
www.hwc.ca/hpb/lcdc/hp_eng.html

WHO Division of Communicable Diseases
www.who.ch/programmes/cds/CDS_Homepage.html

Life's Transitions

The Aging Process

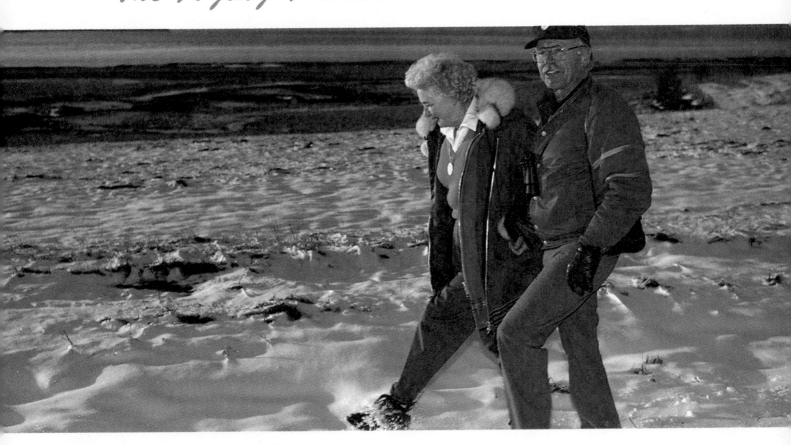

CHAPTER OBJECTIVES

◆ Review the definition of aging, and explain the related concepts of biological age, psychological age, social age, legal age, and functional age.

◆ Explain the impact on society of the growing population of the elderly, including considerations of economics, health care, housing and living arrangements, and ethical and moral issues.

◆ Discuss the biological and psychosocial theories of aging and examine how knowledge of these theories may have an impact on your own aging process.

◆ Identify the major physiological changes that occur as a result of the aging process.

◆ Discuss the unique health challenges faced by the elderly.

◆ Define *death* using different criteria and evaluate why people deny death.

◆ Discuss the stages of the grieving process and describe several strategies for coping more effectively with death.

◆ Review the decisions that are necessary when someone is dying or has died, including hospice care, funeral arrangements, wills, and organ donations.

◆ Describe the ethical concerns that arise from the concepts of the right to die and rational suicide.

Bonnie, aged 82, is a springboard diver. Every morning, she walks ten blocks to the city pool, where she practises her diving and swims to stay in shape. Erin, aged 79, is an internationally recognized expert in family dysfunction. She travels extensively, giving several lectures a week, volunteering her services to community groups, and maintaining an active social life with many close friends. Stewart, aged 83, is a master's level marathoner. He lifts weights regularly, rides a bike, and hikes the hills and valleys around his home when he is not training for his next race. He is a professional writer and has just learned how to run the software programs Word for Windows and Excel on his computer.

■ What do all these people have in common? Do you know any elderly people like them? How do they compare to your own grandparents? What factors do you think have contributed to their healthy aging? Why do you think these people seem atypical? Are they really that unusual?

Every moment of every day, we are involved in a steady aging process. Everything in the universe—animals, plants, mountain peaks, rivers, planets, even atoms—changes over time. This process is commonly referred to as aging. Aging is something that cannot be avoided, despite the perennial human quest for a fountain of youth. Since you can't stop the process, why not resolve to have a positive aging experience by improving your understanding of the various aspects of aging, taking steps toward maximizing your potential, and learning to adapt and develop strengths you can draw upon over a lifetime?

Who you are as you age and the manner in which you view aging (either as a natural part of living or as an inevitable move toward disease and death) are important factors in how successfully you will adapt to life's transitions. If you view these transitions as periods of growth, as changes that will lead to improved mental, emotional, spiritual, and physical phases in your development as a human being, your journey through even the most difficult times may be easier. Explore your own notions about aging in the Rate Yourself box. See how they change after you have read this chapter.

Aging: The patterns of life changes that occur in members of all species as they grow older.

Ageism: Discrimination based on age.

Gerontology: The study of our individual and collective aging processes.

From the moment of conception, we have genetic predispositions that influence our vulnerabilities to many diseases, our physical characteristics, and many other traits that make us unique. Maternal nutrition and health habits influence our health while we are in the womb and during the early months after birth. From the time we are born, we begin to take on characteristics that distinguish us from everyone else. We grow, we change, and we pass through many physical and psychological phases. **Aging** has traditionally been described as the patterns of life changes that occur in members of all species as they grow older. Some believe that it begins at the moment of conception. Others contend that it starts at birth. Still others believe that true aging does not begin until we reach our 40s.

Typically, experts and laypersons alike have used chronological age to assign a person to a particular life-cycle stage. However, people of different chronological ages view age very differently. To the 4-year-old, a university student seems quite old. To the 20-year-old, parents in their 40s are over the hill. Have you ever heard your 65-year-old grandparents talking about "those old people down the street"? Views of aging are also coloured by occupation. For example, a professional linebacker may find himself too old to play football in his mid-30s. Although some baseball players have continued to demonstrate high levels of skills into their 40s, most players are considering other careers by the time they reach 40. Airline pilots and police officers are often retired in their 50s, while professors, senators, and prime ministers may work well into their 70s. Perhaps our traditional definitions of aging need careful reexamination.

What's Your Aging IQ?

Test your knowledge of healthy aging by taking the following test. Answer TRUE or FALSE to each question. Then improve your aging IQ by reading the answers below.

1. Families don't bother with their older relatives.
2. All people become confused or forgetful if they live long enough.
3. You can become too old to exercise.
4. Heart disease is a much bigger problem for older men than for older women.
5. The older you get, the less you sleep.
6. Most older people are depressed. Why shouldn't they be?
7. Older people take more medications than do younger people.
8. People begin to lose interest in sex around age 55.
9. Older people may as well accept urinary accidents as a fact of life.
10. Suicide is mainly a problem for teenagers, not for older people.
11. Falls and injuries just happen to older people.
12. Extremes of heat and cold can be especially dangerous for older people.

Answers

1. False. Most older people live close to their children and see them often. Many live with their spouses. An estimated 80 percent of men and 60 percent of women live in family settings. Only 5 percent of the elderly live in nursing homes.
2. False. Although the confusion and forgetfulness caused by Alzheimer's disease is irreversible, there are at least 100 other problems (head injury, high fever, poor nutrition, adverse drug effects, depression, etc.) that can cause the same symptoms.
3. False. Exercise at any age is beneficial, though the elderly should see a physician for specific guidelines.

4. False. The risk of heart disease after menopause increases dramatically for women. By age 65, both men and women have a 1 in 3 chance of showing symptoms of heart disease.
5. False. In later life, it's the quality of sleep that declines, not total sleep time. As people age, their night sleeping becomes more fragmented and they tend to take more naps during the day.
6. False. Most older people are not depressed. When depression does occur in older people, it is treatable with the same approaches used earlier in the life cycle: family support, psychotherapy, and antidepressant medications.
7. True. Older people often have a combination of conditions that require drugs. Since the chance of adverse reactions to drugs rises with age, careful monitoring is necessary.
8. False. Most older people can lead active, satisfying sex lives.
9. False. Urinary incontinence is a symptom, not a disease. It may be caused by infection, diseases, or the use of certain drugs, and there are many options for treatment.
10. False. Suicide is most prevalent among people age 65 and older. Also, suicide attempts in this group have a higher success rate.
11. False. Falls are the most common cause of injuries among people over 65. Many falls can be avoided by regular vision checks, hearing tests, and improved safety habits in the home. Also important is monitoring the effects of certain medications on balance and coordination.
12. True. The body's thermostat tends to function less efficiently with age, making the older person's body less able to adapt to extreme temperature changes.

Source: Adapted from U.S. Department of Health and Human Services, National Institutes of Health, National Institute on Aging, *What's Your Aging IQ?* (Washington, D.C.: Government Printing Office, 1991).

REDEFINING AGING

Discrimination against people based on age is known as **ageism.** When directed against the elderly, this type of discrimination carries with it social ostracism and negative portrayals of older people. A developmental task approach to life-span changes tends to reduce the potential for ageist or negatively biased perceptions about what occurs as a person ages chronologically.

The study of individual and collective aging processes, known as **gerontology**, explores the reasons for aging and the ways in which people cope with and adapt to this process. Gerontologists have identified several types of age-related characteristics that should be used to determine where a person is in terms of biological, psychological, social, legal, and functional life-stage development:[1]

- *Biological age* refers to the relative age or condition of the person's organs and body systems. Arthritis and other chronic conditions often accelerate the aging process.

- *Psychological age* refers to a person's adaptive capacities, such as coping abilities and intelligence, and to the person's awareness of his or her individual capabilities, self-efficacy, and general ability to adapt to a given situation.

- *Social age* refers to a person's habits and roles relative to society's expectations. People in a particular life stage often share similar tastes in music, television shows, and decor.

- *Legal age,* or chronological age, is probably the most common definition of age in Canada. Legal age is based on chronological years and is used to determine such things as voting rights, driving privileges, drinking age, eligibility for old age security and the Canada Pension Plan and a host of other rights and obligations.

- *Functional age* refers to the ways in which people compare to others of a similar age. It is difficult to separate functional aging from many of the other types of aging, particularly chronological and biological aging.

What Is Normal Aging?

Contemporary gerontologists have begun to analyze the vast majority of people who continue to live full and productive lives throughout their later years. In the past, our youth-oriented society has viewed the onset of the physiological changes that occur with aging as something to be dreaded. The aging process was seen primarily from a pathological (disease) perspective, and therefore as a time of decline; the focus was not on the gains and positive aspects of normal adult development throughout the life span. Many of these positive developments occur in the areas of emotional and social life as older adults learn to cope with and adapt to the many changes and crises that life may hold in store for them.

Gerontologists have devised several categories for specific age-related characteristics. For example, people who reach the age of 65 are considered to fit the general category of old age. They receive special consideration in the

> **Young-old:** People aged 65 to 74.
>
> **Middle-old:** People aged 75 to 84.
>
> **Old-old:** People 85 and over.

form of government assistance programs such as the old age pension. People aged 65 to 74 are viewed as the **young-old**; those aged 75 to 84 are the **middle-old** group; those 85 and over are classified as the **old-old.**

You should note that chronological age is not the only component to be considered when objectively defining *aging.* The question is not how many years a person has lived, but how much life the person has packed into those years. This quality-of-life index, combined with the inevitable chronological process, appears to be the best indicator of the "aging gracefully" phenomenon. The eternal question then becomes "How can I age gracefully?" Most experts today agree that the best way to experience a productive, full, and satisfying old age is to take appropriate action to lead a productive, full, and satisfying life prior to old age. Essentially, older people are the product of their lifelong experiences, molded over years of happiness, heartbreak, and day-to-day existence.

> ### *W*HAT DO YOU THINK?
>
> What factors influence the aging process? Which of these factors do you have the power to change through the behaviours that you engage in right now?

*W*HO ARE THE ELDERLY?

Contrary to popular belief, the elderly are not and never will be the "forgotten minority." The 65-and-over age group will unquestionably be a major force in the future social, political, and economic plans of the nation because of their sheer numbers and buying power. By the year

---

TABLE 14.1 ▪ Canada's Elderly

Canada's total population in 1996 stood at 29 963 000, with 15 118 600 women and 14 845 000 men.

Figures below are in thousands.

Age	Total	Men	Women
65–69	1129.3	536.2	593.1
70–74	979.9	432.8	547.1
75–79	704.3	289.2	415.1
80–84	467.6	174.9	292.7
85–89	240.6	78.3	162.3
90+	120.5	32.5	88.0

Source: Statistics Canada, 1996, **http://www.statcan.ca/english/Pgdb/ People/Population/demo10a.htm.**

2010, a whole generation of 1960s "flower children," who once proclaimed that no one over 30 could be trusted, will begin turning 65. Whereas people aged 65 and older made up 12 percent of the Canadian population in 1992, they are projected to make up 22 percent of the population by 2036 (see Tables 14.1 and 14.2).

A Profile of Today's Elderly

Well over half of these seniors will be women. Because women tend to live longer than men, women comprise relatively large proportions of older age groups. For example, of Canadians currently aged 80 and older, 63 percent are women.

Marital Status. Most men in their 70s and 80s remain married. However, because women tend to outlive their husbands, they are far more likely to be widowed later in life. One consequence is that a relatively large proportion of older women end up living alone.[2]

Financial Security. Family income of elderly families (head over 65) increased in the 1980s from $38 345 to $43 533 in 1989, then decreased to $42 923(in constant 1995 dollars).[3] On the whole, the elderly are doing better today financially than in 1980. In 1980, 34 percent of elderly people had incomes below Statistics Canada's Low-Income Cut-Off (LICO—commonly called the poverty line); in 1994, the figure was 19.3 percent. The rate is higher for unattached elderly people and the decrease only marginal (43 percent poor in 1980, and 40 percent in 1994).[4] People who live by themselves rather than with other family members are more likely to live in "straitened circumstances"; this is particularly so among women. Indeed, of the women aged 65 and over living by themselves, more than half have incomes below the LICOs, and rely rely on old age security (OAS) and the guaranteed income supplement (GIS).

Housing and Living Arrangements. With the costs of owning and maintaining a home slowly moving beyond the reach of the average Canadian, housing problems for low-income elderly people are becoming more acute. Where will the generation of baby-boom elderly find suitable housing? Who will provide the necessary social services, and who will pay the bill? Will the family of the

Learning to cope with challenges and changes early in life develops attitudes and skills that contribute to a full and satisfying old age.

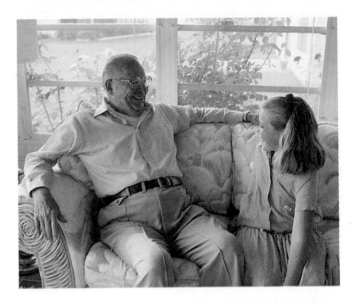

future be forced to coexist with several generations under one roof?

Contrary to popular opinion, most older people do not live in nursing homes. The majority of older people live in family settings until their final days.

Ethical and Moral Considerations. As we have already noted, the "senior boom" of the 1990s and beyond may force us to reexamine many of our present attitudes and practices. At the present time, the implications for an already overburdened health care delivery system are staggering. For example, with our current shortage of donor organs, will we be continually forced to decide whether a 75-year-old should receive a heart transplant instead of a 50-year-old? Questions have already surfaced regarding the efficacy of hooking a terminally ill older person up to costly machines that may prolong life for a few weeks or months but overtax our health care resources. Is the prolongation of life at all costs a moral imperative, or will future generations be forced to devise a set of criteria for deciding who will be helped and who will not? These questions represent potential concerns and problems for all of us.

TABLE 14.2 ■ The Elderly as a Proportion of Total Population, 1951–2036 (Projected)

	1951	1961	1971	1981	1991	2001	2011	2021	2031	2036
Age 65+	7.8%	7.6%	8.1%	9.7%	11.6%	12.9%	14.6%	18.6%	22.7%	23.2%
Age 85+	0.4%	0.4%	0.6%	0.8%	1.0%	1.5%	2.1%	2.3%	2.8%	3.4%

Source: Bertrand Desjardins, "Population Ageing and the Elderly," *Current Demographic Analysis* (Statistics Canada, 1993.)

WHAT DO YOU THINK?

Why are so many people concerned about the greying of Canada? What impact will the boom of elderly people have on society? What actions can we take now to minimize problems in the future?

THEORIES ON AGING

Biological Theories

Of the various theories about the biological causes of aging, the following are among the most commonly accepted.

- *The wear-and-tear theory* states that, like everything else in the universe, the human body wears out. Proponents of the wear-and-tear theory argue that activities such as jogging may actually predispose people to premature bone and joint injuries in later years, particularly in the lower back, hip, and knee areas.

- *The cellular theory* states that at birth we have only a certain number of usable cells, and these cells are genetically programmed to divide or reproduce only a limited number of times. Once these cells reach the end of their reproductive cycle, they begin to die and the organs they make up begin to show signs of deterioration. The rate of deterioration varies from person to person, and the impact of the deterioration depends on the system involved.

- *The autoimmune theory* attributes aging to the decline of the body's immunological system. Studies indicate that as we age, our immune systems become less effective in fighting disease. In some instances, the immune system appears to lose control and to turn its protective mechanisms inward, actually attacking the person's own body. Some gerontologists believe that the condition increases in frequency and severity with age.

- *The genetic mutation theory* proposes that the number of cells exhibiting unusual or different characteristics increases with age. Proponents of this theory believe that aging is related to the amount of mutational damage within the genes. The greater the mutation, the greater the chance that cells will not function properly, leading to eventual dysfunction of body organs and systems.

Psychosocial Theories

Numerous psychological and sociological factors also have a strong influence on the manner in which people age. Psy-

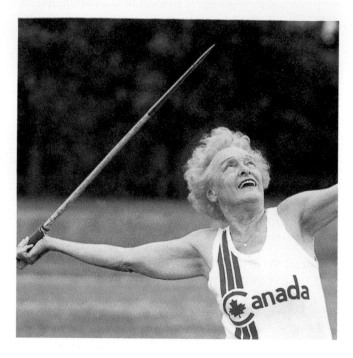

Some people seem to defy many of the theories of aging by remaining fit and even able to participate in competitive sports well into their seventies.

chologists Erik Erikson and Robert Peck have formulated theories of personality development that encompass the human life span. Their theories emphasize adaptation and adjustment as related to self-development. In his developmental model, Erikson states that people must progress through eight critical stages during their lifetimes. If a person does not receive the proper stimulus or develop effective methods of coping with life's turmoil from infancy onward, problems are likely to develop later in life. According to this theory, attitudes, behaviours, and beliefs related to maladjustments in old age are often a result of problems encountered in earlier stages of a person's life.

Peck focusses much of his developmental theory on the crucial issues of middle and old age. He argues that during these periods people face a series of increasingly stressful tasks. Those who are poorly adjusted psychologically or who have not developed appropriate coping skills are likely to undergo a painful aging process.

A key element in the theories of both Erikson and Peck is the incorporation of age-related factors into lifelong behaviour patterns. Both models stress that successful aging involves maintaining emotional as well as physical well-being. Most probably, a combination of psychosocial and biological factors and environmental "trigger mechanisms" causes each of us to age in a unique manner. The question then arises as to what is considered normal in the aging process. How much change is inevitable and how much can be avoided?

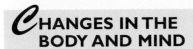

CHANGES IN THE BODY AND MIND

Answers to the question of what is "typical" or "normal" when applied to aging are highly speculative. In order to assess the typical aging process, we should probably ask ourselves what we can reasonably expect to happen to our bodies as we grow older.

Physical Changes

Although the physiological consequences of aging differ in their severity and timing from person to person, there are standard changes that occur as a result of the aging process.

The Skin.   As a normal consequence of aging, the skin becomes thinner and loses elasticity, particularly in the outer surfaces. Fat deposits, which add to the soft lines and shape of the skin, begin to diminish. Starting at about age 30, lines develop on the forehead as a result of smiling, squinting, and other facial expressions. These lines become more pronounced, with added "crow's-feet" around the eyes, during the 40s. During a person's 50s and 60s, the skin begins to sag and lose colour, leading to pallor in the 70s. Body fat in underlying layers of skin continues to be redistributed away from the limbs and extremities into the trunk region of the body. Age spots become more numerous because of excessive pigment accumulation under the skin. The sun tends to increase pigment production, leading to more age spots.

Bones and Joints.   Throughout the life span, your bones are continually changing because of the accumulation and loss of minerals. By the third or fourth decade of life, mineral loss from bones becomes more prevalent than mineral accumulation, resulting in a weakening and porosity (diminishing density) of bony tissue. This loss of minerals (particularly calcium) occurs in both sexes, although it is much more common in females. Loss of calcium can contribute to **osteoporosis**, a condition characterized by weakened, porous, and fractured bones.

Although many people consider osteoporosis a disease of the elderly, it is actually a progressive disorder that may already have begun to affect you. When you hear of osteoporosis, you may envision a slumped over individual with a characteristic "dowager's hump" in the upper back, but this is the rare extreme of the condition. Bone loss occurs over many years and may be without symptoms until actual fractures occur or are diagnosed via X-rays. The spine, hips, and wrists are the most common sites of fractures, though other bones of the body may be involved.[5]

Osteoporotic fractures of the hip, vertebrae, proximal humerus, pelvis, and wrist increase in incidence with age and are more common among women. Moniz estimates

that one in four women aged 60 years and over will have an osteoporotic fracture. About one-third of all women aged 65 and over are afflicted with vertebral osteoporosis. Most hip fractures occur in those aged 80 and over.[6] Several risk factors for developing osteoporosis have been identified:

- *Gender:* Women have a four times greater risk than men have. Their peak bone mass is lower than men's, and they experience an accelerated rate of bone loss after menopause.

- *Age:* After the third and fourth decade of life, all individuals lose bone mass and are more susceptible.

- *Low bone mass:* Low bone mass is one of the strongest predictors of osteoporosis. Measurement of bone density is an important aspect of risk assessment.

- *Early menopause:* The early occurrence of menopause, whether natural or caused by surgery, means that the positive effects of estrogen are lost for a longer period of time. (Decreases in sex hormones—estrogen in females and testosterone in males—appear to increase risk for the disease.) Menstrual disturbances, such as those caused by anorexia or bulimia or excessive exercise, may similarly result in an early loss of bone mass.

- *Thin, small-framed body:* Petite, thin women usually have a relatively low peak bone mass and are therefore at greater risk for osteoporosis. (This is one of the few health areas in which being larger and even slightly overweight is an advantage.)

- *Race:* Whites and Asians are at higher risk of developing osteoporosis than are blacks because blacks have heavier bone density on average. Black women have about one-half the incidence of hip fractures of white women.

- *Lack of calcium:* A lifetime of low calcium intake (well below the RNI and below the natural loss of calcium of 300 to 400 milligrams per day) may result in low peak bone mass and above-average loss of bone mass throughout adulthood.

- *Lack of physical activity:* Immobilized, bedridden, or very inactive people usually have less muscle and bone mass.

- *Cigarette smoking:* Though the mechanism is not clear, smoking is linked to the development of osteoporosis.

- *Alcohol and/or caffeine:* Abuse of these substances is also linked to the development of osteoporosis.

Osteoporosis: A degenerative bone disorder characterized by increasingly porous bones.

- *Heredity:* Unidentified hereditary factors may play a role in the development of osteoporosis.[7]

The goal of both treatment and prevention of osteoporosis is to decrease the likelihood and severity of bone fractures. Currently accepted treatments of established osteoporosis include adequate calcium intake, daily weight-bearing exercises approved by a physician, fall-prevention measures, and use of the hormones estrogen (in those not at high risk for certain forms of cancer) and calcitonin.[8] A recent study has shown that increasing calcium intake to 1380 milligrams per day—an amount that exceeds the current RNI for calcium—both reduces bone loss and increases bone mineralization in women aged 58 to 77.[9] Other therapies for osteoporosis, such as sodium fluoride, various metabolites of vitamin D, and bisphosphonates, are under investigation.[10]

Of these treatments, increasing calcium intake during childhood and young adulthood appears to be quite effective in reducing lifelong risk by promoting denser bone mass.[11] The Canadian RNI for calcium is 800 milligrams per day; in the United States, the Recommended Daily Allowance for people between 19 and 24 years of age is 1200 milligrams. Many experts suggest that the number should be even higher and recommend a standard of 1500 milligrams per day for postmenopausal women.

Yet because they eat less, older women can have difficulty getting the recommended amounts of vitamins and minerals. For instance, in a recent provincial survey, the energy intake of 70 percent of Quebec women aged 65 to 74 years was below 1500 calories per day and 25 percent were consuming less than half the recommended intake of calcium.[12]

Although the vitamin industry would like all of us to take megadoses of calcium every day, the preferred source of calcium is a nutritionally balanced diet.[13] Dairy products, including milk, yoghurt, and cheese, are the best sources of dietary calcium; canned fish, certain dark green leafy vegetables (such as kale and broccoli), legumes, calcium-enriched grain products, and fortified fruit juices may also be good sources.

Regular exercise of weight-bearing joints, maintenance of muscular strength and flexibility, and an adequate intake of calcium are probably your best routes of prevention during early adulthood.

Urinary incontinence: The inability to control urination.

Cataracts: Clouding of the lens that interrupts the focussing of light on the retina, resulting in blurred vision or eventual blindness.

Glaucoma: Elevation of pressure within the eyeball, leading to hardening of the eyeball, impaired vision, and possible blindness.

As you approach menopause or if you have other ailments that could increase your risk, consult an endocrinologist or orthopedic specialist to determine what forms of medical treatment may be most effective for minimizing your risk for osteoporosis.

The Head. With age, features of the head enlarge and become more noticeable. Increased cartilage and fatty tissue cause the nose to grow a half-inch wider and another half-inch longer. Earlobes get thicker and grow longer, while overall head circumference increases one-quarter of an inch per decade, even though the brain itself shrinks. The skull becomes thicker with age.

The Urinary Tract. One problem often associated with aging is **urinary incontinence**, which ranges from passing a few drops of urine while laughing or sneezing to having no control over when and where urination takes place.

However, incontinence is not an inevitable part of the aging process. Most cases are caused by highly treatable underlying neurological problems that affect the central nervous system, medications, infections of the pelvic muscles, weakness in the pelvic walls, or other problems. When the problem is treated, the incontinence usually vanishes.[14]

Incontinence poses major social, physical, and emotional problems for the elderly. Fortunately, there are many treatments for this problem. Drug therapy can slow bladder contractions, increase bladder capacity, contract or relax the bladder sphincter, and increase fluid output. Surgery to repair the pelvic floor is often successful in stress incontinence. Artificial devices that slow urine flow, improvements in access to toilet facilities, rigid schedules for urination, exercises to strengthen the pelvic floor, and many newer treatments have also shown promise.[15]

The Heart and Lungs. Resting heart rate stays about the same during a person's life, but the stroke volume (the amount of blood the muscle pushes out per beat) diminishes as heart muscles deteriorate. Vital capacity, or the amount of air that moves when you inhale and exhale at maximum effort, also declines with age. Exercise can do a great deal to reduce potential deterioration in heart and lung function.

Eyesight. By the age of 30, the lens of the eye begins to harden, causing specific problems by the early 40s. The lens begins to yellow and loses transparency, while the pupil of the eye begins to shrink, allowing less light to penetrate. Activities such as reading become more difficult, particularly in dim light. By age 60, depth perception declines and farsightedness often develops. A need for glasses usually develops in the 40s that evolves into a need for bifocals in the 50s and trifocals in the 60s. **Cataracts** (clouding of the lens) and **glaucoma** (elevation of pressure within the eyeball) become more likely. There may eventually be a tendency toward colour-blindness, especially for shades of blue and green.

Hearing. The ability to hear high-frequency consonants (for example, *s*, *t*, and *z*) diminishes with age. Much of the actual hearing loss is in the ability to distinguish not normal conversational tones but extreme ranges of sound.

Taste. The sense of taste begins to decline as a person gets older. At age 30, each tiny elevation on the tongue (called papilla) has 245 taste buds. By the age of 70, each has only 88 left. The mouth gets drier as salivary glands secrete less fluid. The ability to distinguish sweet, sour, bitter, and salty tastes diminishes. Elderly people often compensate for their diminished sense of taste by adding excessive amounts of salt, sugar, and other flavour enhancers to their food.

Smell and Touch. The sense of smell also diminishes with age. As a result of this loss, coupled with the loss of the sense of taste, food is often less appealing to older people. This lack of appeal may be one factor in the tendency of seniors to be malnourished. Pain receptors also become less effective. The tactile senses decline.

Mobility. Nearly 50 percent of older Canadians report some disability, usually related to mobility and agility; 34 percent require help with housework and shopping. Both incidence and severity of disability increase with age.[16]

Sexual Changes. As men age, they experience notable changes in sexual functioning. Whereas the degree and rate of change vary greatly from person to person, the following changes generally occur:

1. The ability to obtain an erection is slowed.

2. The ability to maintain an erection is diminished.

3. The length of the refractory period between orgasms increases.

4. The angle of the erection declines with age.

5. The orgasm itself grows shorter in duration.

   Women also experience several changes:

1. Menopause usually occurs between the ages of 45 and 55. Women may experience such symptoms as hot flashes, mood swings, weight gain, development of facial hair, and other hormone-related problems.

2. The walls of the vagina become less elastic, and the epithelium thins, making painful intercourse more likely.

3. Vaginal secretions during sexual activity diminish.

4. The breasts decrease in firmness. Loss of fat in various areas leads to fewer curves, with a decrease in the soft lines of the body contours.

Body Comfort. Because of the loss of body fat, thinning of the epithelium, and diminished glandular activity, elderly people experience greater difficulty in regulating body temperature. This change means that their ability to withstand extreme cold or heat may be very limited, thus increasing the risks of hypothermia, heat stroke, and heat exhaustion.

Many elderly retain their intellectual and artistic abilities into old age, despite the inevitable physical declines and progressive diminishment of the sensory functions of sight, sound, taste, smell, and touch.

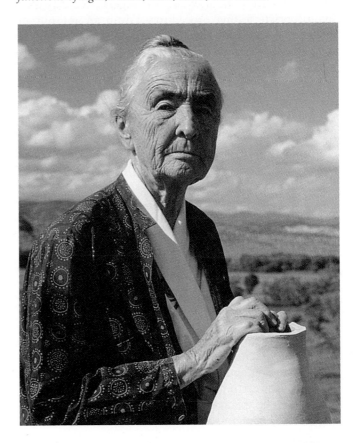

Many of these changes are exacerbated by poor nutrition. For a variety of reasons, getting adequate nutrition is a problem for many seniors. Using assessments based on risk factors associated with malnutrition, 40 to 50 percent of community-dwelling seniors seem to have a moderate to high risk of becoming malnourished, especially among those who live alone. The limited data on frailer seniors suggest that the picture is much worse. Poor nutrition worsens the impact of chronic disease, reduces resistance to infections, slows healing, and increases use of the health care system.

Identifying seniors at risk for malnutrition is key to the empowerment of seniors and their caregivers to strive to maintain an optimal quality of life and to sustain successful aging.[17]

WHAT DO YOU THINK?

Of the health conditions listed in this section, which ones can you prevent? Which ones can you delay? What actions can you take now to protect yourself from these problems?

Mental Changes

Intelligence. Stereotypes concerning inevitable intellectual decline among the elderly have been largely refuted. Recent research has demonstrated that much of our previous knowledge about elderly intelligence was based on inappropriate testing procedures. Given an appropriate length of time, elderly people may learn and develop skills in a similar manner to younger people. Researchers have also determined that what many elderly people lack in speed of learning they make up for in practical knowledge—that is, the "wisdom of age."

Memory. Have you ever wondered why your grandfather seems unable to remember what he did last weekend even though he can graphically depict the details of a social event that occurred 40 years earlier? This phenomenon is not unusual among the elderly. Research indicates that although short-term memory may fluctuate on a daily basis, the ability to remember events from past decades seems to remain largely unchanged in many elderly people.

Flexibility Versus Rigidity. Although it is widely believed that people become more like one another as they age, nothing could be further from the truth. Having lived through a multitude of experiences and having faced diverse joys, sorrows, and obstacles, the typical elderly person has developed unique methods of coping with life. These unique adaptive variations make for interesting differences in how the elderly confront the many changes brought on by the aging process. As a group, the elderly are extremely heterogeneous.

Depression. Most adults continue to lead healthy, fulfilling lives as they grow older. Some research indicates, however, that depression may be the most common psychological problem facing older adults.

Senility. Over the years, the elderly have often been the victims of ageist attitudes. People who were chronologically old were often labelled "senile" whenever they displayed memory failure, errors in judgement, disorientation, or erratic behaviours. Today scientists recognize that these same symptoms can occur at any age and for various reasons, including disease or the use of OTC and prescription drugs. When the underlying problems are corrected, the memory loss and disorientation also improve. Currently, the term **senility** is seldom used except to describe a very small group of organic disorders.

Alzheimer's Disease. Dementias are progressive brain impairments that interfere with memory and normal intellectual functioning. Although there are many types of dementia, one of the most common forms is **Alzheimer's disease.**

Currently, Alzheimer's afflicts an estimated 1 in 20 people between the ages of 65 and 75 and 1 in 5 people over the age of 80. With the Canadian population gradually aging, the total number of Alzheimer's sufferers seems almost certain to increase, representing a real economic burden for the future. While the disease is associated in most people's minds strictly with the elderly, it has been diagnosed in people as young as in their late 40s. In fact, about 5 percent of all cases occur before age 65.

Alzheimer's refers to a degenerative disease of the brain in which nerve cells stop communicating with one another. Ordinarily, brain cells communicate by releasing chemicals that allow the cells to receive and transmit messages for various types of behaviour. In Alzheimer's patients, the brain doesn't produce enough of these chemicals, cells can't communicate, and eventually the cells die.

This degeneration happens in the sections of the brain that affect memory, speech, and personality, leaving the parts that control other bodily functions, such as heartbeat and breathing, working just fine. Thus, the mind begins to go as the body lives on. It all happens in a slow, progressive manner, and it may be as long as 20 years before you notice symptoms.

What are the symptoms of Alzheimer's? Alzheimer's disease is characteristically diagnosed in three stages. During the first stage, symptoms include forgetfulness, memory loss, impaired judgement, increasing inability to handle routine tasks, disorientation, lack of interest in one's surroundings, and depression. These symptoms accelerate in the second stage, which also includes agitation and restlessness (especially at night), loss of sensory perceptions, muscle twitching, and repetitive actions. Many patients become depressed and there is a tendency to be combative and aggressive. In the final stage, disorientation is often complete. The person becomes completely dependent on others for eating, dressing, and other activities. Identity loss and speech problems are common symptoms. Eventually, control of bodily functions may be lost.

Once Alzheimer's disease strikes, the victim's life expectancy is cut in half. Tragically, there is little that can be done at present to treat the disorder. Scientists are experimenting with various drug regimens, but it is unlikely that a drug will be discovered in the immediate future that will undo the damage associated with Alzheimer's disease.

Senility: A term associated with loss of memory and judgement and orientation problems occurring in a small percentage of the elderly.

Alzheimer's disease: A chronic condition involving changes in nerve fibres of the brain that results in mental deterioration.

Alternative Medicine and Older Canadians

Scientific medicine is familiar to us in Canada. What about alternative medicines? What are their techniques? Are they useful for seniors? While a small percentage of seniors currently use them, tomorrow's seniors, people aged 50 to 64, are already using them fairly frequently. Since its creation, the National Advisory Council on Aging (NACA) has encouraged seniors to get as much information as possible about the health care services and drug treatments they are prescribed in order to make informed decisions. This advice remains, whether it concerns traditional or alternative treatment.

Tips

Get information from family and friends. As well, there are numerous publications on the subject of alternative medicines; your municipal library probably has some. Health food stores are also familiar with the resources in your community.

Ask questions. If your alternative medicine practitioner recommends an unusual procedure, think it over. Why is it recommended? Are there any contraindications or side-effects? What results can you hope for?

Ask yourself whether you have confidence in the practitioner. Confidence is important. Do you feel that this person is listening to your needs? Does he or she understand your priorities? Is he or she able to allay your concerns?

Ask yourself whether you are prepared to commit yourself to this process, which may require some major lifestyle changes. Alternative therapies often require significant participation on the part of the patient.

Beware of people who promise you a cureall. There are fads in this field as in others. Inquire about the type of training and experience your practitioner has. As with any other service, reevaluate your commitment to the selected therapy if you do not obtain benefits from it.

Fact File

- In 1994, 12 percent of Canadians consulted both a doctor and an alternative medicine practitioner. Only 2 percent of adults relied exclusively on some form of alternative medicine.

- The use of alternative medicine tends to be more common among women (16 percent) than among men (13 percent).

- A number of studies have shown that it is the most educated and highest-income-earners who make greater use of alternative medicines.

- In a Toronto study of people over the age of 55, 42 of the 240 respondents had consulted an alternative medicine practitioner. They were more likely to take an active part in their health care.

- In a study of self-health techniques among 940 Vancouver residents over the age of 50, the most common techniques were exercise (70 percent), dietary changes (50 percent), stress reduction (50 percent), weight control (50 percent), prayer and meditation (45 percent), and smoking cessation (25 percent). Self-help groups (10 percent) and alternative medicines including plant-based remedies, acupuncture, and massage (15 percent) were the least used.

Sources: National Advisory Council on Aging, "Alternative Medicine and Seniors: an Emphasis on Collaboration," *Expression;* W. Millar and M. P. Beaudet, "Data Taken from the 1994 National Population Health Survey," *Canadian Social Trends,* Spring 1996, 27; M. Kelner, B. Wellman, and B. Wigdor, *The Use of Medical and Alternative Care by Older Adults,* research conducted at the Institute for Human Development, Life Course, and Aging, University of Toronto; B. Mitchell, "Preliminary Results from the First Wave," *North Shore Self Care Study Newsletter,* August 1996, 3, published by the Gerontology Research Centre of Simon Fraser University, British Columbia, K1A 0K9, **http://www.hwc.ca/datahpsb/seniors/index.html**

The results of research into the causes of Alzheimer's disease are inconclusive. Current research is looking into genetic predisposition, malfunction of the immune system, a slow-acting virus, chromosomal or genetic defects, and neurotransmitter imbalance, among other possibilities.

The only known detection test for Alzheimer's was announced in November 1994. Researchers at Harvard Medical School found that people with Alzheimer's appear to be very sensitive to eye drops similar to those used by doctors to dilate the pupils before performing an eye exam. Although many people feel a sensitivity to such eye drops, people with Alzheimer's show reaction with just 1 percent of the normal dose. The test should be available clinically by the end of 1996. Experts hope to use the test to detect Alzheimer's early enough that experimental drugs that may slow progress of the disease will be most effective.[18]

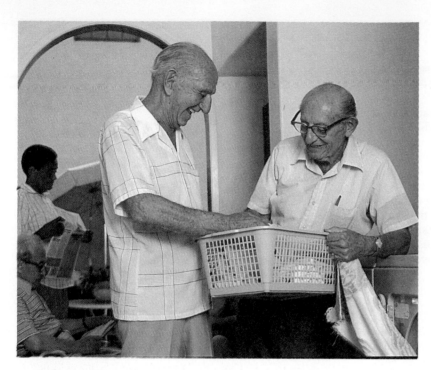

Older people in good health can maintain their independence and find companionship in community housing for the elderly.

$\mathscr{H}$EALTH CHALLENGES OF THE ELDERLY

The elderly are disproportionately victimized by a number of societally-induced problems. Other problems result when people do not develop the ability to cope properly with life's hurdles. Still other problems come from a perceived loss of control over the circumstances of their lives by the elderly—who watch loved ones die, are forced to retire, face problems with personal health, and confront an uncertain economy on a fixed income. If you develop certain skills in your earlier years and acquire strong social supports, you may significantly reduce your risk for problems in old age.

Prescription Drug Use: Unique Problems for the Elderly

It is extremely rare for elderly people to use illicit drugs, but some do overuse, and grow dependent upon, prescription drugs. Beset with numerous aches, pains, and inexplicable as well as diagnosable maladies, some elderly people take between four and six prescription drugs a day. Reported numbers of drugs taken are substantially higher for residents of health care institutions, but this may be because drugs that many of us purchase over the counter, such as ASA, are counted in the total numbers.

Anyone who combines different drugs runs the risk of dangerous drug interactions. The risks of adverse effects are even greater for people with circulation impairments and declining kidney and liver functions. Elderly people displaying symptoms of these drug-induced effects, which may include bizarre behaviour patterns or an appearance of being out of touch, are often misdiagnosed as being senile rather than examined for underlying causes and treated.

Over-the-Counter Remedies

Although today's elderly appear to be more receptive to medical treatment than the elderly of previous generations, a substantial segment of the over-60 population avoid orthodox medical treatment, viewing it as only a last resort. As might be expected, ASA and laxatives head the list of commonly used OTC medications for relief of arthritic pain and the irregular bowel activity sometimes experienced by the elderly.

Vitamins and Mineral Supplements

As with many bodily processes, the digestion of food begins to slow with age. Nevertheless, the body can still use almost all nutrients if they are consumed in moderate quantities and in the right combination. Following are some of the more common vitamin and mineral products often promoted as important to the elderly:

- *Calcium:* Many elderly people do not consume adequate amounts of calcium, or they may take it as an individual supplement without vitamin D, which is necessary for calcium absorption in the body. Research has begun to refute much of the previous thinking about the benefits of calcium supplements versus other treatments after bone and joint deterioration occurs.[19] Adequate calcium intake should be a part of a lifelong regimen of preventive health care.

- *Vitamin E:* Although some gerontologists believe that we should take extra vitamin E because it stops the formation of substances believed to cause aging, this theory is largely unsubstantiated. In fact, evidence suggests that megadoses of any of the fat-soluble vitamins may damage already deteriorating kidneys and livers.

- *Vitamin C:* The likelihood that this vitamin has any appreciable effect on life expectancy is minimal.

- *Vitamin B6 :* Recent research suggests that megadoses of vitamin B6 may cause symptoms similar to multiple sclerosis in some people, making it especially hazardous for the elderly.

Gender Issues: Caring for the Elderly

According to the most recent census data, elderly women fill a disproportionate place in Canadian society. In 1996, for example, there were 2.1 million women and 1.5 million men aged 65 and over. This difference in the number of older women and older men increases with age. Because women live seven years longer then men on average, elderly women are more likely than elderly men to be living alone, and thus to lack the support in the home that helps keep older people independent. The rate of institutionalization is twice as high among older people without a spouse as for married older people; for one thing, a married person has a built-in potential caretaker. Further, women are more likely than men to experience poverty and multiple chronic health problems, a situation referred to as **comorbidity.** Consequently, more elderly women than men are likely to need assistance from children, other relatives, friends, and neighbours.

*U*NDERSTANDING DEATH AND DYING

Death eventually comes to everyone. This is a depressing thought, but each of us must eventually accept the inevitable. Distractions and denial may postpone the reality of death, but they cannot eliminate it. The acceptance of death helps us shape our attitudes about the importance of life. Throughout history, humans have attempted to determine the nature and meaning of death. The questioning continues today. Although we will touch on moral and philosophical questions about death, we will not explore such issues in depth. Rather, our primary focus is to present dying and death as normal components of life and to discuss how we can cope with these events.

Confrontations with death elicit different feelings depending on many factors, including age, religious beliefs, family orientation, health, personal experience with death, and the circumstances of the death itself. To cope effectively with dying, we must address the individual needs of those involved. Why is it that we wish to deny, or even postpone, death? Let's begin by investigating what death means, at least in medical terms.

Defining Death

Dying is the process of decline in body functions resulting in the death of an organism. **Death** can be defined as the "final cessation of the vital functions" and also refers to a state in which these functions are "incapable of being restored."[20] This definition has become more significant as medical and scientific advances have made it increasingly possible to postpone death.

Although irreversible cessation of circulatory and respiratory functions acceptably defines death, irreversible cessation of brain function is also equivalent to death even though the heart continues to beat while the patient is on a respirator.

In 1968, following the publication of the Harvard Criteria for the diagnosis of brain death, the Canadian Medical Association (CMA) provided guidelines that were revised in 1974 and 1975. In 1976, guidelines were established in the United Kingdom, and in 1981, revised guidelines were published in the Journal of the American Medical Association. Brain death must be determined clinically by an experienced physician in accord with accepted medical standards.[21]

The following definitions have evolved to facilitate classification of various phases of biological death:

- *Cell death:* The gradual death of a cell after all metabolic activity has ceased. The rate of cellular death varies according to the type of tissue involved. For example, higher brain cells die five to eight minutes after respiration stops; striated muscle cells die after two to four hours; kidney cells die after about seven hours; and epithelial cells (hair and nails) die after several days. Rigor mortis, the temporary stiffening of muscles, is associated with cell death.

Comorbidity: The presence of a number of diseases at the same time.

Dying: The process of decline in body functions resulting in the death of an organism.

Death: The "final cessation of the vital functions" and the state in which these functions are "incapable of being restored."

- *Local death:* The death of a body part or portion of an organ without the death of the entire organism. For example, a kidney may fail, part of the heart muscle may die, or a limb or section of intestine may die as a result of loss of circulation.

- *Somatic death:* The death of the entire organism, as opposed to death of a part of an organ or an extremity.

- *Apparent death:* The cessation of vital physiologic functions, particularly spontaneous cardiac and respiratory activities, which produces a state simulating actual death but from which recovery is possible through the use of resuscitative efforts.

- *Functional death:* Extensive and irreversible damage to the central nervous system, with respiration and circulatory function maintained only by artificial means.

- *Brain death:* The termination of brain function, as evidenced by loss of all reflexes and electric activity of the brain or by irreversible coma. Brain death is confirmed by an **electroencephalogram (EEG)** reading of electrical activity of brain cells.

The Canadian Medical Association has established the following criteria for the clinical diagnosis of brain death: [22]

1. An etiology has been established that is capable of causing brain death and potentially reversible conditions have been excluded (drug intoxication, treatable metabolic disorders, core temperature less than 32.2°C, shock, and peripheral nerve or muscle dysfunction due to disease or neuromuscular-blocking drugs).

2. The patient is in deep coma and shows no response within the cranial nerve distribution to stimulation of any part of the body. In particular, there should be no motor response within the cranial nerve distribution to stimuli applied to any body regions. There should be no spontaneous or elicited movements arising from the brain. However, various spinal reflexes may persist in brain death.

3. Brain-stem reflexes are absent. Pupillary light and corneal, vestibulo-ocular, and pharyngeal reflexes must be absent. The pupils should be midsize or larger and must be unreactive to light. Care should be taken that atropine or related drugs that could block the pupillary response to light have not been given to the patient.

4. The patient does not breathe when taken off the respirator for an appropriate time.

5. The conditions listed above persist when the patient is reassessed after a suitable interval to ensure that the nonfunctioning state of the brain is persistent and to reduce the possibility of observer error.

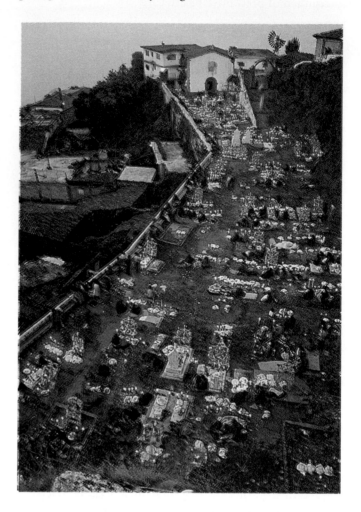

In some cultures death is not feared but viewed as a passage to a better state of being that is to be celebrated.

The CMA also suggests that a physician consult with another experienced physician before determining death.

WHAT DO YOU THINK?

How long do you think you will live? Do you have concerns about the quality of your life up until you die? What can you do now and in the future to help guarantee not only a long life but a healthy quality of life?

Denying Death

We can look at our attitudes toward death as falling on a continuum. At one end of the continuum, death is viewed as the enemy of humankind. Medical science has tended to promote this idea of death. At the other end of the continuum, death is accepted and even welcomed. [23] For people whose attitudes fall at this end, often people with a deep religious faith, death is a passage to a better state of being. But most of us perceive ourselves to be in the middle of this continuum. From this perspective, death is a bewildering mystery that elicits fear and apprehension as well as profoundly influences our attitudes, beliefs, and actions throughout our lives.

In Canada, there is a high level of discomfort associated with death and dying. As a result, we may avoid speaking about death in an effort to limit our own discomfort. You may wish to deny death if you

- avoid people who are grieving after the death of a loved one so you won't have to talk about it

- fail to validate a dying person's frightening situation by talking to the person as if nothing were wrong

- substitute euphemisms for the word *death* (a few examples are "passing away," "kicking the bucket," "no longer with us," "going to heaven," or "going to a better place")

- give false reassurances to people who are dying by saying things like "everything is going to be okay"

- shut off conversation about death by silencing people who are trying to talk about it

- do not touch people who are dying

Although some experts indicate that death denial has always been a predominant characteristic of our society, we must keep in mind that social attitudes change over time. The miraculous feats of science and medicine during the first half of the century created an attitude closer to death-defying than to death-denying. However, the pendulum appears to be swinging back. Today, a growing number of people are rejecting "high-tech" death—death postponed through the use of life-support technology—in favour of more personal, and perhaps more humane, alternatives. The concept of death as an enemy may be giving way to acceptance of dying as a natural part of life.

*7*HE PROCESS OF DYING

Dying is a complex process that includes physical, intellectual, social, spiritual, and emotional dimensions. Accordingly, we must consider the process of dying from several perspectives. Although the preceding section primarily examined the physical indicators of death, consideration of the emotional aspects of dying and "social death" is essential in establishing an appreciation for the multifaceted nature of life and health.

Coping Emotionally with Death

Science and medicine have enabled us to understand changes associated with growth, development, aging, and social roles throughout the life span, but they have not revealed the nature of death. This may partially explain why the transition from life to death evokes so much mystery and emotion. Although emotional reactions to dying vary, there seem to be many similarities in this process.

Much of our knowledge about reactions to dying stems from the work of Elisabeth Kübler-Ross, a major figure in modern **thanatology**, the study of death and dying. In 1969, Kübler-Ross published *On Death and Dying*, a sensitive analysis of the reactions of terminally ill patients. This pioneering work encouraged the development of death education as a discipline and prompted efforts to improve the care of dying patients. In her book, Kübler-Ross identified five psychological stages that terminally ill patients often experience as they approach death: denial, anger, bargaining, depression, and acceptance. The health care profession immediately embraced this "stage theory" and hastily applied it in clinical settings. However, research evidence supporting the concept of stages of grief is neither extensive nor convincing. Although it is normal to grieve when a severe loss has been sustained, some people never go through this process and instead remain emotionally calm. Others may pass back and forth between the stages.

A summation of the five stages follows.

- *Denial:* ("Not me, there must be a mistake.") This is usually the first stage, experienced as a sensation of shock and disbelief. A person intellectually accepts the impending death but rejects it emotionally. The patient is too confused and stunned to comprehend "not being" and thus rejects the idea. Within a relatively short time, the anxiety level may diminish, enabling the patient to sort through the powerful web of emotions.

- *Anger:* ("Why me?") Anger is another common reaction to the realization of imminent death. The person becomes angry at having to face death when others, including loved ones, are healthy and not threatened. The dying person perceives the situation as "unfair" or "senseless" and may be hostile to friends, family, physicians, or the world in general.

Electroencephalogram (EEG): A device that measures the electrical activity of brain cells.

Thanatology: The study of death and dying.

- *Bargaining:* ("If I'm allowed to live, I promise...") This stage generally occurs at about the middle of the progression toward acceptance of death. During this stage, the dying person may resolve to be a better person in return for an extension of life or may secretly pray for a short reprieve from death in order to experience a special event, such as a family wedding or birth.

- *Depression:* ("It's really going to happen to me and I can't do anything about it.") Depression eventually sets in as vitality diminishes and the patient begins to experience distressing symptoms with increasing frequency. The patient's deteriorating condition becomes impossible for him or her to deny, and feelings of doom and tremendous loss may become unbearably pervasive. Feelings of worthlessness and guilt are also common in this depressed state because the dying person may feel responsible for the emotional suffering of loved ones and the arduous but seemingly futile efforts of caregivers.

- *Acceptance:* ("I'm ready.") This is often the final stage. The patient stops battling with emotions and becomes very tired and weak. The need to sleep increases, and wakeful periods become shorter and less frequent. With acceptance, the patient does not "give up" and become sullen or resentfully resigned to death, but rather becomes passive. According to one dying patient, the acceptance stage is "almost void of feelings ... as if the pain had gone, the struggle is over, and there comes a time for the final rest before the long journey."[24] As he or she lets go, the dying person may no longer welcome visitors and may not wish to engage in conversation. Death usually occurs quietly and painlessly while the victim is unconscious.

Some of Kübler-Ross's contemporaries consider her stage theory to be too neat and orderly. Subsequent research has indicated that the experiences of dying people do not fit easily into specific stages and that patterns vary from person to person. A person may move from denial to depression, to anger, to denial again, and so on. Each individual has a distinct mix and process of grieving. Even if it is not accurate in all its particulars, however, Kübler-Ross's theory offers valuable insights for those seeking to understand or deal with the process of dying.

Social Death

The need for recognition and appreciation within a social group is nearly universal. Although the size and nature of the social group may vary widely, the need to belong exists in all of us. Loss of value or of appreciation by others can lead to **social death**, an irreversible situation in which a person is not treated like an active member of society. Dramatic examples of social death include the exile of nonconformists from their native countries or the excommunication of dissident members of religious orders. More often, however, social death is inflicted by avoidance of social interaction. Numerous studies indicate that people are treated differently when they are dying. The isolation that accompanies social death in terminally ill patients may be promoted by the following common behaviours:

- The dying person is referred to as if he or she were already dead.
- The dying person may be inadvertently excluded from conversations.
- Dying patients are often moved to terminal wards and are given minimal care.
- Bereaved family members are avoided, often for extended periods, because friends and neighbours are afraid of feeling uncomfortable in the presence of grief.
- Medical personnel may make degrading comments about patients in their presence.[25]

A decrease in meaningful social interaction often strips dying and bereaved people of recognition as valued members of society at a time when belonging is critical. Some dying people choose not to speak of their inevitable fate in an attempt to make others feel more comfortable and thus preserve vital relationships.

Near-Death Experiences

We cannot speak of the process of dying without mentioning near-death experiences. Thousands of similar reports have been given by people who have almost died or who were actually pronounced dead but subsequently recovered. The descriptions of feelings, perceptions, and visions associated with being near death have many common features. Three phases have been identified in a large number of near-death accounts: resistance, life re-

𝒲HAT DO YOU THINK?

Do you agree with Elisabeth Kübler-Ross's stages of dying? Have you ever lost someone close to you and then experienced any of these stages?

Social death: An irreversible situation in which a person is not treated like an active member of society.

Bereavement: The loss or deprivation experienced by a survivor when a loved one dies.

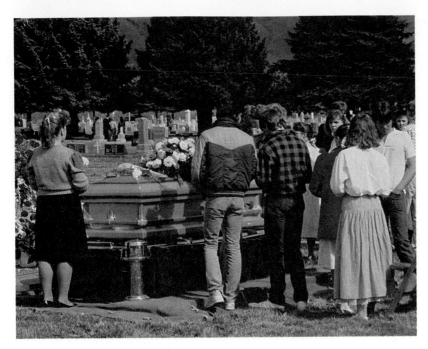

Teenage suicide, a tragically growing cause of death for young people, affects many people, but siblings and friends—who generally have little experience with death—are especially unable to cope with their grief.

view, and transcendence. During the initial phase, resistance, the dying person is aware of extreme danger and struggles desperately to escape from the unseen threat. Many people have reported a sensation of expanding fear. The second phase, life review, has been described as a feeling of being outside one's body and beyond danger. During this period, the dying person feels a sensation of security while observing his or her physical body from an emotionally detached perspective. The dying person's life experiences may also seem to pass by in rapid review. The last phase, transcendence, is characterized by a reported feeling of euphoria, contentment, and even ecstasy. Some people have recalled a sensation of being unified with nature and of having an awareness of infinity.

Coping with Loss

The losses resulting from the death of a loved one may be extremely difficult to cope with. The dying person, as well as close family and friends, frequently suffers emotionally and physically from the impending loss of critical relationships and roles. Words used to describe feelings and behaviour related to losses resulting from death include *bereavement, grief, grief work,* and *mourning.* These terms are related but not identical. An understanding of them may help you to comprehend the emotional processes associated with loss and the cultural constraints that often inhibit normal coping behaviour (see Figure 14.1).

Bereavement is generally defined as the loss or deprivation experienced by a survivor when a loved one dies. Because relationships vary in type and intensity, reactions to losses also vary. The death of a parent, a spouse, a sib-

ling, a child, a friend, or a pet will result in different kinds of feelings. In the lives of the bereaved or of close survivors, "holes" will be left by the loss of loved ones. We can think of bereavement as the awareness of these holes. Time and courage are necessary to fill these spaces.

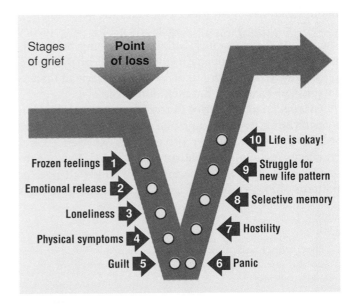

FIGURE 14.1

The diagram shows the stages of grief. People react differently to losses, but most eventually adjust. The common stages of grief and relief are depicted. Generally, the stronger the social support system, the smoother the progression through the stages of grief.

When a person experiences a loss that cannot be openly acknowledged, publicly mourned, or socially supported, coping may be much more difficult. This type of grief is referred to as **disenfranchised grief**.[26] Some examples of loss that may lead to disenfranchised grief include the following:

- *Death of a divorced spouse:* Unresolved anger and hurt along with fond memories are conflicting feelings that may prevent the satisfactory resolution of feelings surrounding the spouse's death.

- *Death of a secret lover:* When a lover dies and no one but the partner knew of the relationship, grief is often hidden. Examples would include a partner in an extramarital relationship or a lover of a gay person who is not openly gay.

- *Death of a gay lover:* Homosexuals may find it difficult to mourn the deaths of their lovers when they themselves are not accepted by their own families or the families of their lovers. The situation can be even more difficult if the lover has died of AIDS because of the unjust stigma and discrimination associated with this disease.

A special case of bereavement occurs in old age. Loss is an intrinsic part of growing old. The longer we live, the more losses we are likely to experience. These losses include physical, social, and emotional losses as our bodies deteriorate and more and more of our loved ones die. The theory of *bereavement overload* has been proposed to explain the effects of multiple losses and the accumulation of sorrow in the lives of some elderly people. This theory suggests that the gloomy outlook, disturbing behaviour patterns, and apparent apathy that characterize these people may be related more to bereavement overload than to intrinsic physiological degeneration in old age.[27]

Grief is a mental state of distress that occurs in reaction to significant loss, including one's own impending death, the death of a loved one, or a quasi-death experience. Grief reactions include any adjustments needed for one to "make it through the day" and may include changes in patterns of eating, sleeping, working, and even thinking.

The term **mourning** is often incorrectly equated with the term *grief*. As we have noted, *grief* refers to a wide variety of feelings and actions that occur in response to bereavement. *Mourning*, in contrast, refers to culturally prescribed and accepted time periods and behaviour patterns for the expression of grief. In Judaism, for example, "sitting *shivah*" is a designated mourning period of seven days that involves prescribed rituals and prayers. Depending on a person's relationship with the deceased, various other rituals may continue for up to a year.

By accepting dying as a part of the continuum of life, many people are able to make necessary readjustments after the death of a loved one. This holistic concept, which accepts dying as a part of the total life experience, is shared by both believers and nonbelievers.

What Is "Normal" Grief?

Grief responses vary widely from person to person. Despite these differences, a classic acute grief syndrome often occurs when a person acknowledges a loss. This common grief reaction can include the following symptoms:

- periodic waves of physical distress lasting from 20 minutes to an hour

- a feeling of tightness in the throat

- choking and shortness of breath

- a frequent need to sigh

- a feeling of emptiness in the abdomen

- a feeling of muscular weakness

- an intense feeling of anxiety that is described as actually painful

Other common symptoms of grief include insomnia, memory lapse, loss of appetite, difficulty in concentrating, a tendency to engage in repetitive or purposeless behaviour, an "observer" sensation or feeling of unreality, difficulty in making decisions, lack of organization, excessive speech, social withdrawal or hostility, guilt feelings, and preoccupation with the image of the deceased. Susceptibility to disease increases with grief and may even be life-threatening in severe and enduring cases.

A bereaved person may suffer emotional pain and may exhibit a variety of grief responses for many months after the death of a loved one. The rate of the healing process depends on the amount and quality of grief work that a person does. **Grief work** is the process of integrating the reality of the loss with everyday life and learning to feel better. Often, the bereaved person must deliberately and systematically work at reducing denial and coping with the pain that results from memories of the deceased. This process takes time and requires emotional effort.

Disenfranchised grief: Grief concerning a loss that cannot be openly acknowledged, publicly mourned, or socially supported.

Grief: The mental state of distress that occurs in reaction to significant loss, including one's own impending death, the death of a loved one, or a quasi-death experience.

Mourning: The culturally prescribed behaviour patterns for the expression of grief.

Grief work: The process of accepting the reality of a person's death and coping with memories of the deceased.

Helping Children Cope with Bereavement

1. *Develop and maintain an open communication pattern with children.* It is difficult and perhaps unrealistic to wait until a crisis situation has developed before including children in the discussion of significant issues. The child who is shunted aside whenever there are "important things" to talk about will have had little opportunity to learn the communication skills that are required to deal with difficult situations. Although limited by their levels of maturation and experience, children observe, think, and make choices. The family in which children feel that they can communicate about anything and everything with their parents and receive a careful and sympathetic hearing is the family that will be able to cope more resourcefully together when faced with bereavement or other stressful life events.

2. *Give children the opportunity to choose attending the funeral.* Adults often assume that children would either not understand funerals or be harmed by the experience. These assumptions may be based on an underestimation of children's cognitive ability as well as their need to be a part of what happens. One set of findings from the Harvard Child Bereavement Study has confirmed that parents tend to give only the illusion of choice: "You don't want to go, do you? No, I know that you don't." As the study also found, children appreciate the opportunity to make their own decisions. In some cases, families encouraged children to make specific recommendations about the funeral, such as, "outside, with lots of flowers, and with bright colors so we can remember all the good things." Furthermore, those who attended the funeral were better able to cope with the loss of the parent. Nevertheless, the child who has decided against attending the funeral should not be forced to do so against his or her wishes.

3. *Encourage the expression of feelings. . . .* The grieving child's thoughts and feelings are a part of reality that cannot be wished away or kept under wraps without adding to the already existing emotional burden. Young children are likely to find valuable means of expression through play and drawings, often accompanied by storytelling. Feelings can also be expressed through a variety of physical activities, including vigorous games through which tension and anger can be discharged. Children of all ages can benefit from open communication with their surviving parent and other empathic adults. An especially valuable way for children to express their feelings is to help comfort others. Even very young children can do this. For example, one child attending a funeral later reported that "at the end while I was crying, my little cousin came up to me and gave me a hug and said it was okay. She was only three." Comforting and altruistic behavior can begin very early in life.

4. *Provide convincing assurance that there will always be somebody to love and look after the child.* The death of a parent arouses or intensifies fears that the surviving parent and other important people may also abandon the child. Verbal assurances are useful, but not likely to be sufficient. Children may become anxious when the surviving parent is out of sight or has not come home at the expected time. Sending the children away for a while is a practice that often intensifies the anxiety of abandonment. Adult relatives and friends who spend time with the children after their bereavement are helping the surviving parent to provide reassurance that there will always be somebody there for them.

5. *Professional counseling should be considered if the bereaved children are at special risk.* The death of both parents, for example, constitutes a special risk, as does a death for which the children might feel that they are somehow [to] blame. There is one special risk that each year rises for thousands of children:

> Mom told us to sit down and she said, "Girls, your Dad died." We both cried right away. We went down to the garage where everybody was. People began holding us and trying to make us feel better. No one knew what to say. We felt like everyone was just staring at us. It was like a big, bad dream. And to make matters worse, we found out from our Mom that Dad had killed himself. . . . It is still hard for us to understand. We were only five and nine years old.

. . . Two girls had to contend—suddenly—with the death of their father and the puzzle and possible stigma of his suicide. Their consuming question was: "If Daddy loved me, why did he leave me?" This became the title of a little book that the girls wrote together over a period of time. In addition to their supportive mother, [they] had the skilled services of a professional counselor, David Dahlke. Every page of the girls' book reflects their personal growth experience as they explored their thoughts, feelings, values, and choices with the counselor's assistance.

Dahlke offers a detailed account of the counseling process along with the girls' own thoughts and comments by the mother. We learn, for example, that the children became afraid that if their mother married again her new husband would also commit suicide. . . .

Other children who suffer parental bereavement under especially traumatic and stressful conditions can also receive valuable assistance from qualified counselors.

Source: Excerpted from Robert J. Kastenbaum, *Death, Society, and Human Experience,* 5th ed., 211–212. © 1995 by Allyn & Bacon. Reprinted by permission.

When an Infant or a Child Dies

The death of a child is terribly painful for the whole family. However, for several reasons, the siblings of the deceased child have a particularly hard time with grief work. Bereaved children usually have limited experience with death and therefore have not yet learned how to deal with major loss. Children may feel uncomfortable talking about death, and they may also receive less social support and sympathy than do the parents of the deceased child. Because so much attention and energy are devoted to the deceased child, the surviving children may also feel emotionally abandoned by their parents. The Building Communication Skills box discusses helping children through the time following a death.

Quasi-Death Experiences

Social and emotional support for the bereaved in the aftermath of death is supported by many cultures. Typically, however, there is little support for many other significant losses in life. Losses that in many ways resemble death and that may carry with them a heavy burden of grief include a child running away from home, an abduction or kidnapping, a divorce, a move to a distant place, a move to a nursing home, the loss of a romance or an intimate friendship, retirement, job termination, finishing a "terminal" academic degree, or ending an athletic career.

These **quasi-death experiences**[28] resemble death in that they involve separation, termination, loss, and a change in identity or self-perception. If grief results from these losses, the pattern of the grief response will probably follow the same course as responses to death. Factors that may complicate the grieving process associated with quasi-death include uncomfortable contact with the object of loss (for example, an ex-spouse) and a lack of adequate social and institutional support.

Quasi-death experiences: Losses or experiences that resemble death in that they involve separation, termination, significant loss, a change of personal identity, and grief.

Hospice: A concept of care for terminally ill patients designed to maximize the quality of life.

Many terminally ill people choose to spend their last days in a hospice where maximum involvement of loved ones is emphasized.

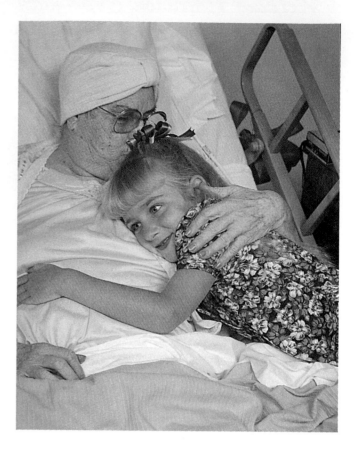

𝒯AKING CARE OF BUSINESS

Caring for dying people and dealing with the practical and legal questions surrounding death can be difficult and painful. The problems of the dying person and the bereaved loved ones involve a wide variety of psychological, legal, social, spiritual, economic, and interpersonal issues. We will now examine some practical problems associated with death and will present a humanitarian alternative that has been offered as a possible solution to many of these problems.

Hospice: An Alternative for the Dying Person

An increasing number of people now consider the hospice philosophy an acceptable alternative to modern "high-tech" death. The objective of **hospice** programs is to maximize the quality of life when doctors determine that death is inevitable. "The Dying Person's Bill of Rights,"

The Dying Person's Bill of Rights

As we face death, what are our rights as human beings? This bill of rights was created at a workshop on "The Terminally Ill Patient and the Helping Person" sponsored by the Southwestern Michigan Insurance Education Council and conducted by Amelia J. Barbus. Its affirmations may help you or a loved one to maintain dignity during the dying process. As a survivor, it may help you understand the patient's needs.

- I have the right to be treated as a living human being until I die.

- I have the right to maintain a sense of hopefulness, however changing its focus may be.

- I have the right to be cared for by those who can maintain a sense of hopefulness, however changing this might be.

- I have the right to express my feelings and emotions about my approaching death in my own way.

- I have the right to participate in decisions concerning my care.

- I have the right to expect continuing medical and nursing attention even though "cure" goals must be changed to "comfort" goals.

- I have the right not to die alone.

- I have the right to be free from pain.

- I have the right to have my questions answered honestly.

- I have the right not to be deceived.

- I have the right to have help from and for my family in accepting my death.

- I have the right to die in peace and dignity.

- I have the right to retain my individuality and not be judged for my decisions, which may be contrary to the beliefs of others.

- I have the right to discuss and enlarge my religious and/or spiritual experiences, whatever these may mean to others.

- I have the right to expect that the sanctity of the human body will be respected after death.

- I have the right to be cared for by caring, sensitive, knowledgeable people who will attempt to understand my needs and will be able to gain some satisfaction in helping me face my death.

Source: Copyright 1975 The American Journal of Nursing Company. Reprinted from H. Whitman, "The Dying Person's Bill of Rights," *American Journal of Nursing,* No. 1 (January 1975): 99. Used with permission. All rights reserved.

---

reprinted in the Skills for Behaviour Change box, reflects the sort of humanitarian philosophy on which the hospice idea is based.

The primary goals of the hospice program are to relieve the dying person's pain, to offer emotional support to the dying person and loved ones, and to restore a sense of control to the dying person, the family, and friends. Although home care with maximum involvement by loved ones is emphasized, hospice programs are under the direction of cooperating physicians, coordinated by specially trained nurses, and fortified with the services of counsellors, clergy, and trained volunteers. Hospital inpatient beds are available if necessary. Hospice programs usually include the following characteristics:

1. The patient and family constitute the unit of care, because the physical, psychological, social, and spiritual problems of dying confront the family as well as the patient.

2. Emphasis is placed on symptom control, primarily the alleviation of pain. Curative treatments are curtailed as requested by the patient, but sound judgement must be applied to avoid a feeling of abandonment.

3. There is overall medical direction of the program, with all health care being provided under the direction of a qualified physician.

4. Services are provided by an interdisciplinary team because no one person can provide all the needed care.

5. Coverage is provided 24 hours a day, seven days a week, with emphasis on the availability of medical and nursing skills.

6. Carefully selected and extensively trained volunteers are an integral part of the health care team, augmenting staff service but not replacing it.

7. Care of the family extends through the bereavement period.

8. Patients are accepted on the basis of their health needs, not their ability to pay.

Despite the growing number of people considering the hospice option, many people prefer to go to a hospital to die. Others choose to die at home, without the intervention of medical staff or life-prolonging equipment. Each dying person and his or her family should decide as early

The Graveyard of Potamia

Potamia is a village in northern Greece not far from Mount Olympus. The 600 people who live there remain in close physical and symbolic contact with the dead. The small cemetery is crowded with twenty or more grave markers that memorialize villagers who have died in the past few years. . . .

By local custom, bodies remain in the graveyard for five years and then are removed to the bone house. During this temporary burial the survivors have ample time to visit their lost loved ones. The survivors' feelings often become expressed with great intensity as the time nears to exhume and transfer the body. Tsiaras recorded a mother's lament:

Eleni, Eleni, you died far from home with no one near you. I've shouted and cried for five years, Eleni, my unlucky one, but you haven't heard me. I don't have the courage to shout any more. Eleni, Eleni, my lost soul. You were a young plant, but they didn't let you blossom. You've been here for five years. Soon you'll leave. Then where will I go? What will I do? Five years ago I put a beautiful bird into the ground, a beautiful partridge. But now what will I take out? What will I find?

In contrast to many cemeteries in the United States, the little graveyard in Potamia is often filled with mourners, usually women. They come not only to express their sorrows through song, speech, and prayer but also to tend the graves. Candles are kept burning at the foot of each grave, and the grounds are tended with scrupulous care. When the gravetending activities have been completed for the day, the women sit and talk to their dead and to each other. The conversation may center on death, and one mourner may seek to comfort another. But the conversation may also include other events and concerns. An important aspect of the village's communal life is mediated through their role as survivors of the dead. For the women especially, the graveyard provides an opportunity to express their *ponos* (the pain of grief). The men find a variety of outlets, but the women are usually expected to be at home and to keep their feelings to themselves. "A woman performs the necessary rites of passage and cares for the graves of the dead 'in order to get everything out of her system.' "

Through their graveside laments and rituals the Greek women attempt to achieve a balance between the dead and the living. The custom of temporary burial has an important role in this process. The deceased can still be treated as an individual and as a member of the community, somebody who retains the right of love, respect, and comfort. In effect, the deceased suffers a second and final death when the grave is destroyed and the physical remains are deposited with the bones of the anonymous dead. It is easier to cope with the symbolic claims of the dead when a definite time limit has been set—in this case a rather generous five-year period. Although the memory of the deceased will continue to be honored, removal of the remains to the bone house represents the reemergence of the life-oriented needs of the survivors.

The survivors are *obliged* to tend the graves and carry out other responsibilities to the deceased. As Tsiaras points out, this process involves a symbolic interaction and continuation between the living and the dead. *The dead have the right to expect it, just as those who are now among the living can expect their survivors to honor their postmortem rights when the time comes.* In Potamia and in many other communities where traditional value systems remain in place, the obligations of the living to the dead are clear, specific, and well known.

Source: Excerpted from Robert J. Kastenbaum, *Death, Society, and Human Experience,* 5th ed., 295–296. © 1995 by Allyn & Bacon. Reprinted by permission.

---

as possible what type of terminal care is most desirable and feasible. This will allow time for necessary emotional and financial preparations. Hospice care may also help the survivors cope better with the death experience.

Making Funeral Arrangements

Anthropological evidence indicates that all cultures throughout history have developed some sort of funeral ritual. For this reason, social scientists agree that funerals somehow assist survivors of the deceased in coping with their loss. The Global Perspectives Box takes a look at how one small town in Greece balances the needs of the living with care for the dead.

In Canada, with its diversity of religious and ethnic customs, funeral patterns vary. Prior to body disposal, the deceased may be displayed to formalize last respects and increase social support to the bereaved. This part of the funeral ritual is referred to as a wake or viewing. The body of the deceased is usually embalmed prior to viewing to retard decomposition and minimize offensive odours. The funeral service may be held in a church, synagogue, or mosque, in a funeral chapel, or at the burial site. Some people choose to replace the funeral service with a simple memorial service held within a few days of the burial. Social interaction associated with funeral and memorial services is valuable in helping survivors cope with their losses.

Common methods of body disposal include burial in the ground, entombment above ground in a mausoleum, cremation, and anatomical donation. Expenses involved in body disposal vary according to the method chosen and the available options. It should be noted that if burial is selected, an additional charge may be assessed for a burial vault. Burial vaults—concrete or metal containers that hold the casket—are required by most cemeteries to limit settling of the gravesite as the casket disintegrates and collapses. (Jewish burials are an exception; Jewish tradition forbids non-biodegradable containers, as well as embalming; the remains are supposed to "return to dust.") The actual container for the body or remains of the dead person is only one of many things that must be dealt with when a person dies. There are many other decisions concerning the funeral ritual that can be burdensome for survivors.

Pressures on Survivors

Stress related to funeral ritual varies culturally as well as individually. In traditional societies, funeral rites and preparation of the body were quite specific. These practices limited the stress on survivors because few decisions had to be made. Bereaved people fully understood their individual roles in funeral customs and even anticipated carrying out expected duties. In contrast, funeral practices in Canada today are extremely varied. A great number of decisions have to be made, usually within 24 hours. These decisions relate to the method and details of body disposal, the type of memorial service, display of the body, the site of burial or body disposition, the cost of funeral options, organ donation decisions, ordering of floral displays, contacting friends and relatives, planning for the arrival of guests, choosing markers, gathering and submitting obituary information to newspapers, printing of memorial folders, as well as numerous other details. Even though funeral directors are available to facilitate decision making, the bereaved may experience undue stress, especially in the event of a sudden death. In our society, people who make their own funeral arrangements can save their loved ones from having to deal with unnecessary problems. Even making the decision regarding the method of body disposal can greatly reduce the stress on survivors.

Wills

The issue of inheritance is a controversial one in some families and should be resolved before the person dies in order to reduce both conflict and needless expense. Unfortunately, many people are so intimidated by the thought of making a will that they never do so and die **intestate** (without a will). This is tragic, especially because the procedure involved in establishing a legal will is relatively simple and inexpensive. In addition, if you don't make up a will before you die, the courts will determine the disposition of your estate, according to certain formulas. Legal issues, rather than your wishes, will preside.

Organ Donation

Canadian doctors performed 1487 organ transplants in 1995, a slight increase from 1993, the Canadian Coalition on Organ Donor Awareness (CCODA) reported. The rate of organ donation has remained relatively stable, increasing from 47.7 transplants per million people in 1991 to 50.7 per million in 1995. In Ontario, each of the province's 11 million residents will receive a new health card during the next five years that will not only ask for consent for organ donation but also retain signed consents on a database. This will ease the burden on families and health care professionals while providing demographic and geographic data for transplant programs. If the Ontario initiative is successful, other provinces may follow suit.[29]

*W*HAT DO YOU THINK?

If you died suddenly, would you get the kind of end-of-life treatment that you want? What can you do to assure that your wishes will be carried out at the time of your death?

*L*IFE-AND-DEATH DECISION MAKING

Life-and-death decisions are serious, complex, and often expensive. We will not attempt to present the "answers" to death-related moral and philosophical questions. Instead, we offer topics for your consideration. We hope that discussion of the needs of the dying person and the bereaved will help you to make difficult decisions in the future. Among problematic or controversial issues are questions concerning the right to die and euthanasia.

Increasingly, Canadians living with terminal or life-threatening diagnoses are demanding to make decisions about their own lives. Options include pain and symptom management, extended palliative care, active and passive forms of euthanasia, and suicide.

Intestate: The situation in which a person dies without having made a will.

Alternatives have accompanied the development of new reproductive technologies, increases in terminal AIDS cases, and a visible increase in public media coverage of actual cases in Canada and the United States. The right to self-determination is situated within the context of society, health and illness, and human rights and freedoms. Considerations of the economic, social, and moral impact of the individual's choice are often involved in decision making. A living will, discussed in the Taking Charge box, is one way in which people may express their wishes about life-and-death choices.

Dyathanasia is a form of "mercy killing" in which someone plays a passive role in the death of a terminally ill person. This passive role may include the withholding of life-prolonging treatments or withdrawal of life-sustaining medical support, thereby allowing the person to die. A recent study shows that withholding food and water from terminally ill patients may actually ease their suffering. **Euthanasia** is the active form of "mercy killing." An example of euthanasia is direct administration of a lethal drug overdose with the objective of hastening the death of a suffering person. Euthanasia is illegal and is viewed as murder. Nevertheless, euthanasia continues to occur. In fact, some experts believe that some doctors induce euthanasia

upon the request of the patient. This type of euthanasia is accomplished by administering large doses of painkillers that depress the central nervous system to the extent that basic life-sustaining regulatory centres cease to function. The heart stops beating, breathing ceases, and total brain death follows shortly.

*W*HAT DO YOU THINK?

Are there any end-of-life situations in which you would ask a physician to help you die? Why or why not?

Dyathanasia: The passive form of "mercy killing" in which life-prolonging treatments or interventions are not offered or are withheld, thereby allowing a terminally ill person to die naturally.

Euthanasia: The active form of "mercy killing" in which a person or organization knowingly acts to hasten the death of a terminally ill person.

TAKING CHARGE

The Living Will

A living will is a written document in which you set out your wishes for health care in the event that, some time in the future, you are unable to consent to treatment. Living wills deal with health care. They do not deal with property or assets. Living wills are only important if you are unable to consent and you have a terminal illness or are seriously injured and unlikely to recover. In such cases medical staff will need to know what measures you would wish them to take to care for you.

There are no guarantees that every term of the living will will be followed. Family members or your proxy in consultation with medical staff will have to make the decision taking in all the existing circumstances, including your expressed wishes. (A proxy is someone you have appointed to make decisions about your health care should you become unable to consent.) A living will may ease the emotional burden from family members or your proxy if they have to make decisions about your health. Many families consider a living will morally binding, especially if you have discussed it with them beforehand.

It is not a request to take positive steps to end your life. Euthanasia, or mercy killing, as it is sometimes called, is the

term used when someone takes positive steps to end your life in order to relieve suffering. Assisted suicide is a term used when someone, at your request, takes positive steps to end your life, because your illness or condition prevents you from committing suicide. Euthanasia and assisted suicide are illegal under Canadian criminal law.

The living will must have your name and address and the date. It will need to set out what kind of life-sustaining treatments you would want in certain circumstances should you be incapable of consenting at the time. You must sign the living will and date it. Your signature should be witnessed by two adults. They should give their address. If you do not already have a proxy, you may also want to include the appointment of someone to consent to treatment on your behalf should you become unable to consent. You should choose someone whom you trust to carry out your wishes. The person must be aged 19 or over but does not have to be your next of kin.

Source: **The Public Legal Education Society of Nova Scotia (PLENS),** *Living Wills.* **http://www.acjnet.org/docs/lvplens.html**

Summary

◆ Aging can be defined in terms of biological age, psychological age, social age, legal age, or functional age.

◆ The rising number of elderly (people age 65 and older) will have a growing impact on our society in terms of economy, health care, housing, and ethical considerations.

◆ Two broad groups of theories—biological and psychosocial—purport to explain the physiological and psychological changes that occur with aging.

◆ Aging changes the body and mind in many ways. Physical changes occur in the skin, bones and joints, head, urinary tract, heart and lungs, senses, mobility, sexual functioning, and temperature regulation. Major physical concerns are osteoporosis and urinary incontinence. Potential mental problems include depression and Alzheimer's disease.

◆ Special challenges for the elderly include prescription drug and OTC interactions, questions about vitamin and mineral supplementation, and issues regarding caregiving.

◆ *Death* can be defined biologically in terms of the final cessation of vital functions. Various classes of death include cell death, local death, somatic death, apparent death, functional death, and brain death.

◆ Death is a multifaceted process and individuals may experience emotional stages of dying including denial, anger, bargaining, depression, and acceptance. Social death results when a person is no longer treated as living. Grief is the state of distress felt after loss. Children, too, need to be helped through the process of grieving.

◆ Practical and legal issues surround dying and death. Many decisions can be made in advance of death through wills and living wills.

◆ The right to die involves ethical, moral, and legal issues. Dyathanasia involves passive help in suicide for a terminally ill patient; euthanasia involves direct help.

Discussion Questions

1. Discuss the various definitions of aging. At what age would you place your parents for each category?

2. As the elderly population grows, what implications are there for you? Would you be willing to pay higher taxes to support government social programs for the elderly?

3. List the major physiological changes that occur with aging. Which of these, if any, can you change?

4. Explain the major health challenges that the elderly may face. What advice would you give to your grandparents before they took a prescription or OTC drug?

5. List the varied definitions of *death*. How do they relate to one another?

6. Discuss why so many of us deny death. How could death become a more acceptable topic to discuss?

7. What are the stages that terminally ill patients theoretically experience? Do you agree with the five-stage theory? Explain why or why not.

8. Compare and contrast the hospital experience with hospice care. What must one consider before arranging for hospice care?

9. Debate whether or not assisted suicide should be legalized for the terminally ill. What restrictions would you include in a law?

Application Exercise

Reread the What Do You Think? scenario at the beginning of the chapter and answer the following questions:

1. Do you think the individuals in the scenario are normal for their age? What is normal for a particular age?

2. What changes have made it easier for elderly people to lead healthy lives? What changes have made it more difficult?

Heart Disease and Stroke in Canada
www.hwc.ca/hpb/lcdc/bcrdd/hdsc/index.html

Canadian Cancer Statistics
www.hwc.ca/hpb/lcdc/bc/stats.html

Seniors Computer Information Project
www.mbnet.mb.ca/crm/

Environmental Health
Thinking Globally, Acting Locally

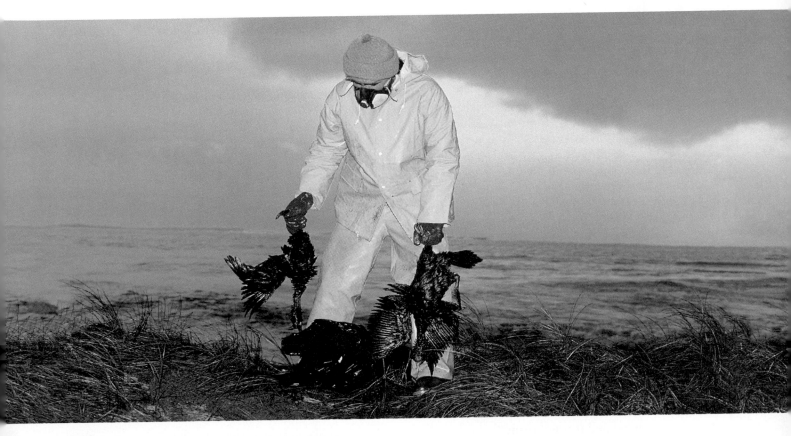

CHAPTER OBJECTIVES

◆ Identify the problems associated with current levels of global population growth.

◆ Discuss the major causes of air pollution, including photochemical smog and acid rain, and the global consequences of the accumulation of greenhouse gases and of ozone depletion.

◆ Identify sources of water pollution and the specific chemical contaminants often found in water.

◆ Describe the physiological consequences of noise pollution.

◆ Distinguish between municipal solid waste and hazardous waste.

◆ Discuss the health concerns associated with ionizing and nonionizing radiation.

In 1971, three friends in Vancouver (Jim Bohlen, Paul Cote, and Irving Stowe) and their wives decided to take a boat to protest a nuclear test by the United States on Amchitka Island in Alaska, located on a major fault line. Initially calling themselves the Don't Make a Wave Committee, they renamed their organization Greenpeace to better proclaim their purpose: to create a green and peaceful world. Although they were arrested, and the bomb was detonated, the opposition to the Amchitka tests became so strong that the president of the United States had to cancel the program the following year. The island was eventually turned into a bird sanctuary. Greenpeace today adheres to the belief that motivated that original voyage: that determined individuals can alter the actions and purposes of even the most powerful by "bearing witness"—that is, by drawing attention to an abuse of the environment through their unwavering presence at the scene, whatever the risk.

■ What can we as individuals do to stop pollution and its attendant problems? What factors put environmental groups at odds with government and industry?

Human health, well-being, and survival are ultimately dependent on the integrity of the planet on which we live. Today the natural world is under attack from the pressure of the enormous numbers of people who live in it, and the wide range of their activities. Even though Canada has made measurable environmental progress in recent years, our environmental achievements allow no room for complacency. An informed citizenry having a strong commitment to care for the environment is essential to the survival of our planet.

Canadians' concern about the environment has intensified since the initial outpouring on the first Earth Day in April 1970. The federal, provincial, and municipal governments share responsibility for the environment. This is supported by thousands of individual Canadians who are changing their habits and working for the environment.

OVERPOPULATION

Our most challenging environmental problem is population growth. The anthropologist Margaret Mead wrote, "Every human society is faced with not one population problem but two: how to beget and rear enough children and how not to beget and rear too many."[1]

In the middle of 1996, world population stood at 5.77 billion persons. Between 1990 and 1995, the world population grew at 1.48 percent per annum, with an average of 81 million persons added each year. This is below the 1.72 percent per annum at which population had been growing between 1975 and 1990, and much below the 87 million persons added each year between 1985 and 1990, which stands now as the peak period in the history of world population growth. Currently, 4.59 billion persons—80 percent of the world's population—live in the less developed regions, and 1.18 billion persons live in the more developed regions. The average annual growth rate is about 1.8 percent in the less developed regions and 0.4 percent in the others.

The per-country population range is from a low in Pitcairn, with 66 residents, to China, with 1.232 billion persons. According to the United Nations, the countries with the largest population size, after China, are India (945 million), the United States (269 million) and Indonesia (200 million). Six other countries have populations of more than 100 million: Brazil (161 million), the Russian Federation (148 million), Pakistan (140 million), Japan (125 million), Bangladesh (120 million), and Nigeria (115 million). Those ten nations are the only ones whose population has

TABLE 15.1 ■ World Population Facts

- The global population in mid-1995 was about 5.7 billion people.
- The current population growth rate of 1.5 percent per annum is the lowest recorded since World War II.
- The population is expected to grow by about 90 million people a year for the next 20 years, dropping to about 50 million a year by 2050.
- The world's 48 least developed countries have a combined population today of about 589 million; this is expected to increase to 1.7 billion by the year 2050.
- In 1995, about 2.6 billion people—45 percent of the global population—were living in urban areas. The proportion is expected to reach 60 percent by the year 2025.
- Twenty years from now, 33 of the world's biggest cities will have a combined population of more than 500 million people.

Source: Fifty Facts from the World Health Report, 1996.

In China, the goal of one child per family is promoted by the government in its effort to reduce the birth rate and gain control of the many problems associated with overpopulation.

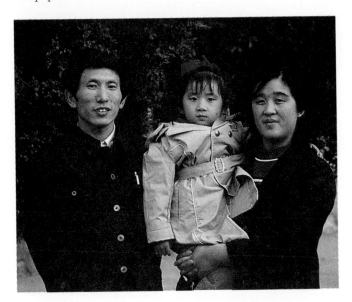

currently exceeded the 100 million mark. According to the medium-fertility variant projection, by the year 2050 seven more countries will have crossed that mark: Ethiopia, Iran, Zaire, Mexico, Philippines, Vietnam and Egypt.[2]

North America and Western Europe have the lowest birth rates. In Canada, the birth rate for 1993 was 1.61. Within Canada, Quebec has the lowest birth rate, at 1.41—well below the replacement rate of 2.1. Countries that can least afford a high birth rate in economic, social, health, and nutritional terms are the ones with the most rapidly expanding populations.

The vast bulk of population growth in developing countries is occurring in urban areas. Third World cities' populations are doubling every 10 to 15 years, overwhelming their governments' attempts to provide clean water, sewage facilities, adequate transportation, and other basic services. As early as 1964, researcher Ronald Wraith described the Third World giant city plagued by pollution and shantytowns as "megalopolis—the city running riot with no one able to control it."[3] In 1950, only three of the world's ten largest cities were in the Third World; by 1980, seven of them were, and this trend is expected to continue into the next century.

As the global population expands, so does the competition for the earth's resources. Environmental degradation caused by loss of topsoil, pesticides, toxic residues, deforestation, global warming, air pollution, and acid rain seriously threatens the food supply and undermines world health.

However, population doesn't tell the whole story. North Americans consume more energy and raw materials per person than do people from other regions of the world. Many of these resources come from other countries, and our consumption is depleting the resource balances of those countries. Therefore, we must start by living environmentally conscious lives.

The concept of zero population growth (ZPG) was born in the 1960s. Proponents of this idea believed that each couple should produce only two offspring. When the parents die, the two offspring are their replacements, and the population stabilizes.

The continued preference for large families in many developing nations is caused by such factors as high infant mortality rates; the traditional view of children as "social security" (they not only work from a young age to assist families in daily survival but also support parents when they are too old to work); the low educational and economic status of women; and the traditional desire for sons that keeps parents of several daughters reproducing until they get male offspring. Moreover, some developing nations feel that overpopulation is not as great a problem as the inequitable distribution of wealth and resources, both within their countries and worldwide. For all these reasons, demographers contend that broad-based social and economic changes will be necessary before a stabilization in population growth rates can occur.

*W*HAT DO YOU THINK?

How would you react to governmentally imposed restriction on family size? Do you favour imposed mandatory limitations in developing nations? What do you think we, as a world community, ought to do about population growth?

*A*IR POLLUTION

As our population has grown, so have the number and volume of the environmental pollutants that we produce. Concern about air quality prompted Parliament to pass the Clean Air Act in 1970. This was consolidated in 1985 into the Canadian Environmental Protection Act.

Sources of Air Pollution

Sulphur Dioxide. **Sulphur dioxide** is a yellowish-brown gas that is a by-product of burning fossil fuels. Electricity

Sulphur dioxide: A yellowish-brown gaseous by-product of the burning of fossil fuels.

It's Not Easy Being Green

Circle the number of each item that describes what you have done or are doing to help the environment.

1. When walking or camping I never leave anything behind.

2. I ride my bike, walk, carpool, or use public transportation whenever possible.

3. I have written my MP or MPP about environmental issues.

4. I avoid turning on the air conditioner or heat whenever possible.

5. My shower has a low-flow shower head.

6. I do not run the water while brushing my teeth, shaving, or handwashing clothes.

7. I take showers instead of baths.

8. My sink taps have aerators installed in them.

9. I have a water displacement device in my toilet.

10. I snip or rip plastic six-pack rings before I throw them out.

11. I choose recycled and recyclable products.

12. I avoid noise pollutants. (I sit away from speakers at concerts, select an apartment away from busy streets or airports, and so on.)

13. I make sure my car is tuned and has functional emission control equipment.

14. I try to avoid known carcinogens such as vinyl chloride, asbestos, benzene, mercury, X-rays, and so on.

15. When shopping, I choose products having the least amount of packaging.

16. I dispose of hazardous materials (old car batteries, used oil, or used antifreeze) at gas stations or other appropriate sites.

17. If I have children or when I have children, I will use cloth rather than disposable diapers.

18. I store food in glass jars and waxed paper rather than in plastic wrap.

19. I use as few paper products as possible.

20. I take my own bag along when I go shopping.

21. I avoid products packaged in plastic and unrecycled aluminum.

22. I recycle newspapers, glass, cans, and other recyclables.

23. I run the clothes dryer only as long as it takes my clothes to dry.

24. I turn off lights and appliances when they are not in use.

Scoring and Interpretation

Count how many items you have circled. Ideally, you can be doing all these things, but if you are trying to do at least some, you can score yourself as follows:

20–24	Good contributions to maintaining the environment.
14–19	Moderate contributions to maintaining the environment.
Below 13	Need to consider the recommendations made in this chapter to help the environment.

---

generating stations, smelters, refineries, and industrial boilers are the main source points. In humans, sulphur dioxide aggravates symptoms of heart and lung disease, obstructs breathing passages, and increases the incidence of such respiratory diseases as colds, asthma, bronchitis, and emphysema. It is toxic to plants, destroys some paint pigments, corrodes metals, impairs visibility, and is a precursor to acid rain, which we discuss later in this chapter.

Particulates. Particulates are tiny solid particles or liquid droplets that are suspended in the air. Cigarette smoke releases particulates. They are also by-products of some industrial processes and the internal combustion engine. Particulates can in and of themselves irritate the lungs and can additionally carry heavy metals and carcinogenic agents deep into the lungs. When combined with sulphur

dioxide, they exacerbate respiratory diseases. Particulates can also corrode metals and obscure visibility.

Carbon Monoxide. Carbon monoxide is an odourless, colourless gas that originates primarily from motor vehicle emissions. Carbon monoxide interferes with the blood's ability to absorb and carry oxygen and can impair thinking, slow reflexes, and cause drowsiness, unconsciousness, and death. When inhaled by pregnant women, it may threaten the growth and mental development of the foetus. Long-term exposure can increase the severity of circulatory and respiratory diseases.

Nitrogen Dioxide. Nitrogen dioxide is an amber-coloured gas emitted by coal-powered electrical utility boilers and by motor vehicles. High concentrations of nitrogen dioxide can be fatal. Lower concentrations increase susceptibility to colds and flu, bronchitis, and pneumonia. Nitrogen dioxide is also toxic to plant life and causes a brown discolouration of the atmosphere. It is a precursor of ozone, and, along with sulphur dioxide, of acid rain.

Ozone. **Ozone** is a form of oxygen that is produced when nitrogen dioxide reacts with hydrogen chloride. These gases release oxygen, which is altered by sunlight to produce ozone. In the lower atmosphere, ozone irritates the mucous membranes of the respiratory system, causing coughing and choking. It can impair lung functioning, reduce resistance to colds and pneumonia, and aggravate heart disease, asthma, bronchitis, and pneumonia. This ozone corrodes rubber and paint and can injure or kill vegetation. It is also one of the irritants found in smog. The natural ozone found in the upper atmosphere, however, serves as a protective membrane against heat and radiation from the sun. We will discuss this atmospheric layer, called the ozone layer, later in the chapter.

Lead. **Lead** is a metal pollutant that is found in the exhaust of motor vehicles powered by fuel containing lead and in the emissions from lead smelters and processing plants. It also often contaminates drinking water systems in homes with plumbing installed before 1930. Lead affects the circulatory, reproductive, and nervous systems. It can also affect the blood and kidneys and can accumulate in bone and other tissues. Lead is particularly detrimental to children and foetuses. It can cause birth defects, behavioural abnormalities, and decreased learning abilities.

Hydrocarbons. Hydrocarbons encompass a wide variety of chemical pollutants in the air. Sometimes known as *volatile organic compounds* (VOCs), **hydrocarbons** are chemical compounds containing different combinations of carbon and hydrogen. The principal source of polluting hydrocarbons is the internal combustion engine. Most automobile engines emit hundreds of different types of hydrocarbon compounds. By themselves, hydrocarbons seem to cause few problems, but when they combine with sunlight and other pollutants, they form such poisons as formaldehyde, various ketones, and peroxyacetylnitrate (PAN), all of which are respiratory irritants. Hydrocarbon combinations such as benzene and benzopyrene are carcinogenic. In addition, hydrocarbons play a major part in the formation of smog.

Photochemical Smog

Photochemical smog is a brown, hazy mix of particulates and gases that forms when oxygen-containing compounds of nitrogen and hydrocarbons react in the presence of sunlight. Photochemical smog is sometimes called *ozone pollution* because ozone is created when vehicle exhaust reacts with sunlight. Such smog is most likely to develop on days when there is little wind and high traffic congestion. In most cases, it forms in areas that experience a **temperature inversion**, a weather condition in which a cool layer of air is trapped under a layer of warmer air, preventing the air from circulating. When gases such as the hydrocarbons and nitrogen oxides are released into the cool air layer, they cannot escape, and thus they remain suspended until wind conditions move away the warmer air layer. Sunlight filtering through the air causes chemical changes in the hydrocarbons and nitrogen oxides, which results in smog. Smog is more likely to be produced in valley regions blocked by hills or mountains—for example, the Los Angeles basin and Tokyo.

The most noticeable adverse effects of exposure to smog are difficulty in breathing, burning eyes, headaches, and nausea. Long-term exposure to smog poses serious health risks, particularly for children, the elderly, pregnant women, and people with chronic respiratory disorders such as asthma and emphysema. According to the Canadian Lung Association, continued exposure accelerates aging of the lungs and increases susceptibility to infections by hindering the functions of the immune system.

Acid Rain

Acid rain is precipitation that has fallen through acidic air pollutants, particularly those containing sulphur dioxides and nitrogen dioxides. This precipitation, in the form of rain, snow, or fog, has a more acidic composition than does unpolluted precipitation. When introduced into lakes and ponds, acid rain gradually acidifies the water. When the acid content of the water reaches a certain level, plant and animal life cannot survive. Ironically, lakes and ponds that are acidified become a crystal-clear deep blue, giving the illusion of beauty and health.

Particulates: Nongaseous air pollutants.

Carbon monoxide: An odourless, colourless gas that originates primarily from motor vehicle emissions.

Nitrogen dioxide: An amber-coloured gas found in smog; can cause eye and respiratory irritations.

Ozone: A gas formed when nitrogen dioxide interacts with hydrogen chloride.

Lead: A metal found in the exhaust of motor vehicles powered by fuel containing lead and in emissions from lead smelters and processing plants.

Hydrocarbons: Chemical compounds that contain carbon and hydrogen.

Photochemical smog: The brownish-yellow haze resulting from the combination of hydrocarbons and nitrogen oxides.

Temperature inversion: A weather condition occurring when a layer of cool air is trapped under a layer of warmer air.

Acid rain: Precipitation contaminated with acidic pollutants.

Acid rain, the result of airborne acid particles from burning fossil fuels, has many harmful effects on the environment, and it poses numerous health hazards, including the risk of cancer from heavy metals that can make their way into the food chain as a result of acid precipitation.

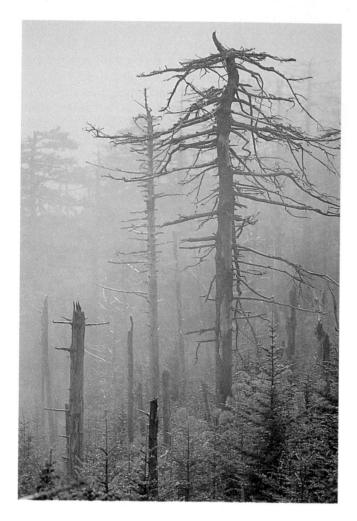

Sources of Acid Rain.   More than 95 percent of acid rain originates in human actions, chiefly the burning of fossil fuels.

When industries burn fuels, the sulphur and nitrogen in the emissions combine with the oxygen and sunlight in the air to become sulphur dioxide and nitrogen oxides (precursors of sulphuric acid and nitric acids, respectively). Small acid particles are then carried by the wind and combine with moisture to produce acidic rain or snow. Because of higher concentrations of sunlight in the summer months, rain is more strongly acidic in the summertime. Additionally, the rain or snow that falls at the beginning of a storm is more acidic than that which falls later.

Southern Ontario experiences some of the highest concentrations of acid aerosols in North America.[4] At present Ontario has no guideline for acid aerosols, such as sulphates.

Effects of Acid Rain.   The damage caused to lake and pond habitats is not the worst of the problems created by acid rain. Each year, it is responsible for the destruction of millions of trees in forests in Europe and North America. Scientists have concluded that 75 percent of Europe's forests are now experiencing damaging levels of sulphur deposition by acid rain. Forests in every country on the continent are affected.[5]

Doctors believe that acid rain also aggravates and may even cause bronchitis, asthma, and other respiratory problems. In Southern Ontario, several air pollution epidemiological studies have demonstrated that increases in acid aerosols and ground level ozone positively correlate with increased hospital admissions due to respiratory problems.[6] People with emphysema and those with a history of heart disease may also suffer from exposure to acid rain. In addition, it may be hazardous to a pregnant woman's unborn child.

Acidic precipitation can cause metals such as aluminum, cadmium, lead, and mercury to **leach** (dissolve and filter) out of the soil. If these metals make their way into water or food supplies (particularly fish), they can cause cancer in humans who consume them.

Acid rain is also responsible for crop damage, which, in turn, contributes to world hunger. Laboratory experiments showed that acid rain can reduce seed yield by up to 23 percent. Actual crop losses are being reported with increasing frequency. In May 1989, China's Hunan Province lost an estimated $260 million worth of crops and seedlings to acid rain. Similar losses have been reported in Chile, Brazil, and Mexico.[7]

A final consequence of acid rain is the destruction of public monuments and structures. Studies in the United States estimate damage to buildings in that country alone to cost more than $5 billion annually.[8]

Indoor Air Pollution

Combatting the problems associated with air pollution begins at home. (See the Focus on Canada box). Indoor air pollution comes primarily from six sources: wood stoves, furnaces, asbestos, passive smoke, formaldehyde, and radon.

Wood Stove Smoke.   Wood stoves emit significant levels of particulates and carbon monoxide in addition to other pollutants, such as sulphur dioxide. If you rely on wood for heating, you should make sure that your stove is properly installed, vented, and maintained. Proper adjustments and emission controls taken to recombust potential pollutants can also help to reduce pollution levels from wood stoves. Burning properly seasoned wood reduces the amount of particulates released into the air.

Furnace Emissions.   People who rely on oil- or gas-fired furnaces also need to make sure that these appliances are properly installed, ventilated, and maintained. Inadequate

Air Quality in Canada: Perceptions

Many people believe that air quality will make them sick:

- Ninety-two percent of Canadians said they were concerned about the impact of pollution on personal health.

- Eight to nine million Canadians believe the air will make them sick.

- One-third of all workers in Canada believe they are somewhat or very likely to experience a health problem as a result of poor air quality in the workplace.

- 62 percent of Canadians believe that their respiratory health has been adversely affected by the environment.

- 50 percent of Ontarians see a direct connection between their health and indoor air quality.

- One-quarter of all workers believe they have already experienced health problems due to air quality.

Sources: Canada Health Monitor, 1992; Decima Research, "An Investigation of the Attitudes of Canadians on Issues Related to Health and the Environment," January 1993; Canadian Lung Association, *The Air You Breathe;* Decima Research, *Report to Health and Welfare Canada,* 1993; Decima Research, *Report to the Canadian Lung Association,* 1994.

---

cleaning and maintenance can lead to a buildup of carbon monoxide in the home, which can be deadly.

Asbestos. **Asbestos** is another indoor air pollutant that poses serious threats to human health. Asbestos is a mineral that was commonly used in insulating materials in buildings constructed before 1970. When bonded to other materials, asbestos is relatively harmless, but if its tiny fibres become loosened and airborne, they can embed themselves in the lungs and cannot be expelled. Their presence leads to cancer of the lungs, stomach, and chest lining, and is the cause of a fatal lung disease called mesothelioma.

Formaldehyde. **Formaldehyde** is a colourless, strong-smelling gas present in some carpets, draperies, furniture, particle board, plywood, wood panelling, countertops, and many adhesives. It is released into the air in a process called outgassing. Outgassing is highest in new products, but the process can continue for many years.

Exposure to formaldehyde can cause respiratory problems, dizziness, fatigue, nausea, and rashes. Long-term exposure can lead to central nervous system disorders and cancer. If you experience symptoms of formaldehyde exposure, have your home tested by a city, county, or state health agency.

Radon. **Radon**, an odourless, colourless gas, is the natural by-product of the decay of uranium and radium in the soil. Radon may penetrate homes through cracks, pipes, sump pits, and other openings in the foundation. At toxic levels, it can cause lung cancer. However, Health Canada considers that radon pollution is not widespread in Canadian homes. Studies indicate that less than one-tenth of one percent of all homes in Canada—fewer than 8000 out of a total of eight million—could have levels of radon sufficiently high to warrant considering a means to

lower the level. Population studies based on a survey of 14 000 homes in 19 Canadian cities did not show a correlation between radon levels in homes and lung cancer.[9]

Household Chemicals. When you use cleansers and other cleaning products, do so in a well-ventilated room. Regular cleanings will reduce the need to use potentially harmful substances. Cut down on drycleaning, as the chemicals used by many cleaners can cause cancer. If your newly cleaned clothes smell of drycleaning chemicals, either return them to the cleaner or hang them in the open air until the smell is gone. Avoid the use of household air freshener products containing the carcinogenic agent dichlorobenzene.

*W*HAT DO YOU THINK?

Has the Canadian government taken strong enough environmental measures to protect citizens? What is the obligation of developing and developed countries regarding the use of fossil fuels? Should the responsibility for curbing their use be equally shared despite disparities in wealth?

Leach: A process by which chemicals dissolve and filter through soil.

Asbestos: A substance that separates into stringy fibres and lodges in lungs, where it can cause various diseases.

Formaldehyde: A colourless, strong-smelling gas released through outgassing; causes respiratory and other health problems.

Radon: A naturally occurring radioactive gas resulting from the decay of certain radioactive elements.

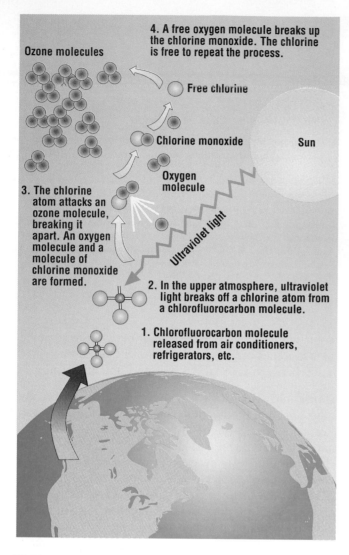

4. A free oxygen molecule breaks up the chlorine monoxide. The chlorine is free to repeat the process.

Ozone molecules

Free chlorine

Chlorine monoxide

Sun

Oxygen molecule

3. The chlorine atom attacks an ozone molecule, breaking it apart. An oxygen molecule and a molecule of chlorine monoxide are formed.

Ultraviolet light

2. In the upper atmosphere, ultraviolet light breaks off a chlorine atom from a chlorofluorocarbon molecule.

1. Chlorofluorocarbon molecule released from air conditioners, refrigerators, etc.

FIGURE 15.1

The diagram shows how the ozone layer is being depleted.

Ozone Layer Depletion

We earlier defined *ozone* as a chemical that is produced when oxygen interacts with sunlight. Close to the earth, ozone poses health problems such as respiratory distress. Farther away from the earth, it forms a protective membrane-like layer in the earth's stratosphere—the highest level of the earth's atmosphere, located from 20 to 50 kilometres above the earth's surface. The ozone layer in the stratosphere protects our planet and its inhabitants from ultraviolet B (UV-B) radiation, a primary cause of skin cancer. Ultraviolet B radiation may also damage DNA and may be linked to weakened immune systems in both humans and animals.

In the early 1970s, scientists began to warn of a depletion of the earth's ozone layer. Special instruments devel-oped to test atmospheric contents indicated that specific chemicals used on earth were contributing to the rapid depletion of this vital protective layer. These chemicals are called **chlorofluorocarbons (CFCs)** (see Figure 15.1).

In 1979, a satellite measurement showing a large hole in the ozone layer over Antarctica shocked scientists. Since then, satellite measurements of the ozone layer have regularly shown increases in the size of the hole.

In September 1987, 24 nations, including Canada, pledged to reduce the use of CFCs by 50 percent by 1999, and to freeze the use of halons by 1992 at their 1986 levels. This agreement, the Montreal Protocol on Substances That Deplete the Ozone Layer, was the first of its kind and set a global precedent. Since then, the Montreal Protocol has been ratified by over 70 countries. The Protocol now calls for the total elimination of CFCs, halons, and carbon tetrachloride by the year 2000 and methyl chloroform by 2005.[10] Canada banned the production of CFCs in 1993 and their importation in 1996. Methyl chloroform was also banned in 1996.

Global Warming

More than 100 years ago, scientists theorized that carbon dioxide emissions from fossil-fuel burning would create a buildup of greenhouse gases in the earth's atmosphere and that this accumulation would have a warming effect on the earth's surface. The century-old predictions are now coming true, with alarming effects. Average global temperatures are higher today than at any time since global temperatures were first recorded, and the change in atmospheric temperature may be taking a heavy toll on human beings and crops. Climate researchers predicted in 1975 that the buildup of greenhouse gases would produce life-threatening natural phenomena, including drought, severe forest fires, flooding, extended heat waves over large areas of the earth, and killer hurricanes.

Greenhouse gases include carbon dioxide, CFCs, ground-level ozone, nitrous oxide, and methane. They become part of a gaseous layer that encircles the earth, allowing solar heat to pass through and then trapping that heat close to the earth's surface. The most predominant of these gases is carbon dioxide, which accounts for 49 percent of all greenhouse gases. Eastern Europe and North America are responsible for approximately half of all carbon dioxide emissions. Since the late nineteenth century, carbon dioxide concentrations in the atmosphere have increased 25 percent, with half of this increase occurring since the 1950s. Not surprisingly, these greater concentrations coincide with world industrial growth.

Rapid deforestation of the tropical rainforests of Central and South America, Africa, and Southeast Asia is also contributing to the rapid rise in the presence of greenhouse gases. Trees take in carbon dioxide, transform it, store the carbon for food, and then release oxygen into the air. As we lose forests, we are losing the capacity to dissipate carbon dioxide.

The potential consequences of global warming are dire. The rising atmospheric concentration of greenhouse gases may be the most economically disruptive and costly change set in motion by our modern industrial society. Estimates in the United States show the costs to their economy, if greenhouse gasses were doubled, to be nearly $60 billion, or roughly 1 percent of U.S. GDP in 1993. In 1990, the Ontario Ministry of Environment and Energy valued crop losses due to ground-level ozone at $70 million.[11] Ozone causes damage to leaf tissue inhibiting photosynthesis, the process by which plants use light energy for growth. Some forest species at risk include northern red oak, eastern white pine, black oak, and sugar maple. Ground-level ozone has been linked to the forest decline observed in Germany and other European countries.[12]

Reducing Air Pollution

Our national air pollution problems are rooted in our energy, transportation, and industrial practices. We must develop comprehensive national strategies to address the problem of air pollution in the 1990s in order to clean the air for the coming century. We must support policies that encourage the use of renewable resources such as solar, wind, and water power as the providers of most of the world's energy.[13] Our atmosphere has no borders.

Most experts agree that shifting away from automobiles as the primary source of transportation is the only way to reduce air pollution significantly. Some cities have taken steps in this direction by setting high parking fees, imposing bans on city driving, and establishing high road-usage tolls. Community governments should be encouraged to provide convenient, inexpensive, and easily accessible public transportation for citizens.

Auto makers must be encouraged to manufacture automobiles that provide good fuel economy and low rates of toxic emissions. Incentives given to manufacturers to produce such cars, tax breaks for purchasers who buy them, and gas-guzzler-taxes on inefficient vehicles are three promising measures in this area.

What can you do to help? Find out in the Building Communication Skills box.

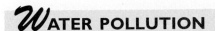

𝒲ATER POLLUTION

Seventy-five percent of the earth is covered with water in the form of oceans, seas, lakes, rivers, streams, and wetlands. Beneath the landmass are reservoirs of groundwater. We draw our drinking water from either this underground source or surface freshwater sources. The status of our water supply reflects the pollution level of our communities and, ultimately, of the whole earth.

The federal government passed the Canada Water Act in 1970 and created the Department of the Environment in 1971, entrusting the Inland Waters Directorate with providing national leadership for freshwater management. Under the Constitution Act (1867), the provinces are "owners" of the water resources and have wide responsibilities in their day-to-day management. The federal government has certain specific responsibilities relating to water, such as fisheries and navigation, as well as exercising certain overall responsibilities such as the conduct of external affairs.[14]

Water Contamination

Any substance that gets into the soil has the potential to get into the water supply. Contaminants from industrial air pollution and acid rain eventually work their way into the soil and then into the groundwater. Pesticides sprayed on crops wash through the soil into the groundwater. Spills of oil and other hazardous wastes flow into local rivers and streams. Underground storage tanks for gasoline may develop leaks. The list continues.

Pollutants can enter waterways by a number of different routes. These routes may be divided into two general categories: *point-source* and *non-point-source*. Pollutants that enter a waterway at a specific point through a pipe, ditch, culvert, or other such conduit are referred to as **point-source pollutants.** The two major sources of this type of pollution are sewage treatment plants and industrial facilities.

Non-point-source pollutants—commonly known as *runoff* and *sedimentation*—run off or seep into waterways

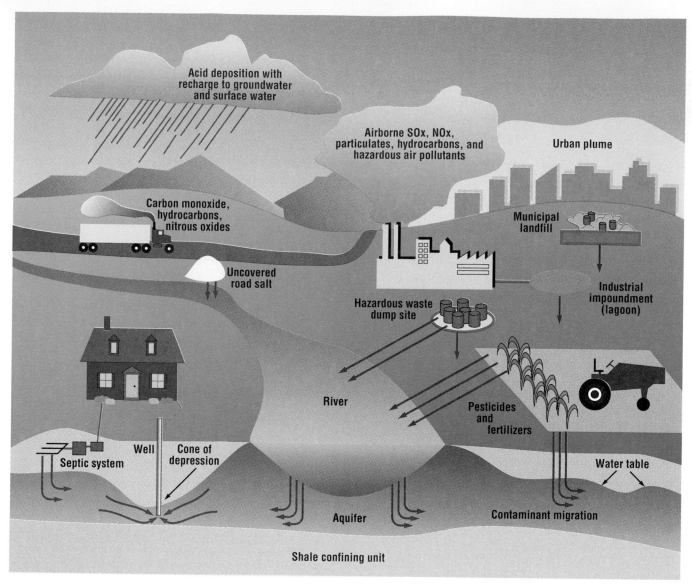

FIGURE 15.2

Sources of Groundwater Contamination

from broad areas of land rather than through a discrete pipe or conduit. It is currently estimated that 99 percent of the sediment in our waterways, 98 percent of the bacterial contaminants, 84 percent of the phosphorus, and 82 percent of the nitrogen come from non-point sources.[15] Non-point-source pollution results from a variety of human land use practices. It includes soil erosion and sedimentation, construction wastes, pesticide and fertilizer runoff, urban street runoff, wastes from engineering projects, acid mine drainage, leakage from septic tanks, and sewage sludge.[16] (See Figure 15.2.)

Septic Systems. Bacteria from human waste can leach into the water supply from improperly installed septic

systems. Toxic chemicals that are disposed of by being dumped into septic systems can also get into the groundwater supply.

Landfills. Landfills and dumps generate a liquid called **leachate**, a mixture of soluble chemicals that come from household garbage, office waste, biological waste, and industrial waste. If a landfill has not been properly lined, leachate trickles through its layers of garbage and eventually into the water supply.

Gasoline and Petroleum Products. Underground storage tanks for gasoline and petroleum products are common; most are located at gasoline filling stations. A number of these underground tanks are thought to be leaking.[17]

Speaking Out on the Environment

There are many ways for individuals to get involved in the crusade against environmental pollution. Here are eight.

- *Monitor legislation.* Several environmental organizations keep tabs on provincial and national laws being considered in order to offer testimony and to generate letter-writing campaigns on behalf of (or against) proposed laws.

- *Write letters.* It may not seem like a potent weapon, but letters to MPs or MPPs on pending bills *do* influence their opinions. When writing to any public official, keep your letter simple. Focus on one subject and identify a particular piece of legislation. Request a specific action and state your reasons for taking your position. If you live or work in the legislator's riding, make sure to say so. Keep the letter to one or two paragraphs, and never write more than one page.

- *Fill out customer comment cards and/or phone toll-free numbers on packages* to let companies know your concerns.

- *Educate others.* You can do this in a variety of ways, from talking to your friends, co-workers, and neighbours to organizing an educational activity.

- *Campaign for environmental candidates.* Look carefully at the environmental positions of candidates at all levels of government.

- *Launch a campaign at school or work.* At one university, for example, members of the law association decided to target the use of plastic foam in the cafeterias. After creating a multi-step, long-term strategy, the students first approached the food services department. The director of food services readily agreed to get rid of foam cups in a matter of days, and the foam food containers as soon as current inventory was depleted. Sometimes all you have to do is ask.

- *Invite speakers to your organization.* Most environmental organizations offer speakers on a wide range of topics who will speak at no charge to your civic, school, religious, or social organization. For maximum impact, consider scheduling a debate or panel discussion among representatives of environmental groups, government agencies, and industry.

- *Get involved with government.* Most communities offer a variety of boards, commissions, and committees that deal with environmental issues: planning commissions, zoning and land-use commissions, parks commissions, transit boards, and so on. Each can play a role in setting policies that affect the quality of the environment in your area.

Source: Adapted from Joel Makower, J. Elkington, and J. Hailes, *The Green Consumer Supermarket Guide,* 260–264, © 1991 by John Elkington, Julia Hailes, and Viking Penguin. Used by permission of Viking Penguin, a division of Penguin Books USA Inc.

Most of these tanks were installed 25 to 30 years ago. They were made of fabricated steel that was unprotected from corrosion. Over time, pinpoint holes develop in the steel and the petroleum products stored in the tanks leak into the groundwater. The most common way to detect the presence of petroleum products in the water supply is to test for benzene, a component of oil and gasoline. Benzene is highly toxic and is associated with the development of cancer.

Chemical Contaminants

Most chemicals designed to dissolve grease and oil are called *organic solvents.* These extremely toxic substances, such as carbon tetrachloride, tetrachloroethylene, and trichloroethylene (TCE), are used to clean clothing, painting equipment, plastics, and metal parts. Many household products, such as stain and spot removers, degreasers, drain cleaners, septic system cleaners, and paint removers, also contain these toxic chemicals.

Organic solvents work their way into the water supply in different ways. Consumers often dump leftover products into the toilet. Industries pour leftovers into large barrels, which are then buried. After a while, the chemicals eat their way out of the barrels and leach into the groundwater system.

A related group of toxic substances contains chlorinated hydrocarbons. The most notorious of these substances are the **polychlorinated biphenyls (PCBs)**, their cousins the *polybromated biphenyls (PBBs),* and the *dioxins.*

Leachate: A liquid consisting of soluble chemicals that come from garbage and industrial waste that seeps into the water supply from landfills and dumps.

Polychlorinated biphenyls (PCBs): Toxic chemicals that were once used as insulating materials in high-voltage electrical equipment.

PCBs. PCBs are fire-resistant and stable at high temperatures and were therefore used for many years as insulating materials in high-voltage electrical equipment such as transformers. PCBs bioaccumulate, meaning that the body does not excrete them but rather stores them in fatty tissues and the liver. PCBs are associated with birth defects, and exposure to them is known to cause cancer. PCBs have not been manufactured in North America since the late 1970s, but millions of kilograms of PCBs have been dumped into landfills and waterways, where they continue to pose an environmental threat.[18]

Dioxins. Dioxins are chlorinated hydrocarbons that are contained in herbicides (chemicals that are used to kill vegetation) and produced during certain industrial processes. Dioxins have the ability to bioaccumulate and are much more toxic than PCBs.

The long-term effects of bioaccumulation of these toxic substances include possible damage to the immune system, increased risk of infection, and elevated risk for cancer. Exposure to high concentrations of PCBs or dioxins for a short period of time can also have severe consequences, including nausea, vomiting, diarrhea, painful rashes and sores, and chloracne, an ailment in which the skin develops hard, black, painful pimples that may never go away.

Pesticides. Pesticides are chemicals that are designed to kill insects, rodents, plants, and fungi. Canadians use millions of kilograms of pesticides each year, but only 10 percent actually reach the targeted organisms. The remaining pesticides settle on the land and in our water supplies. Pesticide residues also cling to many fresh fruits and vegetables and are ingested when people eat these items.

Most pesticides accumulate in the body. Potential hazards associated with long-term exposure to pesticides include birth defects, cancer, liver and kidney damage, and nervous system disorders.

Trihalomethanes. Most Canadians drink water treated with chlorine to kill harmful bacteria. Trihalomethanes (THMs) are synthetic organic chemicals formed at water treatment plants when the added chlorine reacts with natural organic compounds in the water. Any drinking water supply that has been chlorinated is likely to contain THMs, which include such substances as chloroform, bromoform, and dichlorobromomethane. Chloroform in high doses is known to cause liver and kidney disorders, central nervous system problems, birth defects, and cancer. Recent research indicates that THM concentrations can be substantially reduced by adjusting the chlorine dose, improving filtration practices to remove organic material, or adding chlorine after filtration rather than before.[19]

Lead. Lead may be ingested in household water if the house is an older one with lead pipes. Water, particularly acidic water, will leach some of the lead from the pipes.

One way to reduce the possibility of ingesting lead if it does exist in your home's water system is to run the tap water several minutes before taking a drink or cooking with it to flush out water that has been standing overnight in lead-contaminated lines. Although leaded paints and ceramic glazes used to pose health risks, particularly for small children who put painted toys in their mouths, the use of leads in such products has been effectively reduced in recent years.

*W*HAT DO YOU THINK?

What can you do to ensure clean water? What personal actions can you take to conserve water? What measures can you take to avoid excessive exposure to pesticides?

*N*OISE POLLUTION

Loud noise has become commonplace. We are often painfully aware of construction crews in our streets, jet airplanes roaring overhead, stereos blaring next door, and trucks rumbling down nearby freeways. Our bodies have definite physiological responses to noise, and noise can become a source of physical or mental distress.

Prolonged exposure to some noises results in hearing loss. Short-term exposure reduces productivity, concentration levels, and attention spans, and may affect mental and emotional health. Symptoms of noise-related distress include disturbed sleep patterns, headaches, and tension. Physically, our bodies respond to noises in a variety of ways. Blood pressure increases, blood vessels in the brain dilate, and vessels in other parts of the body constrict. The pupils of the eye dilate. Cholesterol levels in the blood rise, and some endocrine glands secrete additional stimulating hormones, such as adrenaline, into the bloodstream.

At this point, it is necessary to distinguish between sound and noise. Sound is anything that can be heard. Noise is sound that can damage the hearing or cause mental or emotional distress. When sounds become distracting or annoying, they become noise.

Unfortunately, despite gradually increasing awareness that noise pollution is more than just a nuisance, noise control programs have been given a low priority by governments. In order to prevent hearing loss, it is important that you take it upon yourself to avoid voluntary and involuntary exposure to excessive noise. Playing stereos in your car and home at reasonable levels, wearing ear plugs when you use power equipment, and establishing barriers (closed windows, etc.) between you and noise will help you keep your hearing intact.

*W*HAT DO YOU THINK?

What do you currently do that places your hearing at risk? What changes can you make in your lifestyle to change these risks?

Health and Environment

Populations in the least developed countries are most at risk from "traditional" environmental health hazards. They include lack of water supply and sanitation, poor housing and shelter, unsafe food, and high prevalence of disease vectors (organisms, such as mosquitos, that carry and transmit diesease-causing microorganisms).

The populations of developing countries undergoing rapid industrialization are at risk both from the "traditional" environmental health hazards and from "modern" hazards such as air and water pollution, hazardous waste, unsafe use of chemicals—including pesticides, workplace hazards, and traffic accidents.

Within cities, mortality and morbidity rates are higher among people in low-income settlements than among people in more affluent areas, because of poor housing, high population density, pollution, lack of basic services, and inadequate social amenities.

Poor environmental quality is directly responsible for around 25 percent of all preventable ill-health in the world today. Heading the list of environmental causes of suffering are diarrheal diseases and acute respiratory infections, which are 100 times higher in undeveloped countries. Malaria, schistosomiasis, other vector-borne diseases, and childhood infections are also strongly influenced by adverse environmental conditions, as are injuries. Deaths due to environmentally related childhood diseases could be virtually eliminated by a combination of environmental improvements, immunization, and proper health care.

By far the highest exposures to air pollution in developing countries occur indoors, where biomass and coal are used for cooking and heating, causing millions of cases of acute and chronic respiratory disease. As many as 1000 million people, mostly women and children, are severely exposed.

Malaria is a major disease transmitted by mosquitoes, the habitat of which is closely linked to climatic and environmental conditions. More than 500 million people in more than 90 countries are affected by malaria. The incidence is increasing, exacerbated by land degradation, deforestation, the expansion of agriculture and mining into new areas, and urbanization. The high rate of malaria in the countries affected is in itself a major impediment to economic development.

There are some promising signs—not yet in terms of environmental improvement, but rather in the national development of policies and infrastructure to address the problems described here. However, the lack of financial and human resources is a major deterrent to progress.

Source: Adapted from World Health Organization, *Health and Environment in Sustainable Development: Five Years after the Earth Summit,* 1997.

LAND POLLUTION

Many areas in North America currently face serious problems in safely and effectively managing their garbage.

Solid Waste

Canadians are generating more trash than ever before. In 1988 Canadians generated 5.41 million tons of packaging waste alone. This particular type of garbage had been reduced by 21 percent by 1992, largely through recycling. By 1993, 91 percent of the population had access to recycling programs. Compostable collection was available in 34 percent of municipalities.[20]

Yet **municipal solid waste** is still outstripping available landfill sites, and the opening of new landfill sites is usually controversial, as people become more aware of the hazards they can pose to nearby land and water. Metropolitan Toronto has had to scramble in the last few years to find communities in other parts of Ontario that would take its overflow garbage.

Part of the answer is increased commitment to recycling, which still diverts a minority of garbage. Experts believe that as much as 90 percent of our garbage is ultimately recyclable. The Skills for Behaviour Change box discusses ways to become a better recycler through better shopping practices.

Dioxins: Highly toxic chlorinated hydrocarbons contained in herbicides and produced during certain industrial processes.

Pesticides: Chemicals that kill pests.

Municipal solid waste: Includes such wastes as durable goods, nondurable goods, containers and packaging, food wastes, yard wastes, and miscellaneous wastes from residential, commercial, institutional, and industrial sources.

Hazardous Waste

The community of Love Canal, New York, has come to symbolize **hazardous waste** dump sites. Love Canal was an abandoned canal that was first used as a chemical dump site by the Hooker Chemical Company in the 1920s. Dumping continued for nearly 30 years. Then the area was filled in by land developers and built up with homes and schools.

In 1976, homeowners began noticing strange seepage in their basements and strong, chemical odours. Babies were born with abnormal hearts and kidneys, two sets of teeth, mental handicaps, epilepsy, liver disease, and abnormal rectal bleeding. The rate of miscarriages was far above normal. Cancer rates were also above normal.

In response to these reports, the New York State Department of Health investigated the area of Love Canal. High concentrations of PCBs were found in the storm sewers near the old canal, but it took the department another two years to order the evacuation of the Love Canal homes. Over 900 families were evacuated, and the state purchased their homes. Finally, in 1978, the expensive process of cleaning up the waste dump began. Many lawsuits for damages are still being litigated.

The large number of hazardous waste dump sites in the United States indicates the severity of the toxic chemical problem in North America. American manufacturers generate more than one tonne of chemical waste per person per year (approximately 250 million tonnes). Three industrial groups produce most of this waste: chemicals and allied products, metal-related industries, and petroleum and coal products.[21]

In Canada, 45 percent of municipalities had hazardous waste programs by 1993. Most of these municipalities (72 percent) had populations of under 30 000. Most programs (96 percent) use a depot system for collection.[22]

The Canadian Environmental Protection Agency (CEPA) has established an overall program to deal with hazardous wastes. The CEPA divides hazardous materials into two groups. Those that are persistent, bioaccumulative, toxic, and primarily the result of human activity, will be targeted for virtual elimination from the environment; substances that do not meet these criteria are candidates for full life-cycle management to prevent or minimize their release into the environment.[23]

Hazardous waste: Solid waste that, due to its toxic properties, poses a hazard to humans or to the environment.

Ionizing radiation: Radiation produced by photons having high enough energy to ionize atoms.

Radiation absorbed doses (rads): Units that measure exposure to radioactivity.

In cooperation with provincial and municipal authorities, the following procedures have been put in place:

- Many wastes are now banned from land disposal or are being treated in such a way that their toxicity is reduced before they become part of land disposal sites.

- Hazardous waste handlers must now clean up contamination resulting from past waste management practices as well as from current activities.

- The CEPA is exploring ways to create economic incentives to encourage ingenuity in waste minimization practices and recycling.

Industry education and cooperation are important in achieving a safer environment.

---

*W*HAT DO YOU THINK?

What do you currently recycle? What are some of the reasons you do not recycle? What concerns would you have about living near a landfill or hazardous waste production or disposal site?

---

*R*ADIATION

A substance is said to be radioactive when it emits high-energy particles from the nuclei of its atoms. There are three types of radiation: alpha particles, beta particles, and gamma rays. Alpha particles are relatively massive particles and are not capable of penetrating human skin. They pose health hazards only when inhaled or ingested. Beta particles are capable of slight penetration of the skin and are harmful if ingested or inhaled. Gamma rays are the most dangerous radioactive particles because they can pass straight through the skin, causing serious damage to organs and other vital structures.

Ionizing Radiation

Exposure to ionizing radiation is an inescapable part of life on this planet. **Ionizing radiation** is caused by the release of particles and electromagnetic rays from atomic nuclei during the normal process of disintegration. Some naturally occurring elements, such as uranium, emit radiation. Other radiation-producing elements, such as deuterium, develop as part of the decay process of uranium or are created by scientists in laboratories. Radiation, whether naturally occurring or human-made, can damage the genetic material in the reproductive cells of living organisms. It can also cause mutations, miscarriages,

Become an Environmental Shopper

Learn the 5 Rs of recycling:

REDUCE the amount of waste you produce.
REUSE as much as possible.
RECYCLE the recyclables.
REJECT overpackaging and products hazardous to the environment.
REACT by joining with other consumers to let manufacturers and governments know your views.

Reduce

- Buy only what you need.
- Buy products having the least amount of packaging.
- Buy products in recycled or recyclable packaging.
- Avoid disposable products that are not recyclable.
- Buy the larger size or in bulk when possible.

Reuse

- Appliances
- Boxes
- Clothing
- Containers
- Grocery bags
- Wrapping paper

Recycle

Learn what is recyclable in your community:

- Aluminum
- Corrugated cardboard
- Glass
- Motor oil
- Newsprint
- Office paper
- Paperboard
- Plastics
- Steel cans

Reject

- Blister packs
- Packaging that promises to disappear
- Products harmful to the environment
- Mixed-material packages
- Supposedly "biodegradable" plastics
- Nonrecyclable packaging
- Overpackaged goods

React

- Write to manufacturers to support environmentally benign packaging and products, and to discourage
  - overpackaging
  - nonrecyclable packaging
  - environmentally harmful products
- Call manufacturers' 800 lines (listed on many packages) to voice your opinion.
- Contact elected officials to request that government at all levels use more recycled products.
- Ask merchants to provide bags made from recycled material or use your own bag.
- Request that your local newspaper use more recycled newsprint.

Source: Johnson County Recycling and Waste Reduction Guide, 4th ed. (1994), 4–6.

---

physical and mental deformities, cancer, eye cataracts, gastrointestinal illnesses, and shortened life expectancies.

Scientists cannot agree on a safe level of radiation. Reactions to radiation differ from person to person. Exposure is measured in **radiation absorbed doses**, or **rads** (also called roentgens). Recommended maximum "safe" dosages range from 0.5 rads to 5 rads per year. Approximately 50 percent of the radiation to which we are exposed comes from natural sources, such as building materials. Another 45 percent comes from medical and dental X-rays. The remaining 5 percent comes from computer display screens, microwave ovens, television sets, luminous watch dials, and radar screens and waves (see Table 15.2). Most of us are exposed to far less radiation than the "safe" maximum dosage per year.

Radiation can cause damage at dosages as low as 100 to 200 rads. At this level, signs of radiation sickness include nausea, diarrhea, fatigue, anemia, sore throat, and hair loss. Death is unlikely at this dosage. At 350 to 500 rads, all these symptoms become more severe, and death may result because the radiation hinders bone marrow production of the white blood cells we need to protect us from disease. Dosages above 600 to 700 rads are invariably fatal. The effects of long-term exposure to relatively low levels of radiation are unknown. Some scientists believe that such exposure can cause lung cancer, leukemia, skin cancer, bone cancer, and skeletal deformities.

Nonionizing Radiation

The lower-energy portions of the electromagnetic spectrum, ranging from lower-energy ultraviolet radiation down through infrared, radar, radio, and the electric and magnetic fields associated with many household appliances

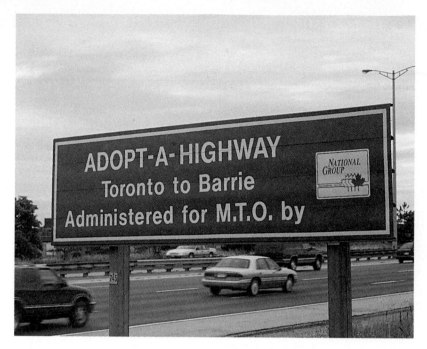

While we may feel that many of the environmental problems facing the world today are beyond our individual control, we can play a significant role in keeping our own little part of it clean, green, and beautiful.

and electric power lines, are **nonionizing radiation.** Although the biological effects of ionizing radiation have been recognized for some time, we still do not know very much about the effects of certain types of nonionizing radiation—in particular, the photons associated with electric and magnetic fields. Techniques for assessing radiation from many such sources are still evolving.[24]

Nuclear Power Plants

One source of radioactive emissions is nuclear power plants. At present, these plants account for less than 1 percent of the total radiation to which we are exposed. Radioactive wastes are produced not only by nuclear power plants but also by medical facilities that use radioactive materials as treatment and diagnostic tools and by nuclear weapons production facilities.

Proponents of nuclear energy believe that it is a safe and efficient way to generate electricity. Initial costs of building nuclear power plants are high, but actual power generation is relatively inexpensive.

Nonionizing radiation: Radiation produced by photons associated with lower-energy portions of the electromagnetic spectrum.

Meltdown: An accident that results when the temperature in the core of a nuclear reactor increases enough to melt the nuclear fuel and the containment vessel housing it.

Nuclear reactors also discharge fewer carbon oxides into the air than do fossil-fuel powered generators. Advocates believe that conversion to nuclear power could help slow the global warming trend.[25]

All these advantages of nuclear energy must be weighed against the disadvantages. First, disposal of nuclear wastes is extremely problematic for the entire world. Additionally, the chances of a reactor core meltdown pose serious threats to a plant's immediate environment and to the world in general.

TABLE 15.2 ■ Doses of Radiation

Source	Rads (per year)
Cosmic rays	0.45
Soil	0.15
Water, food, air	0.25
Air travel (round trip Toronto–London)	0.04
Medical X-rays	0.10
Nuclear power plant in vicinity	0.01
Brick structures	0.50–1.0
Concrete structures	0.70–1.0
Wooden structures	0.30–0.50

Source: Adapted by permission from International Atomic Energy Agency, *Radiation—A Fact of Life,* 1981 ed.

Managing Environmental Pollution

Environmental health begins at home. One celebrant of the 1990 Earth Day stated that in order to save the planet, we will all have to overcome our inertia and make sacrifices that contribute to the good of the planet. By understanding how political and economic issues affect the environment, we can pressure corporations and elected representatives to change policies that are harmful to the environment. For example, environmentalists pressured the World Bank to stop issuing development loans that were leading to the destruction of rainforests. Discussing issues with lawmakers and making decisions at the polls are two ways you can help influence environmental policy.

Making Decisions for You

One of the biggest decisions that we make as consumers is whether to pay more for environmentally safe products. As a student on a tight budget, are you willing to pay 30 to 50 percent more for products such as safer soap and laundry detergent? If not, are you willing to buy a less environmentally unfriendly product? While it's not likely that you can increase your budget enough to buy all environmentally safe products, you can get a start now. Think about the products you buy: Which could you substitute for more environmentally friendly brands?

Checklist for Change: Making Personal Choices

✓ Do you vote? Do you know the difference between rhetoric and reality when it comes to environmental issues?

✓ Do you conserve water? Fix leaky taps quickly. Run washers only with full loads. Don't overwater lawns or gardens.

✓ Do you think before you buy? Do you buy products in recyclable packaging? Do you reuse containers rather than buy new ones?

✓ Do you think before you throw household chemicals away? Make sure you use them up, give them away, or save them for a household hazardous waste collection instead. Consider nonhazardous substitutes.

✓ Do you recycle used oil? Oil dumped down storm drains or on the ground can pollute streams, killing insects, fish, and wildlife.

✓ Do you recycle tin cans, glass, newspaper, paper, plastic, and cardboard?

✓ Have you considered turning in people who litter?

✓ Have you considered walking, riding the bus, using your bike, and/or carpooling whenever possible?

✓ Are you cautious concerning the amount of fertilizers and pesticides you use? If they are overapplied, rain can wash them off lawns and carry them into lakes and streams. Always use low-phosphorus fertilizers.

✓ Do you ask yourself if you really need a product?

✓ Do you consider whether a product is practical and durable, well-made, and of timeless design?

✓ Do you buy used and rebuilt products whenever possible? Do you resell your unused items at yard or garage sales (your trash may be someone else's treasure) or donate them to charities?

✓ Do you compost leaves, clippings, and kitchen scraps?

Checklist for Change: Making Community Choices

✓ Do you work in your community to help create and enforce laws that protect drinking water and that prohibit the manufacture, use, storage, transport, or disposal of hazardous substances in your water supply area?

✓ Do you volunteer to take part in cleanup activities in your community?

✓ Does your community have a hazardous materials ordinance?

Critical Thinking

Your health teacher is leading a protest next week to the corporate headquarters of "one of the country's worst polluters." You are told not only that this company has a terrible record of both point- and non-point-source pollutants, but also that the "corporate bigwigs refuse to do anything about it." After hearing the brief appeal to join the protest, you decide it's your duty as a citizen to go. As your teacher hands out maps to the protest site, you realize that the company in question is your employer! Now you're really confused: your company claims to have spent billions of dollars to reduce pollution and considers itself an innovator in cleaning up sites it polluted in the past. You are upset because only one side of the story is being told. Should you speak up in class?

Using the DECIDE model in Chapter 1, decide what you would do. First, decide why you are upset. Then decide what you would like to accomplish by speaking up. In addition, consider the best setting to communicate your message to your teacher (in class, during office hours, e-mail, etc.).

A **meltdown** occurs when the temperature in the core of a nuclear reactor increases enough to melt both the nuclear fuel and the containment vessel that holds it. Most modern facilities seal their reactors and containment vessels in concrete buildings having pools of cold water on the bottom. If a meltdown occurs, the building and the pool are supposed to prevent the escape of radioactivity.

Opponents of nuclear energy believe that there is no safe place to dispose of, contain, or store our escalating supply of nuclear waste.

Accidents at nuclear power plants are not rare occurrences. In 1985, United States plants experienced nearly 3000 mishaps and 765 emergency shutdowns. At least 18 of the shutdowns were reported to be the result of serious accidents that could have led to reactor core damage.

*W*HAT DO YOU THINK?

How much exposure do you have to ionizing and non-ionizing radiation a year? What measures could you take to reduce this exposure? Do you feel the advantages outweigh the disadvantages of nuclear power? Explain why or why not.

Summary

◆ Population growth is the single largest factor affecting the demands made on the environment. Demand for more food, products, and energy—as well as places to dispose of waste—places great strains on the earth's resources.

◆ The primary constituents of air pollution are sulphur dioxide, particulate matter, carbon monoxide, nitrogen dioxide, ozone, lead, and hydrocarbons. Air pollution takes the forms of photochemical smog and acid rain, among others. Indoor air pollution is caused primarily by wood stove smoke, furnace emissions, asbestos, passive smoke, formaldehyde, and radon. Pollution is depleting the earth's protective ozone layer, causing global warming.

◆ Water pollution can occur either through point sources (direct entry through a pipeline, ditch, etc.) or non-point sources (runoff or seepage from a broad area of land). Major contributors to water pollution include dioxins, pesticides, trihalomethanes, and lead.

◆ Noise pollution affects our hearing and produces other symptoms such as reduced productivity, reduced concentration, headaches, and tension.

◆ Solid waste pollution includes household garbage, plastics, glass, metal products, and paper; limited landfill space creates problems. Hazardous waste is toxic; its improper disposal creates health hazards for those in surrounding communities.

◆ Ionizing radiation results from the natural erosion of atomic nuclei. Nonionizing radiation is caused by the electric and magnetic fields around power lines and household appliances, among other sources. The disposal and storage of radioactive wastes from nuclear power plants and weapons production pose serious potential problems for public health.

Discussion Questions

1. Explain the ways in which the expanding global population affects the environment.

2. List the primary sources of air pollution, acid rain, and indoor air pollution. What can be done to reduce each type of pollution?

3. What are the environmental consequences of global warming? What can we as Canadian citizens do to help slow the deforestation of tropical rainforests?

4. Explain point- and non-point sources of water pollution. Discuss how water pollution can be reduced or prevented altogether. What personal actions can you as a student take?

5. List the loudest sounds you have encountered in the last week (rock concert, construction, airplanes, etc.). How many could have been avoided? What could be done to ease the strain of the unavoidable noises?

6. Given all the open land in Canada, why do you think solid waste disposal is a problem?

7. Are the advantages of nuclear power worth the risks involved with storing nuclear waste? Put another way, if you live near a nuclear power plant, would you be willing to pay two or three times as much for electricity in order to have the nuclear power plant closed? Explain why or why not.

Application Exercise

Reread the What Do You Think? scenario at the beginning of the chapter and answer the following questions:

1. How much progress can be made in the fight against environmental polluters by community action?

Are there alternatives that are more effective?

2. What are an industry's responsibilities to its neighbours?

Health on the Net

C. A. N. DO—The Movement for Clean Air Now
www.web.apc.org/cando/

Atomic Energy Canada Limited
www.aecl.ca/hom_e.htm

Environment Canada, Green Lane Home Page
www.ec.gc.ca/envhome.html

WHO Health and Environment
www.who.ch/programmes/peh/gelnet/hlm97gen.htm

16

*C*onsumerism

Selecting Health Care Products and Services

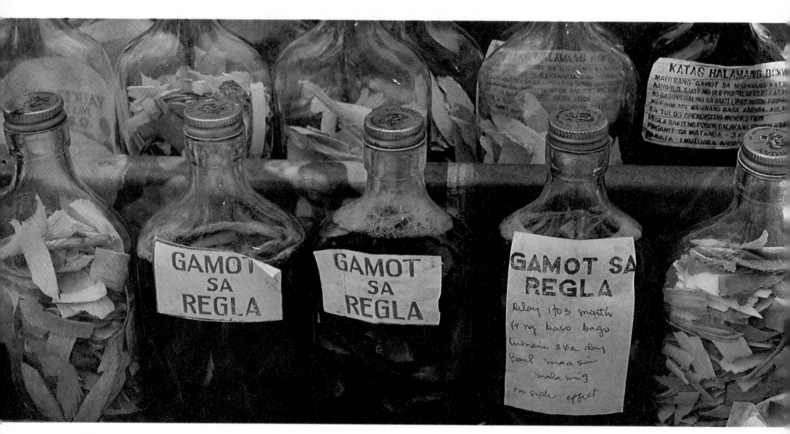

C HAPTER OBJECTIVES

- Discuss the methods advertisers use to attract customers.

- Explain when self-diagnosis and self-care are appropriate, when you should seek medical care, and how to assess health professionals.

- Compare and contrast allopathic and nonallopathic medicine, including the types of treatments that fall into each category.

- Discuss the types of health care available, including types of medical practices, hospitals, and clinics.

- Examine the current problems associated with our health care system, including cost, access, and quality.

- Describe health insurance options, including private insurance coverage, Medicare, and HSOs.

Roberta is a slightly older-than-average college student. She has a history of chronically painful menstrual periods and excessive bleeding. She seeks care from a gynecologist, who immediately states that she must have a hysterectomy. Because she believes that this is the most drastic option and because she has not yet had children and does not wish to go through early menopause, Roberta seeks a second opinion from the first doctor's colleague. Without giving her much of an exam, the second doctor agrees with the first, so she seeks yet another opinion—but this time from a doctor outside the original group's practice. This third doctor adamantly disagrees with the first two and suggests a more conservative treatment not involving surgery.

- Which doctor's advice should Roberta follow? Is it appropriate to seek more than one opinion or more than two? How much say should the patient have in her course of treatment? How can a consumer determine what "quality health care" is?

There are many reasons for you to be an informed health care consumer. Most important, you have only one body, and it is no one's top priority but yours. Doing everything you can to stay healthy and to recover rapidly when you do get sick will enhance every other part of your life. Canada's 300-year history has brought about a commitment to share the liability of illness and injury among the entire population. This is not the case in all countries in the world. Our health care system is based upon shared values of equity, fairness, compassion, and respect for the dignity of all.[1] Even though our society treats health as a social good to which everyone is entitled, you still must be knowledgeable about what resources are available to you and at times you must be assertive in order to obtain services that are in your best interests. As you may already know, medical and health care services are much harder to evaluate than are, say, clothing or fruit and vegetables. In addition, you may seek medical and health services in circumstances of either physical or emotional distress. Thus, your decision-making powers may be compromised and you may find yourself vulnerable when faced with the claims of inferior caregivers or products.

This chapter will help you to become more proactive in making decisions that affect your health and health care. Our health care system includes health care providers, payers (insurance, government, and individuals), and products. In 1996, health care accounted for 9.5 percent of Canada's gross national product. Many different companies aggressively market health products and services to the public. Even medical professionals sometimes feel overwhelmed, confused, and frustrated by the choices. So if you've experienced these feelings, you are not alone. However, there is much you can do to become an informed, responsible consumer of health care products and services.

RESPONSIBLE CONSUMERISM: CHOICES AND CHALLENGES

Perhaps the single greatest difficulty that we face as health consumers is the sheer magnitude of choices available to us. Informed health consumers are aware that there is always more to learn. Because there are so many charlatans competing for a share of the lucrative health market and because misinformation is so common, wise health consumers use every means at their disposal to ensure that they are acting responsibly in their own health choices. Check out your own knowledge in the Rate Yourself self-assessment.

Attracting Consumers' Dollars

Today's marketing specialists can identify a target audience for a given product and carefully go after it with a whole arsenal of gimmicks, subtle persuaders, and sophisticated strategies. Many advertisements present a product as a status symbol that will make you a member of the "in" crowd. In addition, many ads play on your inner fears and insecurities, causing you to wonder whether your deodorant is working, your breath is bad, or your skin is greasy. They may also convince you to purchase the socially correct product.

Other marketing strategies attempt to appeal to your hidden desires. Whatever your desires, countless products and services are available to meet them. Although some marketing tactics are obvious, others are much more

How Good a Health Consumer Are You?

Select the response that best describes your typical health behaviour. After completing this survey, total your points and assess your competence regarding health care products and services.

1 = I never act this way
2 = I sometimes act this way
3 = I act this way most of the time
4 = I always act this way

1. When moving to a new location, I seek recommendations from friends and ask for referrals from physicians who have treated me in the past whom I respect, before I get ill.   1 2 3 4

2. I schedule an interview with health professionals prior to treatment to determine if I am comfortable with them.   1 2 3 4

3. I ask about costs of health care procedures.   1 2 3 4

4. I carefully assess my symptoms and go to the doctor only when necessary.   1 2 3 4

5. I get second opinions when I am unsure of what my physician tells me.   1 2 3 4

6. I ask my physician why a test is being given and what my options are before I allow that test to be performed.   1 2 3 4

7. I follow recommended guidelines for health exams, inoculations, and self-care.   1 2 3 4

8. Whenever I receive a prescription drug, I follow the directions on the bottle exactly, using all medications in the prescribed time period.   1 2 3 4

9. I am aware of differences in prices at various pharmacies and comparison-shop whenever possible.   1 2 3 4

10. When my peers make statements that are obviously incorrect about "health alternatives," I tactfully point out their errors.   1 2 3 4

11. I am aware of my own body and seek medical care quickly when unusual changes occur.   1 2 3 4

12. I attempt to obtain my health information from reputable sources rather than from tabloids.   1 2 3 4

13. I carefully scrutinize health-related advertisements and news items.   1 2 3 4

14. I read the labels of health products and follow instructions carefully.   1 2 3 4

Interpreting Your Score

14–19   Health consumer skills dangerously weak

20–29   Health consumer skills below average

30–44   Health consumer skills about average, not adequate for many situations

45–56   Very good health consumer skills

Beyond Interpretation

In which five areas above do you believe you need improvement?

What can you do to improve in these areas?

---

subtle and difficult to discern. Perfume advertisements that depict passionate embraces and automobile ads that feature expensive sports cars with beautiful women are common. The implied message is that if you purchase a given perfume, your love life will improve, and if you buy that flashy car, attractive people will flock to you.

Many other marketing strategies revolve around "trendy" news items. A good example of this is the current concern about high cholesterol levels. Whereas food ads once focussed heavily on "low calories," the heart-disease scare has prompted advertisements focussing on "low cholesterol" or "low fat."

Why Some False Claims May Seem True

People often fall victim to false health claims because they mistakenly believe that a product or provider has helped them. This belief often arises from two conditions: spontaneous remission and the placebo effect.

Spontaneous Remission. It is commonly said that if you treat a cold, it will disappear in a week, but if you leave it alone, it will last seven days. A **spontaneous remission** from an ailment refers to the disappearance of symptoms without any apparent cause or treatment. Many illnesses, like the common cold and even back strain, are self-limiting and will improve in time, with or without treatment. Other illnesses, such as multiple sclerosis and some cancers, are characterized by alternating periods of severe symptoms and sudden remissions. Because of this phenomenon, people seeking profit may exploit consumers by claiming that their particular treatment, procedure, or drug cured the condition. People experiencing spontaneous remissions can easily attribute their "cure" to a treatment, drug, or provider that had no real effect on the disease or condition.

Placebo Effect. The **placebo effect** is an apparent cure or improved state of health brought about by a substance, product, or procedure that has no therapeutic value. It is not uncommon for patients to report improvements based on what they expect, desire, or were told would happen after taking simple sugar pills that they believed were powerful drugs. About 10 percent of the population is believed to be exceptionally susceptible to the power of suggestion; the remainder may be influenced in varying degrees. Those who are most susceptible may be victimized by aggressive marketing of products and services. Although the placebo effect is often harmless, it does account for the expenditure of millions of dollars on worthless health products and services every year. People who mistakenly use placebos when medical treatment is needed increase their risk for health problems.

$\mathcal{A}$CCEPTING RESPONSIBILITY FOR YOUR HEALTH CARE

As the health care industry has become more sophisticated about seeking your business, so must you become more sophisticated about purchasing its products and services. Apathy and ignorance are not viable options if you want care that serves your own best health interests.

You need to learn how, when, and where to enter the health care system and how to obtain the care you need without incurring unnecessary risk and expense. Acting responsibly in times of illness can be difficult, but the person best able to act on your behalf is you. Being knowledgeable about self-care and its limits is critical for responsible consumerism.

Self-Help or Self-Care

A recent concept in health consumerism is that the patient is the primary health care provider or first line of defense in health. Patients can practise behaviours that promote health, prevent disease, and minimize reliance on the formal medical system. They can also interpret basic changes in their own physical and emotional health and treat minor afflictions without seeking professional help. Self-care consists of knowing your own body and its signals and taking appropriate action to stop the progression of illness or injury or to improve your overall health.

When to Seek Help

Effective self-care requires understanding when you should seek professional medical attention rather than treat a condition by yourself. Surprisingly, people with diagnosed active chronic conditions get professional medical attention for only 5 percent of their episodes or flare-ups and treat the remaining 95 percent themselves.[2] Unfortunately, deciding what conditions warrant professional attention is not always easy. Generally, you should consult a physician if you experience any of the following:

- a serious accident or injury

- sudden or severe chest pains causing breathing difficulties

- trauma to the head or spine accompanied by persistent headache, blurred vision, loss of consciousness, vomiting, convulsions, or paralysis

- sudden high fever or recurring high temperature (over 38.5°C for adults and 39.5°C for children) and/or sweats

- tingling sensation in the arm accompanied by slurred speech or impaired thought processes

- adverse reactions to a drug or insect bite (shortness of breath, severe swelling, dizziness)

- unexplained bleeding or loss of bodily fluid from any body opening

Spontaneous remission: The disappearance of symptoms without any apparent cause or treatment.

Placebo effect: An apparent cure or improved state of health brought about by a substance or product that has no medicinal value.

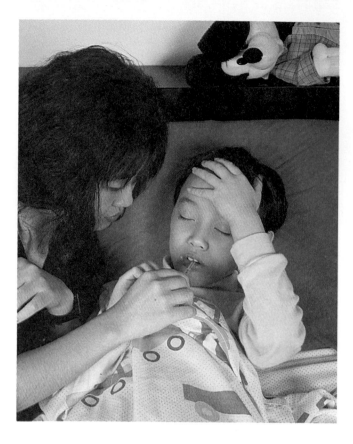

For parents, knowing when to seek help for a sick child is often a challenge since young children are unable to assess their own symptoms and may not be able to describe them adequately.

- unexplained sudden weight loss

- persistent or recurrent diarrhea or vomiting

- blue-coloured lips, eyelids, or nail beds

- any lump, swelling, thickness, or sore that does not subside or that grows for over a month

- any marked change in or pain accompanying bowel or bladder habits

- yellowing of the skin or the whites of the eyes

- any symptom that is unusual and recurs over time

- signs that suggest possible pregnancy

With the vast array of home diagnostic devices currently available, it appears to be relatively easy for most people to take care of themselves. But a strong word of caution is in order here: although many of these devices are valuable for making an initial diagnosis, home health tests cannot fully substitute for regular, complete examinations by a trained practitioner. The Skills for Behaviour Change box offers valuable information about taking an active part in your own health care.

Assessing Health Professionals

Suppose you decide that you do need medical help. You must then identify what type of medical help you need and find out where to obtain it. Initially, selecting a doctor may seem a simple matter, yet many people have no idea how to assess the qualifications of a medical practitioner.

Knowledge of both traditional medical specialties and alternative medicine is critical to making an intelligent selection. You also need to be aware of your own criteria for evaluating a health professional.

Studies indicate that many people's greatest concerns when choosing a doctor have less to do with medical qualifications than with availability and personality. While a warm and caring personality is certainly a valuable attribute, doctors who lack a good bedside manner may, in fact, be better trained and qualified than more cordial practitioners. Carefully consider the following factors about all prospective health care providers:

- What professional educational training have they had? What licence or board certification do they hold?

- Are they affiliated with an accredited medical facility or institution? The Canadian Council on Health Facilities Accreditation requires these institutions to verify all education, licensing, and training claims of their affiliated practitioners.

- Do they indicate clearly how long a given treatment may last, or do they keep you returning week after week with no apparent end in sight?

- Do their diagnoses, treatments, and general statements appear to be consistent with established scientific theory and practice?

- Do they listen to you, and appear to respect you as an individual, and give you time to ask questions?

Asking the right questions at the right time may save you personal suffering. Many patients find that writing their questions down ahead of time helps them to get all their inquiries answered. You should not accept a defensive or hostile response; asking questions is your right as a patient. The Building Communication Skills box discusses finding a personal physician in more detail.

*W*HAT DO YOU THINK?

If you had the choice of seeing a practitioner of your own sex and ethnic background, would you? Why? Do you think it would make a difference in how comfortable you may feel sharing personal or embarrassing but relevant health information? Have you ever had difficulty finding a practitioner with whom you are comfortable?

Being Proactive in Your Health Care

Your personal involvement in your own wellness is critical. Taking a proactive approach to practising preventive behaviours can go a long way toward giving you a long and healthy life. Sometimes, however, regardless of the steps you take to care for yourself, you still get sick. At such a time, it is important that you continue to be actively involved in your care. The more you know about your own body and about factors that can affect your health, the better able you will be to communicate complete information to your doctor. It also helps you to make informed decisions and to recognize when a certain treatment may not be right for you. The following points can help:

- Know your own and your family's medical history.
- Be knowledgeable about your condition—causes, physiological effects, possible treatments, prognosis. Don't rely on the doctor for all this information. Do some research.
- Bring a friend or relative along for medical visits to help you review what the doctor says and possibly write down the doctor's answers to your questions.
- Ask the practitioner to explain the problem and appropriate treatments, tests, and drugs in a clear and understandable way.
- If the doctor prescribes any medications, ask for their generic names so that you can pay less for them.
- Ask for a written summary of the results of your visit and any lab tests.
- If you have any doubt about the doctor's recommended treatment, seek a second opinion.

Afterward:

- Write down an accurate account of what happened and what was said. Be sure to include the names of the doctor and all other people involved in your care, the date, and the place.
- Shop around drugstores for the best prices in the same way that you would when shopping for clothes.
- When filling prescriptions, ask to see the pharmacist's package inserts that list medical considerations concerning the medicines. Request detailed information about any potential drug interactions.
- Have clear instructions written on the label to avoid risk to others who may take the drug in error.

Just like you, doctors are human. Their decisions are based on the best information they have available to them and may be influenced by a number of factors—workload, limited information, personal views. Therefore, in addition to following the practical steps listed above, being proactively involved in your health care also means that you should be aware of your rights as a patient. The following are the basic rights of all individuals seeking care from a health care professional.

1. The right of informed consent. Before receiving any care, you have the right to be fully informed of what is being planned, the risks and potential benefits, and possible alternative forms of treatment, including the option of no treatment. Your consent must be voluntary and without any form of coercion. It is critical that you read any consent forms carefully and amend them as necessary before signing.

2. You have the right to know whether the treatment you are receiving is standard or experimental. In experimental conditions, you have the legal and ethical right to know if the study is one in which some people receive treatment while others do not in order to compare the results and if any drug is being used in the research project for a purpose not approved by the Health Protection Branch of Health Canada.

3. You have the right to privacy, which includes protecting your right to make personal decisions concerning all reproductive matters.

4. You have the legal right to refuse treatment at any time and to cease treatment at any time during its course.

5. You have the right to receive care.

6. You have the right to access all your medical records and to confidentiality of your records.

7. You have the right to seek the opinions of other health care professionals regarding your condition.

CHOICES OF MEDICAL CARE

Familiarizing yourself with the various health professions and health subspecialties will help you choose the right provider for your needs. There are more than 56 000 physicians in Canada today. Those you are most familiar with probably subscribe to allopathic medical procedures.

Most people believe that **allopathic medicine**, or traditional, Western medical practice, is based on scientifically

Allopathic medicine: Traditional, Western medical practice; in theory, based on scientifically validated methods and procedures.

Finding a Personal Physician

Consider the following situation:

Mary wakes one morning with a chest cold. Within several days, the cold has worsened and she thinks she may have developed bronchitis. Mary knows she should see a doctor but she doesn't have a primary care physician, so she decides to let the cold takes its course without seeing someone. The next day, after a night of very laboured breathing, Mary gives in and looks up the name of a doctor in the phone book and calls for an appointment.

Unfortunately, a great many people hesitate about seeking early care because they don't have a physician. The treatment Mary receives will probably be fine. But she will know nothing about the doctor and will be taking a chance on whether she will feel comfortable being treated by this person. Had Mary had a primary care physician, she could have called him or her up as soon as her symptoms had worsened.

One of the most important decisions a person or family has to make is choosing a primary care physician. Your physician plays a critical role in both the prevention and the treatment of illnesses. When you are ill or develop symptoms that need attention, having someone to contact in whom you have confidence can relieve a great deal of anxiety. Yet, despite the importance of identifying and regularly visiting a primary care physician, a great many people wait until they are ill to seek out a doctor. Depending on the severity of the illness, waiting this long can limit a person's options. Selecting a doctor long before the development of an illness allows you the opportunity to identify and interview several doctors in order to find the one that will best fit your needs and with whom you will feel the most comfortable. In Canada, you may have easier access to a primary care physician (general or family practitioner) if another family member visits that practitioner or if you are new to the area. It may be difficult to change doctors if you are remaining in the same locale. This difficulty makes it all the more important to assess a doctor well at the outset.

The following procedure can help you with this process:

- First, consider the following questions:

  - Would you feel more comfortable with a male or female health professional?

  - Is age an important factor to you?

  - Do you have a preexisting condition for which specialization may be helpful?

  - Do you prefer to see primarily one physician or are you comfortable visiting a service having a team of doctors?

- Assemble a list of names of doctors in your area. Names of potential physicians can be identified by:

  - Asking friends and colleagues for recommendations. These are often your best sources of information about a doctor's availability and promptness and overall general concern.

  - Calling the local medical association, local health advocacy groups (many communities provide references as a service), or the local hospital for names of doctors accepting new patients.

  - Researching medical directories at your local library. The Canadian Medical Directory, for example, includes information about every physician who belongs to the CMA.

- Call the offices of the physicians on your list and explain that you are seeking a primary care physician. Ask the receptionist about the doctor's hospital affiliation, office hours, and the kind of coverage the physician has for emergency situations that occur outside normal office hours. Take into consideration the receptionist's tone and how your questions are answered. Find out how much time is allotted for appointments (30 to 45 minutes for a routine physical is average).

- Narrow the list to two or three physicians and make appointments for brief consultations.

- While visiting with each doctor, you should find answers to the following questions:

(continued)

---

validated methods, but you should consider the fact that only about 20 percent of all allopathic treatments have been proven clinically efficacious in scientific trials. Many standard procedures focus on countering a patient's symptoms, not necessarily on curing the root problem. Medical practitioners who adhere to allopathic principles are bound by a professional code of ethics.

Traditional (Allopathic) Medicine

Selecting a **primary care practitioner**—a medical practitioner whom you can go to for routine ailments, pre-

ventive care, general medical advice, and appropriate referrals—is not an easy task. The primary care practitioner for most people is a family practitioner. Others use nontraditional providers as their primary source of care. The common denominator is continuity in services over a period of time. Having a "usual source of care" is important to the quality of care you receive.

Some of what is done in medicine either does not improve health outcomes or creates iatrogenic disease (illness caused by the medical process itself). An essential part of medical care is informed consent. This refers to your right to have explained to you—in nontechnical lan-

- Is the doctor's educational and experiential background appropriate?

- While visiting, do you feel that he or she cares about you as a person?

- Do you feel relaxed in his or her presence?

- Does he or she make you feel rushed?

- Are you encouraged to ask questions and are answers explained clearly?

- Does the physician use a lot of medical jargon, and how do you feel about that?

- Does the doctor use a condescending tone?

- Does the physician attend to you personally or does he or she serve primarily as a "gatekeeper" to specialists?

- Develop some direct questions about treatment that will help to identify the person's philosophy on care. For example, you could ask how the physician would treat a terminally ill patient or about his or her willingness to accommodate your religious feelings.

- Once you choose a physician, get the most from your visits by maintaining an open line of communication. You can do this by:

  - *Always being prepared for an appointment.* Know your medical and family history and be very specific and detailed about any symptoms you may be experiencing.

  - *Being an educated patient.* Expect and insist on a diagnosis explained in a way that you fully understand. Never leave your doctor's office with questions unanswered.

  - *Taking a proactive role in your health care.* Treatment will only work if you follow it. Listen to and follow instructions, find out when you can call with follow-up questions, and be sure that the doctor reports any test results to you promptly.

  - *Communicating your needs to the doctor.* If you have concerns about communication or treatment, speak up.

guage you can understand—all possible side-effects, benefits, and consequences of a specific procedure and treatment regimen as well as available alternatives to it. It also means that you have the right to refuse a specific treatment or to seek a second or even third opinion from unbiased, noninvolved providers.[3]

The legal doctrine of informed consent gives you the right to ask:

- What will happen if I choose not to have a particular test or treatment?

- Can other tests be performed instead? What are their risks?

- How often has the doctor performed this test, surgery, or procedure, and with what proportion of successful outcome?

- Are the risks from the treatment greater than the risks from the condition?

- What are the side-effects of the diagnostic tests? Can these side-effects be treated or reduced?

- Does this procedure require an overnight stay at a hospital or can it be performed in a doctor's office?

- Why has this test been ordered? What is the doctor trying to find or exclude?

- Are these medications necessary? What are their possible side-effects? What will happen if I decide not to take them? What alternatives are available? Is there a generic version that costs less?

- What caused me to have this problem? What can I do to make sure it doesn't happen again?

*W*HAT DO YOU THINK?

Have you ever brought a list of questions to your practitioner's office? If you have, were your questions answered fully? Did you feel at all intimidated or rushed? Do you think patients have the right to question their practitioners' judgement or should they turn over responsibility to the practitioner?

Allied Professionals

The changes in the delivery of health care in recent years have brought far greater attention and responsibility to the roles of a group of health-related professionals long allied with physicians and other health specialists. These include nurses, nurse practitioners, and physician's assistants.

Primary care practitioner: A medical practitioner who treats routine ailments, advises on preventive care, gives general medical advice, and makes appropriate referrals when necessary.

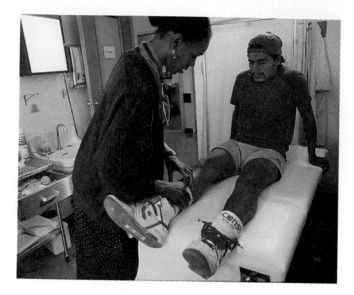

Students frequently turn to health centres, clinics, and hospital emergency rooms for treatment when needed, but those who rely solely on these settings miss out on the benefits of continuity of care by a primary care physician.

Nurses are highly trained and strictly regulated health practitioners who provide a wide range of services for patients and their families, including patient education, counselling, community health and disease prevention information, and administration of medications. They have the designation RN, or registered nurse. Although nurses may work in HSOs, clinics, doctors' offices, student health centres, nursing homes, public health departments, schools, businesses, and other health care settings, many are employed in the hospital setting. There has been an increasing trend away from hospital-based employment as the demand for nurses in other settings has increased.

Nurse practitioners are professional nurses having advanced training obtained through either a master's degree program or a specialized nurse practitioner program. Nurse practitioners have the training and authority to conduct diagnostic tests and prescribe medications. They work in a variety of settings, particularly in hospitals, clinics, and client homes. They have become an increasingly popular source of health care in recent years. Nurses may also earn a bachelor of science and nursing degree (BScN), a masters of science and nursing (MScN), or a research-based Ph.D. in nursing.

Nonallopathic Medicine

While people in other parts of the world consider nonallopathic medicine the "traditional" form of treatment, in North America we tend to think of **nonallopathic medicine** as "alternative medicine." As the government, private payers, and consumers have begun to evaluate the costs, effectiveness, and quality of traditional health care, many have found it wanting. Thus, each year more and more people seek nonallopathic or alternative medical care from providers other than licensed medical doctors. Many nonallopathic practitioners offer effective care at reasonable prices, but because they are not all licensed or regulated, the consumer's job of verifying credentials can be even more difficult than it is in traditional medicine.

There are numerous nonallopathic alternatives. Many people turn to nonallopathic medicine only after more traditional methods have failed to improve their conditions. Because they are often "providers of last resort," these unconventional treatments may appear to produce more negative outcomes overall than does traditional medicine. This has given them a bad reputation in some quarters even though it was the failure of traditional medicine that sent many patients to nonallopathic practitioners in the first place. Although some alternative therapies are controversial and even dangerous, many offer significant benefits.

As with any type of therapy, you must be assertive and directly ask providers of nonallopathic medicine about their training, licensing (if relevant to their field), and affiliations. You should also ask them how many patients suffering from your complaint they have treated. The greatest danger in seeking the assistance of an alternative medical practitioner is usually that it may keep you from obtaining more efficacious conventional treatment (if any is available for your complaint).

Chiropractic Treatment. Chiropractic medicine has been practised for over 100 years. Allopathic medicine and chiropractic medicine were in direct competition over a century ago.[4] Once allopathic medicine became more formally organized and entrenched in society, medical associations exerted their power to restrict the practice of chiropractors, even though there were not many empirical studies at the time proving the safety and efficacy of allopathic medicine. The relationship between medical doctors and doctors of chiropractic has improved since the settlement of a bitter lawsuit in which a group of chiropractors successfully argued that the American Medical Association (AMA) was conspiring to eliminate the practice of chiropractic in the United States.[5] Although there have always been some medical doctors who worked collaboratively with chiropractic doctors, their number has recently increased. Some chiropractic treatments are covered by provincial health insurance and many private insurance companies will now pay for chiropractic treatment if a medical doctor recommends it.

Chiropractic medicine is based on the idea that a life-giving energy flows through the spine via the nervous system. If the spine is subluxated (partly misaligned or dislocated), that force is disrupted. Chiropractors use a variety of techniques to manipulate the spine back into proper alignment so the life-giving energy can flow unimpeded through the nervous system. It has been established that their treatment is effective for chronic low back pain, neck pain, and headaches. In fact, a 1990 *British Medical Journal* article reported that chiropractors were more successful in treating certain types of chronic pain than traditional doctors were.

You should investigate and question a chiropractor as carefully as you would a medical doctor. Be sure to ask whether the chiropractor uses such controversial and unproved practices as colonic flushes, herbal medications, and diet therapies or follows standard chiropractic regimens in treatment. As with many health professionals, you may note vast differences in technique among specialists.

Acupuncture. Acupuncture is the ancient (over 2000 years old) Chinese art of inserting fine needles at points on the skin that fall along 14 major meridians, or pathways of energy (called *qi*), that flow through the body. These points and meridians are thought to be associated with particular internal organs and bodily functions. Proponents of acupuncture believe that the vital forces of life—the yin and the yang—are restored to equilibrium when these points are stimulated. Acupuncture has proved effective for treating chronic pain and for blocking acute pain briefly.[6] Acupuncturists treat complaints as diverse as back and neck pain, menstrual cramps, morning sickness, addiction, asthma, infections, and arthritis. They assist women in labour and can help people quit smoking.

The Acupuncture Foundation of Canada Institute teaches licensed health practitioners about acupuncture. Some licensed M.D.s and chiropractors have trained in acupuncture. If you decide to have acupuncture, it is very important to ascertain whether the needles the acupuncturist uses are disposable or are properly sterilized using an autoclave, because needles reused without proper sterilization can transmit the AIDS virus.

Acupressure is similar to acupuncture, but does not use needles. Instead, the practitioner applies pressure to points critical to balancing yin and yang. Practitioners must have the same basic understanding of energy pathways as do acupuncturists. Acupressure should not be applied by an untrained person to pregnant women or to anyone having a chronic condition.

Herbalists and Homeopaths. Herbalists practise herbal medicine, which is based on the medicinal qualities of plants or herbs. Homeopaths also use herbal medicine (as well as minerals and chemicals), but at the root of their practice is the theory that the administration of extremely diluted doses of potent natural agents that produce disease symptoms in healthy persons will cure the disease in the sick. Herbal and homeopathic medicines are common

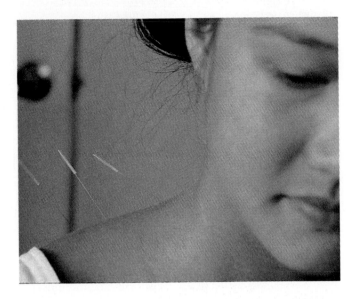

Many have found acupuncture an effective treatment for a variety of complaints.

in Europe and Asia, but are not nearly as accepted in Canada.

Although plants have been used for medicinal purposes for centuries and form the basis of many modern "wonder drugs," herbal medicine is not to be taken lightly. Because something is natural does not necessarily mean that it is safe. Many plants are poisonous, and others can be toxic if used in high doses. One of the greatest dangers with this kind of therapy is that practitioners who mix their own tonics do not use standardized measures. It is therefore imperative that you carefully investigate the chemical properties of herbs yourself before you ingest them.

Naturopathy. Naturopaths believe that illness results from violations of natural principles of life in modern societies. They view diseases as the body's effort to ward off impurities and harmful substances from the environment. Naturopathic treatment uses substances and forces found in nature: water, magnets, gravity, heat, crystals and minerals, herbs, and even the sun. Practitioners argue that returning to a natural, purified state will restore health.

Few naturopathic claims have been substantiated. Although many naturopaths use the title "doctor," the vast

Nurse: Health practitioner who provides many services for patients and who may work in a variety of settings.

Nonallopathic medicine: Medical alternatives to traditional, allopathic medicine.

Chiropractic medicine: A form of medical treatment that emphasizes the manipulation of the spinal column.

An Overview of Medicare in Canada

Prior to the 1940s, private health care predominated in Canada. This meant that access to care was based on ability to pay. By 1961, all ten provinces and two territories had signed agreements to establish public insurance plans to at least provide for universal coverage on in-hospital treatment. The proponents of what was called the "Medicare" scheme held that the private insurance model perpetuated inequality in medical care based on ability to pay rather than need. The then premier of Saskatchewan was an important figure in the fight for universal health care in Canada. As a youngster, he had become ill and had been spared amputation of his leg thanks to the generosity of a physician. His family would have been unable to pay for the treatment the young Tommy Douglas required. Our universal health care plan makes it possible for people to receive needed care regardless of income.

Several factors led to the decision to establish universal health care in Canada:

- the rejection rate of Armed Services recruits in World War II

- the sickness survey of 1951, which verified the poor health of Canadians

- the social and economic cost to Canada in lost production as a result of ill health

- the threat of the Cold War and the possibility that totalitarian regimes would have an appeal because of their professed concern for people

- the signing by the Canadian government of the World Health Organization's constitution, with its humanitarian ideology, which translated into an obligation to introduce universal health insurance.

By 1972 all the provinces and territories had health insurance plans that met the federal guidelines required for funding of health care. These guidelines included:

- public administration (nonprofit and publicly administered and accountable to the provincial government)

- comprehensiveness (in patient care, drugs, supplies, necessary tests, and a broad range of outpatient services and chronic care)

- universality (100 percent of the insured population are entitled, that is, eligible residents)

- accessibility (reasonable access without barriers such as discrimination on the basis of income, age, health status, etc.)

- portability (entitlement when residents move to another province within Canada or when they travel within Canada or abroad; all provinces, however, have some limits on out-of-province coverage and may require prior approval for non-emergency out-of-province care)

Sources: Health Canada, *Canada's Health System* (Ottawa: Public Works and Government Services Canada, 1996) 3; Canada, *Royal Commission on Health Services in Canada,* 1, (Ottawa: Queen's Printer, 1964), 5–6.

---

majority are not M.D.s, and many have not even received a minimum of health training. Thorough training is provided at three naturopathic medical schools in the United States and Canada, and those who receive a naturopathic doctor (N.D.) degree from one of these schools have been through a four-year graduate program that emphasizes humanistically oriented family medicine. If you decide to be treated by a naturopath, you should be exceedingly careful about checking the practitioner's credentials.

Other Alternative Therapies. Many other therapies exist, including reflexology (zone therapy), iridology (light therapy), aromatherapy, and auramassage. Some of these may work, but they have yet to be substantiated scientifically. Others may be harmful to your health or delay you from seeking more efficacious forms of care. Until we can sort through the proliferation of new therapies, it's a good idea to follow the maxim "buyer beware."

WHAT DO YOU THINK?

Should people be allowed to choose any type of practitioner they want—regardless of whether the treatment they advocate has been proven safe or effective? How much should the government spend to investigate new or alternative therapies?

Types of Medical Practices

Many health care providers have found it essential to combine resources into a **group practice**, which can be single- or multispecialty. Physicians share their offices, equipment, utility bills, and staff costs. Proponents of group practice maintain that it reduces unnecessary duplication of equipment and improves the quality of health care through peer review.

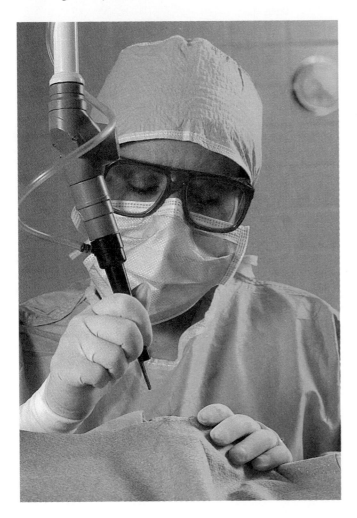

Modern technology has vastly improved the techniques available for treating many illnesses and for saving human life, but it has also played a major role in the escalating costs of medical care.

Solo practitioners are medical providers who practise independently of other practitioners.

Hospitals and Clinics

Both hospitals and clinics provide a range of health care services. These include emergency treatment, diagnostic tests, and inpatient and outpatient (ambulatory) care.

There are several ways to classify hospitals: by profit status (nonprofit or for-profit), by ownership (private, public), by specialty (children's, chronic care, psychiatric, general, acute), by teaching status (teaching-affiliated or not), and by size. **Nonprofit (voluntary) hospitals** have traditionally been run by religious or other humanitarian groups. Before universal health care, such hospitals often cared for patients whether they could pay or not. Today some hospitals retain religious ties and orientations; others are run by independent hospital boards.

For-profit (proprietary) hospitals are few and far between in Canada. They do not receive tax breaks and tend to focus on particular specialties.

More treatments or services, including surgery, are being delivered on an **outpatient (ambulatory) care** basis (care which does not involve an overnight stay) by hospitals, traditional clinics, student health clinics, and nontraditional clinical centres. One type of ambulatory facility that is becoming common is the surgicentre—a place where minor, low-risk procedures such as vasectomies, tubal ligations, tissue biopsies, cosmetic surgery, abortions, and minor eye operations are performed.

Hospitals have made efforts to improve the quality of care and patient outcomes. Many hospitals are now designated as trauma centres. They have helicopters available to transport patients to the hospital quickly, specialty physicians who are in-house (not just on-call) around-the-clock, and specialized diagnostic equipment. This combination of rapid transport and readily available specialty equipment and staff has dramatically reduced mortality rates for trauma patients. However, this same combination means that trauma centres are exceptionally expensive to run.

PROMISES AND PROBLEMS OF OUR HEALTH CARE SYSTEM

Even though we have one of the best health care systems in the world, there are a number of problems with the system. First, there are several levels of government involved in the delivery of health care services. The federal government provides monies that fund health care given that the provinces meet the guidelines (see the Focus on Canada box). The federal government also funds and administers health programs for special groups such as First Nations peoples, war veterans, and prisoners. Using

---

Group practice: A group of physicians who combine resources, sharing offices, equipment, and staff costs, to render care to patients.

Solo practitioner: Physician who renders care to patients independently of other practitioners.

Nonprofit (voluntary) hospitals: Hospitals funded by taxes.

For-profit (proprietary) hospitals: Hospitals that provide a return on earnings to the investors who own them.

Outpatient (ambulatory) care: Treatment that does not involve an overnight stay in a hospital.

federal dollars, the provinces allot monies to health care. As governments struggle to reduce deficits, there is less money available at a time when health care costs continue to rise. Federal and provincial governments have been forced to limit health care spending, resulting in downsizing and restructuring. These organizational divisions and increased fiscal pressures have caused added tension between the federal and provincial governments over power, dollars, and responsibilities.

Physicians and provincial governments also have been in conflict. The provinces have responsibility for medical programs and the allocation of dollars, while physicians control access to programs and institutions. Some provinces provide bonuses for physicians working in remote areas or reduce payments to physicians working in over-serviced areas. As well, other interest groups such as midwives, nurses, and nutritionists vie for financial resources and recognition for their contribution to the health status of Canadians.

Another source of pressure for funding are the many voluntary organizations that assist Canadians, some long-established. For example, the Canadian National Institute for the Blind has been in operation since before Confederation.

Health research is also supported by federal monies. Direct-care health services (hospitals and physicians, for example) must compete for dollars with research and

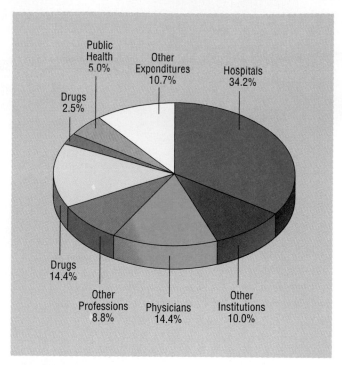

FIGURE 16.1

Distribution of Health Expenditure, Canada, 1996

Source: Health Canada, *Canada's Health System* (Ottawa: Public Works and Government Services Canada, 1996).

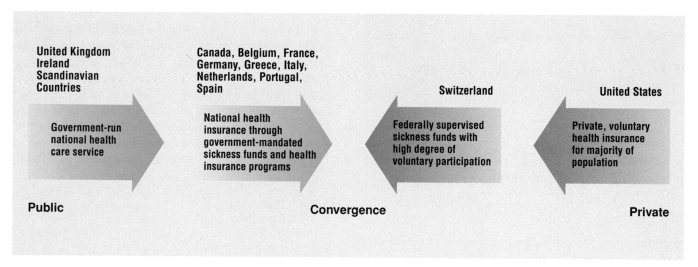

FIGURE 16.2

The Convergence of Public/Private Health Care Systems

Source: Reprinted with permission from Gunter Becher, "European Health Issues," *Employee Benefits Journal,* 38 (March 1993), published by the International Foundation of Employee Benefit Plans, Brookfield, WI.

Health Care: A Global Comparison

How do health care costs in Canada compare with those in the rest of the industrialized world? As the table below shows, they are higher than those in many other countries, but lower than those in the United States, which, with its mostly private system, has the highest health care costs in the world. Presented along with these figures are life expectancies in various countries. Many factors, of course, influence life expectancy. It is interesting to note that, among the relatively better off countries, there is no close relationship between either wealth or health spending and life span.

Life Span, Health, and Wealth

Countries in Order of Life Expectancy	Life Expectancy at Birth, 1992, in Years	Population in Millions, 1992	Real GDP per Capita, 1991	Total Expenditure on Health, % of GDP	Expenditure on Health per Capita, 1991
1 Japan	78.6	124.5	$19 390	6.8	$1 771
4 Sweden	77.7	8.6	17 490	8.8	2 372
5 Spain	77.4	39.1	12 670	6.5	877
6 Greece	77.3	10.2	7 680	4.8	274
7 Canada	77.2	27.4	19 320	9.9	1 847
8 Netherlands	77.2	15.2	16 820	8.7	1 664
11 Australia	76.7	17.6	16 680	8.6	1 466
12 France	76.6	57.1	18 430	9.1	1 912
13 Israel	76.2	5.1	13 460	4.2	509
14 United Kingdom	75.8	57.7	16 340	6.6	1 003
17 Germany	75.6	80.2	19 770	9.1	1 782
18 United States	75.6	255.2	22 330	13.3	2 932
22 Ireland	75.0	3.5	11 430	8.0	886

Source: Table excerpted from Paul Spector, "Failure, by the Numbers," *New York Times*, September 24, 1994, 19. © 1994 by The New York Times Company. Reprinted by permission.

Information in table, titled "Lifespan, Health and Wealth," from U.N. Development Program; Organization for Economic Cooperation and Development.

prevention. Prevention runs a weak third, accounting for only about 5 percent of total health spending in 1996. (See Figure 16.1) The Global Perspectives box compares the health costs of several countries, along with their life expectancies. Figure 16.2 shows Canada's place on a spectrum of public versus private health systems.

Access

Your access to health care is determined by numerous factors, including the supply of providers and facilities and your health status. Doctors are maldistributed by specialty and geographic area. Some rural areas face constant shortages of physicians.

Quality Assurance

The Canadian health care system employs several mechanisms for assuring quality services overall: education, licensure, certification/registration, accreditation, peer review, and, as a last resort, the legal system of malpractice litigation. Some of these mechanisms are mandatory before a professional or organization may provide care, while others are purely voluntary. (Consumers should note that licensure, although provincially mandated for some practitioners and facilities, is only a minimum guarantee of quality.)

Detecting Fraud and Abuse in the System

Becoming knowledgeable and acting responsibly when selecting health care providers and payers will reduce your likelihood of being financially or physically abused. Nevertheless, with the number of options in health products and services available, even the most careful consumer can be victimized. Individual provinces maintain boards for quality assurance in the medical system. If you find yourself in a situation you cannot deal with, remember that the Health Protection Branch of Health Canada, the provincial ministries of health, and the colleges of various professions are responsible for protecting you and other health consumers. Do not hesitate to contact them if you have suspicions about a provider, service, or product.

have been searching for other models that would contain costs while providing improved services and encouraging prevention and shared responsibility. One model that has already been put in place is the Health Service Organization (HSO). The patient registers with the organization, which is funded a set amount per patient per year (capitation), and is responsible for the patient's overall care. The originators of this model believed it would encourage practitioners and patients alike to emphasize prevention. There are currently 87 HSOs in Ontario alone, serving over half a million patients. Many are run by community-based boards. In Ontario, the Community Health Branch of the provincial Ministry of Health is responsible for the HSOs, and defines the program's objectives:

- to create an atmosphere that is supportive of physicians and other health care personnel, and that allows flexibility in responding to health needs

- to develop a coordinated system of health care delivery that makes the most appropriate use of health care resources and that is accessible, efficient, and economical

- to provide special attention to health maintenance and illness prevention

- to decrease institutional health care by giving emphasis to outpatient care, self-care, and home care

HSOs may offer a more comprehensive range of services than the conventional system. For example, counselling is available through HSOs as part of the service. If you live in Ontario, your physician may be a member of an HSO, so that additional services may be available at no cost to you.

𝒲HAT DO YOU THINK?

Do you believe prospective patients should have access to information about practitioners' and facilities' malpractice experience? How about their success and failure rates or outcomes of various procedures?

𝒲HAT DO YOU THINK?

Why is it important that governments cover preventive or lower-level care as well as hospitalization and high-technology interventions? What kinds of incentives cause you to seek early care rather than to delay care?

Health Service Organizations: A New Model of Health Care

The dominant model of medicine in Canada is fee-for-service. A practitioner, most often a physician, performs a service and bills the provincial health plan. Planners

Managing Your Health Care Needs

Throughout this text, we have emphasized behaviours important to keeping you healthy. But now you need to turn your attention to your potential behaviour when you need medical attention. Most people wait until a problem arises to seek medical care and take the first available physician or medical facility. But by looking ahead to future needs, you can take charge of your choices and make positive moves toward getting better health care.

Making Decisions for You

As you have seen in this chapter, many health care decisions are dictated by physicians and government agencies. But many decisions still rest with you.

Checklist for Change: Making Personal Choices

✓ How long did you have to wait before getting an appointment?

✓ How long did you have to wait in the waiting room before being seen?

✓ Does the clerical staff convey their concern for you when delays occur?

✓ Are there educational materials available in the waiting areas?

✓ Are the doctor's credentials clearly displayed?

✓ Does the physician treat you as if he or she is concerned about you?

✓ Do you feel comfortable discussing your problems with the physician?

✓ Are you confident that your doctor knows what he or she is talking about?

✓ Is the doctor willing to talk about issues such as credentials, hospital affiliations, and qualifications of referrals for special needs?

✓ Are you able to understand answers to your questions? Does the doctor seem interested in whether you understand? Seem willing to answer questions? Encourage you to ask questions?

✓ Does the physician tell you why one test is being given rather than another? About risks of the test? About preparation for the tests? About what to expect concerning certain results?

✓ Does the doctor support your obtaining a second opinion, or does he or she seem irritated with such a request?

✓ If you became seriously ill and had to see a lot of this doctor, would you feel comfortable with him or her, or would you rather have someone else?

Checklist for Change: Making Community Choices

✓ What health care services are located in your community?

✓ How long has your doctor been practising in your community?

✓ How many hospitals are within a 30-minute drive from your home? Are any of them teaching hospitals?

Summary

- Advertisers of health care products and services use sophisticated tactics to attract your attention and get your business. Advertising claims sometimes appear to be supported by spontaneous remission (symptoms disappearing without any apparent cause) or the placebo effect (symptoms disappearing because you expect them to).

- Self-care and individual responsibility are key factors involved in reducing rising health care costs and improving health status. But you need to seek medical treatment in situations that are unfamiliar to you or that are emergencies. You should assess health

professionals using their qualifications, their record of treating your specific problem, and their ability to work with you.

- In theory, allopathic ("traditional") medicine is based on scientifically validated methods and procedures. Medical doctors, specialists of various kinds, nurses, and other health professionals practice allopathic medicine. Many nonallopathic ("alternative") forms of health service—including chiropractic treatment, acupuncture, herbalists and homeopaths, and naturopathy—have proven effective for a variety of ailments.

◆ Health care providers may provide services as solo practitioners or in group practices (in which overhead is shared). Hospitals and clinics are classified by profit status, ownership, specialty, and teaching status.

◆ Problems experienced in the Canadian health care system concern demand for scarce dollars, balancing chronic care needs with more acute care facilities, and the shift away from a single-payer approach to a business mentality.

Discussion Questions

1. List some dubious claims made by health care products (such as thigh-reducing creams, hair-growth tonics, muscle-building milkshakes, to name a few). Why do marketers use such claims to attempt to sell their products? Why do consumers buy such products?

2. List some conditions (resulting from illness or accident) for which you don't need to seek medical help. When would you consider each condition to be bad enough to require medical attention? How do you decide to whom and where to go for treatment?

3. What are the differences in education between M.D.s and chiropractors? Under what circumstances would you seek treatment from a nonallopathic practitioner? Which types of nonallopathic medicine seem valid to you? Which seem like quackery?

4. What are the pros and cons of group practices?

5. Discuss the problems of the Canadian health care system. If you were Minister of Health and Welfare, what would you propose as a solution? Which groups might oppose your plan? Which groups might support it?

6. Should governments dictate rates for various medical tests and procedures in an attempt to keep costs down?

Application Exercise

Reread the What Do You Think? scenario at the beginning of the chapter and answer the following question:

1. When you have a medical problem like Roberta's, how do you know if you are getting good advice?

Make up a list of questions for Roberta to ask each physician. Your goal is to give her a better understanding of her diagnosis.

Health on the Net

Canadian Council on Health Services Accreditation
www.cchsa.ca/

Canadian Institute for Health Information
www.cihi.ca

National Forum on Health
www.nfh.hwc.ca

Injury Prevention and Emergency Care

Some of the following information was drawn from First Aid: The Vital Link, *published by The Canadian Red Cross Society.*

Accidents are the leading cause of death for people under the age of 44 and kill more young children than all other causes of death combined. For every person in Canada who dies from an injury, 40 people will be admitted to a hospital for treatment and another 1,300 will visit emergency departments.

Vehicle Safety

Motor vehicle injuries are the leading cause of death of children in Canada. Deaths from motor vehicle accident alone dropped from 25 to 12 per 100 000. But accidents are preventable and more can still be done.

Risk Management Driving. Practicing risk driving management techniques when you drive helps reduce your chances of being involved in a collision. Techniques include:

- **Surround your car with a bubble space.** The rear bumper of the car ahead of you should be three seconds away. To measure your safety bubble, choose a roadside landmark such as a signpost or light pole as a reference point. When the car in front of you passes this point, count "one-one-thousand, two-one-thousand." Make sure you are not passing the reference point before you've finished saying "three-one-thousand."

- **Scan the road ahead of you and to both sides.**

- **Drive with your low beam headlights on.** Being seen is an important safety factor. Driving with your low beam headlights on day or night makes you more visible to other drivers.

In addition:

- Anticipate other drivers' actions.

- Drive refreshed.

- Drive sober.

- Obey all traffic laws.

- Always wear seat belts.

- Ensure children ride in approved and properly installed car seats.

Safety Technology. The last line of defense against a collision is the car itself. How a car is equipped can mean the difference between life and death. When purchasing a car, look for the following features:

- Does the car have airbags? Remember airbags do not eliminate the need for everyone to wear seat belts. Airbags inflate only in the case of frontal crashes.

- Does the car have antilock brakes? Antilock brakes help pump the brakes and prevent them from locking up and, hence, the car from skidding.

- Does the car have impact-absorbing crumple zones?

- Are there strengthened passenger compartment side walls?

- Is there a strong roof support? (The center door post on four-door models gives you an extra roof pillar.)

(Source: Insurance Institute for Highway Safety)

What should I do if my car breaks down?

- Try to get off the road as far as possible.

- Turn on your car's emergency flashers and raise the hood. Set out flares or reflective triangles.

- Stay in the car until police arrive. If others stop to help, ask them to contact the police.

- If you must leave your car, leave a note with the car explaining the problem (as best you can), the time and date, your name, the direction in which you are walking, and what you are wearing. This information will help them look for you if necessary.

- Remove all valuables from the car if you must leave it.

Pedestrian Safety

Each year approximately one-fifth of all motor vehicle deaths involve pedestrians, and another 100,000 are injured each year. The highest death rates involving pedestrians occur in the very young and elderly population. Pedestrian injuries occur most frequently after dark, in urban settings primarily in intersections where pedestrians may walk or dart into traffic. It is not uncommon for alcohol to play a role in the death or injury of a pedestrian. How can you protect yourself from being injured or becoming a fatality?

- Carry or wear reflective material at night to help drivers see you.

- Cross only at crosswalks. Keep to the right in crosswalks.

- Before crossing, look both ways. Be sure the way is clear before you cross.

- Cross only on the proper signal.

- Watch for turning cars.

- Never go into the roadway from between parked cars.

- Where there is no sidewalk, and it is necessary to walk in a roadway, walk on the left side facing traffic.

- Don't wear headphones for a radio or tape player. These may interfere with your ability to hear sounds of motor vehicles.

Cycling Safety

Currently over 17 million Canadians (66% of the population) of all ages cycle for transportation, recreation and fitness. The following are suggestions cyclists should consider following to reduce their risk of injury or death.

- ***Wear a bicycle helmet.***
  - Helmets can reduce bicycle fatalities by 80%.
  - Look for an ANSI (American National Standards Institute), CSA (Canadian Standards Association) or Snell approved helmet.

- ***Cooperate with traffic.***
  - Children should walk their bikes at traffic signals.
  - Be predictable — ride in a straight line; look and signal before turning.
  - Be visible — wear bright clothes (white and yellow are brightest); young children should avoid riding after dark and if riding have a light and reflector.

- ***Practice basic handling skills with your child***
  - Ride with your child and model good riding habits
  - Follow the rules of the road - you have the same rights and responsibilities as the driver of a car.
  - Practice balancing exercises (ride along painted straight lines in a courtyard), turning exercises (shoulder check, use hand signals), stopping/breaking exercises (stop as close as possible to a line without skidding or hitting it. Use both breaks for a safe, quick stop. Practice at different speeds).

Water Safety

Drowning is the second most common cause of injury-related deaths among toddlers, and the majority of these occur in back yard pools. For every toddler who drowns, another 6-10 are hospitalized because of near drowning and 20% of these suffer permanent brain damage. Besides toddlers, the majority of water-related fatalities are occur in the following age groups:

Males 15-24 yrs

Males 45-54 yrs

Elderly over 75 yrs

Use of alcohol is the most common contributing factor in all water-related deaths. Most drownings occur in unsupervised facilities, such as lakes or pools with no lifeguards present. Swimmers should take the following precautions:

- If you are cold and shivering, stop and warm up. Have something hot to drink
- Swim with a buddy
- Refrain from the use of alcohol and other drugs when you are swimming
- Always enter feet first if you do not know the water depth
- Stay within your swimming capabilities
- Watch out for the "dangerous too's": too tired, too cold, too far from safety, too much sun, too much rough play
- Do not chew gum or eat while you swim; you could easily choke
- Give children your undivided attention. Let the phone ring, leave the laundry out in the rain, put off lunch and chores. It only takes a moment for a child to drown.
- Monitor the use of buoyant toys. They are fun, but cannot be rely upon for safety. They may deflate suddenly or be carried by wind or waves into deep water.
- Swim only in a pool where you can see the bottom at the deep end.
- Swim in supervised areas.
- Monitor the weather and environment continually.

If something does go wrong

- Stay calm, do not panic. Call for help.
- Remove yourself from the hazard (such as rough waves) or remove the hazard (such as broken glass on a pool deck).
- Stay in a safe position when performing a reaching assist.
- Use a reaching or throwing assist
- If you fall into the water, use survival positions such as the huddle or help position. If a boat capsizes, stay with the boat.
- Put on a floatation device.
- Follow the lifeguards instructions if there is an emergency.
- Know how to perform first aid.
- Find shelter from the cold or overexposure from the sun.

Home Safety

Falls.   Falls are second only to motor vehicles as a cause of nonviolent fatal injuries. Most falls occur in the home

and take place at floor level rather than at some height. Here are some suggestions to reduce the risk of injury from falls:

- Keep traffic areas well lighted, including stairs.
- Install stairway gates and window barriers to protect children.
- If you use rugs, place a rubber backing underneath the rug to reduce slippage.
- Remove electrical cords from hallways.
- Pick up objects from the floor.
- Clean up water spills on the floor immediately.
- Use nonslip applications on the bathroom tub or shower.
- Outside surfaces should be kept clear of debris, ice, snow, and fallen leaves.
- When using a step ladder, make sure the brace is in the locked position.

Fire.   Fires can be controlled and the resulting damage and injuries reduced by doing the following:

- Install smoke detectors and make sure they are in working order.
- Have two escape routes from each room of your home. Know the emergency procedures in the event of a fire.
- Avoid overloading electrical circuits.
- Replace worn electrical cords.
- Place guards in front of fireplaces, open heaters, and radiators.
- Use flame retardant clothing and blankets for children.
- Do not smoke in bed.

Alcohol Poisoning

Alcohol overdose is considered a medical emergency when one or both of the following occur: an irregular heartbeat or the person is in a coma. The two immediate causes of death in such cases are cardiac arrhythmia and respiratory depression. If a person is seriously uncoordinated and has possibly also taken a depressant, the risk of respiratory failure is serious enough that a physician should be contacted. When dealing with someone who is drunk,

1. Stay calm. Assess the situation.

2. Keep your distance. Before approaching or touching the person, explain what you intend to do.

3. Speak in a clear, firm, reassuring manner.

4. Keep the person still and comfortable.

5. Stay with the drunk person who is vomiting. When lying him/her down, turn their head to the side to prevent the head from falling back. This helps to keep the person from choking on their vomit.

6. Monitor the person's breathing.

In certain situations, it may be necessary to administer first aid. Ideally, first-aid procedures should be performed by someone who has received formal training from the Canadian Red Cross or some other reputable institution. If you do not have such training, contact your physician or call your local emergency medical service (EMS) by dialing 911 or your local emergency number. In life-threatening situations, however, you may not have time to call for outside assistance.

In cases of serious injury or sudden illness, you may need to begin first aid immediately and continue until help arrives. This appendix contains basic information and general steps to follow for various emergency situations. Simply reading these directions, however, may not prepare you fully to handle these situations. For this reason, you may want to enroll in a first-aid course.

Calling for Emergency Assistance

When calling for emergency assistance, be prepared to give exact details. Be clear and thorough, and do not panic. Never hang up until the dispatcher has all the information needed. Be ready to answer the following questions:

1. Where are you and the victim located? This is the most important information the EMS will need.

2. What has happened? How many people are involved?

3. What is the victim's apparent condition?

4. What has been done to help the victim?

5. Are there any life-threatening situations that the EMS should know about (for example, fires, explosions, or fallen electrical lines)?

6. Do you know the victim's name?

7. Is the victim wearing a medic-alert tag (a tag indicating a specific medical problem such as diabetes)?

Are You Liable?

Most of the provinces explicitly encourage bystanders to give first aid with laws called *Good Samaritan laws*. These laws protect citizens and medical professionals who act in good faith to give emergency assistance to ill or injured persons at the scene of an emergency. According to

experts in the field of first aid, the following are reasonable actions:

- You must receive a conscious person's permission before giving care. An exception can be made in the case of a minor when a parent or guardian is not present. If one is present, you must have the consent of the parent or guardian.

- Move a casualty only if the person's life is endangered.

- Call EMS for professional help.

- Check the casualty's airway, breathing, and circulation before providing further care.

- Continue to care for any life-threatening conditions until EMS personnel arrive.

- Use common sense and the skills you have learned and do *not* try to do something beyond your training.

Breathing Emergencies

Immediate first aid for respiratory distress is often crucial in preventing a life-threatening emergency. Respiratory distress can lead to respiratory arrest, which if not immediately cared for, will result in death.

- Do a primary survey and care for life-threatening problems (**A**irways, **B**reathing, **C**irculation or ABC's). Call EMS for help if needed.

- Check for responsiveness, tap or gently shake the person, shout "are you OK?"

- Help the casualty take any prescribed medication for his/her condition (oxygen, inhaler, medicine in an allergy kit).

- If the casualty is conscious but unable to speak, ask yes-no which the casualty can answer by nodding. Try to reduce any anxiety that may contribute to the casualty's breathing difficulty.

- Provide enough air by opening a window. Have people stand back.

- Help the person maintain normal body temperature.

- *Hyperventilation* If the casualty's breathing is rapid and you are certain that it is caused by emotion, such as excitement, give the following first aid:
  - Tell the person to relax and breathe slowly. Reassurance is often enough to correct hyperventilation.
  - **Under no circumstances** should you have the casualty breathe into a bag or other closed container.
  - If the condition does not correct itself within minutes or if the casualty becomes unconscious, call EMS immediately.

- *Respiratory Arrest* Rescue breathing is given to casualties who are not breathing but still have a pulse. It works because the air you breathe into the casualty has enough oxygen to keep the person alive.

  - Roll the person as one unit onto their back if necessary, while supporting their head and neck with one hand.
  - Open the airway by tilting the head back and lifting the chin.
  - Give 2 full breaths - Keep the head tilted back, pinch nose shut, seal your lips tightly around the person's mouth, give 2 full breaths, watch the chest to see that your breaths are going in.
  - Check for pulse - locate Adams apple, slide fingers down into groove of neck on side closer to you, feel for pulse for 5 to 10 seconds. If the person has a pulse, continue rescue breathing. Give 1 breath every 5 seconds. If there is no pulse, begin CPR (if trained).

- *Choking* A person who is choking may have a complete (unable to breathe at all) or partial (some air can get into lungs) airway obstruction.

  - If the person is coughing, encourage and support the coughing. If it persists, call EMS personnel.
  - If the airway is completely or nearly completely blocked, use abdominal thrusts to expel the object.
    - Stand behind the person and wrap your arms around their waist.
    - Make a fist with one hand and place the thumb side of the fist on the middle of the abdomen slightly above the navel and well below the tip of the breast bone.
    - Grasp your fist with the other hand and give quick upward thrusts into the abdomen to dislodge the object. Continue until the coughing stops or the casualty becomes unconscious.
    - If alone and choking, you can give yourself abdominal thrusts in the manner described above, or you can lean forward and press your abdomen over any firm object such as the back of a chair.
    - If casualty is lying down, or has become unconscious, call EMS. Open the airway by grasping the lower jaw and tongue and lifting the jaw. Attempt to dislodge the object by sweeping it out with the finger. Use a hooking action to remove the object.
    - Open airway. Attempt ventilations. If breaths don't go in, re-open the airway and try again. If you still can't get breaths in, give additional thrusts.

- To give abdominal thrusts to an unconscious casualty, straddle the casualty's thighs, position the heel of your hand on the casualty's abdomen just above the navel with your fingers pointing towards the casualty's head, place your other hand on top of the first hand and press into the persons abdomen with upward thrusts.
- If the person continues not breathing, repeat these steps until the person starts to breath or EMS arrives.

- If the casualty is an infant (under 1 year of age), support the infant's head and neck, turn the infant face down on your forearm with head lower than the body. Lower your forearm onto your thigh and give 5 back blows forcefully between infants shoulder blades with the heel of your hand. Support back of infant's head and neck, turn infant onto back on your lap with head supported lower than body. Place middle and index fingers on breastbone between infant's nipples. Quickly compress breastbone 1.3 to 2.5 cms (0.5 to 1 inch) for 5 thrusts. Repeat back blows and chest thrusts until object is coughed up or infant starts to cry, breathe or cough forcefully.

Controlling Bleeding

External Bleeding. Control of external bleeding is an important part of emergency care. Survival is threatened by the loss of 1 litre of blood or more. There are three major procedures for the control of external bleeding: direct pressure, elevation, and use of pressure points.

DIRECT PRESSURE. The best method is to apply firm pressure by covering the wound with a sterile dressing, bandage, or clean cloth. Apply pressure for 5 to 10 minutes to stop bleeding.

ELEVATION. Elevating the wounded section of the body can slow bleeding. For example, a wounded arm or leg should be raised above the level of the victim's heart.

PRESSURE POINTS. Pressure points are sites where an artery that is close to the body's surface lies directly over a bone. Pressing the artery against the bone can limit the flow of blood to the injury. This technique should be used only as a last resort when direct pressure and elevation have failed to stop bleeding.

Knowing where to apply pressure to stop bleeding is critical (see Figure A.1). For serious wounds, seek medical attention immediately.

Internal Bleeding. Although internal bleeding may not be immediately obvious, you should be aware of the following signs and symptoms:

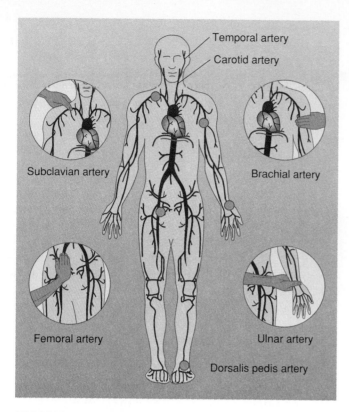

FIGURE A.1

This figure shows pressure points; the points at which pressure can be applied to stop bleeding. Unless absolutely necessary, you should avoid applying pressure to the carotid arteries, which supply blood to the brain. Also, never apply pressure to both carotid arteries at the same time.

- Symptoms of shock (discussed later in this appendix)
- Coughing up or vomiting blood
- Blood in urine
- Black, tarlike stools
- Abdominal discomfort or pain (rigidity or spasms)

In some cases, a person who has suffered an injury (such as a blow to the head, chest, or abdomen) that does not cause external bleeding may experience internal bleeding.

If you suspect that someone is suffering from internal bleeding, follow these steps:

1. Have the person lie on a flat surface with knees bent.

2. Keep the victim warm. Cover the person with a blanket, if possible.

3. Do *not* give the victim any medications or fluids.

4. Send someone to call for emergency medical help immediately.

Nosebleeds. To control a nosebleed, follow these steps:

1. Have the victim sit down and lean slightly forward to prevent blood from running into the throat. Pinch the person's nose firmly closed using the thumb and forefinger. Keep the nose pinched for at least 5 minutes.

2. While the nose is pinched, apply a cold compress to the surrounding area.

3. If pinching does not work, gently pack the nostril with gauze or a clean strip of cloth. Do not use absorbent cotton, which will stick. Be sure that the ends of the gauze or cloth hang out so that it can be easily removed later. Once the nose is packed with gauze, pinch it closed again for another 5 minutes.

4. If the bleeding persists, seek medical attention.

Burn Emergencies

Even after the heat is removed, soft tissue will continue to burn for a few minutes afterwards, causing more damage.

- Do cool burns by flushing with cool water
- Do cover the burn with a moist, or dry non-stick sterile dressing
- Don't touch burns with anything except sterile or clean dressings; do not use absorbent cotton or pull clothes over any burned area.
- Don't remove pieces of cloth that stick to a burned area.
- Don't break blisters.
- Don't use any kind of grease or ointment on severe burns
- Call EMS for second or third degree burns

- *Chemical Burns*
    - The chemical keeps burning as long as it is on the skin. Therefore, wash it from the body as quickly as possible. Continue flushing until EMS arrives.
    - Have the casualty remove clothes that were in contact with the chemical.
    - If an eye is burned by a chemical, flush the eye for 15 minutes or until EMS arrives. Make sure the water flows from the bridge of the nose outward.

- *Electrical Burns* An electrical current running through the body produces heat that can cause a burn. These burns may appear minor but in fact are very severe, because tissues below the skin may be severely damaged. The casualty will have an entrance and an exit wound where the electricity entered and left the body.

- Never approach a casualty of an electrical burn until you are sure the power is turned off. If people are in a car with a downed wire across it, tell them to stay in the vehicle.
- In the primary survey, watch carefully for breathing difficulties or sudden cardiac arrest.
- In the secondary survey, don't forget the exit wound: look for two burn sights. Cover burned areas with a moist, or dry non-stick sterile dressing.
- A casualty of lightning may also have fractures, including spinal fracture, so do not move him or her. Any burns are a lesser problem.

Shock

Shock is usually caused by extensive internal or external bleeding, as the loss of blood leads to low blood volume and decreased oxygen supply to the vital organs. Extensive burns and other fluid loss such as diarrhea and vomiting in children can also cause shock. Symptoms are: *Weakness, Anxiety, Confusion, Pale, cold, clammy skin, Weak, rapid pulse, Drowsiness or unconsciousness.*

- Do a primary survey and care life-threatening problems (ABC's). Call EMS if necessary.
- Do a secondary survey, if needed, and care for other problems (eg be sure the person is warm).
- Keep monitoring ABC's until EMS arrives.
- Help the casualty rest in the most comfortable position and give reassurance.

Poison Emergencies

A poison is any substance that causes injury, illness or death if it enters the body. A poison can enter the body in four ways: ingestion, inhalation, absorbtion through the skin and injection.

- *Ingested poisons*
  - Do a primary care survey for life-threatening problems (ABC's). Call EMS if necessary. Call the poison centre.
  - Keep monitoring the ABC's until EMS arrives.
  - Do not give the casualty anything to drink or eat unless directed by the poison centre. With an unknown poison, if the casualty vomits, save some of the vomit for later medical analysis.
- *Inhaled Poisons*
  - All casualties of inhaled poisons need to breathe oxygen as soon as possible. Remove the person form the gas or fumes only if it is safe for you to do so.
  - Call EMS.
  - Give first aid for the ABC's as needed.

- *Absorbed Poisons*
  - Wash the affected area thoroughly with soap and water.
  - Remove contaminated clothing and avoid contact until it has been laundered.
  - If a rash or weeping lesion develops, apply a paste of baking soda and water to the area several times a day. Lotions such as Calamine® or Caladryl® may be soothing.
  - Antihistamines such as Benadryl® may help dry up the lesions.
- *Injected poisons* Insect and animal stings and bites are common injected poisons.
  - Remove the stinger by scraping it away from the skin with your fingernail or hard plastic like a credit card. Do not use tweezers as the pressure can squeeze more poison into the skin.
  - Wash the area with soap and water and cover to keep it clean.
  - Put ice or a cold pack over the area to reduce pain and swelling.
  - Watch for symptoms of allergic reaction.
  - *Marine life sting* For jellyfish, sea anemone and sting ray stings, bathe the area with sea water. Do not use fresh or hot water. Wear gloves for protection. Remove any tentacles or pieces of the animal. Make a solution of 10 parts water to one part household ammonia, vinegar, baking soda or meat tenderizer and apply to the area. Scrape the area with a razor or knife edge. When dry, apply a topical corticosteroid, antihistamine, local anesthetic cream every 4 hours for several days.
  - *Animal bites* The most serious danger is rabies which is fatal if not treated. Wash the wound (if minor) with soap and water. Control any bleeding and apply a dressing. Watch later for signs of infection. If the wound is bleeding seriously, control the bleeding first - do not clean the wound. Seek medical attention. Call EMS to report the animal bite. They will contact animal control.
  - *Snake bites* Most snakes in Canada are nonpoisonous. They will bite if provoked - treat the bite as a simple wound. The most common venomous snakes in Canada are rattle-snakes. A snakes striking range is about two-thirds of its length forward and one-third upward. If bitten, place the casualty at rest and lower the bitten area below the level of the heart, if practical, to slow the absorption of venom. Reassure the casualty and advise the person not to walk or move around. Death from a snake bite rarely occurs, but the casualty should receive medical assistance as soon as possible. Make sure

the casualty who has difficulty breathing has an open airway. If breathing stops begin rescue breathing along with CPR if heart stops.

Injuries of Joints, Muscles, and Bones

Sprains. Sprains result when ligaments and other tissues around a joint are stretched or torn. The following steps should be taken to treat sprains:

1. Elevate the injured joint to a comfortable position to slow the blood.

2. Apply an ice pack or cold compress to reduce pain and swelling.

3. Wrap the joint firmly with a (roller) bandage.

4. Check the fingers or toes periodically to ensure that blood circulation has not been obstructed. If the bandage is too tight, loosen it.

5. Keep the injured area elevated, and continue ice treatment for 24 hours.

6. Apply heat to the injury after 48 hours if there is no further swelling.

7. If pain and swelling continue or if a fracture is suspected, seek medical attention.

Fractures. Any deformity of an injured body part usually indicates a fracture. A fracture is any break in a bone, including chips, cracks, splinters, and complete breaks. Minor fractures (such as hairline cracks) might be difficult to detect and might be confused with sprains. If there is doubt, treat the injury as a fracture until X-rays have been taken.

Do not move the victim if a fracture of the neck or back is suspected because this could result in a spinal cord injury. If the victim must be moved, splints should be applied to immobilize the fracture, to prevent further damage, and to decrease pain. Following are some basic steps for treating fractures and applying splints to broken limbs:

1. If the person is bleeding, apply direct pressure above the site of the wound,

2. If a broken bone is exposed, do not try to move it back into the wound. This can cause contamination and further injury.

3. Do not try to straighten out a broken limb. Splint the limb as it lies.

4. The following materials are needed for splinting:

   - Splint: wooden board, pillow, or rolled up magazines and newspapers

   - Padding: towels, blankets, socks, or cloth

   - Ties: cloth, rope, or tape

5. Place splints and padding above and below the joint. Never put padding directly over the break. Padding should protect bony areas and the soft tissue of the limb.

6. Tie splints and padding into place.

7. Check the tightness of the splints periodically. Pay attention to the skin color, temperature, and pulse below the fracture to make sure the blood flow is adequate.

8. Elevate the fracture and apply ice packs to prevent swelling and reduce pain.

9. Call EMS.

Head Injuries

A head injury can result from an auto accident, a fall, an assault, or a blow from a blunt object. All head injuries can potentially lead to brain damage, which may result in a cessation of breathing and pulse.

For minor head injuries:

1. For a minor bump on the head resulting in a bruise without bleeding, apply ice to decrease the swelling.

2. If there is bleeding, apply even, moderate pressure. Because there is always the danger that the skull may be fractured, excessive pressure should not be used.

3. Observe the victim for a change in consciousness. Observe the size of pupils and note signs of inability to think clearly. Check for any signs of numbness or paralysis. Allow the victim to sleep, but wake him or her periodically to check for awareness.

For severe head injuries:

1. If the victim is unconscious, check the airway for breathing. If necessary, perform rescue breathing.

2. If the victim is breathing, check the pulse. If it is less than 55 or more than 125 beats per minute, the victim may be in danger.

3. Check for bleeding. If fluid is flowing from the ears or nose, do not stop it.

4. Do not remove any objects imbedded in the victim's skull.

5. Cover the victim with blankets to maintain body temperature, but guard against overheating.

6. Seek medical help as soon as possible.

Temperature Related Emergencies

- *Frostbite* Frostbite is the freezing of body tissues. In superficial frostbite, the skin is frozen but not the tissue below. In deep frostbite, the skin and the underlying tissue is frozen. Both types are serious. The water in and between the body's cells freezes and swells which can damage or destroy the cells. Frostbite can lead to loss of fingers, hands, toes and feet.

- If the casualty shows signs of both frostbite and hypothermia, give first aid for hypothermia (see below).
- Cover the affected area.
- Handle gently, never rub.
- Soak the affected part in water 40.5⁰ C (105⁰ F)
- Do not let the affected part touch the sides or bottom of the container.
- Keep in water until red and warm.
- Bandage with dry, sterile dressing.

- *Hypothermia* The body reacts to cold by contracting blood vessels near the skin to move warm blood to the centre of the body, thus less heat escapes through the skin and the body stays warm. If shivering does not warm the body it cools and if body temperature drops below 35° C, the heart beats unevenly and eventually stops. The air temperature does not have to be below freezing for hypothermia to occur. Elderly people in poorly heated homes, people with poor nutrition, and people who use alcohol and barbiturates can develop hypothermia at temperatures even above freezing, because the body's normal response to cold is impaired.
  - Call EMS personnel
  - Warm body gradually by wrapping in blankets or putting on dry clothing.
  - Apply heat sources (hot water bottle, heating pad if casualty is dry).
  - Give warm liquids to an alert casualty.
  - Do not rewarm too quickly.
  - Handle gently

- *Heat Cramps* Painful spasms of muscles, usually in the calf or abdomen, are caused by fluid and salt loss resulting from heavy exercise or work outdoors in warm or moderate temperatures.
  - Have casualty rest in a cool place.
  - Give cool water or sports drink.
  - Stretch muscle and massage area.

- *Heat related illness* Heat exhaustion is the most common heat illness. Fluid loss from excess sweating is not adequately replaced. This loss leads to low blood volume. Blood flow is reduced to the vital organs as the body tries to give off heat by increasing blood flow to the skin. Heat stroke is much less common and most severe heat emergency. It occurs when heat exhaustion is overlooked. The body cannot cool itself and gradu-

ally stops working. Sweating stops because the body tissues have a lower fluid content, the body temperature rapidly rises and reaches a level where the brain, heart and kidneys cannot function.

- Have casualty rest in a cool place.
- Give cool water.
- Monitor casualty's condition for signals of worsening.
- Loosen tight clothing.
- Remove perspiration soaked clothing.
- Apply cool, wet cloths and fan casualty.
- Call EMS immediately.
- Cool body by any means available (wet towels or sheets, ice packs to groin and armpits).
- Monitor ABC's
- Be prepared to do rescue breathing or CPR.

First Aid Kit

Keep a first aid kit readily available in your home, automobile, workplace and recreation area. Store it in a dry place and replace used and outdated contents regularly. A first aid kit should contain the following:

- Emergency telephone numbers for EMS, your regional poison centre and personal physician. Include the home and office phone numbers of family members, friends or neighbours who can help.
- Sterile gauze pads (dressings), in small and large squares to cover wounds
- Adhesive tape
- Roller and triangular bandages to hold dressings in place or to make an arm sling
- Adhesive bandages in assorted sizes
- Scissors
- Tweezers
- Safety pins
- Ice bag or chemical ice pack
- Disposable gloves such as surgical or examination gloves
- Flashlight with extra batteries in separate bag
- Antiseptic wipes or soap
- Pencil and pad
- Emergency blanket
- Syrup of ipecac
- Eye patches
- Thermometer
- Coins for pay phone
- Red Cross first aid manual

Join Red Cross as we teach you and your family to be safer in, on, and around the water

AquaTots

AquaTots introduces you and your infant or toddler to a new and exciting environment. This three level program focusses on a relaxed approach to water movement for your child and teaches you how to help keep your family safe around the water.

AquaQuest

This program is the choice of more than one million Canadians, ages three and up. Why? Because AquaQuest, a twelve level program, teaches swimming skills and water safety…and water safety is the number one reason parents enroll their children in swimming lessons.

AquaAdults

You are choosing a lifetime of fitness, fun and water safety when you choose AquaAdults. This three level program starts with basic swimming skills and lets you chart your own course…whether it's to stroke improvement, fitness, or water safety skills.

AquaLeader

So you want to teach swimming! Start with our AquaLeader program, which provides you with the basic skills and experience necessary to enter the Water Safety Instructor Program.

Water Safety Instructor

Are you energetic? Enthusiastic? A people person? Do you like getting wet? Then the Canadian Red Cross wants you to take the Water Safety Instructor course. This course certifies candidates 16 years and older to teach AquaTots, AquaQuest, and AquaAdults.

Water Safety Instructor Trainer

Share your experiences and your commitment to the Water Safety Program. This course prepares you to train Water Safety Instructor candidates, and act as a mentor and community resource.

Take a Look at all the Other Ways Red Cross Can Serve You!

ChildSafe Program

Do you live or work with small children? Our special ChildSafe program shows you how to "childproof" your home and heightens your safety awareness to help you create safe environments for children and prevent injuries.

First Responder Program

Are you a professional rescuer? Do you want to know the latest advanced first aid and CPR? The Red Cross can provide you with the knowledge and skills that you need to respond to emergencies with confidence and care.

Automated External Defibrillation Program

Automated external defibrillation can help increase survival rates among people suffering from sudden cardiac arrest. Do you know that the use of an automated external defibrillator only requires 4-6 hours of training and that you only need a Basic Life Support - CPR current certificate prior to this program?

Oxygen Administration Program

Do you want to learn how to use the equipment to administer oxygen to a breathing or a nonbreathing person? In only 2-4 hour anyone can learn how to make appropriate decisions about care to give to someone having difficulty breathing during an emergency situation.

YES YOU CAN: Prevent Disease Transmission Program

This program is geared toward the general public, professionals and others in organizations who need to know about the risk of disease transmission in different settings such as: home, daycare center, office, school, recreational center, highrisk workplace, etc.

First Aid – Vital Link Program

Who can save a life… You can! Take a First Aid or Basic Life Support-CPR course with the Red Cross. It only takes a few hours of you time… and it could mean the difference between life and death for someone you love.

Babysitter's Program

Has your favourite babysitter taken a Red Cross Babysitter's course? This program teaches young adolescents to care for your children, how to do basic first aid, and how to keep the children's environment safe. Give yourself peace of mind when you are away from your children. Ask your babysitter to take this training.

Peoplesavers Program

This 4-level program provides elementary school aged children with viable, confidence building, injury prevention and first aid knowledge and skills. The program can be taught to school students, Scouts & Guides, summer camps, water safety classes, after-school programs or any other group of children.

The Canadian Red Cross offers many other programs and services! For further information, contact your local Red Cross Office or The Canadian Red Cross Society, National Office. 1800 Alta Vista Drive, Ottawa, ON, K1G 4J5 Phone: (613)739-3000 Internet: **www.redcross.ca/fieldops/firstaid**

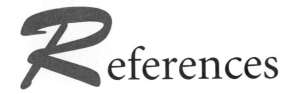

References

CHAPTER 1

1. Statistics Canada, *Canada Year Book 1997* (Ottawa: Minister of Industry, Cat. No. 402-XPE, 1996), 116.
2. C. F. Beckington, "The World Health Organization," in *World Health* (New York: Longman, 1975), 149.
3. World Health Organization, "Constitution of the World Health Organization," *Chronicles of the World Health Organization*, Geneva, Switzerland, 1947.
4. René Dubos, *So Human the Animal* (New York: Scribners, 1968), 15.
5. J. Epp, *Achieving Health for All: A Framework for Health Promotion* (Ottawa: Minister of Supply and Services Canada, 1986).
6. Thomas Stevens and Dawn Fowler Graham, eds., *Canada's Health Promotion Survey 1990: Technical Report* (Ottawa: Minister of Supply and Services, Cat. No. H39-263/2-1990E, 1993).
7. Department of Health and Human Services, *Healthy People 2000: National Health Promotion and Disease Prevention Objectives for the Year 2000* (Washington, D.C.: Government Printing Office, 1990).
8. Lisa Miller, "Medical Schools Put Women in Curricula," *Wall Street Journal*, May 24, 1994, B1, B7.
9. M. Eichler, A. L. Reisman, and E. M. Borins, "Gender Bias in Medical Research," *Women and Therapy*, 12 (1992): 61–70.
10. Carol Tavris, *The Mismeasure of Woman* (New York: Touchstone, 1992), 99.
11. Eichler et al., op. cit., 63.
12. National Cancer Institute of Canada, *Breast Cancer Bulletin* (June 1996), 1.
13. M. DiMatteo, *The Psychology of Health, Illness, and Medical Care: An Individual Perspective* (Pacific Grove, CA: Brooks/Cole, 1994), 101–103.
14. Edward P. Sarafino, *Health Psychology* (New York: John Wiley & Sons, 1990), 189–191.
15. George D. Bishop, *Health Psychology* (Needham Heights, MA: Allyn & Bacon, 1994), 84–86.
16. A. Ellis and M. Bernard, *Clinical Application of Rational-Emotive Therapy* (New York: Plenum, 1985).
17. P. Watson and R. Tharp, *Self-Directed Behavior: Self Modification for Personal Adjustment* (Pacific Grove, CA: Brooks/Cole, 1993), 13.
18. *The Stanford DECIDE Drug Education Curriculum*, Garfield Company, CA.

CHAPTER 2

1. National Mental Health Association, *Mental Health* (Alexandria, VA: National Mental Health Association, 1988), 3–4; W. Menninger, "Emotional Maturity," in *A Psychiatrist for a Troubled World: Selected Papers of William Menninger*, ed. Bernard H. Hall (New York: Viking, 1967), 789–807.
2. Richard Lazarus, *Emotion and Adaptation* (New York: Oxford Press, 1991).
3. Christine Ritter, "Social Supports, Social Networks, and Health Behaviors," in *Health Behavior: Emerging Research Perspectives*, ed. David Gochman (New York: Plenum, 1988).
4. Lester Lefton, *Psychology*, 5th ed. (Boston: Allyn & Bacon, 1994), 626.

5. A. O'Connell and V. O'Connell, *Choice and Change: Psychology of Holistic Growth, Adjustment, and Creativity* (Englewood Cliffs, NJ: Prentice Hall, 1992).
6. C. G. Jung, *Man and His Symbols*, ed. Aniela Jaffe (Garden City, NY: Doubleday, 1963).
7. Ibid., 65.
8. Martin Seligman, *Learned Optimism* (New York: Knopf, 1990).
9. Excerpted by permission from the *University of California at Berkeley Wellness Letter*, July 1992, 3–4. © Health Letter Associates, 1992.
10. D. Grady, "Think Right, Stay Well," *American Health*, xi (1992): 50–54.
11. Ibid., 50–54.
12. Bernie Siegel, *Love, Medicine, and Miracles* (New York: HarperCollins, 1988).
13. Grady, op. cit., 50–54.
14. Ibid., 50–54.
15. Ibid., 50–54.
16. Ibid., 50–54.
17. B. Diverty and M. P. Beaudet, "Depression: An Undertreated Disorder?" *Health Reports* 8 (1997): 9.
18. Adapted by permission of the author from Kathryn Rose Gertz, "Mood Probe: Pinpointing the Crucial Differences Between Emotional Lows and the Gridlock of Depression," *Self*, November 1990, 165–168, 204.
19. G. Terence Wilson, Peter Nathan, K. Daniel O'Leary, and Lee Anna Clark, *Abnormal Psychology* (Boston: Allyn & Bacon, 1996), from Chapter 7.
20. K. L. McEwan, M. Donnelly, D. Robertson, and Clyde Hertzman, *Mental Health Problems Among Canada's Seniors: Demographic and Epidemiologic Considerations* (Ottawa: Minister of Supply and Services, Cat. No. H39-203/1991E, 1991), 17.
21. Lefton, op. cit., 480–482.

CHAPTER 3

1. Hans Selye, *Stress Without Distress* (New York: Lippincott, 1974), 28–29.
2. Charles Morris, *Understanding Psychology* (Englewood Cliffs, NJ: Prentice Hall, 1993), 471–473.
3. Walter Schafer, *Stress Management for Wellness*, 2nd ed. (New York: Harcourt Brace Jovanovich, 1992).
4. R. Ader and S. Cohen, "Psychoneuroimmunology: Conditioning and Stress," *Annual Review of Psychology* 44 (1993): 53–85.
5. N. Cohen, D. Tyrrell, and A. Smith, "Negative Life Events, Perceived Stress, Negative Affect, and Susceptibility to the Common Cold," *Journal of Personality and Social Psychology* (1993): 64 (131–140).
6. Ader and Cohen, op. cit., 53–85.
7. Ibid., 59.
8. Selye, op. cit., 28–29.
9. Thomas Holmes and Richard Rahe, "The Social Readjustment Rating Scale," *Journal of Psychosocial Research* (1967): 213–217.
10. Ibid., 214.
11. Richard Lazarus, "The Trivialization of Distress," *Preventing Health Risk Behaviors and Promoting Coping with Illness*, ed. J. Rosen and L. Solomon (Hanover, NH: University Press of New England, 1985), 279–298.

12. Lester Lefton, *Psychology* (Boston: Allyn & Bacon, 1994), 471.
13. Ibid., 471.
14. R. C. Kessler, K. S. Kendler, A. C. Heath, M. C. Neale, and L. J. Eaves, "Social Support, Depressed Mood, and Adjustment to Stress: A Genetic Epidemiological Investigation," *Journal of Personality and Social Psychology* 62 (1992): 257–272.
15. Charles Morris, op. cit., 447–448.
16. Meyer Friedman and Ray H. Rosenman, *Type A Behavior and Your Heart* (New York: Knopf, 1974).
17. R. Ragland and R. Brand, "Distrust, Rage May Be Toxic Cores That Put Type A Person at Risk," *Journal of the American Medical Association* 261 (1989): 813, 814.
18. Philip L. Rice, *Stress and Health* (Monterey, CA: Brooks/Cole, 1992), 471.
19. Ibid.
20. Robert Eliot, *Is It Worth Dying For?* (New York: Bantam, 1984), 225.

CHAPTER 4

1. van Dijk, Jan J. M., Mayhew, Pat and Killias, Martin, *Experiencing Crime Across the World* (Kluwer Law and Taxation Publishers, 1990) 38.
2. Ibid., 78.
3. J. Frank, "Violent Youth Crime," *Canadian Social Trends*, Autumn 1992, Statistics Canada, 3.
4. W. Gleberzon, *Ethnicity and Violence: Racial Conflict in Vancouver* (unpublished, undated, on file at the Human Rights Library, Fauteux Hall, University of Ottawa) 7-8.
5. K. Adachi, *The Enemy That Never Was: A History of the Japanese Canadians* (Toronto: McClelland and Stewart, 1991).
6. W. Pitman, *Now is Not Too Late* (Submitted to the Council of Metropolitan Toronto by Task Force on Human Relations, Toronto, 1977).
7. M. Suderman and P. Jaffe, *Preventing Violence: School and Community Based Strategies*, Health Canada, 1996.
8. Statistics Canada, *Canadian Crime Statistics* 1995, 5-6.
9. M. Asberg, et al. "Psychology of Suicidal Behaviour," *Annals of the New York Academy of Sciences*, vol 487, (New York: New York Academy of Sciences, 1986).
10. B. L. Tanney, "Mental Disorders, Psychiatric Patients and Suicide," in R. Maris et al. (eds) *Assessment and Prediction of Suicide*, (New York: Guilford Press, 1992).
11. I. Sakinofsky, "The Ecology of Suicide in the Provinces of Canada, 1967-71 to 1979-81", in B. C. Cooper (ed.) *The Epidemiology of Psychiatric Disorders* (Baltimore: Johns Hopkins, 1987).
12. C. Pritchard, "Youth Suicide and Gender in Australia and New Zealand Compared With Countries of the Western World, 1973-87," *Australian and New Zealand Journal of Psychiatry* 26 (4), 1992.
13. Statistics Canada, "Causes of Death 1994," *Mortality: Summary List of Causes*, 1994.
14. Child and Family Canada, *Fact Sheet on Suicide*.
15. J. Frank, op.cit., 9.
16. D. Patel, *Dealing with Interracial Conflict: Policy Alternatives*, Montreal: Institute for Research on Public Policy, 1980.
17. L. McLeod, *Wife Battering in Canada: the Vicious Circle*. Canadian Advisory Council on the Status of Women, 1980.
18. K. Rodgers, "Wife Assault in Canada," *Canadian Social Trends*, Statistics Canada, Autumn 1994, 3.
19. Ibid.
20. Solicitor General, *Family Violence: Not a Private Problem*, RCMP Policy, Public Education Doc.1966.
21. Statistics Canada, *Canadian Crime Statistics*, 1995, 60.
22. Ibid.
23. Statistics Canada, *Family Violence in Canada*, 1994, 42.
24. Statistics Canada, *Violence Against Women Survey, 1993*.
25. A. Joerger et. al. "Why Men Batter: Why Women Stay," *Community Safety Quarterly* 5 (1992): 22-23.
26. N. West, "Crimes against Women," *Community Safety Survey* 5 (1992): 1.
27. H. Pan et al., "Physical Aggression in Early Marriage: Pre-relationship and Relationship Effects," *Journal of Consulting Psychology*.

28. G. Wilson et al., *Abnormal Psychology*, (Boston, MA: Allyn & Bacon, 1996).
29. Ibid.
30. Ibid.
31. *WHO Fact Sheet N150* March 1997, WHO Communications and Public Relations.
32. Ibid.
33. A. Miller, "Newly Recognized Shattering Effects of Child Abuse," *Empathic Parenting*, (1&2, Toronto, 1992).
34. *WHO Fact Sheet N150*, op. cit.
35. *Committee on Sexual Offenses Against Children and Youth - Sexual Offenses Against Children*, Ministry of Supply and Services, 1984.
36. Statistics Canada, "Selected Violations Against the Person, by Gender of Victim and Accused, 1995," *Canadian Crime Statistics, 1995*.
37. *Family Violence in Canada* op. cit. 86.
38. Health Canada, *Dating and Violence - Fact Sheet*, (Ottawa, February 1993).
39. A. Berkowitz, "College Men as Perpetrators of Acquaintance Rape and Sexual Assault: A Review of the Literature," *Journal of American College Health*, 40 (1992): 177.
40. ibid., 178.
41. D. Benson et al., "Acquaintance Rape on Campus: A Literature Review," *Journal of American College Health*, 40 (1992): 158.
42. M. Whittaker, "The Continuum of Violence Against Women: Psychological and Physical Consequenses," *Journal of American College Health*, 40 (1992): 151.
43. A. Mathews, "Campus Crime 101," *Eugene Register Guard*, March, 1993, 2B.
44. T. Schneider, "Rape Prevention," *Community Safety Quarterly* (1992): 8-13.
45. Ibid., 12.
46. Ibid., 13.
47. Ibid.
48. Health Canada, *Health Aspects of Violence Against Women*, Women's Health Forum, Ottawa, 1996.

CHAPTER 5

1. Janet D. Woititz, *Struggle for Intimacy* (Pompano Beach, FL: Health Communications, 1985).
2. Sharon S. Brehm, *Intimate Relationships* (New York: McGraw-Hill, 1992), 4–5.
3. "Vanier Institute on the Family Mission Statement," *Canadian Social Trends*, Summer 1993 (Statistics Canada 11-008E, Ministry of Supply and Services).
4. J. Dunn, "Siblings and Development," *Current Directions in Psychological Science*, 1 (1992): 6–11.
5. J. Turner and L. Rubinson, *Contemporary Human Sexuality* (Englewood Cliffs, NJ: Prentice Hall, 1993), 457.
6. Ibid.
7. G. Levinger, "Can We Picture Love?" in *The Psychology of Love*, ed. R. J. Sternberg and M. Barnes (New Haven: Yale University Press, 1988), 139–159.
8. E. Hatfield, "Passionate and Companionate Love," in *The Psychology of Love*, ed. R. J. Sternberg and M. Barnes (New Haven: Yale University Press, 1988), 191–217.
9. R. A. Baron and D. Byrne, *Social Psychology* (Boston: Allyn & Bacon, 1994), 318.
10. E. Hatfield and G. W. Walster, *A New Look at Love* (Reading, MA: Addison-Wesley, 1981).
11. Helen Fisher, *Anatomy of Love: The Natural History of Monogamy, Adultery, and Divorce* (New York: Norton, 1993).
12. A. Toufexis and P. Gray, "What Is Love? The Right Chemistry," *Time*, 1993, 47–52.
13. Ibid., 51.
14. Ibid., 49.
15. Helen Fisher, op. cit.
16. E. Hatfield, *Love, Sex, and Intimacy: Their Psychology, Biology, and History*, 1993.

17. Deborah Tannen, *You Just Don't Understand: Women and Men in Conversation* (New York: Ballantine, 1990).

18. M. McGill, *The McGill Report on Male Intimacy* (New York: Holt, Rinehart & Winston, 1985), 87–88.

19. Lillian Rubin, *Intimate Strangers* (New York: Harper and Row, 1983).

20. S. Hendricks and C. Hendricks, *Liking, Loving, and Relating*, 2nd ed. (Pacific Grove, CA: Brooks/Cole, 1992).

21. R. Landerman, M. Swartz, and L. George, "The Long-Term Effects of Childhood Exposure to Parental Drinking," paper presented at the annual meeting of the American Public Health Association, Mental Health session, Washington, D.C., 1992. See also A. Diaz, F. Yancovitz, N. Showers, and I. Epstein, "Predictors and Psychological Consequences of Disclosure of Incest by Female Adolescents," paper presented at the annual meeting of the American Public Health Association, Mental Health session, Washington, D.C., 1992.

22. M. Klausner and B. Hasselbring, *Aching for Love: The Sexual Drama of the Adult Child* (New York: Harper and Row, 1990).

23. Statistics Canada, *Canadian Social Trends*, Cat. No. 11-008E, 1994 (Ottawa: Ministry of Supply and Services, 1994).

24. N. Glenn and C. Weaver, "The Changing Relationship of Marital Status to Reported Happiness," *Journal of Marriage and Family* 50 (1988): 317–324. See also W. Wood, N. Rhodes, and M. Whelan, "Sex Differences and Positive Well-Being: A Consideration of Emotional Style and Marital Status," *Psychological Bulletin* 106 (1989): 249–264.

25. Statistics Canada, op. cit.

26. Public Legal Association of Saskatchewan (PLEASASK), *Living Common Law*.

27. R. Friedman and J. Downey, "Homosexuality," *New England Journal of Medicine* 33 (1994): 923–928.

28. Statistics Canada, op. cit.

29. N. Glenn and C. Weaver, op. cit., 318; W. Wood et al., op. cit., 249–252; Sharon S. Brehm, op. cit., 20–23.

30. "Sexuality and Aging: What It Means to Be Sixty or Seventy or Eighty in the '90s," *Mayo Clinic Health Letter*, February 1993.

31. R. C. Friedman and J. I. Downey, "Homosexuality," *JAMA* 331 (1994): 923–930.

32. J. S. Turner and L. Rubinson, *Contemporary Human Sexuality* (Englewood Cliffs, NJ: Prentice Hall, 1993), 251.

33. I. G. Sarason and B. R. Sarason, *Abnormal Psychology*, 6th ed. (Englewood Cliffs, NJ: Prentice Hall, 1989).

34. Martin Weinberg, *Society and the Healthy Homosexual* (New York: Anchor, 1973).

35. A. Bell, M. S. Weinberg, and S. K. Hammersmith, *Sexual Preference: Its Development in Men and Women* (Bloomington: Indiana University Press, 1981).

36. Simon LeVay, "A Difference in Hypothalamic Structure Between Heterosexual and Homosexual Men," *Science*, 253: 1034.

37. N. Bailey and R. Pillard, "Are Some People Born Gay?" *New York Times*, December 17, 1991, 13.

38. R. C. Friedman and J. I. Downey, op. cit., 923–930.

39. Dorothy Tennov, *Love and Limerence* (Chelsea, MI: Scarborough House, 1989), 45–50.

40. Alex Comfort, *The Joy of Sex* (New York: Simon and Schuster, 1972), 14.

41. R. O'Carroll, "Sexual Desire Disorders: A Review of Controlled Treatment Studies," *The Journal of Sex Research*, 28 (19): 607–624.

42. Robert J. Crane, Darwin Goldstein, and Inigo de Tejada, "Impotence," *New England Journal of Medicine*, December 14, 1989, 1648–57.

43. C. Darling and J. Davidson, "Enhancing Relationships: Understanding the Feminine Mystique of Pretending Orgasm," *Journal of Sex and Marital Therapy*, 12 (19): 182–196.

CHAPTER 6

1. Centers for Disease Control, *Contraceptive Options: Increasing Your Awareness* (Washington, D.C.: NAACOG, 1990).

2. University of Southern California School of Medicine, "Noncontraceptive Health Benefits," *Dialogues in Contraception*, 3 (1990): 2.

3. D. E. Greydanus and R. B. Shearin, *Adolescent Sexuality and Gynecology* (Philadelphia: Lea & Febiger, 1990), 107.

4. P. Silva and K. E. Glasser, "Update on Subdermal Contraceptive Implants," *The Female Patient*, 17 (1992): 34–45.

5. Ibid.

6. Planned Parenthood, "Chronology of Court Cases: Dr. Morgentaler and others."

7. Ibid.

8. Childbirth by Choice Trust, *Abortion in Canada Today: The Situation Province by Province* (1995).

9. Planned Parenthood, *Therapeutic Abortions* (1994).

10. Ibid.

11. K. Schmidt, "The Dark Legacy of Fatherhood," *U.S. News and World Report*, December 14, 1992, 94–95.

12. U.S. Department of Health and Human Services, *The Health Benefits of Smoking Cessation: A Report of the Surgeon General*, 1990.

13. American College of Obstetricians and Gynecologists, "Nutrition During Pregnancy," *Patient Education Pamphlet (AP001)*, April 1992.

14. D. Hall and D. Kaufmann, "Effects of Aerobic and Strength Conditioning on Pregnancy Outcomes," *American Journal of Obstetrics and Gynecology*, 157 (1987): 1199–1203.

15. J. D. Forrest, "Contraceptive Needs Through Stages of Women's Reproductive Lives," *Contemporary OB/GYN* (Special Issue on Fertility) (1988): 12–22.

16. W. J. Millar, C. Nair, and S. Wadhera, "Declining Cesarean Section Rates: A Continuing Trend?" *Health Reports*, 8, No. 1 (1996): 17–24.

17. University of Southern California of Medicine, *Dialogues in Contraception*, 3 (1991): 2.

CHAPTER 7

1. J. Beary, Ph.D. dissertatation, Oregon State University, 1994.

2. Health and Welfare Canada, *Food Guide Facts: Background for Educators and Communicators* (Ottawa: Minister of Supply and Services, Cat. No. H39-253/101-1992E, 1992).

3. M. Boyle and G. Zyla, *Personal Nutrition* (St. Paul, MN: West, 1991), 340.

4. Hass, *Staying Healthy with Nutrition* (Berkeley: Celestial Arts, 1992), 31.

5. Janet Christian and Janet Gregor, *Nutrition for Living*, 4th ed. (Benjamin Cummings, 1994), 129.

6. Ibid., 129.

7. R. B. Kanarck and R. Kaufman, *Nutrition and Behavior* (New York: Van Nostrand Reinhold, 1991).

8. *University of California Wellness Letter*, April 1992, 4–6.

9. R. Mensink and M. Katan, "Effect of Dietary Trans-Fatty Acids on High-Density and Low-Density Lipoprotein and Cholesterol Levels in Healthy Subjects," *New England Journal of Medicine*, August 16, 1990.

10. G. Ruoff, "Reducing Fat Intake with Fat Substitutes," *American Family Physician*, 43 (1991): 1235–42.

11. F. Mattson, "A Changing Role for Dietary Monounsaturated Fatty Acids," *Journal of American Dietetic Association* (1989): 387–391.

12. Walter Willet and Albert Ascherio, "Trans-Fatty Acids: Are the Effects Only Marginal?" *American Journal of Public Health*, 84 (1994): 722–724.

13. Janet Christian and Janet Gregor, op. cit., 56.

14. Haas, op. cit., 165.

15. Health and Welfare Canada, *Action Toward Healthy Eating: Technical Report* (Ottawa: Ministry of Supply and Services, Cat. No. H39 166/1-1990E, 1990).

16. L. Katzenstein, "Food Irradiation: The Story Behind the Scare," *American Health*, 60–80.

17. A. Hechtt, "Preventing Food-Borne Illnesses," *FDA Consumer Magazine*.

18. "Diagnosing Food Allergies," *University of California at Berkeley Wellness Letter*, May 1992, 7.

19. Ibid., 7.

20. Ibid., 7.

CHAPTER 8

1. Federal, Provincial, and Territorial Advisory Committee on Population Health, *Report on the Health of Canadians,* for the Meeting of Ministers of Health, Toronto, September 11, 1996 (Ottawa: Minister of Supply and Services, 1996).

2. Philip Elmer-Dewitt, "Fat Times," *Time,* January 16, 1995, 60.

3. Ibid., 60.

4. M. Lavery et al., "Long-Term Follow-up of Weight Status of Subjects in a Behavioral Weight Control Program," *Journal of the American Dietetic Association,* 89 (1989): 1259–64; J. Schlosber, "The Demographics of Dieting," *American Demographics,* 9 (1987): 35–62.

5. W. Sheldon, S. Stevens, and W. Tucker, *The Varieties of Human Physique* (New York: Harper and Row, 1940), 104.

6. A. Stunkard, *Psychiatric Update: American Psychiatric Association* (New York: Harper and Row, 1985), 87.

7. Claude Bouchard et al., "The Response to Long-Term Overfeeding in Identical Twins," *New England Journal of Medicine,* 322 (1990): 1477–88.

8. Ibid.

9. Albert Stunkard et al., "The Body-Mass Index of Twins Who Have Been Raised Apart," *New England Journal of Medicine,* 322 (1990): 1483–87.

10. P. Jaret, "The Way to Lose Weight," *Health,* January/February 1995, 52–59.

11. Ibid., 55.

12. F. Katch and W. McArdle, *Introduction to Nutrition, Exercise, and Health,* 4th ed. (Philadelphia: Lea & Febiger, 1992), 77.

13. Philip Elmer-DeWitt, op. cit., 61.

14. Ibid., 61.

15. Ibid., 61.

16. S. Lichman et al., "Discrepancy Between Self-Reported and Actual Caloric Intake and Exercise in Obese Subjects," *New England Journal of Medicine,* 327 (1992): 1894–97.

17. Kelly Brownell, "Comments on the Latest Study on Yo-Yo Diets by Steven N. Blair of the Institute for Aerobics Research in Dallas," paper presented at the annual research meeting of the American Heart Association, Monterey, CA, January 1993.

18. Thomas Stephens and Dawn Fowler, eds., *Canada's Health Promotion Survey, Technical Report* (Minister of Supply and Services Canada, 1993), Cat. No. H39-263-2-1990E.

19. M. Boyle and G. Zyla, *Personal Nutrition* (St. Paul, MN: West Publishing, 1991), 21.

20. J. Robison et al., "Obesity, Weight Loss, and Health," *Journal of the American Dietetic Association,* 93 (1993): 448.

21. Ibid., 448.

22. Simone French and R. Jeffery, "Consequences of Dieting to Lose Weight: Effects on Physical and Mental Health," *Health Psychology,* 13, No. 3 (1994): 195–212; G. Wilson, "Relation of Dieting and Voluntary Weight Loss to Psychological Functioning and Binge Eating," *Annals of Internal Medicine,* 119 (1993): 727–730.

23. Simone French and R. Jeffrey, op. cit., 195–96.

24. L. Lissner et al., "Variabilities in Body Weight and Health Outcomes in the Framingham Study," *New England Journal of Medicine,* 324 (1991): 1839–44; ibid., 197–98.

25. J. Horm and K. Anderson, "Who in America Is Trying to Lose Weight," *Annals of Internal Medicine,* 119 (1993): 672–676; and ibid., 203.

26. "Jury Still Out on Olestra," *Montreal Gazette,* April 2, 1997, CA.

27. G. Terrence Wilson, Peter Nathan, K. Daniel O'Leary, and Lee Anna Clark, *Abnormal Psychology* (Boston: Allyn & Bacon, 1996).

28. Ibid.

29. Ibid.

30. Ibid.

CHAPTER 9

1. B. A. Dennison, J. H. Straus, E. D. Mellits, et al., "Childhood Physical Fitness Tests: Predictor of Adult Physical Activity Levels?" *Pediatrics,* 82 (1988): 324–330; K. E. Powell and W. Dy-singer, "Childhood Participation in Organized School Sports and Physical Education as Precursors of Adult Physical Activity," *American Journal of Preventive Medicine,* 3 (1987): 276–281.

2. U.S. Department of Health and Human Services, *Healthy People 2000: National Health Promotion and Disease Prevention Objectives* (DHHS [PHS] Publication No. 91-50213) (Washington, D.C.: U.S. Government Printing Office, 1991).

3. R. Gates, "Fitness Is Changing the World: For Women," *IDEA Today,* July/August 1992, 58.

4. C. J. Caspersen, K. E. Powell, G. M. Christianson, "Physical Activity, Exercise, and Physical Fitness: Definitions and Distinctions for Health-Related Research," *Public Health Report,* 100 (1985): 126–131.

5. L. Kravitz and R. Robergs, "To Be Active or Not to Be Active," *IDEA Today,* March 1993, 47–53.

6. T. Baranowski, C. Bouchard, O. Bar-Or, et al., "Assessment, Prevalence, and Cardiovascular Benefits of Physical Activity and Fitness in Youth," *Medicine and Science in Sports and Exercise,* 24, No. 6, supplement (1992): S237–S247.

7. L. Bernstein et al., "Adolescent Exercise Reduces Risk of Breast Cancer in Younger Women," *Journal of the National Cancer Institute,* September 1994.

8. T. Baranowski et al., op. cit.

9. R. S. Gibson, C. A. MacDonald, and P. D. Smit Vanderkooy, "Dietary Fat Patterns of Some Canadian Preschool Children in Relation to Indices of Growth, Iron, Zinc, and Dietary Status," *Journal of Canadian Dietary Association,* 54, No. 1 (1993): 33–37.

10. V. H. Heyward, *Advanced Fitness Assessment and Exercise Prescription,* 2nd ed. (Champaign, IL: Human Kinetics Publishers, 1991).

11. W. L. Haskell, A. S. Leon, C. J. Caspersen, et al., "Cardiovascular Benefits and Assessment of Physical Activity and Physical Fitness in Adults," *Medicine and Science in Sports and Exercise,* 24, No. 6, supplement (1992): S201–S220.

12. Ibid.

13. W. H. Ettinger, Jr., and R. F. Afable, "Physical Disability from Knee Osteoarthritis: The Role of Exercise as an Intervention," *Medicine and Science in Sports and Exercise,* 26 (1994): 1435–1440.

14. P. A. Kovar, J. P. Allegrante, C. R. MacKenzie, et al., "Supervised Fitness Walking in Patients with Osteoarthritis of the Knee: A Randomized, Controlled Trial," *Annals of Internal Medicine,* 116 (1992): 529–534; D. T. Felson, Y. Zhang, J. M. Anthony, et al., "Weight Loss Reduces the Risk of Symptomatic Knee Osteoarthritis in Women: The Framingham Study," *Annals of Internal Medicine,* 116 (1992): 535–539.

15. B. L. Drinkwater, "Does Physical Activity Play a Role in Preventing Osteoporosis?" *Research Quarterly for Exercise and Sport,* 65 (1994): 197–206.

16. H. M. Frost, "Skeletal Structural Adaptations to Mechanical Usage (SATMU)—1. Redefining Wolff's Law: The Bone Remodeling Problem," *The Anatomical Record,* 226 (1990): 403–413.

17. B. L. Drinkwater, op. cit.

18. National Institutes of Health, "Consensus Development Conference Statement on Diet and Exercise in Non-Insulin-Dependent Diabetes Mellitus," *Diabetes Care,* 10 (1987): 639–644.

19. S. P. Helmrich, D. R. Ragland, and R. S. Paffenbarger, Jr., "Prevention of Non-Insulin-Dependent Diabetes Mellitus with Physical Activity," *Medicine and Science in Sports and Exercise,* 26 (1994): 824–830.

20. S. N. Blair, H. W. Kohl III, R. S. Paffenbarger, et al., "Physical Fitness and All-Cause Mortality: A Prospective Study of Healthy Men and Women," *JAMA,* 262, No. 17 (1989): 2395–2401.

21. E. R. Eichner, "Infection, Immunity, and Exercise: What to Tell Patients?" *Physician and Sportsmedicine,* January 1993, 125–135.

22. D. C. Nieman, "Exercise, Immunity and Respiratory Infections," *Sports Science Exchange,* August 1992.

23. D. C. Nieman, L. M. Johanssen, J. W. Lee, et al., "Infectious Episodes in Runners Before and After the Los Angeles Marathon," *Journal of Sports Medicine and Physical Fitness,* 30 (1990): 316–328.

24. E. R. Eichner, op. cit.

25. Ibid.

26. R. Gates, op. cit., 58.

27. C. J. Casperson et al., op. cit.

28. T. Baranowski et al., op. cit.

29. E. T. Howley, and D. B. Franks, *Health Fitness Instructor's Handbook,* 2nd ed. (Champaign, IL: Human Kinetics Books, 1992).

30. B. Stamford, "Tracking Your Heart Rate for Fitness," *Physician and Sportsmedicine,* March 1993.

31. U.S. Centers for Disease Control and Prevention and American College of Sports Medicine, "Summary Statement: Workshop on Physical Activity and Public Health," *Sports Medicine Bulletin,* 28, No. 4 (1993): 7.

32. G. A. Klug and J. Lettunich, *Wellness: Exercise and Physical Fitness* (Guilford, CT: Dushkin, 1992).

33. P. D. Wood, "Physical Activity, Diet, and Health: Independent and Interactive Effects," *Medicine and Science in Sports and Exercise,* 26 (1994): 838–843.

34. S. J. Hartley-O'Brien, "Six Mobilization Exercises for Active Range of Hip Motion," *Research Quarterly for Exercise and Sport,* 51 (1980): 625–635.

35. R. A. Schmidt, *Motor Control and Learning,* 2nd ed. (Champaign, IL: Human Kinetics, 1988).

36. P. A. Sienna, *One Rep Max: A Guide to Beginning Weight Training* (Indianapolis: Benchmark, 1989).

37. Ibid.

38. H. G. Knuttgen and W. J. Kraemer, "Terminology and Measurement in Exercise Performance," *Journal of Applied Sport Science Research,* 1 (1987): 1–10.

39. W. J. Kraemer, "Involvement of Eccentric Muscle Action May Optimize Adaptations to Resistance Training," *Sports Science Exchange,* November 1992.

40. P. A. Sienna, op. cit.

41. W. L. Westcott, "Muscular Strength and Endurance," *Personal Trainer Manual—The Resource for Fitness Instructors* (San Diego: American Council on Exercise, 1991), 235–274.

42. D. M. Brody, "Running Injuries: Prevention and Management," *Clinical Symposia,* 39 (1987).

43. Ibid.

44. J. C. Erie, "Eye Injuries: Prevention, Evaluation, and Treatment," *Physician and Sportsmedicine,* November 1991, 108–122.

45. J. G. Stock and M. F. Cornell, "Prevention of Sports-Related Eye Injury," *American Family Practice,* August 1991, 515–520.

46. R. C. Wasserman and R. V. Buccini, "Helmet Protection from Head Injuries Among Recreational Bicyclists," *American Journal of Sports Medicine,* 18 (1990): 96–97.

47. J. Andrish and J. A. Work, "How I Manage Shin Splints," *Physician and Sportsmedicine,* December 1990, 113–114.

48. D. M. Brody, op. cit.

49. American Academy of Orthopedic Surgeons, *Athletic Training and Sports Medicine,* 2nd ed. (Park Ridge, IL: AAOS, 1991).

50. B. Q. Hafen and K. J. Karren, *Prehospital Emergency Care and Crisis Intervention,* 4th ed. (Englewood Cliffs, NJ: Prentice-Hall, 1992).

51. J. S. Thornton, "Hypothermia Shouldn't Freeze Out Cold-Weather Athletes," *Physician and Sportsmedicine,* January 1990, 109–113.

CHAPTER 10

1. Addiction Foundation of Manitoba, *Mission Statement.*

2. H. F. Doweiko, *Concepts of Chemical Dependency* (Pacific Grove, CA: Brooks/Cole, 1993), 9.

3. C. Nakken, *The Addictive Personality* (Center City, MN: Hazelden, 1988), 23.

4. V. Johnson, *Intervention: Helping Someone Who Doesn't Want Help* (Minneapolis, MN: Johnson Institute, 1986), 16–35.

5. Health Canada, Drug Costs in Canada. Updated: 06/18/97. **http://www.hcsc.qc.ca/main/hc/web/datapcb/datahesa/drugs/Edrugs /htm**

6. Eric Single, Anne MacLennan, and Patricia MacNeill, "Alcohol and Other Drug Use in Canada," in Health Promotion Directorate, Health Canada, and the Canadian Centre on Substance Abuse, *Horizons 1994.*

7. Ibid.

8. Ibid.

9. Canadian Foundation for Drug Policy, *Canada Drug Legislation Update* (Ottawa: 1997).

10. Canadian Centre on Substance Abuse/Addiction Research Foundation, *Canadian Profile, 1997.*

11. Canadian Centre on Substance Abuse, *Substance Abuse Policy in Canada,* presentation to the House Standing Committee on Health, October 8, 1996.

12. Canadian Centre on Substance Abuse/Addiction Research Foundation, *Canadian Profile, 1997.*

13. "Substance Abuse Policy in Canada," a presentation to the House Standing Committee on Health, October 8, 1996.

14. Ibid.

15. Addiction Research Foundation, "Cocaine Fact Sheet," 1995.

16. National Drug Survey, *Canadian Profile, 1992.*

17. National Institute on Drug Abuse, *NIDA Capsules,* April 1989, 18–19.

18. Addiction Research Foundation, *Drug Abuse Update,* "Drugs and Driving," Spring 1991.

19. M. A. Learner, "The Fire of Ice," *Newsweek,* November 27, 1989, 37–38.

20. Ibid.

21. National Institute on Drug Abuse, *NIDA Capsules: Designer Drugs,* August 1989, 17–21.

22. Ibid.

23. "The History of Synthetic Testosterone," *Scientific American,* February 1995, 80.

24. CCSD, *Canadian Profile 1997: Alcohol, Tobacco & Other Drugs.*

25. *Business Quarterly* (Winter 1996).

CHAPTER 11

1. Canadian Council on Substance Abuse and Addiction Research Foundation, *Canadian Drug Profile* (1994): 51–54.

2. Statistics Canada, *National Population Health Survey Overview,* 10.

3. Addiction Research Foundation, *Facts About Alcohol.*

4. Ibid.

5. *Canadian Profile, 1997: Alcohol, Tobacco and Other Drugs.*

6. Addiction Research Foundation, Statistical Information Service.

7. C. Presley and P. Meilman, *Alcohol and Drugs on American College Campuses: A Report to College Presidents* (Carbondale, IL: Southern Illinois University Press, 1992), 9.

8. *Canadian Profile,* op. cit.

9. Addiction Research Foundation, op. cit.

10. R. D. Moore and T. A. Pearsons, "Moderate Alcohol Consumption and Coronary Heart Disease: A Review," *Medicine* 65 (1986): 242–67; Y. Okamota et al., "Role of Liver in Alcohol-Induced Alteration of High Density Lipoprotein Metabolism," *Journal of Laboratory Clinical Medicine* 111 (1988): 484–485.

11. W. C. Willett et al., "Moderate Alcohol Consumption and the Risk of Breast Cancer," *New England Journal of Medicine* 316 (1987): 1174–80.

12. Statistics Canada, *Mortality: Summary List of Causes, 1995,* Cat. No. 84-209, 14–15.

13. *Canadian Profile,* op. cit.

14. CCSD/Addiction Research Foundation, *1994 Canadian Profile, Canadian Profile 1997: Alcohol, Tobacco and Other Drugs.*

15. F. K. Goodwin and E. M. Gause, "Alcohol, Drug Abuse, and Mental Health Administration," *Prevention Pipeline* 3 (1990): 19.

16. S. I. Benowitz, "Studies Help Scientists Home In on Genetics of Alcoholism," *Science News,* September 29, 1984, 17.

17. Kenneth Blum et al., "Allelic Association of Human Dopamine D2 Receptor Gene in Alcoholism," *AMA* 262 (1990): 2055–59.

18. Ray and Ksir, *Drugs, Society, and Human Behavior* (St. Louis: Times Mirror/Mosby, 1990).

19. Eric Single, Lynda Robson, Xiaodi Xie, and Jürgen Rehm, *The Costs of Substance Abuse in Canada* (Canadian Centre on Substance Abuse, 1996).

20. J. Kinney and G. Leaton, *Loosening the Grip: A Handbook of Alcohol Information,* 4th ed. (St. Louis: Times Mirror/Mosby, 1991).

21. Ibid.

22. Canadian Centre on Substance Abuse, *Treatment: Canadian Directory of Substance Abuse Services.* Order from the Centre, 75 Albert St., Ste. 300, Ottawa K1P 5E7 Phone: (613) 235-4048 ext. 231. Toll-free order line: 1-800-214-4788. Fax: (613) 235-8101.

23. Health Canada, January 1996.
24. L. Brown, ed., *The State of the World, 1990* (New York: Norton, 1990), 100–102.
25. U.S. DHHS/Office on Smoking & Health, "Psychosocial Risk Factors for Initiating Tobacco Use," in *Preventing Tobacco Use Among Young People: A Report of the Surgeon General* (Atlanta: 1994); U.S. DHHS/OSH, "Changes in Knowledge About the Determinants of Smoking Behaviour," in *Reducing the Health Consequences of Smoking: 25 Years of Progress* (Washington: 1989), 329–376; E. Fisher, Jr., E. Lichtenstein, and D. Haire-Joshu, "Multiple Determinants of Tobacco Use and Cessation," in C. T. Orleans and J. Slade, Jr., *Nicotine Addiction: Principles & Management* (New York: Oxford, 1993), 59–88; S. Spoke and associates, *A Literature Review on Smoking: The Social, Psychological and Physiological Influencers Affecting Decisions and Behaviour* (Health Canada, OTC/HPB, March 1996).
26. Canadian Centre on Substance Abuse, *The Cost of Substance Abuse in Canada* (1997).
27. World Health Organizations, *Breaking Free from Tobacco Company Sponsorship* (1996).
28. Health Canada, January 1996.
29. Health Canada, "1994 Health Canada Study," *Canadian Journal of Public Health* (1995): 62.
30. Environmental Protection Agency, *Secondhand Smoke Report*, 1993.
31. P. Hilts, "Wide Peril Is Seen in Passive Smoking," *The New York Times*, May 9, 1990, A25.
32. P. Hilts, op. cit., A25.
33. R. D. Tollison, op. cit., 7.
34. M. Dewey, *Smoke in the Workplace* (Toronto: N.C. Press, 1986), 14.
35. Health Canada, *Caffeine and You*.
36. Ibid.

CHAPTER 12

1. *Heart Disease and Stroke in Canada*, 1995.
2. American Heart Association, *Heart and Stroke Facts 1995* (Dallas, TX: American Heart Association, 1995), 1.
3. Ibid., 2.
4. Ibid., 2.
5. Ibid., 2.
6. Ibid., 3.
7. Ibid., 3.
8. Ibid., 4.
9. Ibid., 32.
10. *Health Reports*, 3 (1991), No. 4.
11. American Heart Association, op. cit., 19.
12. American Heart Association, Twentieth Science Writers Conference, January 1993.
13. American Heart Association, Monterey Meeting, January 1993.
14. World Health Organization, cardiac study.
15. American Heart Association, *Heart and Stroke Facts 1995*, 20.
16. Ibid., 20.
17. Ibid., 21.
18. Ibid., 21.
19. R. Eliot, "Changing Behavior: A New Comprehensive and Quantitative Approach," keynote address at the annual meeting of the American College of Cardiology on Stress and the Heart, Jackson Hole, WY, July 3, 1987.
20. Statistics Canada, *Summary List of Causes*, 1995, 84–209.
21. "Cardiovascular Diseases in Women," in *Heart Disease and Stroke in Canada*, 1995.
22. *JAMA*, January 18, 1995.
23. *Heart and Stroke Facts 1995*, 12.
24. Ibid., 12.
25. L. A. Green and M. T. Ruffin, "A Closer Examination of Sex Bias in the Treatment of Ischemic Cardiac Disease," *Journal of Family Practice*, October 1994, 331–336.
26. *Heart and Stroke Facts 1995*, 10.
27. *New Study: Effectiveness of Bypass vs. Aggressive Use of Medications*.

28. J. E. Willard, R. A. Lange, and D. L. Hillis, "The Use of Aspirin in Ischemic Heart Disease," *New England Journal of Medicine*, 327 (1992): 175–179.
29. *Heart and Stroke Facts 1995*, 10.
30. Statistics Canada, "Cancer Incidence and Mortality, 1997". *Health Reports 1997*, 8, No. 4.
31. Ibid.
32. Statistics Canada, "Cancer Incidence and Mortality, 1997". *Health Reports 1997*, 8, No. 4.
33. T. G. Krontirus, "The Emerging Genetics of Human Cancer," *New England Journal of Medicine* 309 (1983): 404; and A. G. Knudson, "Genetics of Human Cancer," *Annual Review of Genetics* 20 (1986): 23.
34. American Cancer Society, *Cancer Facts & Figures—1994* (Atlanta: American Cancer Society, 1995), 1.
35. Ibid., 20.
36. Ibid., 12.
37. Ibid., 9.
38. National Cancer Institute statistics, in "Breast Cancer Risk," *Health*, May/June 1994, 14.
39. Statistics Canada, "Cancer Incidence and Mortality, 1997," *Health Reports, 1997*, 8, No. 4.
40. American Cancer Society, op. cit., 10.
41. Ibid., 10; and K. C. Allison, "Eat to Beat Cancer," *American Health*, October 1993, 72–78.
42. American Cancer Society, op. cit., 10.
43. Leslie Bernstein, Brian E. Henderson, Rosemarie Hanisch, Jane Sullivan-Halley, and Ronald K. Ross, "Physical Exercise and Reduced Risk of Breast Cancer in Young Women," *Journal of the National Cancer Institute* 86, No. 18, (September 21, 1994): 1403–1408.
44. American Cancer Society, op. cit., 9.
45. Ibid., 9.
46. Statistics Canada, "Cancer Incidence and Mortality, 1997," *Health Reports, 1997*, 8, No. 4.
47. American Cancer Society, op. cit., 11–12.
48. Ibid., 15.
49. Ibid., 15–16.
50. Ibid., 16.
51. Harvey A. Risch, Meera Jain, Loraine D. Marrett, and Geoffrey R. Howe, "Dietary Fat Intake and Risk of Epithelial Ovarian Cancer," *Journal of the National Cancer Institute* 86, No. 18 (September 1994): 1409–1415.
52. American Cancer Society, op. cit., 16.
53. Ibid., 12–13.
54. Ibid., 13.
55. Ibid., 13.
56. Ibid., 14.
57. Ibid., 14.
58. Ibid., 21.
59. Ibid., 2.
60. Ibid., 2.

CHAPTER 13

1. H. Sheldon, *Boyd's Introduction to Human Disease* (Philadelphia: Lea and Febiger, 1992).
2. The World Health Organization, *World Health Report 1996: Fighting Disease, Fostering Development*.
3. Health Canada, *Prevention and Management of Infectious Diseases*, (July 1995).
4. T. Shulman, J. Phair, and H. Sommers, *The Biological and Clinical Basis of Infectious Disease* (Philadelphia: W. B. Saunders, 1992); and A. Benenson, *Control of Communicable Diseases in Man* (Washington, DC: American Public Health Association, 1990).
5. *Canada Communicable Disease Report, 22-18*, (Sept. 15, 1996).
6. Health Canada, *Understanding Tuberculosis* (1995).
7. *Canada Communicable Disease Report*, Supp. 21S4 (November, 1995).
8. "PID: Guidelines for Prevention, Detection, and Management," *Clinical Courier* 10 (1992): 1–5.

9. P. Marchbanks, N. Lee, and H. Peterson, "Cigarette Smoking as a Risk Factor for PID," *American Journal of Obstetrics and Gynecology* 162 (1990): 639–644, J. Kahn, C. Walker, and A. Washington, "Diagnosing Pelvic Inflammatory Disease," *Journal of the American Medical Association* 226 (1991): 2594–2604, and "Sexually Transmitted Diseases in the 1990's," op. cit., 8.

10. Health Canada, *Canada Communicable Diseases Report,* 23–12 (June 15, 1997).

11. *Canada Communicable Diseases Report,* 23–12, (June 15, 1997).

12. World Health Organization, *Weekly Epidemiological Record, 70* (2) (Jan. 13, 1995), cited in *Canadian Social Trends* (Summer, 1995).

13. Gerald J. Stine, *Acquired Immune Deficiency Syndrome: Biological, Medical, Social and Legal Issues* (Englewood Cliffs, NJ: Prentice Hall, 1993), 125–146.

14. Ibid., 125.

15. Ibid., 147–148

16. J. Allen, "Oh, My Aching Head," *Life,* 1994, 66–76.

17. Ibid., 70.

18. Ibid., 72.

19. Kristen Rottensten Monograph Series on Aging-related Diseases IX. *Osteoarthritis.* Vol. 17, No. 3/4—1996 Health Canada.

20. New Study of Back Pain Treatment.

CHAPTER 14

1. B. Hayslip and P. Panek, *Adult Development and Aging* (New York: Harper and Row), 1992, 21.

2. Centre for International Statistics, Canadian Council on Social Development, 1996.

3. Statistics Canada 1996. **http://www.statcan.ca/english/Pgdb/People/Families/famil105.htm**

4. Statistics Canada, Cat. No. 13–207.

5. National Osteoporosis Foundation, *Physicians' Resource Manual on Osteoporosis: A Decision-Making Guide,* 2nd ed. (National Osteoporosis Foundation, 1991), and National Dairy Council, "Calcium and Osteoporosis: New Insights," *Dairy Council Digest,* 63 (1992): 1–6.

6. Mary Gordon and Julie Huang, *Monograph Series on Aging-Related Disorders: VI. Osteoporosis,* Vol. 16, No. 1 (Health Canada, 1995).

7. U.S. Department of Health and Human Services, Public Health Service, National Institutes of Health, *Osteoporosis Research, Education, and Health Promotion* (NIH Publication No. 91-3216, September 1991), 2.

8. National Dairy Council, *Calcium and Osteoporosis,* 3, and Food and Nutrition Board, *Subcommittee on the 10th Edition of the FDA's Recommended Dietary Allowances,* 10th ed. (Washington, D.C.: National Academy Press, 1989).

9. Ibid., 6.

10. U.S. Department of Health and Human Services, op. cit., 21–25.

11. Ibid., 6.

12. National Institute of Nutrition, *Food and Nutrition Opportunities in the Seniors' Market: A Situation Analysis—Executive Summary,* March 1996.

13. U.S. Department of Health and Human Services, op. cit., 7.

14. A. Ferrini and R. Ferrini, *Health in the Later Years* (Madison, WI: Brown and Benchmark, 1993), 281.

15. Ibid., 283.

16. National Institute of Nutrition, op. cit.

17. Ibid.

18. Gina Kolata, "Researchers Discover Simple Eyedrop Test to Detect Alzheimer's," *New York Times,* November 11, 1994.

19. N. Watts et al., "Intermittent Cyclical Etidronate Treatment of Postmenopausal Osteoporosis," *New England Journal of Medicine,* 323 (1990): 73–80.

20. *Oxford English Dictionary* (Oxford: Oxford University Press, 1969), 72, 334, 735.

21. Canadian Medical Association, "Guidelines for the Diagnosis of Brain Death," *Canadian Medical Association Journal,* 136 (1987): 200A.

22. Ibid.

23. Lewis R. Aiken, *Dying, Death, and Bereavement,* 3rd ed. (Boston: Allyn & Bacon, 1994), 4.

24. Elisabeth Kübler-Ross, *On Death and Dying* (New York: Macmillan, 1969), 113.

25. Robert J. Kastenbaum, *Death, Society, and Human Experience,* 5th ed. (Boston: Allyn & Bacon, 1995), 95.

26. K. J. Doka, ed., *Disenfranchised Grief: Recognizing Hidden Sorrow* (Lexington, MA: Lexington Books, 1989).

27. Kastenbaum, op. cit., 336–337.

28. The term *quasi-death experience* was coined by J. B. Kamerman; see J. B. Kamerman, *Death in the Midst of Life* (Englewood Cliffs, NJ: Prentice Hall, 1988), 71.

29. "Organ Donor Awareness Week Held This Month," *Canadian Medical Association Journal,* 152 (1995): 1279.

CHAPTER 15

1. R. Caplan, *Our Earth, Ourselves* (New York: Bantam, 1990), 247.

2. United Nations, "1996 Pop/626/Rev. 1," press release.

3. M. Lowe, "Shaping Cities," in *State of the World,* ed. Lester Brown (New York: Norton, 1992).

4. Canadian Lung Association, *Why Care About the Air You Breathe?* (1991).

5. Lester Brown, "A New Era Unfolds," in *State of the World, 1993,* ed. Lester Brown (New York: Norton, 1993).

6. Canadian Lung Association, op. cit.

7. H. F. French, "Clearing the Air," in *State of the World, 1990,* 109.

8. L. Pringle, *Rain of Troubles* (New York: Macmillan, 1988), 78.

9. Health Canada, "Radon Information Sheet" (Minister of Supply and Services, 1989).

10. "Thinning of the Ozone Layer" (Minister of Supply and Services, 1992).

11. Canadian Council of Ministers of the Environment, *Management Plan For Nitrogen Oxides and Volatile Organic Compounds* (Ottawa: 1990).

12. Canadian Lung Association, op. cit.

13. H. F. French, op. cit., 110.

14. Environment Canada, *Water Policy in Canada—Canada's Water* (March 1997).

15. A. Nadakavukaren, *Man and Environment: A Health Perspective* (Prospect Heights, IL: Waveland, 1990), 412–414.

16. R. Griffin, Jr., "Introducing NPS Water Pollution," *EPA Journal,* 17 (1991): 6–9.

17. J. Naar, *Design for a Livable Planet* (New York: Harper and Row, 1990), 68.

18. A. Nadakavukaren, op. cit., 183.

19. Ibid., 447.

20. Statistics Canada, *Household Waste Management in the 90s, Environmental Perspectives,* Cat. No. 11-528E, No. 2.

21. A. Nadakavukaren, op. cit., 415.

22. Statistics Canada, op. cit.

23. Environment Canada, *Toxic Substances Management Policy* (Government of Canada, June 1995).

24. D. W. Moeller, *Environmental Health* (Cambridge, MA: Harvard University Press, 1992), 31.

25. C. Flavin, "Slowing Global Warming," in *State of the World, 1990.*

CHAPTER 16

1. Canadian Institute for Health Information, *Canada's Health System* (1996).

2. K. J. Egan and W. J. Katon, "Responses to Illness and Health in Chronic Pain Patients and Healthy Adults," *Psychosomatic Medicine,* 49 (1987): 470–481.

3. G. Annas, *The Rights of Patients: The Basic ACLU Guide to Patient Rights,* 2nd ed. (Chicago: Southern Illinois University Press, 1989), 105, and J. A. Robertson, *The Rights of the Critically Ill* (New York: Bantam, 1983), 32–77.

4. P. Starr, *The Social Transformation of American Medicine* (New York: Basic Books, 1982), 127, 229.

5. J. Drawbridge, "Medical Report: The Chiropractic Cure," *Glamour,* April 1993, 61–62.

6. A. Toufexis, "Dr. Jacob's Alternative Mission: A New NIH Office Will Put Unconventional Medicine to the Test," *Time,* March 1, 1993, 43–44, 64–66.

Photo Credits

p. 1, Bachmann/The Image Works; p. 3, David Coleman/Stock Boston; p. 4, Canapress/Jon Murray; p. 21, Richard Clintsman/Tony Stone Worldwide; p.22, Elena Dorfman/Offshoot Stock; p. 25 Terry Vine/Tony Stone Worldwide; p. 28, Lori Adamski Peek/Tony Stone Worldwide; p.36, Mark Richards/Photo Edit; p.37, David Young-Wolff/Photo Edit; p. 38, Acey Harper/Reportage Stock; p. 41, CBC/Fred Phipps; p. 48, John Running; p. 50, Ben Barhart/Offshoot Stock; p. 53, David Young-Wolff/Photo Edit; p. 62, Marko Shark; p. 67, Shumsky/The Image Works; p. 69, Reinstein/The Image Works; p. 73, Todd Bigelow/Black Star; p. 74, Jacques Chenet/Woodfin Camp and Associates; p. 80, Ellie Herwig/Stock Boston; p. 85, W. Hill/The Image Works; p. 87, Robert Brenner/Photo Edit; p. 94, Cary Wolinsky/Tony Stone Worldwide; p. 100, First Light; p. 101, Bill Gillette/Stock Boston; p. 110, Lisa Quinones/Black Star; p. 111, W.P. Wittman Ltd.; p. 117, Michel Tcherevkoff/The Image Bank; p. 118, Charles Thatcher/Tony Stone Wordwide; p. 134, Bruce Ayres/Tony Stone Worldwide; p. 135, Julie Marcotte/Stock Boston; p. 138, Tom McCarthy/Photo Edit; p. 141, The Slide Farm/Al Harvey; p. 148, Mark Lewis/Tony Stone Worldwide; p. 150, J. De Cunha Petit Format/Photo Researchers; p. 156, A. Neste; p. 159, B. Daemmrich/The Image Works; p. 172, Will & Deni McIntyre/Photo Researchers; p. 176, J. Sohm/The Image Works; p. 177, David Madison/Tony Stone Worldwide; p. 181, David Young-Wolff/Photo Edit; p. 182, Elena Dorfman/Offshoot Stock; p. 188, Frank Siteman/Tony Stone Worldwide; p. 197, Biophoto Associates/Photo Researchers; p. 203, The Slide Farm/Al Harvey; p. 205, Robert E. Daemmrich/Tony Stone Worldwide; p. 211, David R. Frazier/Tony Stone Worldwide; p. 215, Bob Daemmrich/Stock Boston; p. 216, The Slide Farm/Al Harvey; p. 220, Jean Francois Causse/Tony Stone Worldwide; p. 227, R. Campillo/The Stock Market; p. 233 James Prince/Photo Researchers; p. 247, Earl Young/Tony Stone Worldwide; p. Greg Weiner/Liaison International; p. 252, Bonnie Kamin; p. 255, Timothy Shonnard/Tony Stone Worldwide; p. 257, Jeff Isaac Greenberg/Photo Edit; p. 258, Marko Shark; p. 265, Le Duc/Monkmeyer Press Photo; p. 275, Michael Newman/Photo Edit; p. 276, Tony Freeman/Photo Edit; p. 277, Mark C. Burnett/Stock Boston; p. 283, Courtesy of Health Corp.; p. 287, Dorothy Greco/The Image Works; p. 302, Stacy Pick/Stock Boston; p. 308, Elena Dorfman/Offshoot Stock; p. 314, Toronto Sun/Craig Robertson; p. 333, Okonewski/The Image Works; p.338, Chuck Woody/Canapress; p. 342, Elena Dorfman/Offshoot Stock; p. 347, James A. Martin/Offshoot Stock; p. 353, The Slide Farm/Al Harvey; p. 357, W. P. Wittman Ltd; p. 358, Toronto Sun/Wanda Goodwin; p. 361, Joe Monroe/Photo Researchers; p. 364, S. Gazin/The Image Works; p. 366, Michael Townsend/Tony Stone Worldwide; p. 369, Michael Grecco/Stock Boston; p. 372, Spencer Grant/Stock Boston; p. 379, David Woodfall/Tony Stone Worldwide; p. 381, John McDermott/Tony Stone Worldwide; p. 384, Will & Deni McIntyre/Photo Researchers; p. 394, Marko Shark; p. 398, Alain Evrard/Photo Researchers; p. 402, Esbin-Anderson/The Image Works; p. 406, Andy Levin/Photo Researchers; p. 407, W. Hill Jr./The Image Works; p. 409, Mulvehill/The Image Works.

$\mathcal{I}$ndex*

*Numbers followed by the letter f refer to figures; numbers followed by the letter t refer to tables; numbers in bold refer to marginal definitions.

Amniotic sac, 138, **139**
Amphetamines, **235,** 243
  teratogenic effects of, 134t
Amping, 243
Amyl nitrite, **250,** 251
Anabolic steroids, **250,** 251, 252
Anacin, interactions with alcohol, 262t
Anal intercourse, **111**
Analgesics, **236**
  over-the-counter, 236
Anaprox, 236
Anatomy, reproductive
  female, 103–106
  male, 106–107
Anatomy of an Illness, 37
Anatomy of Love, 90
Androgyny, **102**
Anemia, **167**
Aneurysm, **288**
Anger
  at death, 367
  management of, 61
Angina pectoris, **287**
Angiography, **296**
Angioplasty, **298**
Animal-borne pathogens, 321
Anorexia nervosa, 180, **199**
Antabuse, 233, 271
  interactions with alcohol, 262t
Antacids
  drug interactions of, 233
  side effects of, 238t
Antagonism, drug, 233
Antecedents
  of behaviour, 21
  defined, 21
Anti-abortion protests, 130
Anti-Chinese riots, 71
Antibiotics, **236**
  drug interactions of, 233
  interactions with alcohol, 262t
  to treat STDs, 332, 333
Antibodies, defined, **323**
Anticholinergics, 237
Antidepressants, 39, **236**
  interactions with alcohol, 262t
Antifungal drugs, 334
Antigen, defined, **322**
Antihistamines, 237
  drug interactions of, 232
  interactions with alcohol, 262t
Antitussives, 237
Anxiety, controlling, 27
Anxiety disorders, **40–41**
Aortic valve, 288
Apparent death, 366
Appetite, 148–149, **187**
Appetite suppressants, 237
Approval, need for, 86
Aromatherapy, 408
Arousal, 108
Arrhythmia, 288
Arteries, **286**
Arterioles, **286**
Arteriosclerosis, **286**
Arthritis, **348–349**
Asbestos, 386, **387**
Ascherio, Albert, 162

Ascorbic acid. *See* Vitamin C
Aspirin
  drug interactions of, 233
  function of, 236
  interactions with alcohol, 262t
  side effects of, 238t
  teratogenic effects of, 134t
Assault
  prevention of, 77–82
  sexual, 74
Association of Canadian Distillers, 265
Asthma, **341**
  medications for, 237
Atherosclerosis, 160, **289–290**
Athletic performance, carbohydrates and, 158–159
Ativan, interactions with alcohol, 262t
Atria, **286**
Attachment, as component of love, 90
Attitudes
  defined, **15**
  influencing behaviour, 15–17
Attraction, as component of love, 90
Auramassage, 408
Australia
  emotional expression in, 42
  life expectancy in, 411
Autoerotic behaviour, **111**
Autoimmune diseases, 323
Autoinnoculation, **317**
Autoimmune theory of aging, 358
Autonomic nervous system (ANS)
  defined, **53**
  role in stress response, 52
Autonomy, **98**
Awlad 'Ali people, 42
AZT (zidovudine), 339

B-cells, 323
Background distressors, 57–58
Bacteria
  defined, **316**–317
  types of, 316–317
Badgley Committee, 81
Bailey, N., 109
Bandura, Albert, 32
Barbiturates
  drug interactions of, 234
  teratogenic effects of, 134t
Barbus, Amelia, 373
Bargaining, at death, 368
Bartlett's Familiar Quotations, 89
Basal metabolic rate
  (BMR), **187,** 190
Basis, of behaviour, 21
Battered But Not Beaten; Preventing Wife Battering in Canada, 81
Battering, 72
Bedouin people, 42
Behaviour, as stressor, 54
Behaviour change
  analysis of, 21
  beliefs and attitudes and, 15–17
  checklists for, 23
  decision making for, 22
  factors influencing, 14–15, 14f
  facilitating, 19
  goal-setting in, 22–24

  intentions of, 18
  readiness for, 16
  reinforcement for, 1–20
  self-assessment and, 21
  significant others and, 18
  social factors in, 18–19
  techniques of, 19–21
Behaviour change skills
  avoiding skin cancer, 301
  cutting fat from the diet, 163
  dying person's bill of rights, 372
  environmental shopping, 393
  fighting addiction, 244
  health care consumerism, 400
  preventing date rape, 79
  quitting smoking, 279
  readiness to change, 16
  sexual health, 103
  strength training, 217
  test-taking, 59
  trusting, 29
  weight control, 196
Behavioural interdependence, 86
Behavioural psychology, defined, **32**
Belief
  defined, **15–16**
  influencing behaviour, 15–16
Bell, A., 109
Benign, defined, **298**
Bennett, William, 185
Benzedrine, 243
Bereavement, 369–370
  helping children with, 371
Bereavement overload, **371**
Beta blockers, **288**
Beta particles, 392
Bias, crimes caused by, 68–69
Biceps, 215–216
Bill C-8, 239
Bill C-43, 130
Binge drinking, **257**
Binge eating disorder (BED), **199**
Bioelectric impedance analysis (BIA), 182, **183**
Biofeedback, to treat stress, **63**
Biological age, 356
Biopsy, **298**
Biotin, 164t
Birthing centers, 139
Bisexuality, **108,** 109
Black tar, 246, **247**
Blocking, 21
Blood alcohol concentration (BAC), **259–260**
  effects of, 260f
Blood, circulation of, 285
Blood pressure, 291
Blood vessels, disorders of, 291
Body image, 180–181
Body mass index (BMI), **183**
Body temperature method of contraception, **127**
Body weight resistance, 215
Bohlen, Jim, 381
Bones
  acute injury to, 427–428
  age-related changes to, 360
Boston Veterans Affairs Medical Centre, 348
Bradycardia, 291
Brain death, 366
Brazil, acid rain in, 384

Oral ingestion, of drug, **232**
Oral-genital contact, 111–112, 119
Organ donation, 375
Organic foods, **173**
Organic solvents, 393
    drug effects of, 250
Organizational supports, for health, 8
Orgasm, 107
    disorders of, 113
Orgasmic phase, 108
Osteoarthritis, **205, 348**
Osteoporosis, **205**
    exercise to prevent, 205,
    incidence of, **361**
    risk factors for, 361–362
Ottawa Charter for Health Promotion, 83
Outercourse, as contraceptive, 119
Outpatient care, **411**
Ovarian cancer, 309–310
Ovarian follicles, 104, **105**
Ovaries, **104,** 105f
Over-the-counter (OTC) drugs, 237–238
    elderly use of, 364
    side effects of, 238t
    types of, 237
Overload, 56, **57**
Overload principle, 214
Overpopulation, 380–381
Overuse injuries, **219–220**
Overweight. *See* Obesity
Ovo-vegetarians, 170
Ovulation, **105**
Oxytocin, 91
Ozone, 386
    layer, 386f
    pollution, 385

Pain, 323
Paint thinner, drug effects of, 250
Pancreas, 346
    alcohol effects on, 264
Panic attacks, **40**
Pap test, **307**
Parasitic diseases, 325
Parasympathetic nervous system, defined, **53**
    role in stress response, 52
Parenting, 98–99
Parents
    as models of relationships, 91, 97
    role of, 88
Parkinson's disease, 351t
Particulates, **383**
Partnering scripts, 97
Partners, 89
Passion, as component of love, 90
Passionate love, 89
Passive smoking, 275, 292–293
Pathogen
    defined, **316**
    routes of entry of, 316–317
    types of, 316–322
PBBs (polybrominated biphenyls), 389
PCBs (polychlorinated biphenyls), 389
PCP (phencyclidine), **249**
Peck, Robert, 350
Pedophilia, 113
Pelvic inflammatory disease (PID), **142,** 43, **331**
Penicillin, **318**

interactions with alcohol, 262t
Penis, **106**
Pentamidine, 340
Peptic ulcer, **345**
Percodan, 246
Pergonal, 143
Perineum, 103, **139**
Periodontal diseases, **318–319**
Personal control, 32
Pesco-vegetarians, 17169
Pesticides, **390**
    as water pollutant, 392
PET scan, 41, 296
Petit mal, 342
Petroleum, pollution from, 388
Peyote, **248**
Phencyclidine, **250**
Phenobarbital, 235
    drug interactions of, 233
Phenylethylamine (PEA), 89
    adverse reactions to, 176
Phenylpropanolamine, 238
Phobias, **40**–41
Phosphourus, 164t,
Photochemical smog, **383**
Physical abuse, 93
Physical activity, 205
Physical attraction, 92
Physical fitness
    benefits of, 205–208
    cardiovascular, 209–212
    components of, 209t
    defined, 208, **209**
Physical health, 3
    self-assessment of, 7
    and self-esteem, 36
Physicians
    assessment of, 402
    choosing, 403–404
Physiological needs, 33
Physiology
    female, 102–106
    male, 106–107
Pill, the, 120–121
    failure rate of, 120t
Pillard, R., 109
Pinch test, 182, **183**
Pinworms, 321
Pituitary gland, **101, 104**
Placebo effect, **401**
Placenta, **137,** 139
Placidyl, interactions with alcohol, 262t
Plantar fasciitis, 219–220
Plaque, **289**–290
    atherosclerotic, **160,** 161
Plateau, defined, **185**
Plateau phase, 108
Platelet adhesiveness, **275**–276
PMS. *See* Premenstrual syndrome
Pneumonia, **318,** 340
Point source pollutants, **387**
Polio, immunization against, 324t
Pollution
    air, 381–387
    land, 391–392
    management of, 397–398
    noise, 390
    radiation as, 392–396

water, 387–390
Polychlorinated biphenyls. *See* PCBs
Polydrug use, **234**
Polysaccharides, 158, **159**
Polyunsaturated fat, 161
Population explosion, 382–383
Positive reinforcement, **19,** 20
Positivity, 27
Positron emission tomography (PET), 41, **291**
Possessional reinforcers, 19
Postpartum depression, **140**
Postpartum period, 140
Posttraumatic stress disorder (PTSD), 41
Potamia, graveyard of, 374
Potassium, 164t,
Potentiation, 232
Poverty, and access to exercise, 208
Prader-Willi syndrome, 132
Preconception care, **132**
Precontemplation, of behaviour change, 17
Predictability, 29
    in relationship, 98
Predisposing factors, defined, 14
Pregnancy
    alcohol and, 264
    avoiding. *See* Contraception
    contingency planning for, 133
    ectopic, 142
    emotional issues in, 132
    finances and, 132–133
    maternal health and, 132
    nutrition in, 134–135
    paternal health and, 132
    prenatal care for, 133–135
    process of, 136–137
    signs of, 136
    smoking and, 277
    testing for, 136
    timing of, 135–136
    trimesters of, 136–137
    weight gain in, 135
Prejudice, 30, **31**
Premature ejaculation, **113**
Premenstrual syndrome (PMS), 42–43, 105,
    345–346
Prenatal care, 133–135
Prenatal testing, 137–138
Preorgasmic, **113**
Preparation, of behaviour change, 17
Prescription drugs, 235–237
    types of, 234–235
Pressure, as stressor, 54
Prevalence, defined, 9
Prevention, defined, **7**
Primary care practitioner, 404
Primary prevention, defined, **7**
Primary syphilis, 329
Prochaska, James, 17
Prodromal, defined, 335
Progesterone, **104**
Progestin-only pills, 122
Proliferative phase, 105
Proof, defined, **259**
Proprietary hospitals, 409
Prostaglandin inhibitors, **236,**
Prostate, 105, **106,**107
Prostate cancer, 304–305
Prostate-specific antigen (PSA), 311